Principles and Practice of

GERIATRIC MEDICINE

for Postgraduate and Practitioner

Principles and Practice of

GERIATRIC MEDICINE

for Postgraduate and Practitioner

Editor

Prasun Chatterjee

MD(Geriatric Medicine) FRCP(Edinburgh)

Chief Geriatric Medicine and Longevity Science
Artemis Hospitals, Gurugram and New Delhi
Member, Technical Advisory Group for Measurement, Monitoring and Evaluation, WHO
UN Decade of Healthy Ageing
Former Professor, AIIMS, Department of Geriatric Medicine, New Delhi
Vice President – Indian Academy of Geriatrics

Foreword

AB Dey

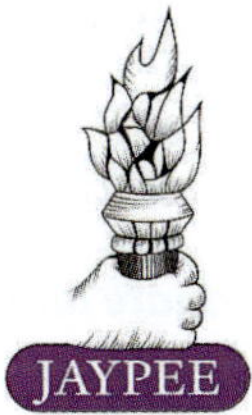

JAYPEE BROTHERS MEDICAL PUBLISHERS

The Health Sciences Publisher

New Delhi | London

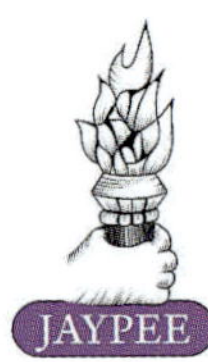

JAYPEE Jaypee Brothers Medical Publishers (P) Ltd

Headquarters
EMCA House, 23/23-B
Ansari Road, Daryaganj
New Delhi 110 002, India
Landline: +91-11-23272143, +91-11-23272703
+91-11-23282021, +91-11-23245672
e-mail: jaypee@jaypeebrothers.com

Corporate Office
4838/24, Ansari Road, Daryaganj
New Delhi 110 002, India
Phone: +91-11-43574357
Fax: +91-11-43574314
e-mail: jaypee@jaypeebrothers.com

Overseas Office
JP Medical Ltd.
83, Victoria Street, London
SW1H 0HW (UK)
Phone: +44-20 3170 8910
e-mail: info@jpmedpub.com

EU GPSR Authorised Representative
Logos Europe, 9 rue Nicolas Poussin
17000, La Rochelle, France
Phone: +33 (0) 6 67 93 73 78
e-mail: contact@logoseurope.eu

Website: www.jaypeebrothers.com
Website: www.jaypeedigital.com

***Principles and Practice of Geriatric Medicine for Postgraduate and Practitioner* / Prasun Chatterjee**

First Edition: **2026**

ISBN: 978-93-6616-223-2

Printed at: Samrat Offset Pvt. Ltd.

CONTRIBUTORS

Abhijith Rajaram Rao MD(Geriatric Medicine) (AIIMS, New Delhi) Fellowship Geriatric Oncology(TMC, Mumbai)
Assistant Professor
Department of Geriatric Medicine
National Centre for Ageing (NCA)
AIIMS
New Delhi, India

Akshata Rao MBBS MD MRCP
Senior Resident
Department of Geriatric Medicine
AIIMS
New Delhi, India

Ambica Singh MD(Geriatric Medicine)
Assistant Professor
Department of Geriatric Medicine
National Centre for Ageing (NCA)
AIIMS
New Delhi, India

Ananta Aryal MD(Geriatric Medicine) (AIIMS, New Delhi)
Consultant Geriatrician
Department of Geriatrics
NAMS, Bir Hospital
Kathmandu, Nepal

Ananya Parampalli Ravindra MD(Ophthalmology) FICO(UK)
Senior Resident
Department of Ophthalmology
Dr Rajendra Prasad Centre for Ophthalmic Sciences (RPC)
AIIMS
New Delhi, India

Anoop Aggarwal MPT(Sports Medicine) PhD(Physiotherapy)
Senior Physiotherapist
Pt. Deendayal Upadhyaya National Institute for Persons with Physical Disabilities
New Delhi, India

Anupa Pillai MD(Geriatric Medicine)
Senior Resident (Academic)
Department of Medical Oncology
Tata Memorial Hospital, Mumbai
Homi Bhabha National Institute
Mumbai, Maharashtra, India

Anup Singh MD(Internal Medicine)
Professor and Head
Department of Geriatric Medicine
Banaras Hindu University
Varanasi, Uttar Pradesh, India

Arunansu Talukdar MBBS MD(Internal Medicine)
Professor
Department of Geriatric Medicine
Medical College
Kolkata, West Bengal, India

Arun Kumar Choudhary MD(PMR) Fellowship in Pain Medine
Assistant Professor
Department of PMR
AIIMS
New Delhi, India

Ashish Goel MD(Medicine) MPH
Professor and Head
Department of General Medicine
Dr BR Ambedkar State Institute of Medical Sciences (AIMS), Mohali
Sahibzada Ajit Singh Nagar, Punjab, India

Avinash Chakrawarty MD(General Medicine)
Additional Professor
Department of Geriatric Medicine
AIIMS
New Delhi, India

Baldeep Kaur MBBS MD(Medicine)
Assistant Professor
Department of General Medicine
Dr BR Ambedkar State Institute of Medical Sciences (AIMS), Mohali
Sahibzada Ajit Singh Nagar, Punjab, India

Bharathi Purohit PhD
Assistant Professor
Division of Public Health Dentistry
Centre for Dental Education and Research
AIIMS
New Delhi, India

Lt Col Sumit Bhaskar MD(Medicine) PG Diploma(Geriatrics)
Associate Professor
Department of Geriatric Medicine
Armed Forces Medical College (AFMC)
Pune, Maharashtra, India

Dhruvendra Lal MBBS MD
Assistant Professor
Department of Community Medicine
Dr BR Ambedkar State Institute of Medical Sciences (AIMS), Mohali
Sahibzada Ajit Singh Nagar, Punjab, India

Gaurav Sharma MD(Geriatric Medicine) (AIIMS, New Delhi)
Consultant
Department of Geriatrics
AIG Hospital
Hyderabad, Telangana, India

Gevesh Chand Dewangan MBBS MD(Geriatric Medicine) MRCP(UK)
Specialist Consultant
Department of General Medicine
ESIC Hospital
Raipur, Chhattisgarh, India

Kapil Sikka MS DNB FACS
Professor
Department of Otorhinolaryngology and Head–Neck Surgery
AIIMS
New Delhi, India

Laxmi Kant Goyal MD(Internal Medicine) FRCP(Edinburgh)
Professor and Head
Department of Geriatric Medicine
SMS Medical College
Jaipur, Rajasthan, India

Madhulatha Alexander MBBS MD
Professor
Department of Obstetrics and Gynecology
Osmania Medical College
Hyderabad, Telangana, India

Mala Kapur Shankardass PhD(Medical Sociology) Postdoctorate(Ageing Studies) Diploma in Gerontology
International Consultant, Founder Member and Managing Trustee
Development, Welfare and Research Foundation (DWRF)
Retired Senior Faculty
University of Delhi
New Delhi, India
Asia Representative: International Network for Prevention of Elder Abuse

Mamta Saini MBBS MD(Geriatric Medicine)
Consultant
Department of Geriatric Medicine
Mahavir Jaipuriya Rajasthan Hospital
Jaipur, Rajasthan, India

Mangala Suresh Borkar MD(Internal Medicine)
Professor
Department of Geriatrics
Government Medical College
Chatrapati Sambhajinagar, Aurangabad, Maharashtra, India

Mayank Shrivastava MD(Medicine)
Associate Professor
Department of Geriatric Medicine
JLN Medical College
Ajmer, Rajasthan, India

Meenal Thakral MBBS MD(Geriatric Medicine)
Attending Consultant
Department of Geriatric Medicine
Artemis Hospital
Gurugram, Haryana, India

Meenaxi Sharda MD(Medicine) DCH FIAE FICP
Senior Professor and Head
Department of General Medicine
Government Medical College
Kota, Rajasthan, India

Minakshi Dhar MD(Internal Medicine)
Professor and Head
Department of Geriatric Medicine
AIIMS
Rishikesh, Uttarakhand, India

Monika Devi Sharma MD(Geriatric Medicine)
Senior Resident
Department of Geriatric Medicine
AIIMS
New Delhi, India

Namrata Makkar DNB(MHA)
Assistant Professor
Department of Geriatric Medicine
National Centre for Ageing (NCA)
AIIMS
New Delhi, India

Neethu Susan Abraham MD(Palliative Medicine)
Consultant
Department of Palliative Medicine
St Gregorios Medical Mission
Multi-Speciality Hospital, Parumala
Thiruvalla, Kerala, India

Nidhi Soni MD(Geriatric Medicine)
Assistant Professor
Department of Geriatric Medicine
National Centre for Ageing (NCA)
AIIMS
New Delhi, India

NN Prem MD(Geriatric Medicine)
Chief Consultant Geriatrician
Elderly Care Specialist Physician
Department of Geriatric Medicine
Jaslok Hospital and Research Centre
Mumbai, Maharashtra, India

Pragya Tyagi MASLP
Audiologist and Speech Language Pathologist
Department of Otorhinolaryngology and Head–Neck Surgery
AIIMS
New Delhi, India

Prakash Kumar MOT PhD(KGMU, Lucknow) MSc(TCD, Ireland)
Principal and Professor
Department of Occupational Therapy
Mahatma Gandhi University of Medical Sciences and Technology
Jaipur, Rajasthan, India

Pramod Kumar Mehta MD(Geriatric Medicine)
Assistant Professor
Department of Geriatric Medicine
AIIMS
New Delhi, India

Prasun Chatterjee MD(Geriatric Medicine) FRCP(Edinburgh)
Chief Geriatric Medicine and Longevity Science
Artemis Hospitals, Gurugram and New Delhi
Member, Technical Advisory Group for Measurement, Monitoring and Evaluation, WHO
UN Decade of Healthy Ageing
Former Professor
Department of Geriatric Medicine
AIIMS, New Delhi, India
Vice President – Indian Academy of Geriatrics

Preethy Kathiresan MD(Psychiatry) DNB(Psychiatry) DM(Addiction Psychiatry)
Assistant Professor
Department of Psychiatry
AIIMS
New Delhi, India

Lt Col Pritam Priyansu Purohit MD DNB(Medicine, Subspecialty Residency in Geriatrics)
Classified Specialist Medicine and Geriatrician
Medical Division, Command Hospital
Armed Forces Medical College (AFMC)
Pune, Maharashtra, India

Radhika Tandon MD DNB FRCSEd FRCOphth
Chief, Department of Ophthalmology
Dr Rajendra Prasad Centre for Ophthalmic Sciences
AIIMS
New Delhi, India

Raja Babu Ramawat MD(Psychiatry)
Research Scientist II (Medical)
National Drug Dependence Treatment Centre (NDDTC)
AIIMS
New Delhi, India

Rajesh Malhotra MS FRCS FACS FICS FIMSA FAMS FNASc
Clinical Lead and Senior Consultant Orthopedics
Indraprastha Apollo Hospitals
Former Head
Department of Orthopedics
AIIMS
New Delhi, India

Raj Kumar Tata MD(Geriatric Medicine)
Senior Resident
Department of Geriatric Medicine
National Centre for Ageing (NCA)
AIIMS
New Delhi, India

Rashi Jain PhD
Research Scientist
Department of Geriatric Medicine
AIIMS
New Delhi, India

Rasika Panwar MSc(Psychology)
Psychologist
Department of Psychology
AIIMS
New Delhi, India

Ritu Duggal MDS(Orthodontics)
Chief and Professor
Department of Orthodontics
Centre for Dental Education and Research (CDER)
AIIMS
New Delhi, India

Ruchika Madan MPT(Musculoskeletal)
Physiotherapist
Department of Geriatric Medicine
National Centre for Ageing (NCA)
AIIMS
New Delhi, India

Sahil Batra MBBS MS
Assistant Professor
Department of Orthopedics
AIIMS
New Delhi, India

Sankha Shubra Chakrabarti MD(Internal Medicine)
Professor
Department of Geriatric Medicine
Institute of Medical Sciences
Adjunct Faculty, Interdisciplinary School of Life Sciences
Banaras Hindu University
Varanasi, Uttar Pradesh, India

Saumyarup Pal MD(Geriatric Medicine)
Senior Resident(Academic)
Department of Hospital Medicine and Critical Care
AIIMS
Rishikesh, Uttrakhand, India

Shakti Kruti MD(Geriatric Medicine)
Senior Resident
Department of Geriatric Medicine
National Centre for Ageing (NCA)
AIIMS
New Delhi, India

Shreya Biswal MD(Geriatric Medicine)
Senior Resident
Department of Geriatric Medicine
AIIMS
New Delhi, India

Sudeep Mathew George MD(Geriatrics)
Senior Resident
Department of Geriatric Medicine
National Centre for Ageing (NCA)
AIIMS
New Delhi, India

Sumit Jaiswal MD
Geriatrician
Department of Geriatric Medicine
Banaras Hindu University
Varanasi, Uttar Pradesh, India

Sunil Jyani MBBS MD
Assistant Professor
Department of Geriatric Medicine
Mahatma Gandhi Medical College and Hospital
Jaipur, Rajasthan, India

Sunny Singhal MD(Geriatric Medicine) MRCP(UK)
Assistant Professor
Department of Geriatric Medicine
Sawai Man Singh (SMS) Medical College
Jaipur, Rajasthan, India

Surekha Viggeswarpu MD(Medicine) FRCP
Senior Professor
Department of Geriatrics
Christian Medical College
Vellore, Tamil Nadu, India

Sushma Bhatnagar MD(Anesthesia)
Senior Consultant and Lead, Pain and Palliative Medicine
Department of Pain and Palliative Medicine
Indraprastha Apollo Hospital
New Delhi, India

Swarup Das MBBS MD(Geriatric Medicine) (AIIMS New Delhi)
Senior Resident
Department of Geriatric Medicine
National Centre for Ageing (NCA)
AIIMS
New Delhi, India

Sweta Kedia PhD
Assistant Professor
Department of Clinical Psychology
AIIMS
New Delhi, India

Tilotma Jamwal DNB(MHA)
Assistant Professor
Hospital Administration
National Centre for Ageing (NCA)
AIIMS
New Delhi, India

Vasu Digra MD(Geriatric Medicine)
Senior Resident
Department of Geriatric Medicine
National Centre for Ageing (NCA)
AIIMS
New Delhi, India

Yamini Ajmera MD(Geriatric Medicine)
Consultant
Department of Geriatric Medicine
Artemis Hospitals
Gurugram, Haryana, India

Yogesh Poonia MD(Geriatric Medicine)
Senior Resident
Department of Geriatric Medicine
National Centre for Ageing (NCA)
AIIMS
New Delhi, India

Yogita Gupta MD DNB FRCSEd
Faculty
Department of Ophthalmology
Deen Dayal Upadhyay Hospital
New Delhi, India

FOREWORD

It gives me great pleasure to write the foreword for *"Principles and Practice of Geriatric Medicine for Postgraduate and Practitioner"* in India, a multiauthor publication edited by the eminent Indian Geriatrician Professor Prasun Chatterjee.

This monograph comes at a time when most predictions on global demographic transitions indicate that by the year 2050, there will be over 2 billion people aged 60 years and the number of persons aged 80 years is expected to reach 426 million. This demographic is also coupled with an epidemiological transition to preponderance of noncommunicable diseases from communicable disease. The health systems in most countries are under stress to cater to the unique needs of older people. The need for a robust and integrated healthcare system catering to this demographic is more urgent than ever.

Geriatric medicine is not merely an extension of internal medicine for older people but a specialized field that recognizes the unique and interconnected health challenges faced by older adults. The multidimensional nature of aging brings forth complexities such as multimorbidity, frailty, dementia, depression, and other geriatric syndromes. Addressing these requires a multidisciplinary approach that transcends organ-specific care. It calls for a paradigm shift from disease-centric treatment to integrated, person-centered care—a philosophy that forms the cornerstone of geriatric practice.

The author's vision for this book—to equip postgraduate students and practitioners with a systematic approach to geriatric care—is both timely and essential. By incorporating case vignettes and discussions, this book not only bridges the gap in existing literature but also provides a practical roadmap for delivering evidence-based care to older adults. It emphasizes the importance of improving functionality and quality of life, which should always be the ultimate goal of geriatric medicine.

I commend the authors and contributing experts for their commitment to advancing geriatric education and practice. This book will undoubtedly serve as an invaluable resource for students, clinicians, and all those dedicated to improving the lives of our older population. I am confident that this book will inspire a new generation of healthcare professionals to view aging not as a challenge but as an opportunity to transform the health system to care for all ages.

AB Dey
Former Professor
AIIMS, New Delhi

PREFACE

With India's population of 80+ individuals rising at an unprecedented rate, it is imperative to have a comprehensive, context-specific reference in Geriatric Medicine. "*Principles and Practice of Geriatric Medicine for Postgraduate and Practitioner*" in India has been developed as a quick reference for postgraduate students, family physicians, and clinicians, offering an up-to-date overview of aging and age-related disorders in the Indian context.

This book represents a nationwide collaboration of eminent experts from AIIMS, CMC Vellore, Calcutta Medical College, Armed Forces Medical College, Banaras Hindu University, and leading institutions across India, including contributions from regional centers in Jaipur, Kota, and beyond. This collective effort ensures both academic depth and practical applicability across diverse healthcare settings.

This book would be the first of its kind to feature a multidisciplinary collaboration in geriatric practice, addressing clinical, social, psychological, and biological aspects of aging. It emphasizes syndromes such as frailty, sarcopenia, falls, cognitive decline, multimorbidity, and end-of-life care through various emerging allied specialties like ortho-geriatrics, geriatric psychiatry, geriatric dentistry, geriatric oncology, rehabilitation, nutrition, palliative care, and spirituality.

A notable feature is the inclusion of Geroscience and Regenerative Medicine, highlighting the connection between biological aging and clinical intervention. Aimed at bridging evidence and experience, this book seeks to provide readers with both scientific knowledge and clinical wisdom, promoting a comprehensive, capacity-focused approach to elderly care throughout India.

Prasun Chatterjee

ACKNOWLEDGMENT

As per the will of the Almighty and the blessings of my parents, we have completed this timely and relevant book, "*Principles and Practice of Geriatric Medicine for Postgraduate and Practitioner*", which will serve as a comprehensive, evidence-based reference for clinicians, students, and researchers dedicated to the care of older adults in India.

I sincerely appreciate all the esteemed contributors from across the country, whose chapters add valuable insight through their wisdom and clinical experience. Their commitment has turned this into a truly national academic achievement and a significant milestone in the development of geriatric medicine in India.

I must thank my colleagues, Dr Abhijith, Dr Akshata, Dr Raj Kumar, Dr Avinash, and the students at the Department of Geriatric Medicine, AIIMS, New Delhi, for dedicating their valuable time to help to complete this project.

I remain indebted to my mentors, Dr AB Dey, teachers, and collaborators at national and international institutions, including the World Health Organization, whose guidance has continually shaped my journey as a geriatrician.

My heartfelt thanks to the editorial and publishing teams of M/s Jaypee Brothers Medical Publishers (P) Ltd., New Delhi, India, for their professionalism, patience, and support throughout this process.

Finally, I dedicate this work to the elderly population of our country—the true inspiration behind every page of this book. I am equally grateful to my family, especially my wife, for her constant encouragement, understanding, and unconditional support, which have been my greatest strength in pursuing this endeavor.

Prasun Chatterjee

CONTENTS

SECTION 1: PRINCIPLES OF GERIATRICS AND GERONTOLOGY

SECTION 2: GERIATRIC SPECIFICS

SECTION 3: PREVENTIVE AND SOCIAL GERIATRICS

SECTION 1

Principles of Geriatrics and Gerontology

CHAPTER 1

Global Demography and India's Perspective

Meenaxi Sharda, Mayank Shrivastava, Akshata Rao

INTRODUCTION

Understanding the world's demographics is of paramount importance in the field of geriatric medicine as aging brings unique challenges and opportunities. The impact of the aging population on healthcare systems, economies, and societies is profound. This chapter aims to provide a comprehensive overview of global demographic trends, focusing on India, as there is a rapid increase in its elderly population. This shift presents unique challenges for India, including developing robust healthcare and social support systems to cater to the aging population. Additionally, the cultural, social, and economic factors influencing the aging process in India add layers of complexity to the issue.

GLOBAL DEMOGRAPHIC TRENDS

The four global demographic "megatrends" are: (1) population growth, (2) population aging, (3) international migration, and (4) urbanization. Trends in population aging are particularly relevant and have continued and lasting impacts on Sustainable Development Goals.

Global Trends in Population Aging

The demographic shift of the population toward older ages is known as population aging. The global population aged 65+ years is projected to grow from 703 million in 2019 to 1.5 billion by 2050, with one in six people over 65 years, according to World Population Prospects 2019. By the 2070s, individuals aged 65+ years are expected to reach 2.2 billion, surpassing children under 18 years. By the mid-2030s, those aged 80+ years will exceed 265 million, outnumbering infants under 1 year. As per the World Population Prospects 2024, the countries are at different stages of the demographic transition. In 63 countries, including China, Germany, Japan, and the Russian Federation, which is 28% area, the population is expected to peak in size before or during 2024. In 48 countries containing 10% of the world's population, such as Brazil, the Islamic Republic of Iran, and Vietnam, it is expected to peak between 2025 and 2054. In the remaining 126 countries and areas, including India, Indonesia, and Nigeria, the population growth will likely continue through 2054, and possibly peak after 2100. It also includes countries such as Australia, Canada, and the United States of America **(Fig. 1)**.

As populations age, the shares of working-age adults (25–64 years) and older adults (65+ years) will increase, while those of children (0–14 years) and youth (15–24 years) will decline **(Fig. 2 and Table 1)**.

Regional Trends

Eastern and Southeastern Asia had the largest older population (260 million) in 2019, projected to rise to 573 million by 2050 (+312 million). Europe and Northern America, home to over 200 million elderly, rank second, but the growth rate is expected to be the slowest (+48%). Northern Africa and Western Asia are expected to see the fastest growth, from 29 million in 2019 to 96 million in 2050 (+226%), followed by sub-Saharan Africa, rising from 32 to 101 million (+218%). By the year 2050, less developed countries will be home to two-thirds of the world's elderly population (1.1 billion), and the least developed countries will have the highest growth rate (+226%) **(Table 2)**.

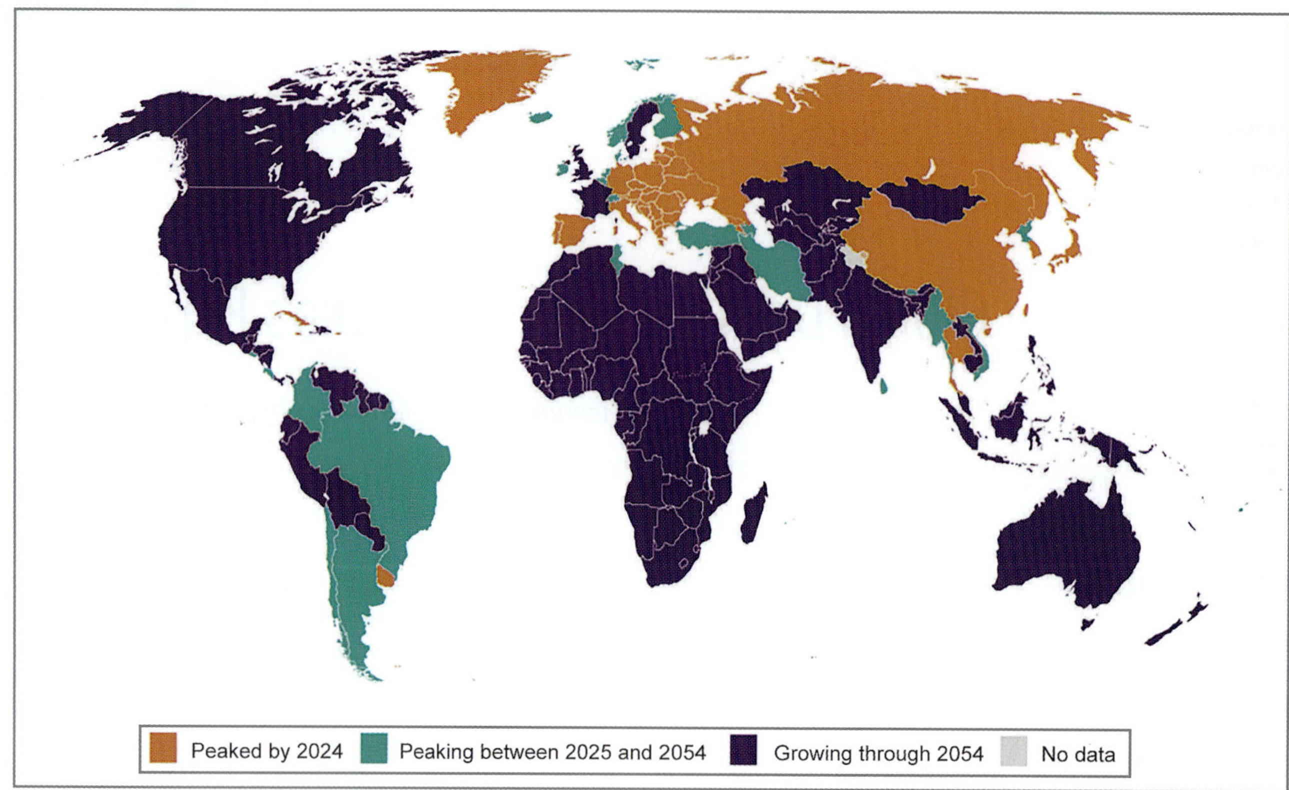

FIG. 1: Countries and areas by timing of the observed or projected population peak.

Source: United Nations. (2024). World Population Prospects 2024. [online] Available from https://population.un.org/wpp/ [Last accessed May, 2025].

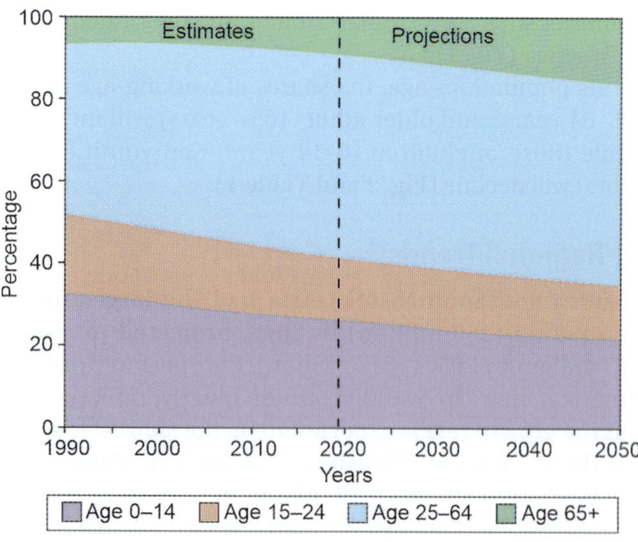

FIG. 2: Global population by broad age groups, 1990–2050 (percentage).

Source: United Nations. (2019). World Population Prospects 2019. [online] Available from https://www.un.org/development/desa/pd/news/world-population-prospects-2019-0 [Last accessed May, 2025].

TABLE 1: Effect of population aging on the distribution of population.

Age group	Population in 2019 (%)	Population in 2050 (%)
Children (0–14 years)	33	21
Youth (15–24 years)	19	14
Working age (25–64 years)	42	49
Older (65+ years)	6	16

Factors Contributing to Population Aging

Population aging is driven by a significant decline in fertility rates, increased life expectancy at birth, and more rapid gains in life expectancy at older ages. The demographic transition occurs in stages. In the early stage, population growth rises due to declining mortality rates, while fertility remains high. In the intermediate stage, fertility declines, but population growth continues due to more births than deaths. Eventually, birth and death

TABLE 2: Number of persons aged 65 years or over by geographic region, 2019 and 2050.

Region	Number of persons aged 65 years or over in 2019 (millions)	Number of persons aged 65 years or over in 2050 (millions)	Percentage change between 2019 and 2050
World	702.9	1548.9	120
Sub-Saharan Africa	31.9	101.4	218
Northern Africa and Western Asia	29.4	95.8	226
Central and Southern Asia	119.0	328.1	176
Eastern and Southeastern Asia	260.6	572.5	120
Latin America and the Caribbean	56.4	144.6	156
Australia and New Zealand	4.8	8.8	84
Oceania, excluding Australia and New Zealand	0.5	1.5	190
Europe and Northern America	200.4	296.2	48

Source: United Nations. (2019). World Population Prospects 2019. [online] Available from https://www.un.org/development/desa/pd/news/world-population-prospects-2019-0 [Last accessed May, 2025].

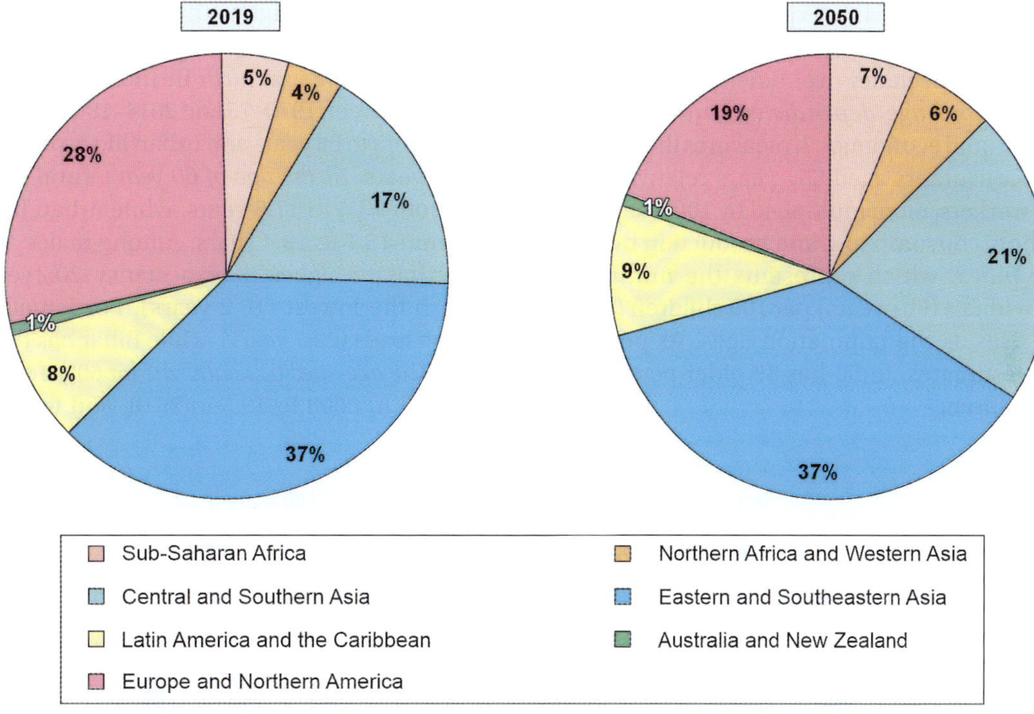

FIG. 3: Distribution of population aged 65 years or over by region, 2019 and 2050 (percentage).

Source: United Nations. (2019). World Population Prospects 2019. [online] Available from https://www.un.org/development/desa/pd/news/world-population-prospects-2019-0 [Last accessed May, 2025].

rate balance at low levels, slowing population growth. In the final stage, growth halts or becomes negative, leading to population stabilization or decline **(Fig. 3)**. Globally, life expectancy at birth rose by 7.7 years (12%) from 1990–1995 to 2015–2020 and is expected to increase by another 4.5 years (6%) by 2045–2050. Sub-Saharan Africa saw the largest rise, from 49.1 years in 1990–1995 to 60.5 years in 2015–2020, with an additional projected gain of 7.6 years by 2045–2050.

Life expectancy at age 65 years is the additional years a person can expect to live after 65 years, based on age-specific mortality rates. Globally, it was 17 years from

2015 to 2020 and is projected to increase to 19 years by 2045–2050. Australia and New Zealand currently lead with 17.5 years at age 65 years, expected to rise to 23.9 years by 2050 due to better healthcare and living conditions. Women tend to outlive men; in 2015–2020, women at 65 years were expected to live 18 more years, while men were expected to live 16 years. By 2050, 54% of the global population aged 65+ years is projected to be women.

Measures of Population Aging

- The *old-age dependency ratio (OADR)* is the number of people aged 65+ years per 100 working-age individuals (20–64 years), indicating economic dependency. This ratio is projected to increase from 16 to 28 per 100 by 2050.
- The *prospective old-age dependency ratio (POADR)* measures old age based on a remaining life expectancy of 15 years. It calculates the people above the age closest to a remaining life expectancy of 15 years relative to those aged 20 years and older, capturing increases in life expectancy over time.
- The *economic old-age dependency ratio* considers demographics and economics. It measures the effective number of consumers aged 65+ years relative to the number of workers, often multiplied by 100, using data on population, consumption, and production by age.
- The *aging index,* which represents the number of elderly individuals (60+ years) per 100 children (under 15 years), rises as the population ages. As per 2021 population estimates, India has 39 older persons for every 100 children.

INDIAN SCENARIO

Demographic Profile of Older Adults in India

India is experiencing moderate population aging. In 1961, 5.6% of the population was aged 60+ years, rising to 10.1% in 2021 and projected to reach 13.1% in 2031 and 19.5% (319 million) by 2050, with 36.1% by 2100. By 2050, one in five Indians will be elderly. The elderly population in 2021 was around 138 million, comprising 67 million males and 71 million females, growing at an annual rate of 3.28%, and the growth rate of the elderly was 36% in the last two decades, compared to 12.4% for the general population from 2011 to 2021. Interstate variations exist, with southern and northern states such as Himachal Pradesh and Punjab, having higher shares of elderly than the national average, a trend expected to continue by 2036. States with higher fertility, such as Bihar and Uttar Pradesh, will see a lower increase in elderly population share but will still rise by 2036. The sex ratio of the elderly (1,065 in 2021) is higher than the general population's (948), projected to reach 1085 by 2031 **(Fig. 4)**.

Life expectancy at birth in India has increased significantly. Between 1970–75 and 2014–18, rural life expectancy rose from 48 to 68 years and urban life expectancy from 58.9 to 72.6 years. *At the age of 60 years,* rural life expectancy grew from 13.5 to 17.6 years, while urban life expectancy rose from 15.7 to 19.4 years. Among males aged 60 years, Punjab has the highest life expectancy (20.2 years) and Uttar Pradesh the lowest (16.2 years). For females, Himachal Pradesh leads (22.7 years), while Bihar has the lowest (16.3 years). The *age-specific death rate* for 60–64 years decreased from 22.5 in 2008 to 19.5 in 2018, and for 65–69 years, it

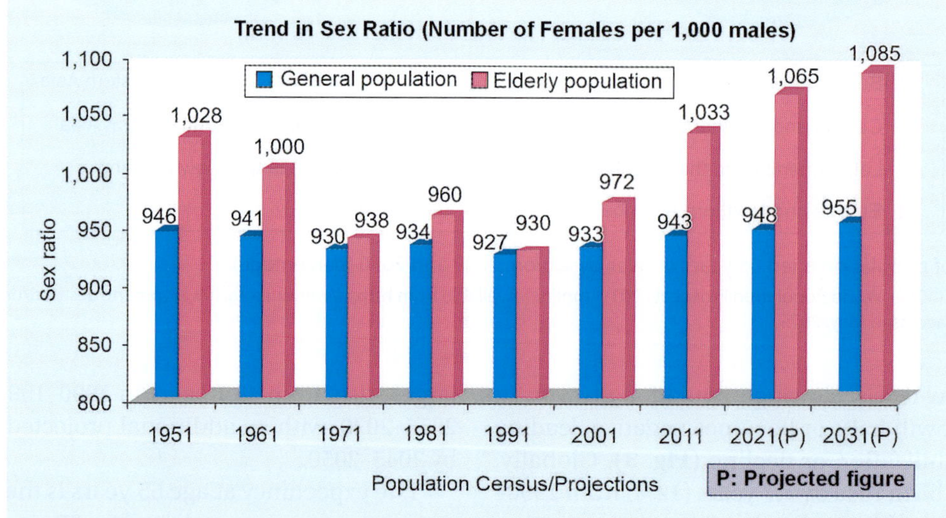

FIG. 4: Sex ratio trends in general and elderly population (number of females per 1,000 males).

Source: Government of India. (2021). Elderly in India 2021. [online] Available from https://mospi.gov.in/sites/default/files/publication_reports/Elderly%20in%20India%202021.pdf. [Last accessed May, 2025].

declined from 33.5 to 31.3. The *old-age dependency ratio* increased from 10.9% in 1961 to 14.2% in 2011, projected to reach 15.7% in 2021 and 20.1% by 2031, with ratios of 15.1 for rural and 12.4 for urban areas in 2011 **(Fig. 5)**.

CHALLENGES SPECIFIC TO INDIA

Feminization: Gender disparities persist across all ages but intensify in old age, as older women are often widowed, living alone, without income or assets, and reliant on family for support.

Ruralization: According to the 2011 Census, 71% of older adults in India live in rural areas, where remoteness, income insecurity, limited healthcare access, and isolation are more pronounced than in urban regions.

The 2020 *Longitudinal Aging Study in India (LASI)* surveyed over 72,000 people aged 45+ years, for *health, lifestyle factors, economic, and social well-being* of India's aging population, revealing significant issues. Many older adults suffer from chronic conditions such as hypertension and diabetes, with 27% aged 60+ years reporting functional limitations. Mental health concerns, including depression, are common, and over 75% lack health insurance. Socioeconomic disparities heavily influence health outcomes and access to care.

AGING-RELATED POLICIES AND PROGRAMS

International Policy Frameworks on Aging

- United Nations principles for older persons
- *International Day of Older Persons*: Established by the UN General Assembly on October 1, 1990.
- *WHO Decade of Healthy Aging (2021–2030)*: Aims to improve older individuals' well-being through age-friendly environments, combating agism, integrated care, and building long-term care systems.

Policy Response to Aging in India

- National Policy on Older Persons (NPOP) and National Program for Health Care of the Elderly (NPHCE)
- Maintenance and Welfare of Parents and Senior Citizens Act (2007)
- *Social security and welfare schemes*: *Antodaya Anna Yojana, Varishtha Pension Bima Yojana*, Indira Gandhi National Old Age Pension Scheme (IGNOAPS), and senior citizen concessions, including concessional loans for small businesses.
- *Programs for the elderly: Atal Vayo Abhyuday Yojana*

COMPARATIVE ANALYSIS: INDIA VERSUS GLOBAL TRENDS

- *Demographic trends*: Both worldwide and in India, demographic changes include population aging, rising life expectancy, declining fertility rates, and increased urbanization.
- *Health and socioeconomic implications*: Globally, noncommunicable diseases (NCDs) are the primary healthcare focus, while India faces a dual burden of communicable and NCDs. Aging populations impact national finances, necessitating robust retirement policies and pension schemes, especially in India. While traditional joint family caregiving in India is declining, it still offers more support compared to

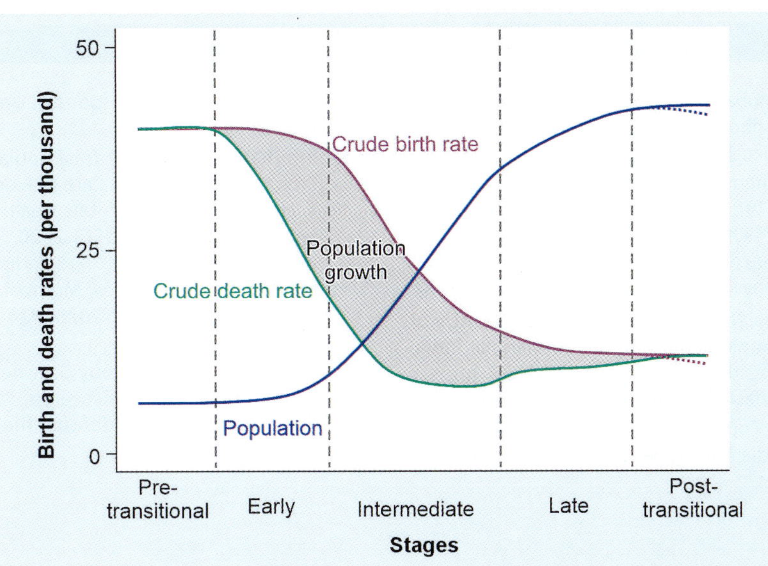

FIG. 5: Schematic representation of the demographic transition.
Source: United Nations. (2024). World Population Prospects 2024. [online] Available from https://population.un.org/wpp/. [Last accessed May, 2025].

developed countries. Societies worldwide are working on age-friendly environments and social support.

- *Policy and programmatic responses*: Comprehensive healthcare policies focusing on elderly care, late retirement, and employment are being adopted globally and in India. However, these programs need better coverage, implementation, and monitoring.
- *Innovations and best practices*: Technologies such as telemedicine, health monitoring devices, and digital health platforms are improving elderly care. Smart homes and assistive technology enhance the quality of life for seniors.
- *Lessons and opportunities:* India, with its large population, could adopt models such as universal healthcare coverage (Japan, Norway), long-term care insurance (Germany, South Korea), and age-friendly cities (Canada, the Netherlands). India's community-based care, telemedicine, and nongovernmental organization (NGO)/private sector involvement offer valuable insights for low-resource global communities.

CONCLUSION

The integration of demographic insights into geriatric medicine is crucial for addressing the evolving needs, preparedness for the future, and developing strategies to improve the quality of life for the elderly population. Comparing India's situation with global trends reveals both similarities and differences. The challenges of an aging population are universal, but the solutions must be context and country-specific.

Self-Assessment Questionnaire

Q1. What are the global demographic "megatrends," and why is population aging particularly significant for sustainable development?

Q2. What are the key factors driving population aging?

Q3. Compare the regional trends in population aging between Eastern/Southeastern Asia and Europe/Northern America.

Q4. Explain the concept and importance of the old-age dependency ratio (OADR).

Q5. What is the aging index, and what does a higher index indicate about a country's demographic profile?

Q6. Outline the major demographic changes in India's elderly population from 1961 to 2050.

Q7. Discuss the challenges of feminization and ruralization of aging in India. How do these factors impact elderly health and social security?

Q8. Suggest at least two global best practices or innovations in elderly care that India could adapt to strengthen its geriatric care.

FURTHER READINGS

1. Bloom DE, Luca DL. The global demography of aging. In: Piggott J, Woodland A, (Eds). Handbook of the Economics of Population Aging. Netherlands: Elsevier; 2016. pp. 3-56.
2. United Nations, Department of Economic and Social Affairs, Population Division (2019). World Population Ageing 2019: Highlights (ST/ESA/SER.A/430).
3. United Nations (2024). World Population Prospects 2024: Summary of Results. UN DESA/POP/2024/TR/NO. 9. New York: United Nations.
4. NSO (2021), Elderly in India, National Statistical Office, Ministry of Statistics & Programme Implementation, Government of India, New Delhi. Ageing and health. Accessed June 27, 2025. https://www.who.int/news-room/fact-sheets/detail/ageing-and-health
5. International Institute for Population Sciences & United Nations Population Fund 2023. India Ageing Report 2023, Caring for Our Elders: Institutional Responses. United Nations Population Fund, New Delhi.
6. International Institute for Population Sciences (IIPS), National Programme for Health Care of Elderly (NPHCE), MoHFW, Harvard T. H. Chan School of Public Health (HSPH) and the University of Southern California (USC) 2020. Longitudinal Ageing Study in India (LASI) Wave 1, 2017-18, India Report, International Institute for Population Sciences, Mumbai. https://india.unfpa.org/sites/default/files/pub-pdf/20230926_india_ageing_report_2023_web_version_.pdf
7. Sanderson WC, Scherbov S. A new perspective on population aging. Demographic Research. 2017;16(2):27-58. https://www.iipsindia.ac.in/sites/default/files/LASI_India_Report_2020_compressed.pdf

CHAPTER 2

Theories of Aging

Pramod Kumar Mehta

INTRODUCTION

Aging and age-related diseases are currently among the most prominent medical challenges. The developments in the field of medicine have significantly increased life expectancy worldwide in the last few decades. However, with this increasing life expectancy, there has also been a significant increase in the burden of degenerative diseases that puts considerable stress on the healthcare system of the countries. Slowing down or preventing the aging process has been linked with preventing these age-related degenerative diseases (a phenomenon known as the longevity dividend). Hence, a better understanding of the aging process and theories of aging is of utmost importance in the current scenario.

Aging Definition

It is said that "aging" is easy to recognize but difficult to define. There is not one universally accepted definition. Most definitions indicate that "aging is a process associated with decline in the structure and function, impaired maintenance and repair systems, increased susceptibility to disease and death, and a reduced reproductive capacity." Bernard and Strehler defined aging by the means of four postulates:

1. *Aging is universal*: The process of aging occurs in different degrees in all the individuals of the species.
2. *Aging must be intrinsic*: The factors attributing to aging are endogenous and not dependent on extrinsic factors. They may, however, be modified by extrinsic factors.
3. *Aging must be progressive*: Changes leading to aging progress continuously throughout the lifespan
4. *Aging must be deleterious*: The process of aging negatively impacts the structure and function across different systems.

AGING THEORIES

Since the dawn of the previous century, scientists have tried to solve the mystery of the aging process. Multiple theories have been proposed by different researchers, with a few standing the tide of time. In this section, we discuss the most important and accepted theories and hallmarks of aging available in the current literature.

Evolutionary Theories

Evolutionary theories of aging delve into the evolutionary forces shaping lifespan and aging patterns across species. Most evolutionary theories are linked to two main strategies: (1) Reproduction and (2) longevity and the interaction between the two. Over the course of evolution, early reproductive success with a finite lifespan gained prominence over longevity and immortality for maintaining the existence of the species. In the evolutionary process, the survival after the reproductive period takes a backseat, and the individual goes through a number of degenerative processes resulting in aging. The process of aging after reproductive age can be rapid (programmed death seen in annual plants and Pacific salmon), gradual (as seen in most species from yeast to humans), or very negligent (e.g., Rougheye rockfish and Bristlecone pine). Some of the main classical evolutionary theories are mentioned below:

- *Programmed cell death*: This is one of the earliest aging theories, proposed by Weissman in 1882. According to this theory, the process of aging and death is genetically programmed to occur. It has evolved so that older animals are removed from the population and the natural resources are available for younger members of the species.

- *Mutation accumulation*: This theory given by Medawar states that natural selection favors traits that are beneficial for reproduction but in turn fails to prevent the accumulation of mutations that are deleterious in late life.
- *Antagonistic pleiotropy*: This is one of the most accepted evolutionary theories and was proposed by George C Williams. It extends the mutation accumulation theory and proposes that the genes that confer benefits early in life (contributing to fertility and other essential components) may also have detrimental effects in late life. As a result, the benefits of enhanced fertility early in life come at the cost of the deterioration of the body in later life.
- *Disposable soma theory*: This theory was proposed by Kirkwood and Holliday in 1979. It suggests that resources allocated to somatic maintenance compete with those invested in reproduction, resulting in a tradeoff between longevity and reproductive success. The somatic cells are disposable from an evolutionary perspective and hence accumulate the damages that cause aging. At the same time, resources are preferentially diverted to the maintenance and repair of germ cells.

  All these theories assume that the natural selection has a negligible or negative influence on aging. Some theories also propose the positive aspects of the aging process in evolution.
- *Grandmother hypothesis*: Hamilton gave this theory explaining how evolution can enhance old age. According to this theory, the long-lived grandparents take care of the young grandchildren and have a significant impact on their survival. They also share genes, including those that cause increased longevity. This phenomenon is observed across multiple species, including humans.
- *Adaptive senectitude*: It has been observed that traits that are harmful in younger humans, such as obesity and hypertension, paradoxically appear to be associated with greater survival and function in very old age. This might represent an adaptive senectitude or reverse antagonistic pleiotropy, where some traits harmful in young adults may become beneficial in older adults.

Biological Theories: Hallmarks of Aging

The process of aging is characterized by a set of hallmarks that meet three criteria: (1) They are observed with age, (2) their progression can be experimentally accelerated, and (3) they can potentially be slowed down, halted, or reversed through therapeutic interventions. There are 12 hallmarks of aging: (1) Genomic instability, (2) telomere shortening, (3) epigenetic changes, (4) loss of proteostasis, (5) impaired macroautophagy, (6) disrupted nutrient sensing, (7) mitochondrial dysfunction, (8) cellular senescence, (9) depletion of stem cells, (10) altered intercellular communication, (11) chronic inflammation, and (12) dysbiosis **(Fig. 1)**.

The interconnectedness of aging hallmarks implies that modifying one specific hallmark typically impacts others as well. This highlights the complexity of aging, emphasizing the need to consider it as a comprehensive process rather than focusing solely on individual aspects. Below, we discuss some essential biological theories of aging. These theories incorporate the 12 hallmarks of aging mentioned above.

Primary

Genomic Instability

It arises from a variety of internal and external factors that damage DNA, including replication errors, oxidative stress, and environmental agents. This damage leads to mutations, chromosomal rearrangements, and telomere shortening, contributing to aging and age-related diseases. Cells counter these effects with DNA repair mechanisms, yet these systems weaken over time, increasing the accumulation of mutations. In nuclear DNA, such damage can disrupt essential genes, impairing stem cell function and accelerating tissue aging. Studies suggest that animals with better DNA repair tend to live longer, with proteins such as SIRT6 and enzymes for oxidative DNA repair possibly playing roles in promoting longevity.

Mitochondrial DNA (mtDNA) is also affected, accumulating mutations due to its high replication rate and lack of protective proteins. While the exact impact of mtDNA damage on aging is unclear, mutations in mitochondrial genes in animal models have been linked to accelerated aging. Additionally, structural changes in the nuclear lamina, crucial for chromatin organization, lead to instability and premature aging syndromes such as Hutchinson–Gilford progeria. Experimental treatments targeting these factors show promise in delaying aging in certain cases, although further research is needed to confirm these interventions' effects on normal aging.

Oxidative stress, resulting from an imbalance between reactive oxygen species (ROS) and antioxidant defenses, is implicated in aging and age-related diseases. Harman's free radical theory of aging suggests that oxygen-derived free radicals are accountable for age-related damage. Despite the presence of antioxidant systems, they cannot

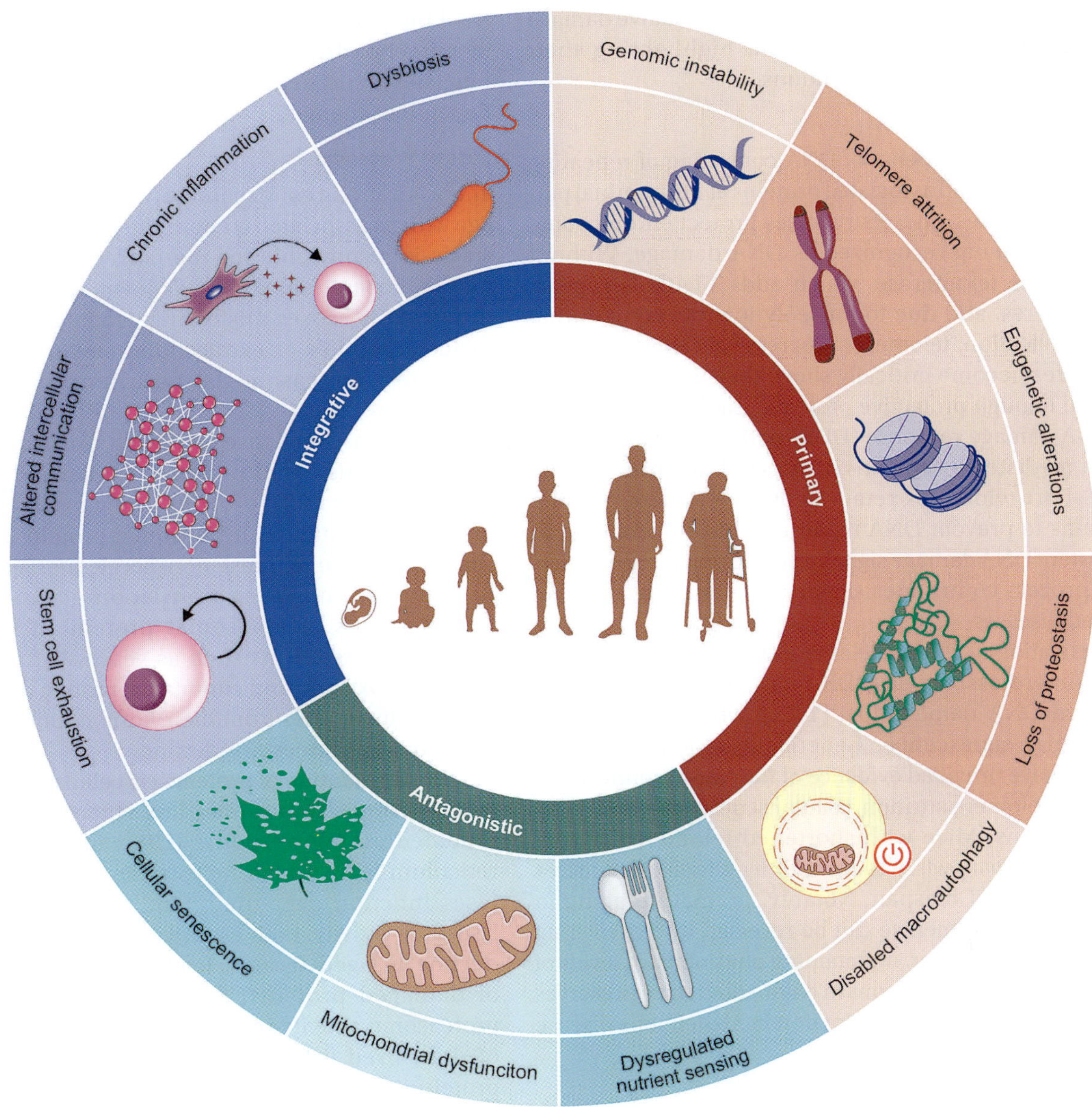

FIG. 1: Twelve hallmarks of aging.
Source: López-Otín C, Blasco MA, Partridge L, Serrano M, Kroemer G. Hallmarks of ageing: an expanding universe. Cell. 2023;186(2): 243-78.

completely neutralize all the free radicals produced throughout the cell's lifespan. Consequently, cells and tissues suffer oxidative damage, contributing to cellular senescence, DNA mutations, and protein dysfunction, accelerating the aging process. Enhancing antioxidant defenses leads to a rise in average lifespan. Lifespan has been seen to be affected by not only resistance to oxidative stress but also targeted alterations to the antioxidant pool.

Miquel et al. proposed that senescence results from ROS damaging the mitochondrial genome in postmitotic cells. The constant ROS production by mitochondria throughout life induces chronic oxidative stress associated with aging, playing a pivotal role in the aging process. Elderly animals exhibit a greater oxidation level than their younger counterparts, accumulating oxidized proteins, DNA forms, and lipids. Moreover, short-lived species exhibit a significantly higher rate of oxidant production by mitochondria compared to longer lived species.

Assessing biomarkers of oxidative stress appears more appropriate than measuring the rate of oxidant production. DNA is identified as a key target for oxidative damage associated with aging. mtDNA, in particular, shows much higher levels of oxidation with age compared to nuclear DNA. Both endogenous and exogenous antioxidants play a crucial role in mitigating oxidative damage and preserving cellular function, highlighting their potential as antiaging interventions.

Telomere Attrition

Telomeres are segments of DNA consisting of repeating TTAGGG units and associated proteins at the terminal part of chromosomes. These structures protect chromosome ends from being recognized as DNA damage. Without the enzyme telomerase, which adds TTAGGG repeats to telomeres, and due to nucleolytic processing during DNA replication, telomeres progressively shorten. When telomeres become critically short, they lose their ability to bind enough protective proteins, leading to activation of DNA damage response (DDR) pathways and cell cycle arrest mediated by proteins such as p21 and p16. Despite this, short telomeres retain enough telomere-binding proteins to prevent DNA repair and fusion, resulting in persistent DNA damage signaling and cellular senescence. This process contributes significantly to aging and age-related diseases.

Activation of DDR at telomeres leads to the formation of telomere-associated DDR foci (TAFs) or telomere-induced DNA damage foci (TIFs), which are markers of cellular senescence. Genetically modified animal models have provided evidence of the causal connections between telomere attrition, cellular senescence, and aging in organisms. Mice with shortened telomeres exhibit reduced lifespan, while those with lengthened telomeres show increased lifespan. Notably, premature aging in mice lacking telomerase can be reversed by reactivating telomerase. Moreover, maintaining physiological levels of telomerase in adult neurons in engineered mice preserves cell survival and cognitive function in Alzheimer's disease models.

Epigenetic Alterations

The epigenetic clock theory proposes that age-related changes, such as DNA methylation, histone modifications, and regulation by noncoding RNA, serve as molecular signatures of aging, allowing for the precise estimation of chronological age and prediction of lifespan. Specific genomic sites experience increased methylation as individuals age. Histone demethylases modify the insulin and insulin-like growth factor-1 (IGF-1) signaling pathway which are directly correlated with longevity.

Epigenetic clocks provide valuable insights into the biological aging process and hold promise as biomarkers for monitoring aging-related changes and assessing the efficacy of antiaging interventions. Sirtuins play a significant part in repairing DNA and keeping the genome stable by coordinating signals of DNA damage with the activation of repair enzymes. Drugs such as resveratrol have the potential to trigger the sirtuins and reduce ROS in mitochondria. This action enhances mitochondrial biogenesis and function, leading to the reversal of age-dependent changes.

Loss of Proteostasis

There is a strong connection between proteostasis and old age with its associated comorbidities. The protein homeostasis is responsible for the correct protein molecule folding, reparation, and breakdown. A disruption of the proteostasis causes misfolding, leading to intracellular inclusion bodies or extracellular amyloid plaques and ultimately increasing the occurrence of age-related pathologies.

Proteostasis collapse can result from increased production of misfolded proteins, oxidative damage, and mutations that make proteins prone to aggregation. For instance, a mutation in ribosomal protein RPS9, which causes error-prone translation, accelerates aging in mice. In contrast, improving translation accuracy through modifications to ribosomal protein RPS23 extends lifespan in organisms such as yeast, worms, and flies. Slowed translation and cumulative protein damage divert cellular chaperones from their normal functions, further exacerbating proteostasis decline.

The degradation of proteins via cellular quality control mechanisms also becomes less efficient with age. The unfolded protein response (UPR) in the endoplasmic reticulum (ER), which helps maintain protein folding, loses function over time. Similarly, proteasome and lysosome activity, both essential for protein degradation, decline in aged tissues, leading to the accumulation of damaged proteins. Studies have shown reduced proteasome activity in aging organs, such as the brains of short-lived fish, and the buildup of ubiquitinylated proteins in various species, including flies, mice, and humans.

Chaperone-mediated autophagy (CMA), a specific lysosomal degradation pathway, also diminishes with age. In mice, restoring CMA by re-expressing LAMP2A, a key component, has been shown to reduce liver aging. Enhancing autophagy through pharmacological or genetic interventions has been identified as a possible approach to remove protein aggregates, prolong lifespan, and postpone the development of neurodegenerative disorders.

Disabled Macroautophagy

Autophagy, or macroautophagy, is a process where cytoplasmic material is enclosed in double-membrane vesicles called autophagosomes, which later fuse with lysosomes to digest their contents. This process not only manages protein degradation (proteostasis) but also eliminates nonprotein materials, such as lipids, glycogen, and even entire organelles such as damaged mitochondria (mitophagy). Autophagy plays a crucial role in maintaining cellular health by removing dysfunctional components and invading pathogens. However, with aging, the efficiency of autophagy declines, contributing to the accumulation of damaged organelles and protein aggregates, reduced pathogen elimination, and increased inflammation, all of which promote age-related diseases.

In humans, autophagy-related genes such as *ATG5*, *ATG7*, and *BECN1* show decreased expression with age. Reduced autophagy in immune cells (such as T and B lymphocytes) is linked to lower levels of proautophagic metabolites such as spermidine. This decline in autophagy accelerates aging and contributes to conditions such as neurodegeneration, cardiovascular disease, and cancer. Animal studies demonstrate that inhibiting autophagy speeds up aging, leading to early organ degeneration and increased inflammation, but restoring autophagy reverses some of these effects and enhances lifespan.

Stimulating autophagy has been shown to extend lifespan in model organisms. For example, increasing autophagy in specific tissues of flies or mice leads to improved metabolic health and motor function. Spermidine supplementation in mice promotes autophagy, extending lifespan and reducing cardiac aging. Autophagy-inducing compounds such as NAD+ precursors and urolithin A have shown positive effects on health span in clinical trials, improving muscle strength and reducing inflammation, offering promising avenues for delaying aging and preventing age-related diseases.

Antagonistic

Dysregulated Nutrient Sensing

Diet significantly impacts aging across all species. Among the most influential nutritional strategies affecting aging is caloric restriction (CR). Prolonged CR not only extends lifespan but also postpones the onset of various age-related illnesses. Multiple interconnected pathways are involved in mediating the effects of nutrition and CR on aging. To mimic the benefits of CR, drugs called CR mimetics have been developed to target these pathways.

One of the nutrient-sensing pathways includes insulin and IGF-1 signaling pathway, and a downregulation of this pathway has been found to increase the lifespan. Growth hormone deficiency and genetic variation in the FOXO (forkhead box O) family of transcription factors have also been associated with a long life. Another pathway is the mTOR pathway which when deactivated by reduced protein intake or rapamycin delays aging.

Research has shown that NAD+ availability declines with age, leading to decreased activity of sirtuins. This reduction affects communication between the nucleus and mitochondria within cells and between the hypothalamus and adipose tissue at a systemic level. These changes in cellular and systemic processes likely play a role in age-related functional decline and the development of aging-related diseases. Adenosine monophosphate (AMP)-activated protein kinase (AMPK) activity and fibroblast growth factor 21 (FGF21) levels increase with dietary restriction and increase lifespan.

Mitochondrial Dysfunction

Mitochondrial dysfunction, linked to aging, results from accumulating mtDNA mutations, impaired proteostasis, reduced mitochondrial turnover, and altered dynamics. This deterioration hampers energy production, increases ROS, and triggers inflammation and cell death, all of which contribute to aging. Strategies targeting mitochondrial health, such as L-carnitine supplementation, have shown potential in enhancing energy production in aging populations. Interestingly, mild mitochondrial inhibition can promote "mitohormesis," a stress response that may extend lifespan in animals by activating the mitochondrial unfolded protein response (UPRmt).

Interventions such as metformin and partial mitochondrial uncoupling can improve metabolic health, but whether such strategies enhance human lifespan remains uncertain. Increased mitochondrial membrane permeability (MMP), linked to shortened lifespan, can be countered by compounds such as elamipretide, which has shown promise in mitigating mitochondrial-related aging effects. Additionally, antioxidant compounds (e.g., MitoQ, SkQ1) are being explored for their antiaging potential.

Mitochondria also produce microproteins such as humanin and MOTS-c, which decline with age. Elevated levels of these proteins in centenarians correlate with reduced inflammation and better metabolic health, highlighting their potential as antiaging agents that support cellular health and systemic balance.

Cellular Senescence

At the heart of cellular senescence theory lies the notion that aging is driven by the gradual deterioration of individual cells. Over time, cells undergo oxidative stress damage, DNA mutations, and metabolic dysfunction. This damage triggers a state of senescence, where cells cease to divide and function properly, contributing to tissue degeneration and, ultimately, organismal aging. Key players in this theory include telomeres, the protective caps at the end of chromosomes, whose shortening acts as a molecular clock marking cellular aging.

Senescent cells undergo specific gene expression changes, primarily involving cell-cycle and metabolism-related genes, as well as genes related to the senescence-associated secretory phenotype (SASP). The SASP, which includes soluble signaling factors, secreted proteases, and insoluble proteins/extracellular matrix (ECM) components, influencing neighboring cells by activating receptors and signal pathways. This can lead to various aging-associated diseases. The cellular senescence is also affected by the expression of mediators of aging, such as the INK4a/ARF coregulatory molecules. Genetic modifications and certain drugs such as dasatinib, quercetin, and fisetin have been found to remove the senescent cells expressing INK4 and, hence, delay aging.

As individuals age, the stem cell reservoir may decline due to several factors. One reason could be the diminished ability of these cells to self-renew and instead undergo terminal differentiation, exiting the stem cell pool. Alternatively, exposure to cellular stress might trigger apoptosis or senescence, further contributing to the depletion of the stem cell population. Stem cell transplantation from young mice into old ones and inhibition of the p38 mitogen-AMPK signaling pathway have been found to improve lifespan.

Integrative

Stem Cell Exhaustion

Aging is characterized by a decline in tissue renewal and repair, with each organ utilizing its own strategy. For instance, skeletal muscle relies on satellite cells for both renewal and repair, while the skin's epidermis has multiple stem cell niches near hair follicles. In organs such as the liver, lung, and pancreas, low rates of renewal during normal conditions are replaced by injury-induced dedifferentiation, where non-stem cells reacquire stem-like properties to aid tissue repair. This injury-induced plasticity becomes impaired with aging and may be more significant for aging than resident stem cell plasticity under normal conditions.

To counteract aging-related declines in stem cell function, researchers focus on "cellular reprogramming," which transforms adult cells into induced pluripotent stem cells (iPSCs) by using transcription factors such as OCT4, SOX2, KLF4, and MYC (OSKM). This process reverses cellular aging characteristics, including the resetting of the DNA methylation clock and telomere lengthening. Interestingly, reprogramming can be halted midway, allowing cells to rejuvenate without fully losing their identity. This "partial reprogramming" resets aging markers without fully erasing cell-specific functions.

Partial reprogramming has shown promising results in enhancing tissue repair in aged mice, improving regeneration in organs such as the pancreas, muscles, nerves, eyes, skin, heart, and liver. It has also reversed aging-related dysfunctions such as reduced neurogenesis and visual acuity. This approach mimics natural tissue repair processes, where cells temporarily dedifferentiate before regenerating, effectively rejuvenating tissues. Additionally, factors such as FOXM1, which promote dedifferentiation during tissue injury repair, may further support strategies for enhancing tissue repair and combating aging in humans. Ultimately, partial reprogramming offers a potential pathway for restoring tissue repair capacity and delaying aging-related decline.

Altered Intercellular Communication

Aging is associated with alterations in intercellular communication, affecting neural, hormonal, and neuroendocrine signaling pathways. These changes disrupt homeostasis, promoting chronic inflammation, impaired immunosurveillance, and dysbiosis. One focus of aging research is identifying bloodborne factors that either promote or counteract aging. For example, transfusions of old blood into young mice induce aging, while diluting old blood can rejuvenate tissues. Key proaging factors include CCL11, β2-microglobulin, and IL-6, while factors such as TIMP2 and GDF11 show antiaging effects, although GDF11 may also cause tissue fibrosis.

Long-range and short-range communication mechanisms, including signals from organs such as the heart, liver, and muscles, are crucial in regulating aging. These signals can be altered with age, contributing to systemic aging effects. Additionally, the ECM undergoes significant changes with age, such as elastin fragmentation and collagen crosslinking, leading to tissue fibrosis. This stiffening of the ECM impacts cell function, promotes fibrosis, and accelerates aging. The ECM also influences the behavior of senescent cells, which secrete enzymes that further damage the matrix, amplifying proaging signals.

Research has shown that manipulating ECM properties can influence aging. Inhibiting the mechanosensitive ion channel PIEZO1 or sustaining YAP/TAZ signaling can rejuvenate old cells and prevent age-related changes. Moreover, compounds such as chondroitin sulfate and hyaluronic acid have been found to restore collagen in the ECM and extend lifespan in certain models. These findings suggest that targeting ECM stiffness and related pathways may be a promising approach for improving tissue health and delaying aging.

There are various changes in the functioning of the nervous and endocrine systems with aging. These changes produce a negative effect on the body's response to stimuli, reproductive capacity, and other physiological processes.

The hypothalamic–pituitary–adrenal (HPA) axis is seen as the master regulator, orchestrating life stages through physiological adjustments. Hormones regulate metabolism, immune function, and tissue repair, and their decline with age can lead to impaired physiological function and increased vulnerability to age-related diseases. Chronic stress exposure can weaken adaptation capacity, leading to "diseases of adaptation," that are linked to or partially triggered by prolonged physiological or psychological responses to stress, eventually contributing to aging and characterized by decreased stress survival ability.

The interaction between and within the neuroendocrine and immune systems is facilitated by the neuropeptides and cytokines. Additionally, cytokines can reciprocally influence neuroendocrine functions.

Chronic Inflammation

Chronic low-grade inflammation, or inflammaging, is a hallmark of aging and is implicated in the pathogenesis of age-related diseases. Chronic inflammation can stem from the persistent release of reactive molecules by immune cells, leading to tissue damage; production of cytokines by damaged cells and activated immune cells, altering tissue function; and interference with "anabolic signaling," inhibiting insulin and growth factor pathways postmeal or exercise. The inflammaging theory posits that dysregulation of the immune system with age leads to sustained inflammatory responses, contributing to tissue damage, dysfunction, and aging-related phenotypes.

Inflammaging arises from various sources:

- From the accumulation of damaged macromolecules and cells due to increased production and inadequate elimination with age
- Harmful byproducts from microbial constituents, such as oral or gut microbiota, can infiltrate surrounding tissues and circulation.
- Cellular senescence contributes to inflammaging.
- Increased activation of the coagulation system with age may lead to heightened inflammation, possibly contributing to arterial and venous thrombosis in the elderly.
- Age-related changes to the immune system, termed immunosenescence, play a role in inflammaging. Adaptive immunity declines while innate immunity may become mildly hyperactive.
- Defective regulation of the complement pathway can induce local inflammatory reactions.

Inflammatory mediators are crucial in driving inflammaging and represent potential targets for interventions aimed at attenuating age-related inflammation and promoting healthy aging.

Dysbiosis

The gut microbiome is increasingly recognized as essential for a wide range of physiological functions. It aids in nutrient breakdown, defends against harmful pathogens, and produces vital metabolites, including vitamins and short-chain fatty acids (SCFAs). Beyond local digestive roles, the gut microbiota also communicates with the nervous system and other distant organs, exerting a significant influence on overall health and well-being. When this delicate communication is disrupted, leading to an imbalanced microbiome, or dysbiosis, it has been linked to several chronic conditions, including obesity, type 2 diabetes, neurological disorders, cardiovascular diseases, and certain cancers. These connections suggest that the gut microbiome is not only central to digestion but also plays a broader role in regulating systemic health and disease risk. Recent studies have focused on gut microbiota alterations in aging, as changes in this bacterial community are linked to age-related diseases.

Aging impacts gut microbiota, leading to a general decline in microbial diversity. Studies on centenarians show reduced levels of certain core bacteria, such as *Bacteroides* and *Roseburia*, and an increase in genera such as *Bifidobacterium* and *Akkermansia*, which may have prolongevity effects. Research on over 9,000 individuals aged 18–101 years revealed that gut microbiomes become increasingly distinctive to a person with increasing age and are directly related to their health. Healthier individuals continue shifting toward unique microbial compositions, while those in poorer health do not.

Fecal microbiota transplantation (FMT) studies demonstrate that dysbiosis contributes to chronic inflammation and immune decline in aging. It has been seen in animal studies that transferring gut microbiota has prevented neurodegenerative disorders. Other interventions, such as probiotics and dietary changes, can restore beneficial bacteria such as *Akkermansia*, improving age-related conditions such as insulin resistance and inflammation.

Overall, restoring a youthful gut microbiome holds promise for extending health span and lifespan by mitigating age-related microbial imbalances.

CONCLUSION

The quest to unravel the mysteries of aging continues to inspire scientific inquiry and innovation. From cellular mechanisms to evolutionary dynamics, theories of aging offer diverse perspectives on this complex phenomenon. By elucidating the underlying mechanisms driving aging, researchers aim at increasing longevity and ultimately enhancing the quality of life for individuals across the lifespan.

Self-Assessment Questionnaire

Q1. Define "aging" and explain the four postulates proposed by Bernard and Strehler.

Q2. How does the disposable soma theory explain the trade-off between longevity and reproduction?

Q3. Discuss the key differences among programmed cell death, mutation accumulation, and antagonistic pleiotropy theories.

Q4. What are the 12 hallmarks of aging, and how are they interrelated?

Q5. Explain the epigenetic clock theory and its relevance in estimating biological age.

Q6. What is inflammaging, and how does it contribute to age-related diseases?

Q7. Describe the concept of stem cell exhaustion and the role of partial reprogramming in reversing age-related decline.

Q8. Define dysbiosis and explain its association with systemic inflammation and longevity.

FURTHER READINGS

1. Loscalzo J, Fauci AS, Kasper DL, Hauser S, Longo D, Jameson JL. Harrison's Principles of Internal Medicine, 21st edition. New York: McGraw Hill Education; 2022.
2. Halter JB, Ouslander JG, Studenski S, High KP, Asthana S, Supiano MA, et al. Hazzard's Geriatric Medicine and Gerontology, 8th edition. Noida: McGraw Hill; 2022.
3. Viña J, Borrás C, Miquel J. Theories of ageing. IUBMB Life. 2007; 59(4-5):249-54.
4. da Costa JP, Vitorino R, Silva GM, Vogel C, Duarte AC, Rocha-Santos T. A synopsis on ageing-theories, mechanisms and future prospects. Ageing Res Rev. 2016;29:90-112.
5. López-Otín C, Blasco MA, Partridge L, Serrano M, Kroemer G. Hallmarks of ageing: an expanding universe. Cell. 2023;186(2): 243-78.
6. Franceschi C, Campisi J. Chronic inflammation (inflammageing) and its potential contribution to age-associated diseases. J Gerontol A Biol Sci Med Sci. 2014;69 Suppl 1:S4-9.
7. Miquel MDC, Sánchez Cuervo M, Delgado Silveira E, Machuca IS, González-Blazquez S, Errasquin BM, et al. Potentially inappropriate drug prescription in older subjects across health care settings. Eur Geriatr Med. 2010;1(1):9-14.

CHAPTER 3

Physiological Changes with Aging

Sunny Singhal

INTRODUCTION

Similar to reproduction, aging is also one of the basic characteristics shown by almost all multicellular living organisms. Though easy to recognize, it is difficult to define. In simple words, aging is the process of becoming older. However, old age itself is not a disease but a normal, universal, and inevitable biological phenomenon. Aging can therefore be defined in terms of either simpler chronological age numbers or more complex biological changes.

Biological aging though difficult to define is more accurate and based on the physiological changes that reduce the efficiency of the organ systems. Being old does not mean just an increase in the years of age. It means accumulation of harmful changes in our body, thus causing a decrease in our physiological fitness. This in turn leads to increased risks of illness and death. Thus, aging can be defined as a complex, coordinated, and progressive process which is associated with a decline in structure and function causing a decrease in the maintenance and repair capacity of an organism and thereby increasing its susceptibility to disease and death.

Therefore, knowing these physiological changes is of paramount importance and key to understanding biological aging. In this chapter, we will discuss the physiological changes seen in various organ systems.

HEMATOLOGICAL SYSTEM

Hematopoietic cells in the body are a precursor to all blood cell lineages. However, with age there is a change in the number and differentiation of these cells **(Flowchart 1)**. The most common finding seen in marrow is decreased cellularity as a result of age-related necrosis, fibrosis, and fatty tissue infiltration. Marrow cellularity decreases from 100% at birth to 70% at 65 years. Though there is a replacement of active bone marrow by adipose tissue, the number of hematopoietic stem cells (HSCs) increase in number. However, the HSCs show age-related changes such as increased DNA damage, cell cycle defects, telomere attrition, and epigenetic dysregulation. HSCs also exhibit a bias favoring increased differentiation into myeloid progenitor cells (granulocytes, monocytes, erythrocytes, and platelets) and decreased lymphocyte progenitors (lymphocytes and natural killer cells). The increase in myeloid progenitors has been linked to the increased prevalence of myeloproliferative disorders in older adults.

The HSCs or early progenitor cells also show increased clonal hematopoiesis in older age. Clonal hematopoiesis refers to the phenomenon where a subset of blood cells is derived from a single cell and shares identical DNA. Thus, these are clones of a common blood cell progenitor and this phenomenon is known as "clonal hematopoiesis of indeterminate potential" (CHIP). Recent studies have shown CHIP to be an age-related phenomenon with its prevalence increasing from <1% in a 40-year-old to 10–20% in a 70-year-old. CHIP is associated with a higher risk of development of hematological malignancy and inflammatory state as well as coronary heart disease and ischemic stroke.

Anemia is commonly seen in older adults which may be due to nutritional deficiency, chronic disease (kidney disease, etc.), myelodysplasia, or other causes. However, about one-third of these older patients do not have any underlying cause despite extensive blood and marrow workup. This unexplained anemia (UA), which is usually mild and normocytic with a low reticulocyte count, has been hypothesized due to a number of factors such as inflammaging (described later) and occult myelodysplasia. White blood cell count does not show

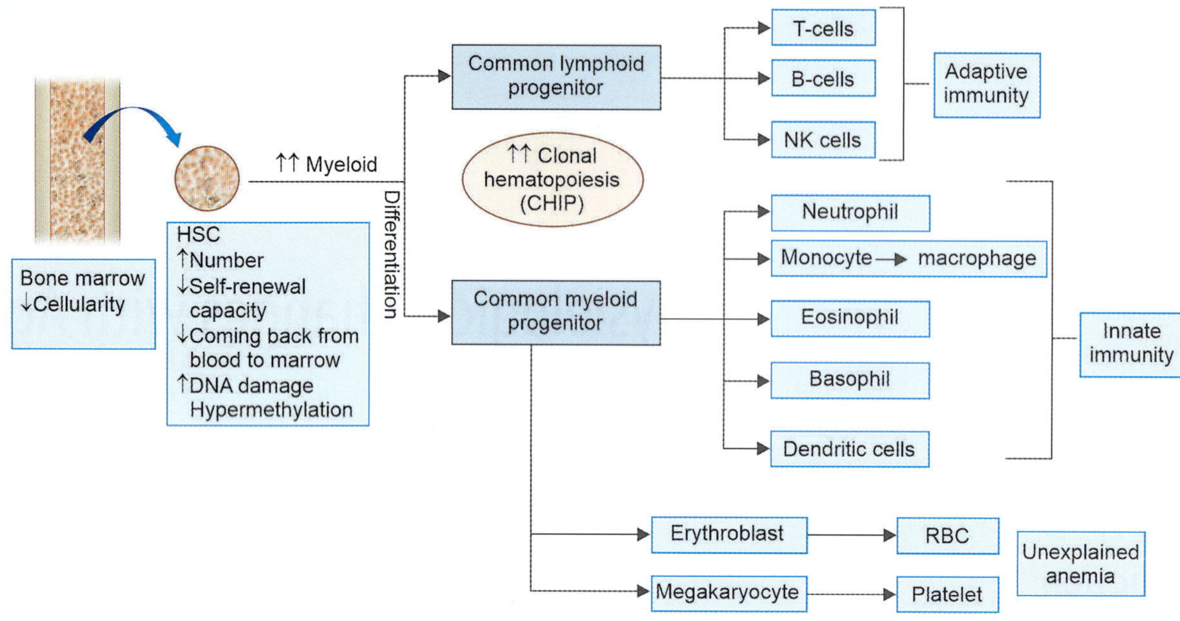

FLOWCHART 1: Aging and the hematopoietic system.

any significant change with aging; however, an increased neutrophil count may be seen in frail elderly. Due to the limited research, not much change is seen or known in platelet number and function in older people.

Aging is considered a prothrombotic state. The incidence of venous thrombosis and pulmonary thromboemboli is higher in older population. Older people have higher levels of procoagulant markers such as fibrinogen, D-dimer, and factor VIII. These markers are also associated with the pathogenesis of atherosclerosis and cardiovascular disease. However, the bleeding complications from warfarin and other anticoagulants also increase in older people. Hence, the current guidelines do not recommend use of anticoagulants as primary prophylaxis in older people who do not have any other risk factors.

IMMUNE SYSTEM

Aging is associated with increased susceptibility to infections and poor outcomes in an older adult. This may be partially attributed to the various changes occurring in the immune system with aging. This age-related immune dysregulation is known as immunosenescence. Aging is associated with alterations in both innate and adaptive immunity leading to an increased risk of acquiring new infections, reactivation of latent infections, increased mortality, and decreased efficacy of vaccines.

The immune system of the body can be divided into two broad categories, i.e., innate and adaptive immunity. The innate immune system which provides an early response to an infection or vaccine is mediated by tissues (skin and mucous membranes), cells (dendritic cells, natural killer cells, neutrophils, monocytes, basophils, and eosinophils), and biochemical factors (complements and cytokines). On the other hand, adaptive immunity which provides delayed but more specific response is mediated by B and T lymphocytes.

The cells of the innate immune system show decreased function with age. They show decreased response to chemotactic stimuli (chemotaxis) and decreased production of cytokines. Further, there is a decrease in the phagocytic capacity of neutrophils and macrophages and cytotoxicity of natural killer cells. There is also a decrease in the expression of costimulatory molecules on antigen presenting cells (APCs), thus affecting T-cell recruitment and activation.

Involution of thymus with age significantly reduces T-cell lymphopoiesis in older adults and therefore, T-cell pool is then maintained by the division of preexisting T-cells. Thus, there is a decreased number of naïve T-cells and an increased number of memory T-cells. There is also significantly decreased expression of costimulatory protein CD28 from the surface of CD8+ cytotoxic T-cells, thus affecting T-cell activation. Monoclonal plasma cells increase with age leading to monoclonal gammopathy in older people. However, the antibody response to infection or immunization is impaired. Older adults have lower peak titers of antibodies and faster decline of titers after vaccination. Further, there is a loss of T- and

B-cell repertoire diversity with age. Finally, there is an impairment in the negative selection, thus generating autoreactive lymphocytes and autoantibodies.

As discussed earlier, there are changes in cytokine production with aging. While there is a decrease in the secretion of interleukin 2 (IL-2) and IL-12, there is an increase in the secretion of proinflammatory cytokines such as IL-6 and tumor necrosis factor α (TNF-α). There is also an increase in acute-phase reactants such as C-reactive protein (CRP) and plasma clotting factors. Additionally, other age-associated changes such as decreased sex hormones leading to increased IL-6 production and dysregulated mitochondrial function causing increased reactive oxygen species can further contribute. This proinflammatory state associated with aging is known as "inflammaging". The increase in the level of proinflammatory cytokines, especially IL-6, has been associated with an increased risk of frailty and mortality in older adults and has further been linked to the pathogenesis of other age-related disorders such as atherosclerosis, diabetes, Alzheimer's disease, sarcopenia, osteoporosis, etc.

CARDIOVASCULAR SYSTEM

Have you wondered why cardiovascular diseases such as hypertension, coronary artery disease, or heart failure are common in older people? We know atherosclerosis as one of the key culprits but is it the only cause or does aging also has a role in it?

Though older age is one of the risk factors for atherosclerosis, age-related changes in arteries are different from atherosclerosis. Large elastic arteries like aorta have increased stiffness of the vessel wall and increased lumen **(Fig. 1A)**. This is in contrast to atherosclerosis where the lumen of a blood vessel decreases. The aortic lumen diameter and length increase with age. However, since it is fixed at both ends, this increase in length results in tortuous, ectatic, and rightward-shifted aorta seen often on chest X-rays of older persons.

Vascular endothelium in older adults shows decreased NO (vasodilator) levels and increased endothelin-1 (vasoconstrictor) levels. This endothelial dysfunction leads to increased tonic contraction of old arteries, thus making them stiff and less compliant. The aortic stiffness increases systolic blood pressure, widens pulse pressure, and may also cause hypertrophy and fibrosis of the left ventricle. All these changes increase the risk of heart disease, stroke, and kidney disease.

Cardiac aging is associated with death of cardiac myocytes with compensatory cellular hypertrophy. It is accompanied by fibrosis and collagen accumulation in myocardium. Heart undergoes structural changes with age such as increased septal wall thickness, mild decrease in left ventricle diameter, left atrial (LA) dilatation, dilatation, and rightward shifting of the aortic root. **(Fig. 1B)**. These changes can be normal with age and should be considered while interpreting an echocardiograph of an older adult. However, they can also have significant consequences as an increase in the LA size may lead to an increased risk of atrial fibrillation and subsequently stroke and death in elderly.

There are significant valvular changes in an aging heart. By the age of 80 years, 90% of the apparently healthy subjects have multivalvular regurgitation, the most common being the aortic regurgitation. Age-related collagen deposition,

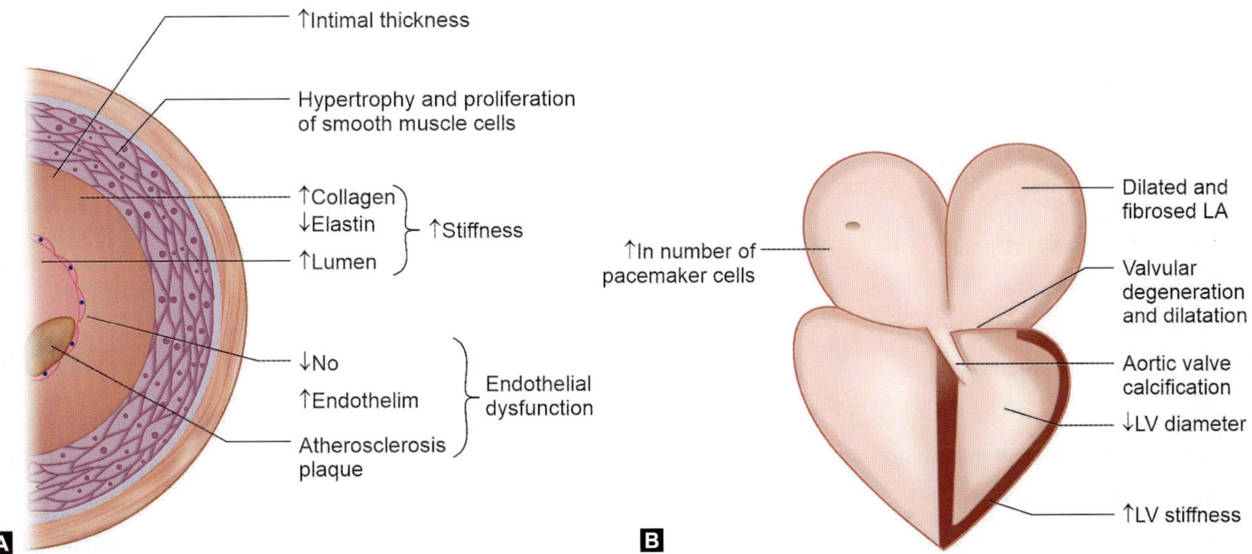

FIGS. 1A AND B: Age-related changes in the (A) blood vessels and (B) heart.

lipid accumulation, and focal dystrophic calcification can lead to annular dilatation of all the four valves (semilunar > atrioventricular) leading to valvular regurgitation. Most of the time, these are mild and clinically insignificant; however, sometimes these changes may exacerbate and can lead to severe regurgitation such as severe aortic regurgitation. Similarly, age-related degenerative changes may lead to thickening of aortic valve leaflets causing aortic sclerosis which is generally considered benign. However, degenerative changes can also lead to significant aortic stenosis requiring valve replacement. A senile calcification syndrome is seen in elderly, especially in end-stage kidney disease involving a triad of calcifications of aortic cusps, mitral annulus, and coronary arteries.

There is also a decrease in the sensitivity of the heart to sympathetic stimulation with age. Though the baseline heart rate and cardiac output remain the same, the older hearts are not able to achieve the same peak heart rate and cardiac output during exercise as in their younger age. There are increased atrial and ventricular ectopics which are normal for older age. While systolic function remains the same with age, the diastolic function is significantly reduced. Older healthy adults show a different pattern of Doppler diastolic left ventricular (LV) filling with decreased early atrial and increased late atrial flow velocities. While this pattern may be considered impaired or abnormal in younger adults, it is normal for older adults. However, this altered diastolic LV filling in addition to the vascular changes (such as hypertension) increases the risk of heart failure with preserved ejection fraction (HFpEF) in elderly. **Table 1** summarizes the key structural and functional age-related changes in the cardiovascular system.

NEUROLOGICAL SYSTEM

Older adults show a number of structural and functional changes with age. Structural changes seen in brain are diffuse and include thinning of the cortex and loss of gray matter. However, rather than a decrease in the number of neurons, morphological changes of neurons **(Fig. 2)** are more responsible for the age-related cognitive decline. There is a reduction in the number of dendrites and its synaptic connections. Synaptic plasticity, i.e., ability of the brain to reorganize the existing or develop new neural pathways, also decreases with age. Additionally, the neurons undergo segmental demyelination followed by remyelination, thus resulting in decreased conduction velocity along axons and thereby affecting reaction time. Similar to other parts of the body, the brain also shows a proinflammatory state with increased reactivity and dysfunction of glial cells (astrocytes and microglia). Further, vascular changes (decreased perfusion and impaired autoregulation), decreased cerebral metabolism, and altered neurotransmitter activity contribute to changes in the older brain. As discussed later, an increased level of adrenal glucocorticoids due to adrenal aging causes damage to the hippocampus which may cause memory loss.

Cognitive decline is commonly seen in older adults. It is difficult to accurately draw a line between the normal age-related changes and the pathological dementia-related changes in brain. However, the normal age-related changes in elderly are usually considered to be subtle which do not interfere with their activities of daily living. There is a decline in the processing speed with age, thereby causing psychomotor slowing. While normal elderly are

TABLE 1: Structural and functional changes in the cardiovascular system with age.

Structural changes	Functional changes
Vascular changes	
↑Intimal thickness	↑Atherosclerosis
↑Stiffness and ↓compliance	Systolic hypertension and increased pulse pressure
Increased aortic lumen and length	Tortuous and rightward shift of aorta on chest X-ray (unfolding of aorta)
↓NO and ↑endothelin-1	↑ Tonic contraction of arteries causing stiffness
Cardiac changes	
LA fibrosis and hypertrophy	↑ Risk of atrial fibrillation
↑ LV stiffness	↑ Risk of diastolic dysfunction and heart failure with preserved ejection fraction
Aortic valve calcification and thickening	Aortic sclerosis and stenosis
Degenerative annular dilatation	Valvular regurgitation
↓ β-adrenergic sensitivity	↓ Ability to increase heart rate and contractility in response to exercise and β-agonists (↓ peak heart rate and cardiac output)

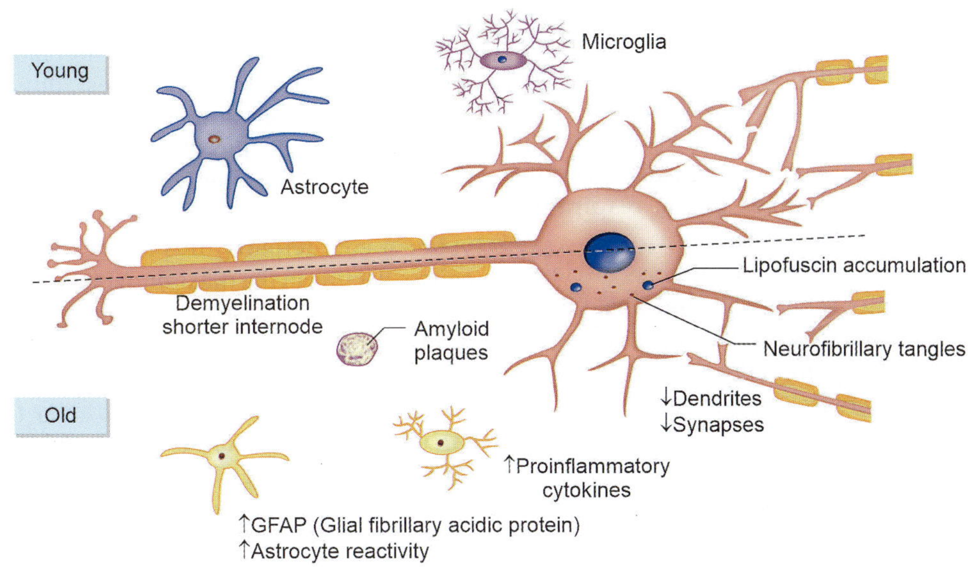

FIG. 2: Neuronal and glial changes with age.

able to remember old memories, they have difficulty in retaining and recalling of new information. Similarly, though the language abilities remain unimpaired, they can sometimes struggle with spontaneous word finding. This "tip-of-the-tongue" phenomenon seen in normal people is different from dysnomia seen in dementia.

Healthy older adults typically show slowing of alpha rhythm in EEG. As people age, the sleep/wake circadian rhythm becomes less synchronized, no longer producing the same response to external cues, resulting in less-consistent sleep/wake periods across the 24-hour day.

The most common change seen in the peripheral nervous system is loss of spinal motor neurons. This coupled with other musculoskeletal changes leads to decreased muscle bulk and strength, a condition known as sarcopenia. Further, there can be slowness in motor activities. Reflexes, particularly superficial reflexes, may be also decreased in advance age. The most common sensory tract affected in older adults is dorsal column with older adults commonly having decreased vibratory and proprioceptive sensations. Additionally, thermal sensitivity is also reduced, thus making them feel colder. Autonomic dysfunction also increases with age, thus increasing the prevalence of orthostatic hypotension in older adults.

MUSCULOSKELETAL SYSTEM

Aging musculoskeletal system causes significant changes in bones, muscles, and joints, thus making them susceptible to the development of osteopenia/osteoporosis, sarcopenia, and osteoarthritis. Older adults often complain of muscle weakness, joint pain, and fragility fractures. Though they are found to be common in elderly, they should not be considered normal and should undergo further investigation, treatment, and rehabilitation.

Aging is associated with a decrease in both bone mass and bone mineralization. The increased bone loss in older age can be attributed to increased osteoclastic activity and decreased osteoblastic activity. There is also increased differentiation of stromal cells toward adipocytes instead of osteoblasts. Hormonal changes, especially decreased estrogen levels in postmenopausal women, along with decreased vitamin D levels and increased parathyroid hormone (PTH) activity further accelerate the bone loss.

This muscle atrophy in older people can be attributed to both neurological and muscular reasons. Aging is associated with both loss of spinal motor neurons and their firing activity. The changes seen in muscle include decreased protein synthesis, increased apoptosis, dysfunctional excitation-contraction coupling, and increased inflammatory cytokines. All these can lead to a decrease in muscle mass and function which is known as sarcopenia.

Articular cartilage in older adults is associated with decreased hydration, increased cross-linking and stiffness of collagen, and accumulation of advanced glycosylation end products (AGEs). Further, the chondrocytes and their proliferative capacity are reduced. This causes a decrease in the cartilage's tensile strength, stiffness, and fatigue resistance. Intervertebral disks also show similar degenerative changes leading to disk herniation and prolapse.

PULMONARY SYSTEM

Lung function is an important determinant of vitality and intrinsic capacity in older adults and is affected by both intrinsic aging and cumulative extrinsic or environmental factors (smoking, pollution, etc.). Aging causes various structural and functional changes to the respiratory system as well as in the control of breathing.

The major structural changes include loss of elastic recoil of alveoli, stiffening of chest wall, and weakness of the respiratory muscles. The structural changes are mostly seen in smaller airways rather than the large airways. The alveolar surface area decreases progressively after the age of 30–40 years due to the age-related enlargement of alveoli and alveolar airways. This leads to an increase in the tendency of small airways to collapse while expiration leading to air-trapping and subsequently hyperinflation. This age-related hyperinflation is known as "senile emphysema". The other significant change is seen in the chest wall itself. The ossification of costal cartilages and calcification of rib articulating surfaces increase chest wall stiffness. The loss of intervertebral space and osteoporotic collapse of vertebral bodies increase kyphosis and anteroposterior diameter of chest, thus creating the so-called barrel chest and further reducing compliance of the chest wall. Finally, with age there is weakness of respiratory muscles with diaphragm showing 25% decreased strength in older persons as compared to their younger counterparts. This age-related muscle weakness causes decline in the maximum inspiratory and expiratory pressures in otherwise healthy older adults.

As a result of the structural changes, pulmonary function tests (PFTs) show some changes **(Figs. 3A to C)**. The expiratory flows, peak expiratory flow rate (PEFR), forced expiratory volume in 1 second (FEV_1), and forced vital capacity (FVC) decrease with age. However, the decline in FEV_1 is more than FVC, thus also decreasing the ratio of FEV_1/FVC. This can be visualized in flow–volume curve where the expiratory limb becomes more concave in older people. As mentioned earlier, the loss of elastic recoil of lung tissue causes an increase in the total lung capacity (TLC). However, this increase is counteracted

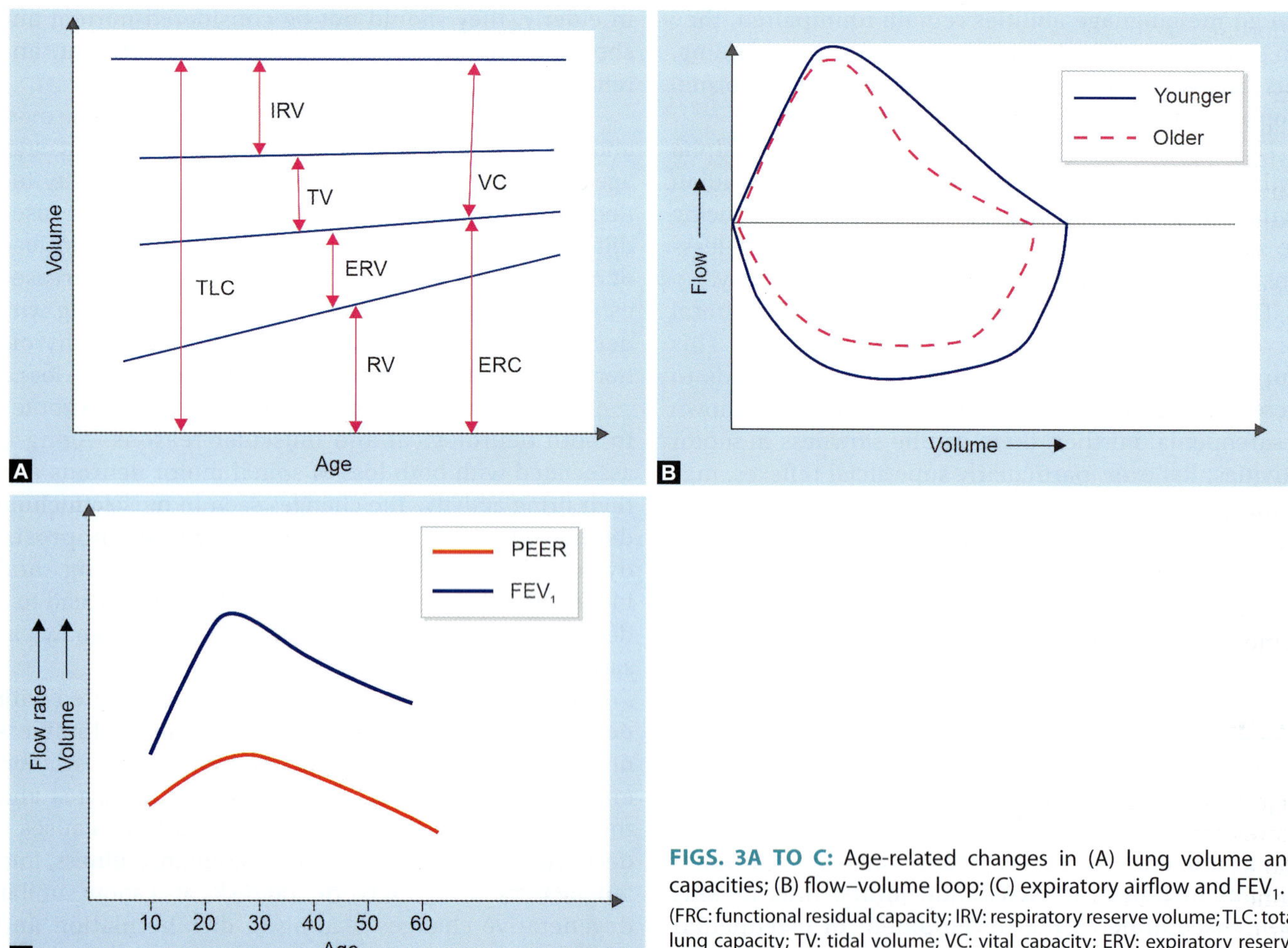

FIGS. 3A TO C: Age-related changes in (A) lung volume and capacities; (B) flow–volume loop; (C) expiratory airflow and FEV_1.
(FRC: functional residual capacity; IRV: respiratory reserve volume; TLC: total lung capacity; TV: tidal volume; VC: vital capacity; ERV: expiratory reserve volume; RV: residual volume)

by increased stiffness of chest wall, thus overall keeping TLC unchanged with age. However, the reduced elastic recoil increases the residual volume (RV) and functional residual capacity (FRC). Abnormally high RV/TLC can be seen as hyperinflation on chest X-ray similar to that seen in a patient with chronic obstructive pulmonary disease (COPD). As you can see, unchanged TLC and increased FRC will mean a decrease in tidal volume in an older adult. However, they breathe at a higher respiratory rate to compensate for a similar minute ventilation.

Decreased FEV_1/FVC ratio and increased RV also decrease ventilation at the lung bases, thus causing ventilation-perfusion (V/Q) mismatch at the bases. The V/Q mismatch causes reduced arterial oxygen tension (PaO_2) which is sufficient for adequate hemoglobin saturation unless there is a coexistent lung disease. Further, the V/Q mismatch and the reduced alveolar area decrease the diffusion capacity (DL_{CO}) or gas transfer (TL_{CO}). The exercise capacity of older adults as indicated by peak oxygen uptake (VO_{2max}) also decreases with age as a result of both cardiac and respiratory changes.

Older individuals also show decreased ventilatory responses to both hypoxia and hypercapnia. These differences in responses of older adults are due to a lesser increase in tidal volume, while the ventilatory rate increases normally. This reduced responsiveness of tidal volume is considered to be the result of decreased ventilatory drive or neural output by the respiratory center. The older adults are less sensitive to β_2 adrenergic agonists on its airways while showing more sensitivity to respiratory depression by opioids and sedatives. Another commonly under-reported condition is sleep-disordered breathing which is more common in older subjects with more prevalence seen in patients of heart failure and Alzheimer dementia.

As discussed earlier, immune function also decreases with age. This immunosenescence along with various chronic immunosuppressive conditions such as malnutrition, diabetes, or renal failure predisposes the older adult to a higher risk of respiratory infections. Additionally, they are at a higher risk of aspiration pneumonia due to neurological illnesses such as dementia, stroke, Parkinson's disease.

URINARY SYSTEM

The kidney changes with aging are related to many factors such as decreased Sirtuin production, reduced Klotho expression, increased angiotensin II receptor signaling, and other factors. Older age is associated with reduced kidney size with one study estimating a decrease of 10% per decade. However, the decreased cortical volume is compensated by an increase in the medullary volume, thereby keeping the overall renal parenchymal volume stable. The number of kidney cysts also increases; however, they are usually benign.

Microscopically, there is a gradual and continuous decrease in nephron number primarily because of the loss of podocytes. This is accompanied with age-related glomerulosclerosis, which is focal and global. This is different from the pathological glomerulosclerosis, which is focal, segmental, and with solidification. The tubules of these glomeruli also undergo atrophy. However, the remaining nephrons show compensatory tubular enlargement. Renal arteries are arterioles that show thickening (arteriosclerosis) and hyalin deposition and are associated with atherosclerosis. Further, interstitial fibrosis is also seen thus creating a picture of age-related nephrosclerosis (glomerulosclerosis, tubular atrophy, arteriosclerosis, and interstitial fibrosis).

As a result of the structural changes, glomerular filtration rate (GFR) decreases with age in healthy people at the rate of 6–8 mL/min/1.73 m^2 per decade **(Fig. 4)**. However, this is not a universal finding as many people (around one-third) do not show any GFR decline with age. Additionally, the circadian variation of GFR seen in younger population is blunted in older age. However, despite the decrease in GFR, proteinuria is not normally present, and presence of proteinuria should be considered pathologic. The renal function reserve, which is a measure of the ability of the kidneys to acutely increase its GFR in response to high protein load, remains unimpaired with age. The tubular function also reduces with age with its decreased ability to handle water, sodium, potassium, bicarbonate, and other electrolytes.

Renal plasma flow (RPF) decreases with age with the vessels exhibiting diminished responsiveness to atrial

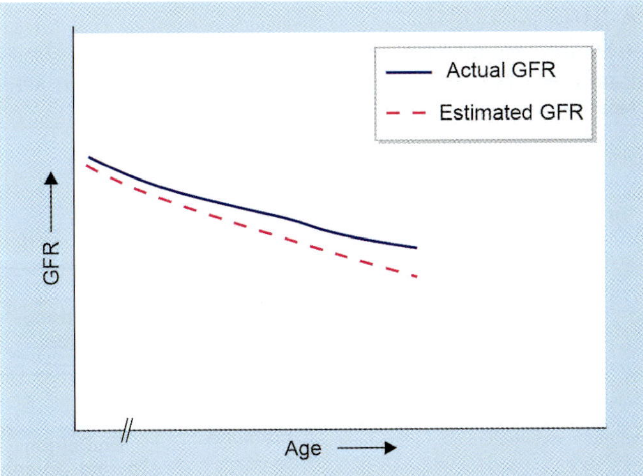

FIG. 4: Glomerular function rate (GFR) declines with age. Estimated GFR (eGFR) is calculated indirectly using various equations (e.g., Cockcroft–Gault).

natriuretic peptide (ANP) and vasodilators. The renin-angiotensin-aldosterone system (RAAS) decreases with age with reduced plasma renin activity and serum aldosterone levels. The RAAS system also shows reduced responsiveness to hypovolemia, hyponatremia, and hyperkalemia.

Similarly, older age is also associated with increased lower urinary tract symptoms (LUTS) and urinary incontinence. Detrusor muscle overactivity seen in older adults can reduce the bladder's functional capacity. Further, they also show diminished sensitivity to bladder volume. This delays the bladder filling sensation, thereby narrowing the time gap between the first urge to void and urinary leakage. Prostatic enlargement and pelvic organ prolapse seen in older males and females, respectively, can further increase symptoms. Various mechanisms and types of urinary incontinence have been discussed in detail separately in Chapter 16. **Box 1** summarizes various age-related changes in upper and lower urinary systems.

BOX 1 Changes in the urinary system with age.

Upper urinary tract:
- Glomeruli: Age-associated glomerulosclerosis, ↓GFR, no proteinuria
- Tubules: Tubular atrophy and compensatory hypertrophy; ↓concentrating and dilutional capacity; impaired acidification; impaired handling of sodium, potassium, calcium, phosphorus, and magnesium
- Vascular: Arteriosclerosis and hyalinosis; ↓RPF

Lower urinary tract:
- Detrusor muscle overactivity
- ↓ Bladder sensitivity
- Prostate enlargement (males)/pelvic organ prolapses (females)
- ↑LUTS
- Urinary incontinence

(GFR: glomerular filtration rate; LUTS: lower urinary tract symptoms; RPF: renal plasma flow)

ENDOCRINE SYSTEM

The role of hormones in aging has fascinated scientists for a long period. This led to emergence of the concept of hormonal fountain of youth in the early 20th century and use of various hormones such as growth hormones, testosterone, and estrogen as antiaging medicines. Though widely discredited now, it is still being used by quacks to fool naïve people.

Table 2 provides a brief summary of changes seen in various endocrine systems with age. Aging is associated with multiple hormonal changes such as changes in its activity, transport, receptor interaction, and clearance. As shown in **Figure 5**, the circadian rhythm is also affected with aging which causes a change in the secretion of releasing hormones from the hypothalamus. This further decreases the level of pituitary hormones and subsequently the level of end-organ hormone. This decreased hormone level then acts on the hypothalamus and pituitary via the feedback mechanism. Basal plasma concentrations of most of the hormones do not change significantly with normal aging. However, decreased homeostatic reserve and increased risk of autoimmune diseases and malignancy in older age can affect hormone levels.

Aging increases the risk of adenomas and empty sella in pituitary which can be seen as incidental findings on

TABLE 2: Age-related changes in various endocrine organs.

Pituitary	↓GH; ↓prolactin; ↓melatonin; ↓nocturnal increase of ADH
Thyroid	↑TSH; ↔free T4; ↓T3 and ↑rT3 seen in very old
Adrenal	↑Cortisol levels; ↓HPA axis sensitivity to glucocorticoid feedback; ↓aldosterone and adrenal androgens; ↑noradrenaline
Gonads	↓Estrogen; ↓testosterone

(ADH: antidiuretic hormone; GH: growth hormone; HPA: hypothalamic–pituitary–adrenal; rT3: reverse triiodothyronine; T4: thyroxine; T3: triiodothyronine; TSH: thyroid-stimulating hormone)

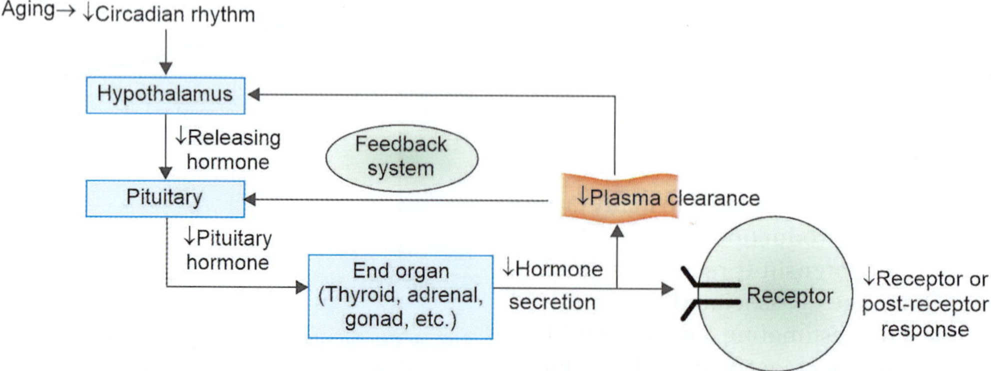

FIG. 5: Changes in the hormonal system with age.

MRI. The decreased nocturnal secretion of melatonin is associated with sleep-wake rhythm disturbances in older adults, especially in patients with Alzheimer disease. Hence, melatonin and melatonin agonists can show some improvement in sleep. Vasopressin or antidiuretic hormone (ADH) decreases with age, thus leading to nocturia and further increasing the risk of hyponatremia in older adults.

Like the pituitary gland, the thyroid gland also shows a higher risk of neoplasms with age. There is an increase in the nodularity and fibrosis of the thyroid gland. Though there is a mild increase in thyroid-stimulating hormone (TSH) levels (thus increasing the prevalence of subclinical hypothyroidism), free thyroxine (T4) levels remain unchanged in the absence of any underlying thyroid disease. In very old age, there is a decrease in triiodothyronine (T3) levels and an increase in rT3 levels. Due to a decreased clearance rate, older hypothyroid patients require a lower dose of T4.

Adrenal aging is associated with increased activity of the hypothalamic-pituitary-adrenal (HPA) axis leading to increased cortisol levels. Additionally, there is a decrease in the sensitivity of HPA axis to glucocorticoid feedback. This chronic cortisol increase is associated with poor cognition, depression, anxiety, sarcopenia, frailty, osteoporosis, decreased immunity, diabetes, hypertension, and also increased mortality in older adults. However, there is also decreased secretion of adrenal androgens. The ratio of serum cortisol to dehydroepiandrosterone sulfate (DHEAS) shows a gradual increase with age and higher values are associated with neurodegenerative illnesses such as dementia. As discussed earlier, aging is associated with decreased renin and aldosterone levels. Aging is also associated with increased sympathetic tone due to increased noradrenaline release. However, despite the increased tone, there is decreased receptor sensitivity to noradrenaline in older patients, thus attenuating its physiological effects.

Indian women undergo menopause earlier as compared to the western counterparts at the age of 40–50 years. However, postmenopausal symptoms such as hot flashes, night sweats, sleep disturbances, etc., may last for few years after menopause. The decreased estrogen level has also been linked with postmenopausal cognitive impairment and is a potential area of further research. Unlike abrupt and complete cessation of ovarian function, testicular function declines gradually and only partially. Total testosterone declines at the rate of 1% per year in older men. Though sometimes used, andropause is a misnomer and inaccurate to define this age-related testosterone decline. This "partial androgen deficiency of the aging male" is found to be associated with lower hemoglobin, cognitive performance, muscle strength, sarcopenia, bone mineral density, and frailty.

SEXUALITY AND SEXUAL FUNCTION

Sexuality in older adults is considered a taboo subject and older people are generally considered asexual. Physicians often avoid discussing the sexual issues of older people. However, it is a real problem in Indian elderly which can cause marital problems and mental health issues in the older age too. Hence, it is essential for geriatricians to know regarding changes in the sexual function of older adults.

Surprisingly, sex can be helpful for older couples in the form of good exercise, thus improving their circulation and providing them with a feeling of closeness and even relieving arthritic pain. The subsequent release of endorphins also alleviates their mood making them happy and less depressed.

However, besides the social stigma and prejudice, the sex life of older people has many problems and challenges associated with it. The first one is decreased libido. Decreasing sex-hormone levels with age (testosterone in men and estrogen in women) coupled with psychological issues can lead to decreased sexual desire and arousal in older people. On the other hand, they may also exhibit inappropriate sexual behaviors or disinhibition which can be secondary to dementia, delirium, or psychosis.

The decreased estrogen and testosterone level in older women and men leads to changes in their sexual response cycle **(Table 3)**. Besides these age-related changes, older men and women have sexual dysfunction disorders too such as erectile dysfunction in men and sexual pain disorder in women.

Besides the hormonal changes, there are physical and psychological issues too. Depression, anxiety, and dementia can also affect libido and sexual function. Similarly, arthritis makes it difficult for them to maintain proper sexual position. Other conditions such as heart disease, urinary incontinence, and uterine prolapse and the side effects of various medications (thiazides, beta blockers, etc.) also prevent them from enjoying a healthy and fulfilling sex-life.

GASTROINTESTINAL SYSTEM

Though aging leads to some structural changes in the alimentary tract, there are no significant changes in its function. This can be attributed to the considerable reserve of the GI tract. Hence, most of the GI disorders are usually the result of superimposed effects of other factors (genetics, diseases, toxins, drugs, etc.). Common changes seen are decreased gut blood flow, impaired mucosal immunity, and dysfunctional myenteric plexus.

Older adults often complain of dry mouth due to decreased salivary secretion. Delayed relaxation of the upper esophageal sphincter coupled with oropharyngeal

TABLE 3: Changes in the sexual response cycle with age.

Females	Males
Decreased blood flow to vagina and clitoris and less intense genital engorgement	Decreased penile rigidity
Reduced and less intense vaginal contractions	Fewer and less forceful contractions of the urethra
Longer excitement and plateau phase while shortened orgasmic phase	Longer excitement and plateau phase while shortened ejaculatory and orgasmic phase
Vaginal dryness, atrophy, and shortening with narrowing of introitus causing pain during intercourse	Lower ejaculatory volume
Decreased breast vasocongestion and nipple stimulation	Increased refractory period between two erections

muscle weakness can predispose older adults to dysphasia and aspiration. Dyspepsia and gastroesophageal reflux disease (GERD) are other common complaints seen in older adults. Aging is associated with both decreased acid secretion and gastric mucosal cytoprotective prostaglandins. There is also increased prevalence of *Helicobacter pylori* colonization. Further, there is delayed gastric emptying of liquids, while solid foods emptying remain normal. Digestive and absorptive functions of the small intestine remain normal. Loss of enteric neurons in myenteric plexus leads to increased colon transit, thus increasing the risk of constipation. Aging is associated with altered metabolism and clearance of some drugs. However, overall hepatobiliary and pancreatic function does not show much change.

OTHER ORGANS

Skin, the largest organ of the body, undergoes a multitude of changes. These changes are secondary to the free-radical damage, progressive telomere shortening, and chronic UV-induced damage. This leads to thickened, hyperpigmented skin making it wrinkly, saggy, and leathery type. The thermoregulation of older adults is also altered, thereby making them more sensitive to cold and decreasing their sweat response to hot temperature. Additionally, the wound-healing capacity is reduced leading to chronic ulceration and delayed healing.

Vision impairment is one of the common disabilities in older adults leading to further complications such as falls, dementia, and depression. The vision impairment can be secondary to both age-related changes and diseases. Older adults have decreased accommodation, visual acuity, visual field, contrast sensitivity, depth and motion perception, color discrimination, dark adaptation, processing speed, and increased sensitivity to glare. The pupils in older adults are smaller in size and less reactive to light and accommodation. With aging, the lens also loses its elasticity and therefore the ability to become more rounded, which is required while focusing on nearby objects. This loss of accommodative ability of lens impairs near-vision of an older adult and is known as presbyopia and is different from hypermetropia seen in younger people. There is also a restriction of upward gaze eye movement causing difficulty for them to read street signs or traffic lights while driving. On the other hand, diseases such as cataract, glaucoma, diabetic retinopathy, and age-related macular derangement can cause a further decrease in the vision of older generation.

Hearing impairment is another common disability seen in the elderly. Unlike younger people, hearing impairment in the older people is mostly of sensorineural type secondary to degeneration of hair cells at the base of organ of Corti and loss of afferent neurons. This age-related hearing impairment which affects predominantly higher frequencies is known as presbycusis. Additionally, they have difficulty in speech discrimination and impaired vestibular function, thus causing balance difficulties. Increased thirst, decreased smell, and altered taste sensation are the other common changes seen with age.

CONCLUSION

In this chapter, we tried to understand aging and its related biological changes. Though there is no universal definition, it is commonly understood as declining physiological fitness leading to increased susceptibility to diseases and death.

Biological aging is associated with various changes in the different physiological systems. While some organ systems, such as the gastrointestinal system, do not show significant change, others such as the renal system are significantly affected. Similarly, not all structural changes will translate to functional decline. For example, a decrease in marrow cellularity with age does not significantly decrease its hematopoietic ability. On the other hand, changes in our visual and auditory systems significantly decrease our seeing and hearing capability.

Hence, it is important for a clinician to know about normal physiological age-related changes. While managing an older patient, one should be able to identify and differentiate between normal and abnormal changes so as to make an appropriate diagnosis and treatment plan.

Self-Assessment Questionnaire

Q1. What is UA of old age?

Q2. What is inflammaging and what is its significance?

Q3. What are the changes seen in the left ventricle with aging?

Q4. What are structural changes seen in neuron in older people?

Q5. What is sarcopenia?

Q6. What are the differences seen in PFTs of a healthy older subject as compared to a healthy young adult?

Q7. What is age-related nephrosclerosis?

Q8. What is adrenal aging?

Q9. What are the various barriers to healthy sex life in older adults?

Q10. What is the difference between presbyopia and presbycusis?

FURTHER READINGS

1. Halter JB, Ouslander JG, Studenski S, High KP, Asthana S, Supiano MA, et al (Eds.) Hazzard's Geriatric Medicine and Gerontology, 7th edition. New York: McGraw-Hill Education; 2017.
2. Fillit H, Rockwood K, Young J (Eds). Brocklehurst's Textbook of Geriatric Medicine and Gerontology, 8th edition. Philaldelphia, PA: Elsevier, Inc.; 2017.
3. Sinclair AJ, Morley JE, Vellas B (Eds). The physiology of ageing. In: Pathy's Principles and Practice of Geriatric Medicine. Chichester: Wiley; 2012. pp. 33-42.

CHAPTER 4

Immunology of Aging

Monika Devi Sharma

INTRODUCTION

Aging is a complex and multifaceted process that profoundly affects blood cell development and function. The concept of cellular senescence, first established by Hayflick and Moorhead in 1961, reveals that normal somatic cells can divide only a limited number of times before entering an irreversible growth arrest. This understanding is crucial for exploring age-related changes in hematopoietic stem cells (HSCs), which play a vital role in blood cell production.

With the rise in human life expectancy, the aging population encounters greater risks for age-related conditions, such as tumors, as well as higher rates of immunotherapy failure and increased cancer recurrence. This process, referred to as immunosenescence and first introduced by Roy Walford, involves the degradation and reorganization of immune organ structures due to aging, resulting in compromised function of both the innate and adaptive immune systems. Consequently, older adults often have less effective vaccination responses and heightened vulnerability to infections, age-related diseases, and cancers. Since the 1980s, research has illuminated the mechanisms of immunosenescence, revealing that age-related declines in immune response and increases in proinflammatory status, termed "inflammaging," are central features. Inflammaging, proposed by Claudio Franceschi in 2000, arises from constant antigen exposure and stressors. Additionally, thymic involution represents a critical alteration in the aging immune landscape. Immunosenescence affects all lineages of the immune system, resulting in altered innate and adaptive immune responses and a greater incidence of infections. For example, older adults are at an increased risk for the development of reactivation tuberculosis and varicella zoster virus (VZV) infection; age is also an independent risk factor for mortality and impaired functional outcome from sepsis and infection with the severe acute respiratory syndrome coronavirus 2 (SARS-CoV-2), the cause of COVID-19. Immune system aging also contributes to impaired responses to vaccines against influenza and other pathogens.

Understanding the molecular mechanisms underlying these age-related changes is essential for developing targeted therapeutic strategies to mitigate the effects of aging on blood cell function and overall health. As the global population of older adults continues to rise, research in this area will play a pivotal role in addressing the challenges associated with aging and immune health. This chapter will provide an updated overview of the aging blood cells, focusing on the interplay between genetic, epigenetic, and environmental factors that influence hematopoiesis and immune function in the elderly.

EFFECTS OF AGING ON HEMATOPOIESIS

Hematopoietic stem cells are crucial for sustaining blood production throughout an organism's life. Their ability to self-renew and differentiate is vital for maintaining the homeostasis of the hematopoietic system. However, aging significantly impacts the intrinsic characteristics of HSCs, leading to a decline in their functionality, independent of external microenvironmental factors. Recent studies reveal that while DNA damage was historically seen as the primary factor in HSC aging, a broader array of biological processes also deteriorate with age. Key areas of focus include epigenetic modifications, chromatin architecture, autophagy, proteostasis, and metabolic changes. These interconnected processes are essential for understanding the intrinsic aging mechanisms of HSCs.

Given the increasing elderly population and the correlation between aging and various hematologic disorders, such as myelodysplastic syndromes and acute myeloid leukemia, exploring HSC aging is of paramount importance. Research into the intrinsic mechanisms of HSC aging may unveil new molecular targets for potential interventions aimed at ameliorating or delaying the aging process in the hematopoietic system, ultimately improving outcomes for older patients with hematologic conditions.

Increase in Phenotypic Hematopoietic Stem Cells Number and Decrease in Regenerative Capacity

The quantity and frequency of HSCs in the bone marrow of both mice and humans tend to rise with age, yet their regenerative ability, as assessed through transplantation assays, significantly diminishes. Researchers largely attribute this phenomenon to cell-intrinsic mechanisms, although the aging microenvironment can also contribute to the decline **(Fig. 1)**.

Myeloid Skewing

Hematopoietic stem cells in older individuals tend to have an increased differentiation capacity for the myeloid lineage, while their ability to differentiate into the lymphoid lineage is diminished. Moreover, even though there is a greater number of myeloid cells, their quality is negatively affected **(Fig. 2)**.

DNA Damage

Aging significantly impacts HSCs, particularly through the accumulation of DNA damage. This damage arises from both internal processes, such as DNA replication and mitochondrial activity, and external factors such as radiation and chemotherapy. As HSCs age, they exhibit a two- to threefold increase in DNA damage markers, such as γH2AX foci, indicating a decline in genomic integrity. This accumulation of DNA lesions can lead to mutations, contributing to clonal hematopoiesis and increasing the risk of hematological malignancies.

Epigenetic Drift

The epigenetic landscape and chromatin organization of HSCs change significantly with age. Aged HSCs display specific differences in DNA methylation, distinct histone modifications, and alterations in chromatin arrangement compared to younger HSCs.

Cell Polarity

In young HSCs, various molecules display a polarized arrangement in both the cytoplasm and nucleus, a characteristic that diminishes in aged HSCs. Recent research has indicated that the decline in HSCs' function and stem cell potential associated with aging is directly linked to the loss of polarity in specific biomolecules within the cells.

Metabolic Changes and Autophagy Dysfunction in Hematopoietic Stem Cells

Hematopoietic stem cells typically exhibit a low metabolic rate, primarily relying on glycolysis while in a quiescent state. Upon activation, young HSCs transition to a more

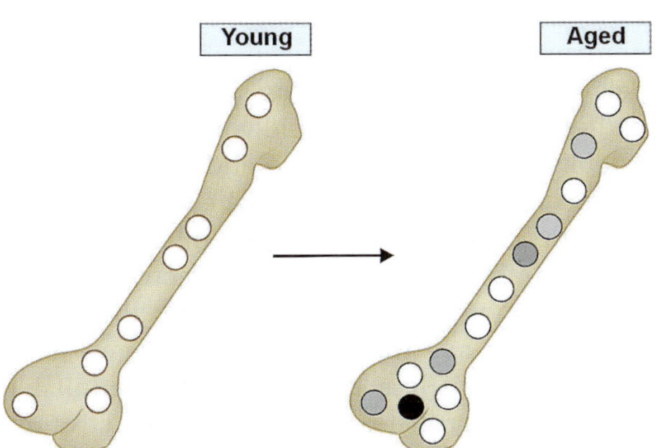

FIG. 1: In aged mice, the absolute number of cells with regenerative potential increases, but the extent to which individual aged cells contribute to blood cell production becomes highly variable. The relative frequency of stem cells with high regenerative potential (white) compared with cells with low regenerative potential (gray and black) thus decreases upon aging.

Source: de Haan G, Lazare SS. Aging of hematopoietic stem cells. Blood. 2018; 131(5):479-87.

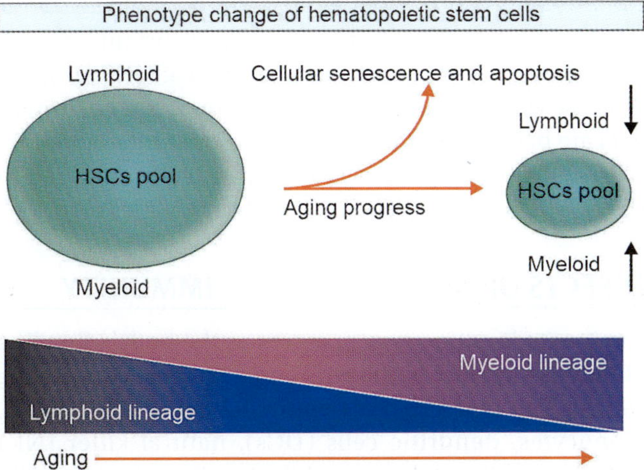

FIG. 2: Change in HSC phenotype during the aging process. Since lymphoid genes are decreased and myeloid genes are increased by aging, the phenotypic shift from the lymphoid to the myeloid lineage in aged HSCs ultimately contributes to immune dysfunction and the decline of adaptive immunity.

(HSCs: hematopoietic stem cells)

Source: Kim MJ, Kim MH, Kim SA, Chang JS. Age-related deterioration of hematopoietic stem cells. Int J Stem Cells. 2008;1(1):55-63.

oxidative metabolic state, which can revert to glycolysis when they return to quiescence. In contrast, aged HSCs demonstrate a persistent increase in oxidative metabolism, leading to elevated levels of reactive oxygen species (ROS). This increase in ROS contributes to oxidative stress, which is associated with a diminished regenerative capacity.

Metabolic stress can activate autophagy, a critical cellular process that degrades and recycles damaged cellular components. Autophagy involves the encapsulation of organelles or cytosolic portions within double-membrane vesicles, which subsequently fuse with lysosomes for degradation. However, autophagy becomes deregulated with aging, resulting in impaired cellular maintenance and contributing to age-related diseases, including cancer. The decline in autophagic activity in aged HSCs is linked to the accumulation of damaged organelles and proteins, exacerbating the functional decline of these cells. This relationship underscores the importance of autophagy in maintaining cellular homeostasis and its potential role in the aging process and related pathologies **(Figs. 3A and B)**.

Altered Proteostasis

Proteostasis refers to the equilibrium between protein production and degradation, facilitated by various cellular mechanisms, including autophagy and the ubiquitin-proteasome system (UPS). In aged HSCs, these protective mechanisms are weakened, leading to increased protein stress and a loss of regenerative ability **(Fig. 4)**.

Signaling Pathways and Hematopoietic Stem Cell Aging

Key signaling pathways, including transforming growth factor-beta (TGF-β), Notch, nuclear factor-κB (NF-κB), and Wnt, are vital for regulating the hematopoiesis, ensuring a delicate balance between quiescence and differentiation. With aging, these pathways are intrinsically modified in HSCs, which affects their functional capabilities **(Fig. 5)**.

EFFECTS OF AGING ON INNATE IMMUNITY

The innate immune system serves as the body's first line of defense against pathogens and vaccines, comprising various cell types such as epithelial cells, neutrophils, monocytes, dendritic cells (DCs), natural killer (NK) cells, basophils, and eosinophils. It utilizes biochemical components such as complement proteins, antimicrobial peptides (e.g., defensins), proinflammatory cytokines, and antiviral interferons (IFNs). Key functions include pathogen clearance through intracellular killing by neutrophils and macrophages, destruction of infected or cancerous cells by NK cells, and the lysis of extracellular pathogens via complement activation.

Neutrophils

Neutrophils are a vital component of the innate immune system, serving as the first line of defense against infections caused by rapidly dividing bacteria, yeast, and fungi. They utilize various microbicidal mechanisms to combat pathogens, including:

- *Reactive oxygen and nitrogen species production:* Neutrophils generate ROS and reactive nitrogen species (RNS) that are toxic to microbes.
- *Release of proteolytic enzymes and peptides:* Neutrophils can release enzymes and microbicidal peptides from cytoplasmic granules, which help to break down pathogens.
- *Neutrophil extracellular traps (NETs):* Neutrophils can also expel NETs, which are networks of fibers that trap and kill microbes outside the cell.

Age-related Changes in Neutrophil Function

While neutrophil numbers do not decline with age, their functionality is significantly impacted. The key findings related to age and neutrophil activity are given in the following text.

- *Neutrophil generation:* Neutrophils originate from HSCs, which differentiate into either lymphoid or myeloid lineages. Research has shown that with advancing age, there is a shift toward myeloid progenitors, often at the expense of lymphoid progenitors. This phenomenon is partly due to the clonal expansion of myeloid-biased HSCs, indicating a stable pool of neutrophils even in older adults.
- *Compromised microbicidal activity:* Although neutrophil counts remain constant, their functional capabilities diminish with age. For instance, older neutrophils exhibit reduced chemotaxis, which delays their arrival at infection sites. This delay allows pathogens, particularly rapidly dividing bacteria, to establish a stronger foothold and increases the risk of infection. However, diminished chemotaxis can result in not only reduced neutrophil migration to the sites of inflammation but also defective neutrophil egress from inflamed tissues. Notably, the clearance of apoptotic neutrophils by macrophages—termed *efferocytosis*—is less efficient in older adults. This inefficiency correlates with heightened activation of macrophage p38 mitogen-activated protein (MAP) kinase. Interestingly, administering a p38 inhibitor has been shown to restore efferocytosis and promote inflammatory resolution, suggesting potential therapeutic avenues for addressing age-related dysregulation of inflammation.
- *Impact on tissue damage and inflammation:* The impaired chemotactic response also contributes

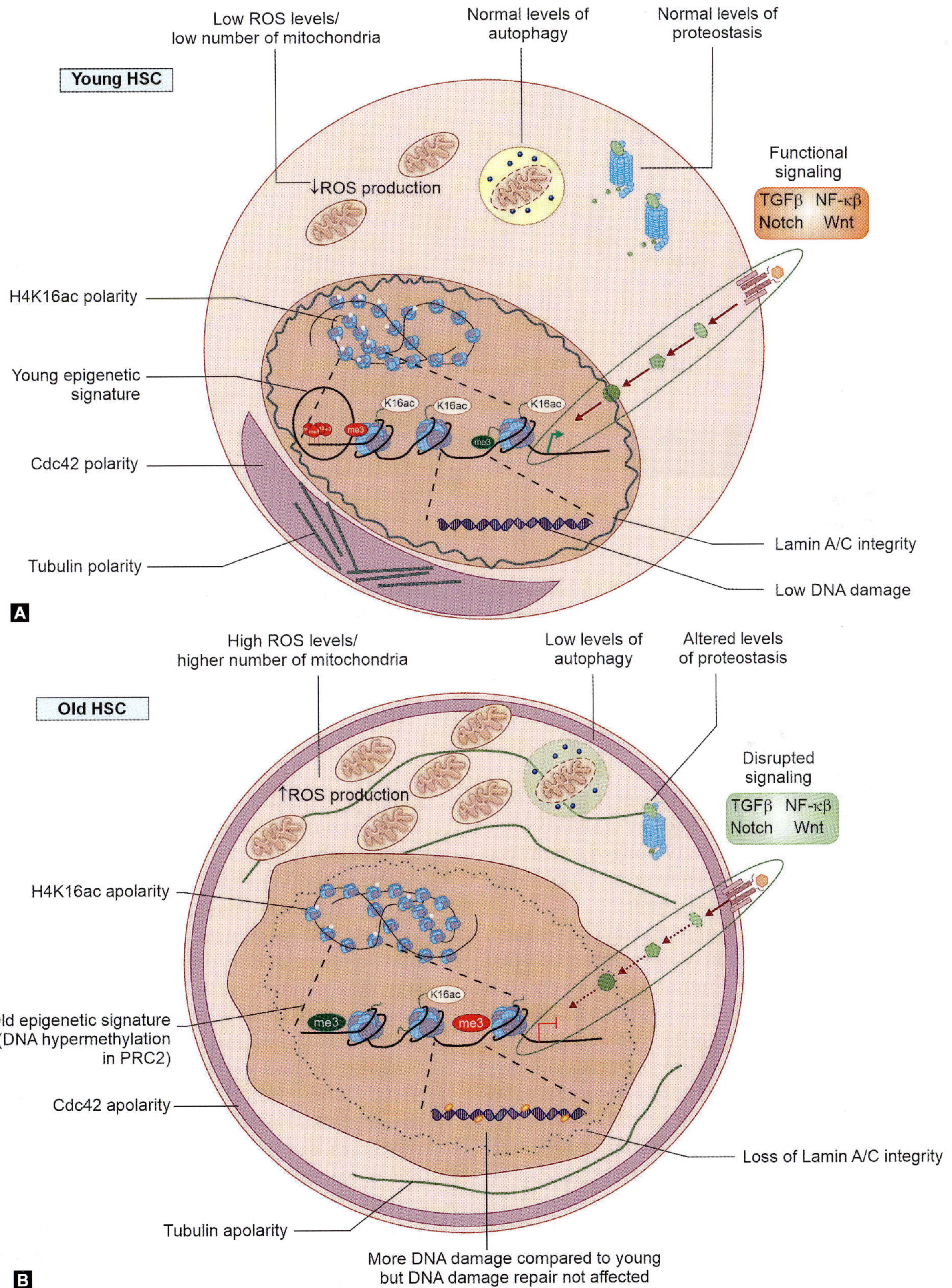

FIGS. 3A AND B: Intrinsic hallmarks of hematopoietic stem cells (HSC) aging. (A) Representative features of young HSC; (B) Representative features of aged HSC.

(green me3: H3K4me3; K16ac: H4K16ac; met: DNA methylated; PRC2: polycomb repressive complex 2; red me3: H3K27me3; ROS: reactive oxygen species)

Source: Mejia-Ramirez E, Florian MC. Understanding intrinsic hematopoietic stem cell aging. Haematologica. 2020;105(1):22-37.

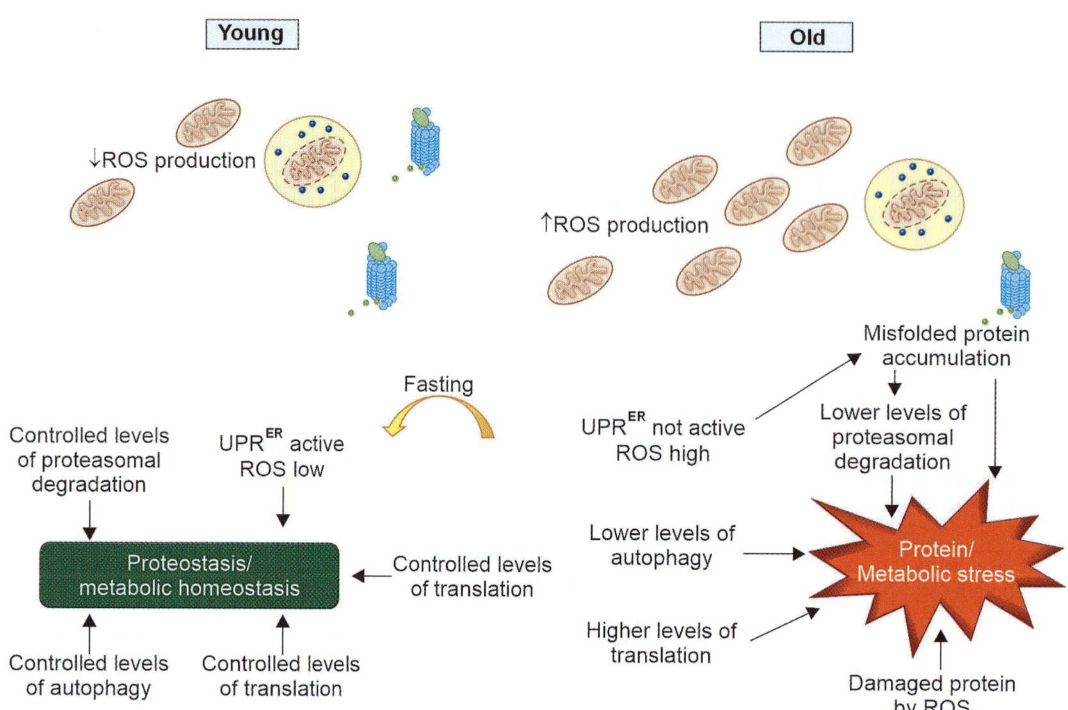

FIG. 4: Metabolic homeostasis and proteostasis during aging in hematopoietic stem cells (HSC). Young HSCs fine-tune several biological processes: They maintain a low metabolic rate, control protein degradation, and regulate autophagy. Aged HSCs show an unbalanced scenario where these processes lose their metabolic homeostasis and proteostasis, converging into a status of metabolic and protein stress. Fasting is able to restore at least partially the activity of the UPRER and proteostasis in aged HSC.

(ROS: reactive oxygen species; UPRER: unfolded protein response)

Source: Mejia-Ramirez E, Florian MC. Understanding intrinsic hematopoietic stem cell aging. Haematologica. 2020;105(1):22-37.

to increased tissue damage, as neutrophils may secrete proteolytic enzymes (such as elastase) while navigating through tissues. This prolonged activity can extend inflammation and hinder its resolution, leading to further complications in older adults.

- *Neutrophil accumulation in injury models:* In research involving burn injury in mice, it was observed that although neutrophil accumulation rates did not differ between young and old mice, the resolution of inflammation was significantly delayed in older mice. This finding underscores the greater tissue damage and prolonged inflammatory response in the aging population.
- *Reduced phagocytosis:* Neutrophils from older adults exhibit reduced phagocytic activity against opsonized *Escherichia coli* and *Streptococcus pneumoniae*, alongside a compromised ability to kill these pathogens. This decline may be linked to lower levels of dehydroepiandrosterone sulfate (DHEAS), a steroid that enhances superoxide production in neutrophils. Additionally, age-related impairments in intracellular bacteria killing could stem from altered signaling pathways, affecting the respiratory burst and apoptotic responses, ultimately leading to decreased protection against infections.
- *Altered signaling pathways:* Aging seems to disrupt various cellular signaling processes in neutrophils. Despite the unaltered expression of receptors that mediate neutrophil activation, downstream signaling events—including calcium mobilization, phosphoinositide-3 kinase (PI-3K) pathways, MAP kinase, protein kinase B, Janus kinase-signal transducers and activators of transcription (JAK-STAT), and SHP-1 signaling—are affected. This suggests that broader changes in generic signaling processes are likely responsible for the observed functional decline in neutrophils with age.
- In conclusion, while neutrophils remain present in sufficient numbers as we age, their functional capacity diminishes, leading to increased susceptibility to infections and prolonged inflammation. Understanding these changes can provide insights into potential therapeutic approaches to bolster immune function in older adults.

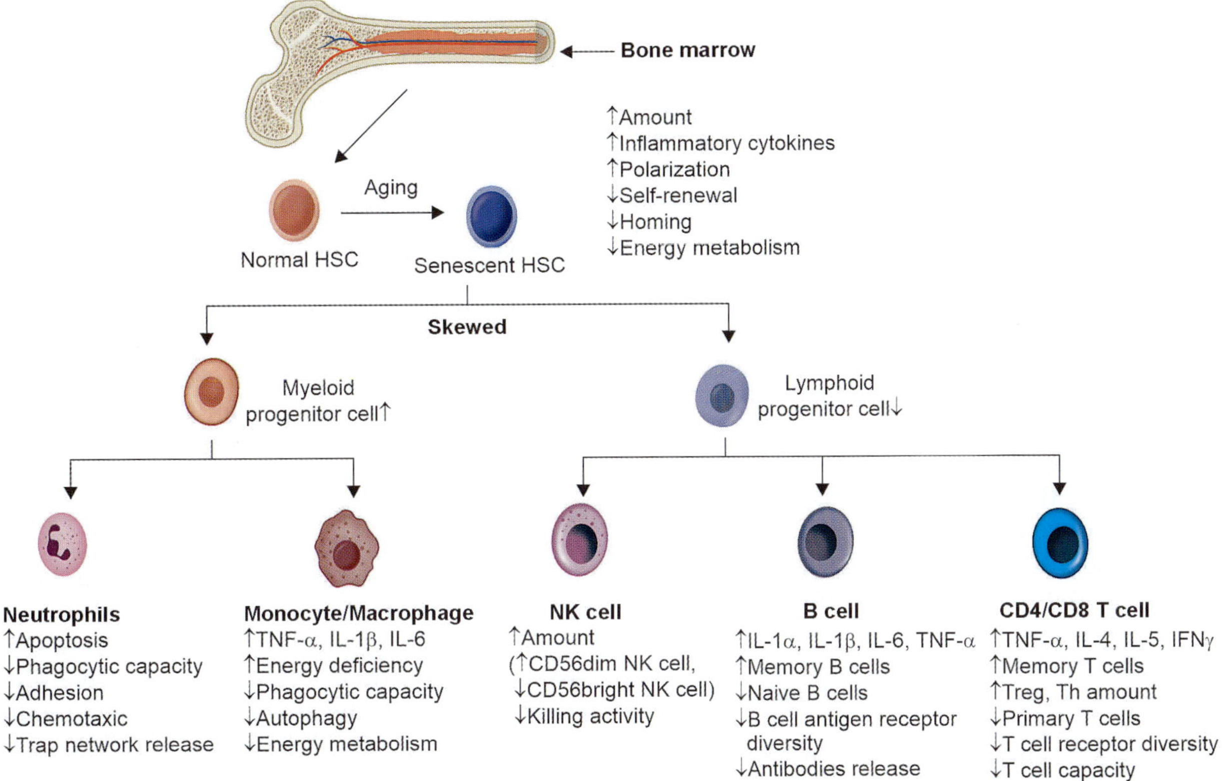

FIG. 5: Characterization of HSC differentiation into immune cells during aging. Inflammation in senescent bone marrow impairs the function of HSCs. HSCs differentiate into various immune cells, and their senescence leads to changes in the number and functions of immune cells. Common features of immune cell senescence include a decline in performing immune functions and an increase in the release of inflammatory factors.
(IFN: interferon; IL: interleukin; NK cell: natural killer cell; TNF: tumor necrosis factor)
Source: Li X, Li C, Zhang W, Wang Y, Qian P, Huang H. Inflammation and aging: signaling pathways and intervention therapies. Signal Transduct Target Ther. 2023;8(1):239.

Natural Killer Cells

Natural killer cells, crucial components of the innate immune system, play a key role in eliminating virus-infected and malignant cells. Hyporesponsiveness of NK cells has been observed in certain conditions, such as Chédiak-Higashi syndrome, a rare autosomal recessive disorder. This syndrome is characterized by the fusion of cytoplasmic granules and impaired degranulation of lysosomes in neutrophils, leading to compromised immune responses.

Key mechanisms of NK cell function are as follows:

- *Cytotoxic mechanisms*: NK cells utilize proteases called granzymes stored in cytoplasmic granules to induce cell death in target cells. They release perforin, a protein that creates pores in the membranes of infected or cancerous cells, allowing granzymes to enter and trigger apoptosis. NK cells possess surface receptors that recognize major histocompatibility complex (MHC) class I molecules on host cells. These receptors prevent NK cells from initiating apoptosis. However, tumor cells often downregulate MHC class I expression to evade T-cell responses, making them vulnerable to NK cell-mediated killing, which helps maintain immune surveillance.
- *Antibody-dependent cytotoxicity*: NK cells can also recognize the Fc region of antibodies, allowing them to kill target cells that have been tagged by immunoglobulins (Ig). This process enhances the immune response against pathogens.

Age-related Changes in Natural Killer Cells

- In humans, NK cells are categorized into two main populations: (1) NK cells specialized for cytotoxicity (CD56low—low CD56 adhesion protein expression) and (2) NK cells specialized for cytokine production (CD56hi—high CD56 expression). The CD56hi population decreases with age, leading to reduced cytokine secretion. Although there is an expansion of the CD56low cytotoxic NK cell subset in older adults, their cytotoxic capability per cell is diminished. This decline may be partly due to reduced recruitment of perforin to target cells, which impairs their ability to induce apoptosis effectively. These age-associated alterations in NK function may result in part from changes in zinc homeostasis in older individuals, and there is evidence that NK cell function can be improved with zinc supplementation. In aged mice, NK cells exhibit reduced ability to kill infected cells, lower infiltration into the lungs, and diminished production of IFN-γ during influenza virus infection compared to younger counterparts. In an ectromelia poxvirus model, NK cells from older mice displayed intrinsic migration defects to lymph nodes. Additionally, type I IFNs appear less effective in enhancing NK cell cytotoxicity and IFN-γ and granzyme B production in older subjects, indicating a decline in NK cell functionality with age.

- Understanding the aging of NK cells has significant clinical relevance. Research indicates that both NK cell counts and their functional measures correlate with mortality rates in critical illnesses, such as sepsis. Additionally, older adults, particularly those in nursing homes, show increased rates of infections and mortality associated with compromised NK cell activity.
- Classical NKT cells, characterized by their CD1d-restricted T-cell receptors (Vα14/Vβ8.2 in mice and Vα24/Vβ11 in humans), are a unique subset of "innate immune lymphocytes." Research in mice has shown that the number of NKT cells increases with age, and their functionality is also heightened. A study by Stout-Delgado et al. investigated the role of NKT cells in modulating the inflammatory response during viral infections using a herpes simplex virus-2 (HSV-2) model. The findings revealed significantly higher levels of IL-17A in older mice compared to younger ones, which correlated with increased neutrophil recruitment to the liver and enhanced chemokine production. Importantly, NKT cells from aged mice produced more IL-17A than their younger counterparts. Furthermore, transferring aged NKT cells into young mice led to hepatic damage. This notion of an intensified inflammatory response with aging has also been linked to heightened IL-17-dependent T-cell allogeneic reactions and increased expression of the IL-23/p19 gene in bone marrow-derived dendritic cells from aged mice. Such hyperinflammatory responses may contribute to the negative outcomes associated with infections or sepsis in older populations.

Monocytes and Macrophages

Monocytes and macrophages are critical components of the innate immune system. Monocytes can differentiate into macrophages and DCs upon responding to inflammation. With aging, there is an increase in monocyte numbers, which correlates with clinical frailty. However, this increase contrasts with a decline in macrophage functionality, particularly regarding toll-like receptor (TLR) activation.

Age-related Changes in Monocytes

Research shows that aging is associated with reduced cytokine production in response to TLR activation. For instance, studies on mice (C57BL/6 and Balb/c strains) have documented decreased levels of proinflammatory cytokines such as IL-6 and tumor necrosis factor α (TNF-α) following TLR activation, which appears to be linked to decreased TLR gene expression or impaired signal transduction pathways, such as MAP and JNK kinases.

In humans, similar declines in TLR function have been observed. Older individuals show reduced TLR1/2-induced cytokine production, likely due to decreased surface expression of TLR1. This impairment is further associated with a reduced ability to express CD80, a costimulatory protein critical for adaptive immune responses, such as the antibody response to influenza vaccination.

Age-related Changes in Macrophages

Macrophage functionality also declines with age. A recent study evaluating delayed-type hypersensitivity (DTH) responses to Candida antigens revealed significant decreases in TNF-α, IL-6, and IFN-γ levels in older individuals compared to younger ones. The diminished intracellular production of TNF-α in dermal macrophages may hinder T-cell migration during antigen challenges. Notably, while aged dermal macrophages can still produce TNF-α ex vivo, their dysfunction likely reflects changes in the skin microenvironment. These findings highlight the implications for both cutaneous innate immunity and clinical applications such as tuberculin skin testing, emphasizing that age-related changes in monocyte and macrophage function can significantly impact immune responses.

Dendritic Cells

Human DCs comprise various subsets, primarily myeloid DCs and plasmacytoid DCs (pDCs). Myeloid DCs are versatile and can develop into either macrophages or specialized tissue DCs. In contrast, pDCs are less effective as antigen-presenting cells (APCs) but are highly efficient at producing type I IFN (IFN-α) in response to viral infections. The maturation of DCs is influenced by interactions between cells and soluble factors in their environment. They secrete chemokines that attract other immune cells. When DCs encounter bacterial components, viral antigens, or danger signals from damaged host cells, these infectious agents bind to specific TLRs. This binding activates DCs, leading to the release of cytokines and chemokines that stimulate the innate immune system and recruit T and B cells for adaptive immune responses. Plasmacytoid DCs play a crucial role in antiviral defenses. They produce high levels of IFN-α, which not only enhances the ability of NK cells to eliminate infected cells but also helps T cells mature into cytotoxic killers.

Age-related Changes in Dendritic Cells

Dendritic cells are crucial for linking the innate and adaptive immune systems. They efficiently process and present antigens to initiate immune responses, utilizing specialized molecules that facilitate their functions.

- *Reduced numbers and functionality*:
  - Aging studies have shown a decrease in the number of DCs, particularly Langerhans cells, and impaired migration to lymph nodes.
  - There is a decline in the expression of costimulatory molecules, which are essential for effective antigen presentation and immune activation. Aging hampers the ability of DCs to prime T cells effectively, leading to reduced immune responses.
- *Altered antigen processing:* The ability of DCs to process and present antigens declines due to reduced autophagy, which is essential for generating peptides for antigen presentation.
- *Impaired cytokines signaling*: Aged DCs often secrete higher levels of proinflammatory cytokines but have a diminished capacity to produce anti-inflammatory cytokines such as IL-10. This imbalance contributes to chronic inflammation and loss of self-tolerance. Aged DCs become more reactive to self-antigens due to heightened activation states, which can lead to autoimmune conditions.
- *Defects in plasmacytoid DCs:* pDCs, which are important for producing type I IFNs in response to infections, show decreased functionality with age. Aged pDCs produce lower levels of IFN-α when stimulated by pathogens compared to their younger counterparts, weakening the immune defense against viral infections.

Overall, aging adversely affects dendritic cell populations, leading to decreased numbers, impaired antigen processing, and reduced immune responses. Understanding these changes is crucial for developing better vaccines and therapies for older adults, who are more vulnerable to infections **(Fig. 6)**.

Pattern Recognition Receptors

Pattern recognition receptors (PRRs) play a crucial role in the immune system, comprising several major families, including transmembrane proteins such as TLRs and C-type lectin receptors (CLRs), as well as cytoplasmic proteins such as retinoic acid–inducible gene (RIG)-1-like receptors (RLRs) and NOD-like receptors (NLRs). Connections between the innate and adaptive immune systems are facilitated by proteins such as lipopolysaccharide (LPS)-binding protein and TLRs, which signal the production of cytokines and the activation of T and B lymphocytes. Among humans, 11 TLRs have been identified, and their activation triggers a series of intracellular events that lead to the destruction of infected cells and immune response initiation. Meanwhile, NLRs and RLRs, which are intracellular sensors, form inflammasomes that activate inflammatory responses in reaction to pathogen-associated molecular patterns (PAMPs). Mutations in inflammasome components can lead to chronic inflammation and increase the risk of various diseases, including autoinflammatory syndromes and crystallopathies such as gout.

Aging and Pattern Recognition Receptors Signal Transduction

Alterations in Toll-like Receptors Expression

Aging is associated with impaired signaling through PRRs, particularly TLRs. Research indicates that innate immune cells from older adults show decreased TLR expression compared to younger individuals. For example, diminished surface expression of TLR1 in human monocytes correlates with reduced TLR1–TLR2-induced cytokine production. Other age-related decreases in TLR expression have been documented, including TLR3 and TLR8 in monocyte-derived DCs (mDCs) and TLR7 and TLR9 in plasmacytoid DCs (pDCs). In mice, a general decrease in TLR gene expression has been observed, but the pattern is more variable in humans, suggesting potential post-transcriptional mechanisms affecting TLR protein levels. Notably, while total TLR1 protein expression is comparable in young and older human monocytes, surface levels are lower in older adults, likely due to altered transport mechanisms.

Toll-like Receptors Signaling and Cytokine Production in Aged Monocytes and Macrophages

Toll-like receptor signaling is essential for linking innate and adaptive immune responses through the production of costimulatory molecules and proinflammatory cytokines. Studies in aged mice show a generalized decline in TLR gene expression and reduced TLR-induced production of cytokines such as TNF and IL-6 in macrophages. However,

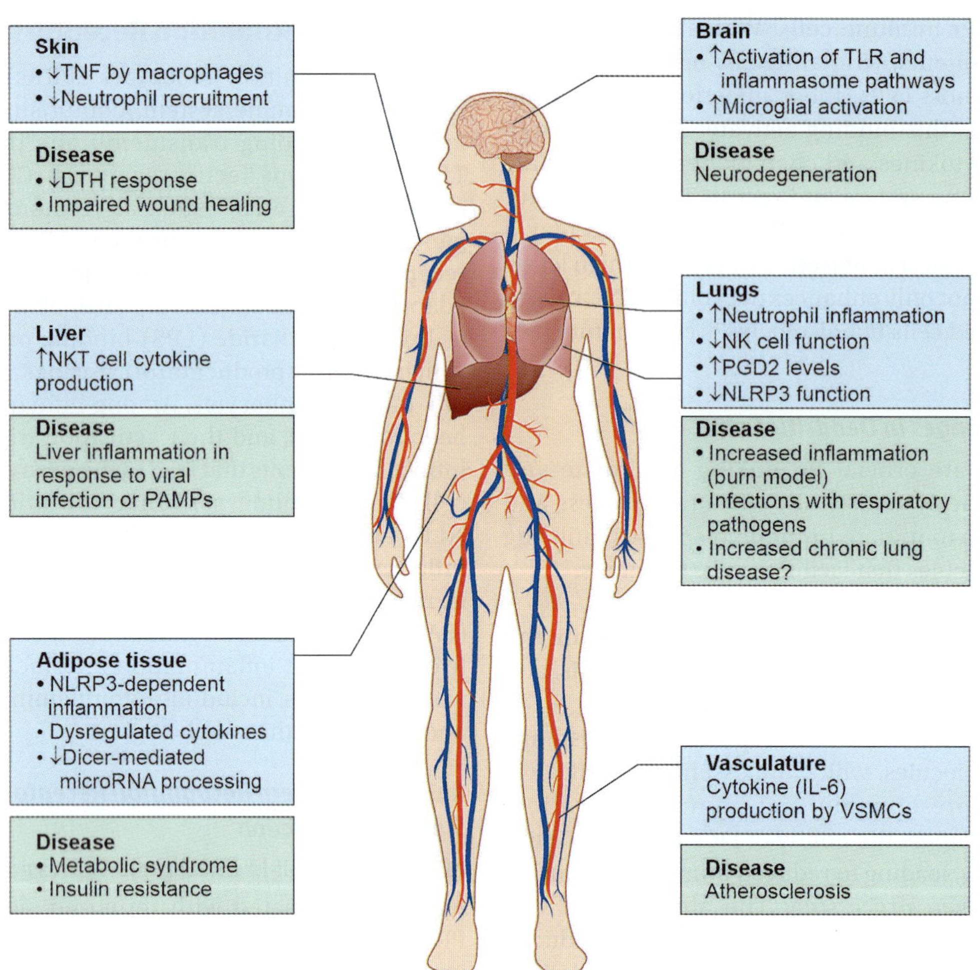

FIG. 6: Organ-specific changes of the innate immune system associated with aging and disease. The effects of aging in various organ systems are depicted. Diminished innate immune responses are found in some cases, such as in the skin, in which a decrease in tumor necrosis factor (TNF) production by macrophages results in decreased endothelial cell activation and diminished delayed-type hypersensitivity (DTH) responses. In addition, studies in mice have linked diminished neutrophil recruitment to impaired wound healing. Decreased natural killer (NK) cell function and induced NLRP3 (NOD, LRR-, and pyrin domain-containing 3) function in response to the influenza virus limit protective responses to infection in the lungs. However, there are also instances of dysregulated inflammatory responses found in aging; for example, there is increased neutrophil recruitment in the lungs following burn injury in a mouse model. In the liver, there is experimental data showing that NKT cells show exaggerated inflammatory responses that contribute to immune pathology during viral infection or to toll-like receptor (TLR) activation. In the brain, TLR and inflammasome signaling are increased with aging and are associated with microglial activation. Signaling via the NLRP3 inflammasome also contributes to increased age-associated inflammation in adipose tissue. Finally, in the vasculature, increased basal production of interleukin-6 (IL-6) by vascular smooth muscle cells (VSMCs) has been found in aged rodents and nonhuman primates and may provide a potential explanation for the increased prevalence of atherosclerosis with aging.

(PAMPs: pathogen-associated molecular patterns; PGD2: prostaglandin D2)

Source: Shaw AC, Goldstein DR, Montgomery RR. Age-dependent dysregulation of innate immunity. Nat Rev Immunol. 2013;13(12):875-87.

the effects vary by mouse strain; for instance, while aged C57BL/6 mice exhibited decreased TLR expression, aged BALB/c mice had unchanged surface TLR2 and TLR4 levels but still showed reduced cytokine production, potentially linked to decreased p38 MAPK expression. Similar trends have been observed in aged rhesus macaques and human monocytes, where TLR1–TLR2 stimulation results in lower TNF and IL-6 production due to decreased MAPK signaling.

Aging also affects the expression of costimulatory molecules CD80 and CD86 in monocytes, which can influence the efficiency of antigen presentation and correlate with antibody responses to vaccines. Despite diminished function, there is evidence of dysregulated inflammatory responses in older individuals, such as increased TNF production in specific monocyte subsets with age.

Toll-like Receptor Signaling and Cytokine Production in Aged Dendritic Cells

In contrast to macrophages and monocytes, DCs in mice may retain their functional capacity with age. However, there is evidence of reduced type I IFN production by pDCs in aged mice following viral challenge. This dysfunction is associated with decreased nuclear translocation of IRF7. Moreover, aged bone marrow-derived DCs (BMDCs) show increased IL-23 production, which could lead to a bias toward TH17 cell responses, potentially contributing to increased inflammation in older adults.

In human studies, aged primary DCs show reduced IL-12 production after TLR4 stimulation and decreased TLR-induced cytokine responses. This is accompanied by a generalized decline in TLR function, correlating with poorer antibody responses to influenza vaccination. Basal cytokine levels in mDCs and pDCs also increase with age, which may reflect chronic TLR activation and contribute to inadequate responses to pathogens and vaccines.

Signaling Downstream of Other Pattern Recognition Receptors

The effects of aging on other PRRs, such as NOD-like receptors (NLRs) and RLRs, remain to be fully understood. Evidence suggests that the NLRP3 inflammasome is involved in age-associated inflammation, particularly in adipose tissue and the brain. However, older mice may show reduced production of proinflammatory cytokines such as IL-1β and IL-18 in response to NLRP3 activation during infections, indicating failures in innate immune activation amid dysregulated inflammation.

Pattern recognition receptors signaling also intersects with macroautophagy, which tends to be defective in aged organisms. Impaired autophagy may influence PRR function and ROS production, potentially complicating the immune response in older individuals.

Toll-like Receptor Agonists as Vaccine Boosters for Older Adults

Certain TLR activators, such as lipid A from bacteria, are being explored to improve vaccine responses in older adults. These activators can help stimulate the production of proinflammatory cytokines, which can boost the activity of CD4+ T cells in older individuals.

For instance, using flagellin, a TLR5 ligand, has been linked to stronger immune responses in aged mice and specific human cells. A vaccine that included flagellin and peptides from the influenza virus protected older mice from lung infections, although their protection was not as strong as that seen in younger mice, likely due to weaker adaptive immune responses in older mice. In a clinical study, a similar vaccine showed a strong antibody response in people over 65 years without significant side effects.

Additionally, TLR9 ligands, like CpG oligonucleotides, have been tested alongside other agents to improve vaccine effectiveness against influenza and pneumonia in both young and aged mice. These combinations helped restore specific antibody responses in older mice.

A recent study found that a TLR4 agonist, glucopyranosyl lipid, boosted the ability of myeloid dendritic cells (mDCs) to fight the influenza virus in laboratory tests by increasing their production of granzyme B.

Overall, these findings suggest that TLR activators can enhance vaccine responses in older adults. However, it is important to use them carefully, as different TLR activators may have unique effects on the immune systems of older individuals **(Fig. 7)**.

INFLAMMAGING

The aging process leads to a complex interplay of innate immune responses characterized by heightened levels of proinflammatory cytokines (such as IL-6 and TNF-α), acute phase reactants (such as C-reactive protein), and clotting factors, collectively referred to as "inflammaging". This chronic inflammatory state is associated with increased mortality risk and decreased muscle mass and strength in older adults, and it plays a significant role in various age-related diseases, including cardiovascular disease, diabetes, Alzheimer's disease, and osteoporosis. The mechanisms behind inflammaging are not fully understood but are thought to involve the activation of PRRs by pathogen-associated molecular patterns (PAMPs) from chronic infections, as well as the accumulation of damage-associated molecular patterns (DAMPs) such as non-cell-associated nucleic acids, mitochondria, ATP, urate crystals, heat shock proteins, ceramide, hyaluronan, amyloid, and others resulting from cellular or tissue damage. Defects in autophagy associated with aging lead to a diminished capacity for clearing damaged cellular components, which exacerbates chronic inflammation. This chronic inflammatory state, often referred to as inflammaging, is linked to the senescence-associated secretory phenotype (SASP), characterized by the release of proinflammatory cytokines such as IL-6 and IL-8 from senescent cells. The accumulation of these damaged cells and their secretions creates a feedback loop that perpetuates inflammation, further impairing autophagic processes. Hormonal changes, such as reduced testosterone and estrogen levels, also elevate cytokine production, while increased mitochondrial activity and oxidative stress in aging may further exacerbate this proinflammatory environment **(Figs. 8 and 9)**.

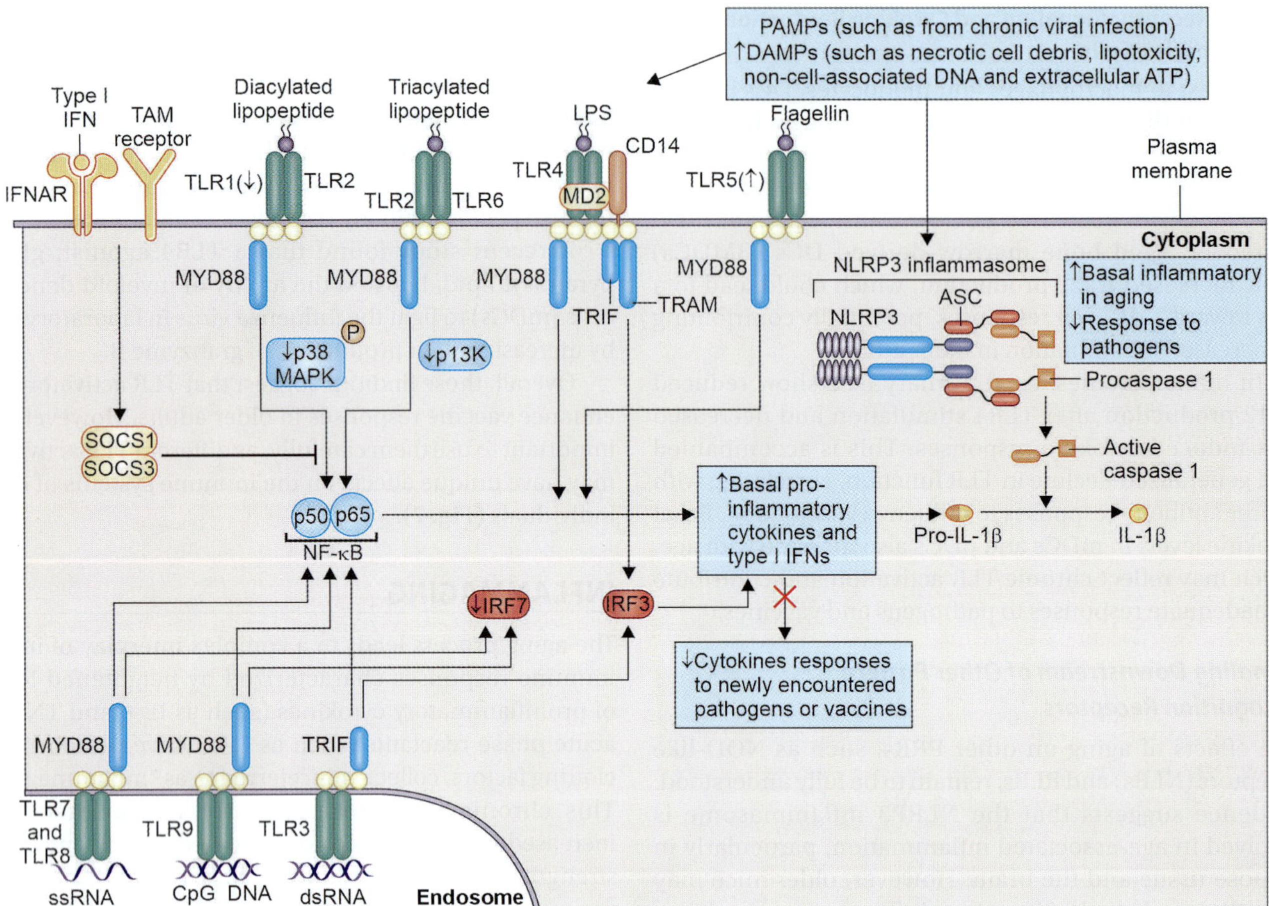

FIG. 7: Effects of aging on innate immune PRR signaling. Toll-like receptor (TLR) and NLRP3 (NOD-, LRR-, and pyrin domain-containing 3) signaling pathways are depicted. With aging, elevated levels of pattern recognition receptor (PRR) ligands [pathogen-associated molecular patterns (PAMPs) and damage-associated molecular patterns (DAMPs)], which could arise from chronic viral infection (such as with CMV) or from cell damage, respectively, contribute to an elevated proinflammatory state, as manifested by increased basal levels of proinflammatory cytokines that may result partly from TLR signaling and partly from NLRP3 signaling. Such basal activation may restrict responsiveness to new pathogens or vaccines, resulting in innate immune failure and impaired adaptive immune responses. Changes in protein expression of TLR1 and TLR5 in humans are indicated; results in mice suggest that there is either a widespread decrease in *TLR* gene expression or unchanged expression levels, but that there are alterations in intracellular signaling proteins [such as decreased levels of p38 mitogen-activated protein kinase (MAPK)].

(CMV: cytomegalovirus; dsRNA: double-stranded RNA; IFN: interferon; IFNAR: IFNα/β receptor; IL-1β: interleukin-1β; IRF: IFN-regulatory factor; LPS: lipopolysaccharide; MD2: myeloid differentiation factor 2; MYD88: myeloid differentiation primary-response protein 88; NF-κB: nuclear factor-κB; PI3K: phosphoinositide 3-kinase; SOCS: suppressor of cytokine signaling; ssRNA: single-stranded RNA; TAM: TYRO3, AXL and MER; TRAM: TRIF-related adaptor molecule; TRIF: TIR-domain-containing adaptor protein inducing IFNβ)

Source: Shaw AC, Goldstein DR, Montgomery RR. Age-dependent dysregulation of innate immunity. Nat Rev Immunol. 2013;13(12):875-87.

ADAPTIVE IMMUNE SYSTEM

Adaptive immunity is characterized by antigen-specific responses to a foreign antigen or pathogen. A key feature of adaptive immunity is that following the initial contact with an antigen (*immunologic priming*), subsequent antigen exposure leads to more rapid and vigorous immune responses (*immunologic memory*). It comprises two main components: (1) Cellular immunity, primarily mediated by T lymphocytes, and (2) humoral immunity, driven by B lymphocytes, both of which originate from a common stem cell in the bone marrow. Bone marrow serves as the primary site for the maturation of B cells, monocytes, macrophages, DCs, and granulocytes, containing pluripotent stem cells that can differentiate into all hematopoietic cell types under the influence of colony-stimulating factors. T-cell precursors also arise from HSCs and migrate to the thymus for maturation. Once mature, T lymphocytes, B lymphocytes, monocytes, and DCs enter circulation and home to peripheral lymphoid organs such as lymph nodes and spleen, as well as mucosal-associated lymphoid tissues in the gut and

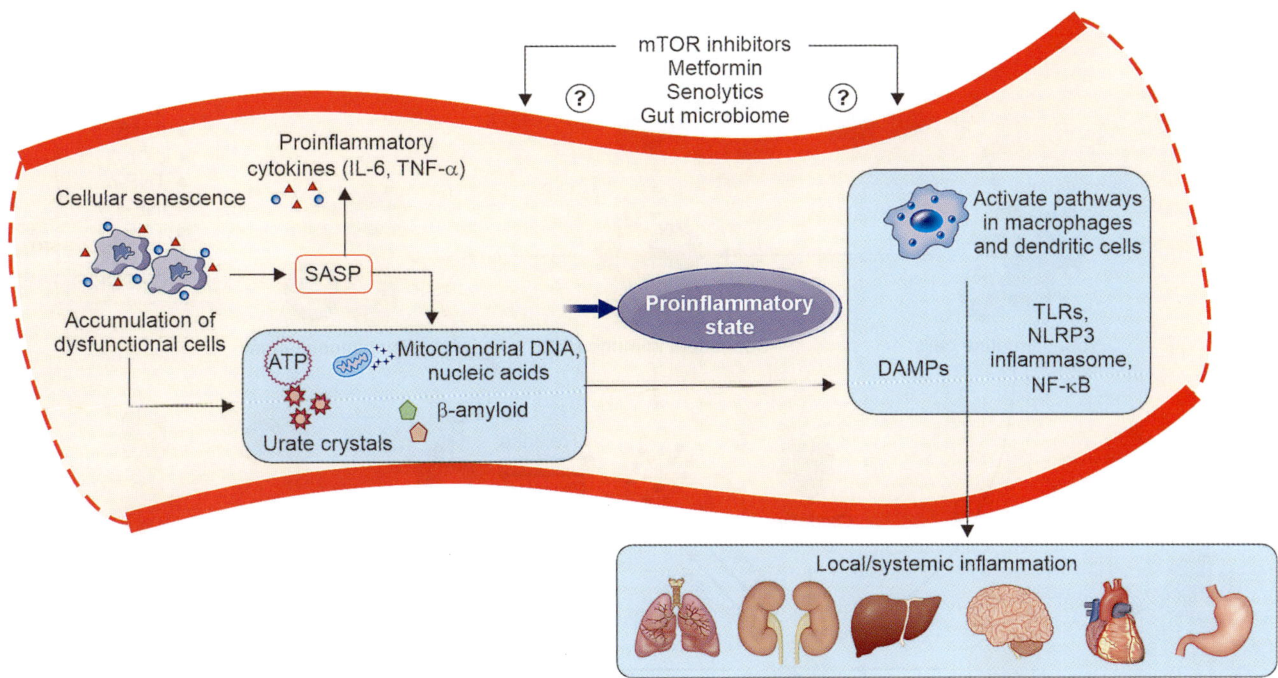

FIG. 8: Depiction of potential factors that contribute to age-associated chronic inflammation.
(SASP: senescence-associated secretory phenotype)
Source: Halter JB, Ouslander JG, Studenski S, High KP, Asthana S, Supiano MA, et al. Hazzard's Geriatric Medicine and Gerontology, 8th edition. New York: McGraw Hill; 2022.

genitourinary and respiratory tracts, where they await activation by foreign antigens.

T Cells

T cells, essential for cell-mediated immunity, originate from CD34+ pro-T cells in the bone marrow and mature in the thymus, where they undergo a rigorous selection process to establish a functional T-cell repertoire. The thymus exports about 2% of thymocytes daily, with production declining by 3% per year over the first four decades of life. Mature T cells comprise 70–80% of peripheral blood lymphocytes and are categorized into CD4+ and CD8+ subsets, with CD4+ helper T cells that assist in B-cell and CD8+ T-cell development, while CD8+ cytotoxic T cells are responsible for lysing virus-infected or foreign cells. Long-lived memory T cells are divided into effector memory T cells, which reside in nonlymphoid organs and respond rapidly to infections, and central memory T cells, which reside in lymphoid organs. T cells undergo a selection process in the thymus to ensure self-tolerance and the ability to recognize foreign antigens. Thymocyte selection includes positive selection for TCRs that weakly bind to self-peptides and negative selection to eliminate autoreactive T cells. Following maturation, T cells migrate to peripheral tissues, where memory subsets can respond quickly to infections **(Fig. 10)**.

T-cell Antigen Recognition: Molecular Mechanism

The T-cell receptor (TCR) is a disulfide-linked heterodimeric protein, composed of either αβ or γδ chains, which are noncovalently attached to a complex of five CD3 subunits (γ, δ, ε, ζ, and η). In humans, the majority of T cells express a TCR composed of alpha (α) and beta (β) chains (95%), and a smaller subset of T cells express a TCR with gamma (γ) and delta (δ) chains. TCR-αβ or TCR-γδ must be associated with CD3 molecules to properly integrate into the T-cell membrane. The CD3 molecules play a key role in mediating the T-cell activation signals through the TCRs, while the combination of TCR-α and -β or -γ and -δ forms the site for antigen binding.

The TCR for antigen molecules, which includes α, β, γ, and δ chains, shares structural and sequence similarities with Ig heavy and light chains, categorizing it within the *Ig gene superfamily*. The genes encoding TCRs are organized as clusters of gene segments that rearrange during T-cell maturation, facilitating the diversity needed for effective antigen recognition. The TCR-α chain is located on chromosome 14 and comprises variable (V), joining (J), and constant (C) regions, while the TCR-β chain on chromosome 7 includes multiple V, D (diversity), J, and C segments. The TCR-γ chain is also on chromosome 7, and the TCR-δ chain is found within the TCR-α locus on chromosome 14. TCR diversity arises from the various

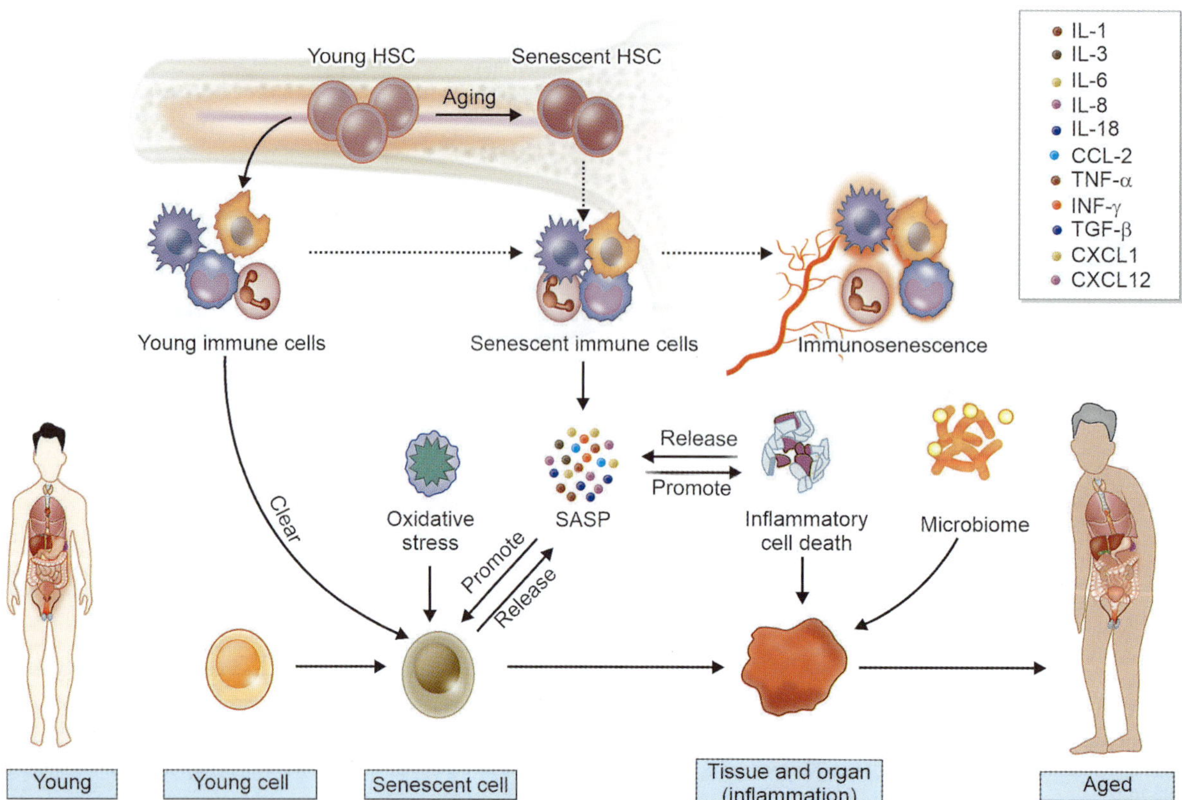

FIG. 9: Inflammaging at the molecular, cellular, and organ levels. During the aging process, almost all cells in the body undergo senescence, a state characterized by a dysfunctional state and senescence-associated secretory phenotype (SASP). While immune cells play a crucial role in recognizing and eliminating these senescent cells, they are also affected by SASP, leading to a phenomenon called immunosenescence. Immunosenescence can impair the immunity to respond to infections and diseases, making the organism more vulnerable to illnesses. Moreover, the accumulation of senescent cells can trigger inflammation in organs, leading to organ damage and an increased risk of age-related diseases. This process is exacerbated by positive feedback loops that drive the accumulation of inflammation and organ damage, leading to further inflammation and an even higher risk of aging-related diseases.

Source: Li X, Li C, Zhang W, Wang Y, Qian P, Huang H. Inflammation and aging: signaling pathways and intervention therapies. Signal Transduct Target Ther. 2023;8(1):239.

combinations of V, D, and J segments, as well as from nucleotide additions at rearrangement junctions, and the pairing of individual chains to form TCR dimers **(Fig. 11)**.

T-cell receptor-αβ cells specifically recognize short peptide fragments (~9–13 amino acids) derived from protein antigens, rather than native proteins or carbohydrates. These foreign antigens can be taken up by APCs through endocytosis into acidified vesicles or by phagocytosis, where they are degraded into small peptides that associate with MHC class II molecules in the *exogenous antigen-presentation pathway*. Intracellular vesicles containing MHC class II molecules fuse with peptide-containing vesicles, allowing the peptides to bind to MHC class II and subsequently be transported to the cell surface for recognition by CD4+ T cells. Alternatively, antigens that originate endogenously in the cytosol, such as from replicating viruses, are processed via the *endogenous antigen-presentation pathway*, where they are cleaved into peptides by the proteasome and transported into the endoplasmic reticulum by TAP proteins to associate with MHC class I molecules. MHC I-peptide complexes are then transported to the cell surface for recognition by CD8+ T cells. CD4 and CD8 molecules stabilize these TCR-antigen interactions by directly binding to MHC class II and I molecules, respectively, enhancing T-cell activation.

When a mature T-cell TCR binds to a foreign peptide presented by self-MHC class I or II molecules, adhesion ligands such as CD54-CD11/CD18 and CD58-CD2 stabilize this interaction and enhance their expression. This binding triggers lipid rafts in the T-cell membrane, concentrating signaling molecules such as the TCR/CD3 complex, CD28, LAT, src family PTKs and ZAP-70, facilitating essential phosphorylation events that transmit activation signals to the nucleus, leading to gene expression for T-cell functions such as IL-2 secretion.

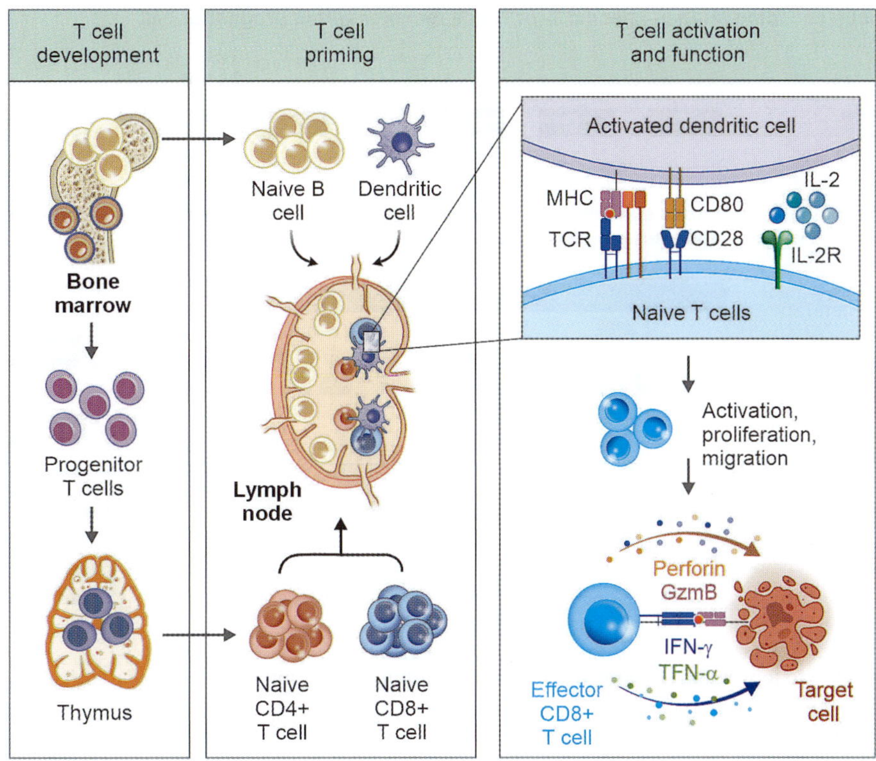

FIG. 10: A brief overview of T-cell development and activation. T-cell development begins in the bone marrow with hematopoietic stem cells that acquire a lymphoid progenitor state. These cells migrate to the thymus, a specialized primary lymphoid organ, to undergo additional maturation and selection against self-reactive T-cell clones. During this process, progenitor T cells differentiate into either mature CD4+ or CD8+ T cells and exit the thymus. These antigen-naive T cells can be activated in the lymph node by dendritic cells that provide TCR, costimulatory, and cytokine signaling for the acquisition of effector T-cell functions.

Source: Han S, Georgiev P, Ringel AE, Sharpe AH, Haigis MC. Age-associated remodeling of T cell immunity and metabolism. Cell Metab. 2023;35(1):36-55.

Age-related Changes in T Cells

The aging adaptive immune system is characterized by a gradual decline in functionality and an increase in autoimmune disorders. This deterioration results in a heightened risk of infections and cancer, as well as a reduced effectiveness of vaccinations. Key hallmarks of T-cell aging include four primary features: Thymic involution, which reduces the production of new T cells; mitochondrial dysfunction, leading to impaired energy metabolism; genetic and epigenetic alterations that disrupt normal cellular functions; and loss of proteostasis, which affects protein maintenance. Additionally, there are four secondary hallmarks: (1) A reduction in the diversity of the TCR repertoire; (2) an imbalance between naïve and memory T cells; (3) T-cell senescence, marked by diminished proliferative capacity; and (4) a lack of effector plasticity, limiting the ability of T cells to adapt to new challenges. Together, these hallmarks contribute to two integrative features of aging: (1) Immunodeficiency and (2) inflammaging. Notably, these aspects of T-cell aging are interrelated, progressing simultaneously and influencing one another, which results in common characteristics seen in the immune system of older individuals.

Thymic Involution

A significant change in the immune system with aging is thymic involution, where the thymus, crucial for generating a diverse T-cell repertoire, gradually decreases in function. This process begins in childhood and peaks around puberty in humans **(Fig. 12)**.

Thymic involution leads to disrupted tissue architecture, reduced thymic mass, and a decline in thymocyte numbers, resulting in fewer naïve T cells reaching circulation and a compensatory expansion of memory T cells. This diminishes the diversity of the peripheral T-cell repertoire, compromising the immune response to pathogens.

Mitochondrial Dysfunction

Older T cells have a higher abundance of mitochondrial proteins but show impaired oxidative phosphorylation, likely due to ineffective recycling of dysfunctional

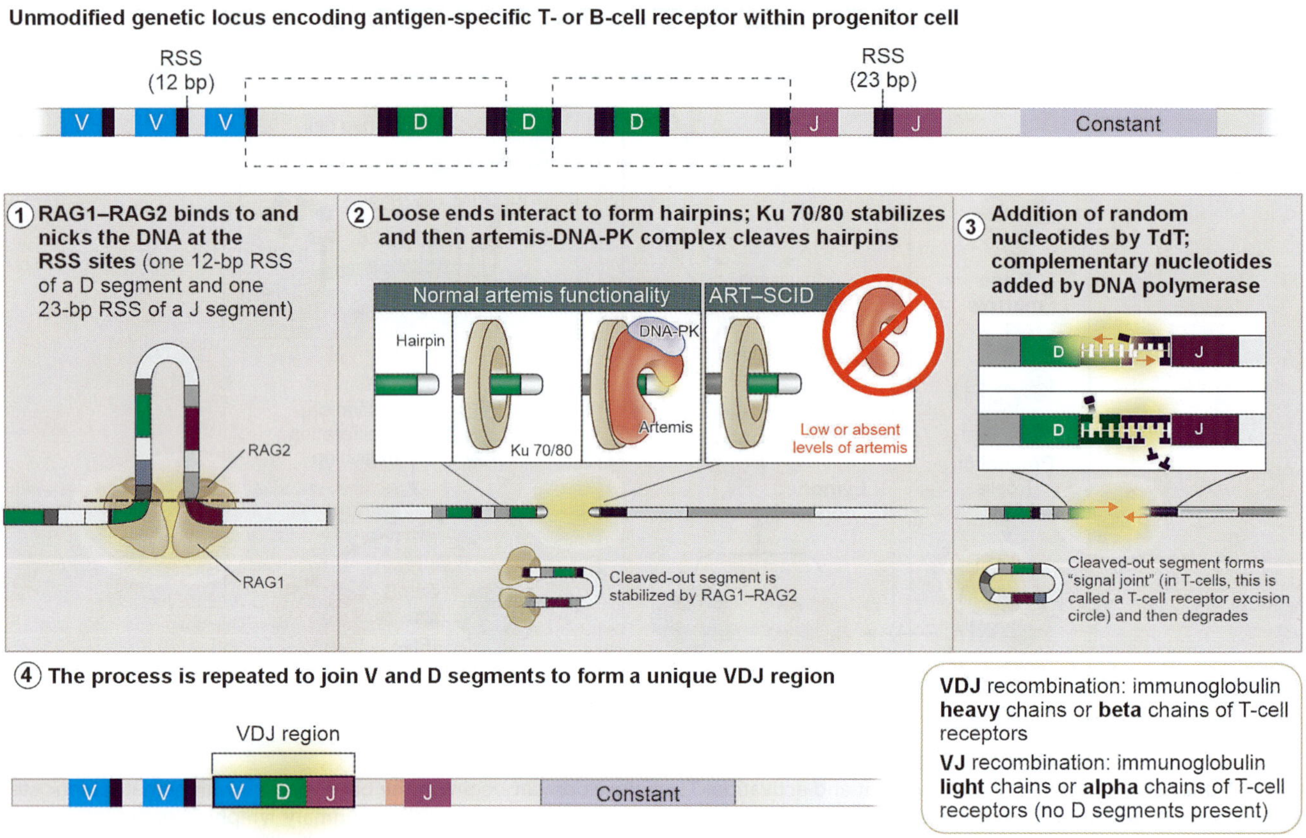

FIG. 11: VDJ recombination.
(V: variable; D: diversity; J: joint)
Source: NEJM. Illustrated glossary. N Engl J Med [Internet]. 2002 [cited 2025 May]. Available from: https://illustrated-glossary.nejm.t/

mitochondria via autophagy. This impairment is further exacerbated by persistent antigenic stimulation from chronic viral infections.

Mitochondria play crucial roles beyond energy metabolism; they act as signaling hubs that manage ROS and calcium spikes. However, in aged T cells, these signaling pathways become dysregulated, leading to a proinflammatory phenotype. This shift occurs through various mechanisms, including the accumulation of inflammatory metabolites, epigenetic changes, post-transcriptional protein modifications, and the release of mitochondrial DNA (mtDNA) into the cytoplasm, which activates the cGAS-STING pathway. This cascade triggers inflammasome activation and upregulates proinflammatory cytokine genes.

Additionally, glycolytic metabolism in aged T cells enhances inflammatory responses by activating PI3K-AKT-FOXO signaling. These cells also show increased basal activity of PI3K-AKT-mTOR and MAPK signaling pathways.

Overall, age-associated mitochondrial decline in T lymphocytes is linked to the development of a senescent phenotype, underscoring the significance of mitochondrial health in immune function during aging.

Genetic and Epigenetic Alterations

Aging T lymphocytes experience various genetic and epigenetic alterations that impact their function and health. Chromosomal changes accumulate over time, increasing the risk of T-cell leukemias, particularly influenced by mutations in HSCs. Genomic instability arises from mitochondrial stress and telomere shortening, which is exacerbated by factors such as chronic viral infections. Notably, the downregulation of repair enzymes such as MRE11A contributes to telomere damage and upregulates senescence markers. Epigenetically, aging is associated with modifications in DNA methylation and histone codes, leading to functional changes in T-cell signaling pathways. Additionally, there is a decline in specific microRNAs, such as miR-181a and miR-146,

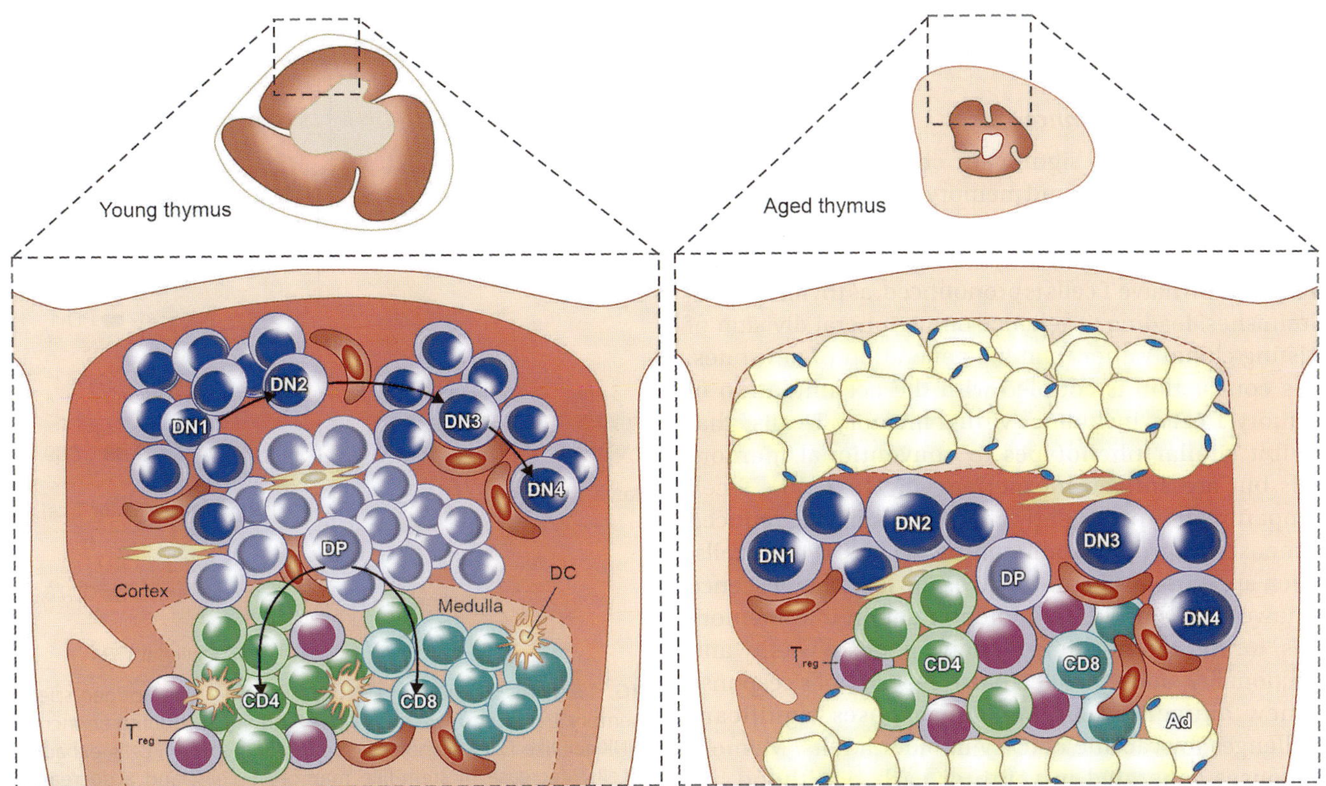

FIG. 12: Thymus involution. With age, thymic cellularity gradually declines, commensurate with disruption of tissue architecture, reduced production of naive T cells, and reduction in the peripheral TCR repertoire.

(Ad: adipocyte; DC: dendritic cell; DN: double-negative CD4–CD8–thymocytes; DP: double-positive CD4+CD8+ thymocytes)

Source: Mittelbrunn M, Kroemer G. Hallmarks of T cell aging. Nat Immunol. 2021;22(6):687-98.

which further disrupts T-cell expansion and immune responses. Collectively, these alterations in aging T cells significantly affect immune function and overall health.

Loss of Proteostasis

With aging, T cells experience a significant loss of proteostasis, primarily due to decreased activity of proteolytic systems such as *proteasomes* and *autophagy*. In older individuals, the expression of calpains and tripeptidyl peptidase II (TPPII) declines, with TPPII deficiency linked to premature immunosenescence of CD8+ T cells. Additionally, the activation of the proteasome through TCR signaling diminishes in aged CD4+ T cells, leading to increased senescence markers such as PD-1. Autophagy, responsible for recycling protein aggregates and organelles, also becomes insufficient due to factors such as increased nutrients (glucose and free fatty acids) and growth factors (insulin and IGF1) that accompany metabolic syndrome, in particular in the context of obesity, overactivate the autophagy-inhibitory mTORC1 pathway, reduce activation of nutrient sensors such as sirtuin-1, lower levels of spermidine that are required for the translation of proautophagic proteins, and reduce activation of proautophagic transfection factor cascades such as the FOXO1-TFEB axis. This decline in autophagy particularly affects memory T cells and Treg cells, which rely on oxidative phosphorylation and mitochondrial quality control, likely because autophagy plays an essential role in mitochondrial quality control, contributing to a loss of immunological memory and tolerance. Restoring autophagy through caloric restriction, NAD precursor supplementation, and mTORC1 inhibitor rapamycin or dietary spermidine can enhance T-cell function and health span.

Reduction of T-cell Receptor Repertoire

The TCR repertoire undergoes notable shifts with aging, influenced by various factors such as reduced generation of naïve T cells from the thymus, clonal hematopoiesis that favors certain T cells regardless of their antigen recognition, and persistent selection by peripheral antigens, particularly from chronic infections such as cytomegalovirus (CMV), which can result in "memory inflation." Furthermore, recent studies indicate that the pool of CD4+ human stem cell memory T lymphocytes (TSCM) declines with age, linked to diminished Wnt/βcatenin signaling and an increase in Dickkopf-related protein 1, a natural inhibitor of this pathway.

Naive–memory Imbalance

As individuals' age, significant changes occur in the balance between naive and memory T cells, primarily due to thymic involution, persistent antigen stimulation, and an increasingly inflammatory environment. In humans, the decline in naive T cells is pronounced, as thymic output diminishes, leading to reliance on peripheral division of existing clones rather than the generation of new ones. This contraction is coupled with the accumulation of memory T cells, including "virtual memory T cells" that exhibit similar phenotypes to conventional memory cells but are antigen inexperienced. The CD8+ T-cell compartment is particularly affected, displaying reduced homeostatic proliferation compared to CD4+ T cells, which are more resilient with age. The loss of quiescence in naive T cells drives their differentiation into memory cells, further diminishing the naive pool's diversity and functionality, and limits the naive T-cell pool's response to new antigens. This imbalance poses significant challenges for vaccine efficacy in older adults. Memory responses generated in youth or early adulthood are generally more durable than those produced in older age, highlighting the implications of age-related T-cell dynamics for immunological health **(Fig. 13)**.

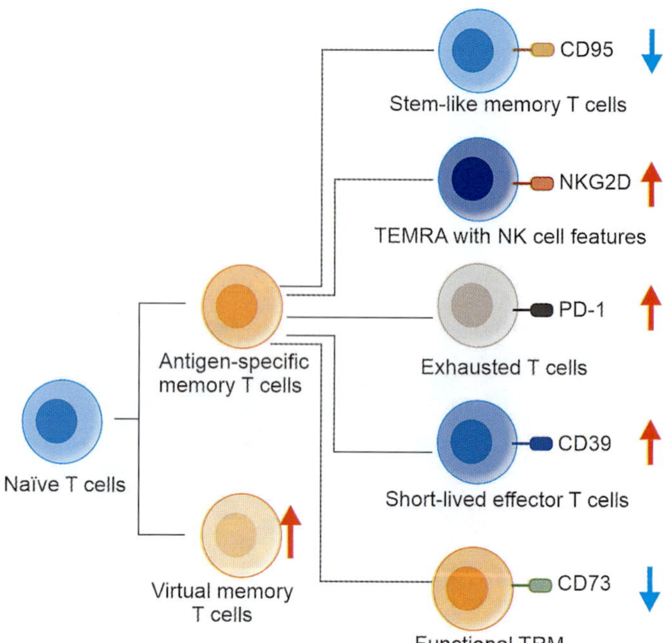

FIG. 13: Fates of memory T cells with age. The antigen-specific memory T cells adopt several fates with age, including an increase in NK cell-like TEMRA, short-lived effector memory T cells, exhausted T cells, decrease in stem-like memory T cells, and a decrease in tissue-residing T memory cells. Virtual memory T cells without prior experience of antigen encounter also increase with age.

(TEMRA: terminally differentiated CD8+ T cells; TRM: tissue-resident memory T cells)

Source: Zhang H, Weyand CM, Goronzy JJ. Hallmarks of the aging T-cell system. FEBS J. 2021;288(24):7123-42.

T-cell Senescence

Aging is marked by the accumulation of dysfunctional, terminally differentiated T cells that acquire a senescent or exhausted phenotype due to persistent antigen stimulation, particularly from chronic infections. While both senescent and exhausted T cells exhibit defects in TCR-triggered proliferation, they differ in molecular signaling and secretory profiles, with senescent T cells secreting proinflammatory factors typical of the SASP. Features of senescent T cells include low telomerase activity, short telomeres, signs of DNA damage, resistance to apoptosis, and the loss of costimulatory molecules such as CD27 and CD28, along with the upregulation of terminal-differentiation markers such as KLRG1 and CD57. CD8+ T cells tend to acquire senescence faster than CD4+ T cells. Factors such as menin, mTORC1 signaling, PI3K, p38 MAPK signaling, and sestrins play crucial roles in regulating T-cell senescence. Additionally, regulatory T cells (Tregs) experience more severe senescence than effector T cells, impacting their function and proliferation. Chronic viral infections can accelerate this process by inducing telomere attrition and DNA damage. Senescent T cells have been implicated in age-related diseases such as cardiovascular, metabolic, and neurodegenerative disorders. Strategies to deplete senescent T cells (senolysis) may offer therapeutic avenues for mitigating aging and its associated diseases **(Fig. 14)**.

Lack of Effector Plasticity

CD4+ T lymphocytes have long been classified into distinct subtypes such as TH1, TH2, TH9, TH17, TH22, TFH, and Treg cells. With advancing age, T cells often lose their quiescent state and shift into a terminally differentiated phase, which can lead to biased lineage commitments and a reduction in their plasticity. This diminishment in adaptability compromises the immune system's capability to tackle new antigenic threats **(Figs. 15 and 16)**.

B-cells

B cells are classified into various subsets, primarily B-1 and B-2 cells, each with unique developmental pathways and functions. B-1 cells, predominantly found in neonates, develop from fetal liver progenitor cells. B-2 cells make up the majority of adult B cells and rely on BAFF-BAFFR signaling for development and

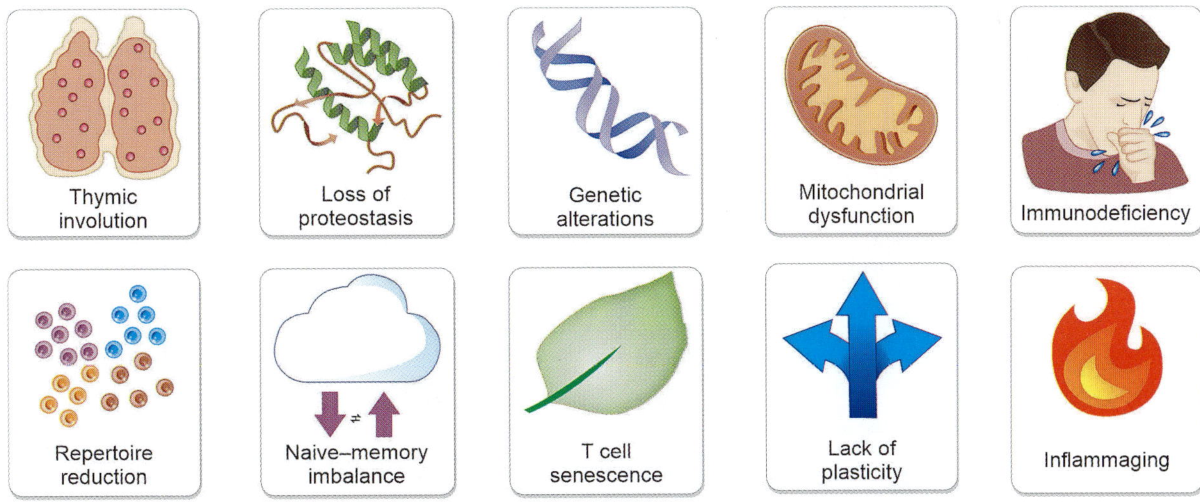

FIG. 14: Hallmarks of T-cell aging. The scheme enumerates the molecular hallmarks that define T-cell aging.
Source: Mittelbrunn M, Kroemer G. Hallmarks of T cell aging. Nat Immunol. 2021;22(6):687-98.

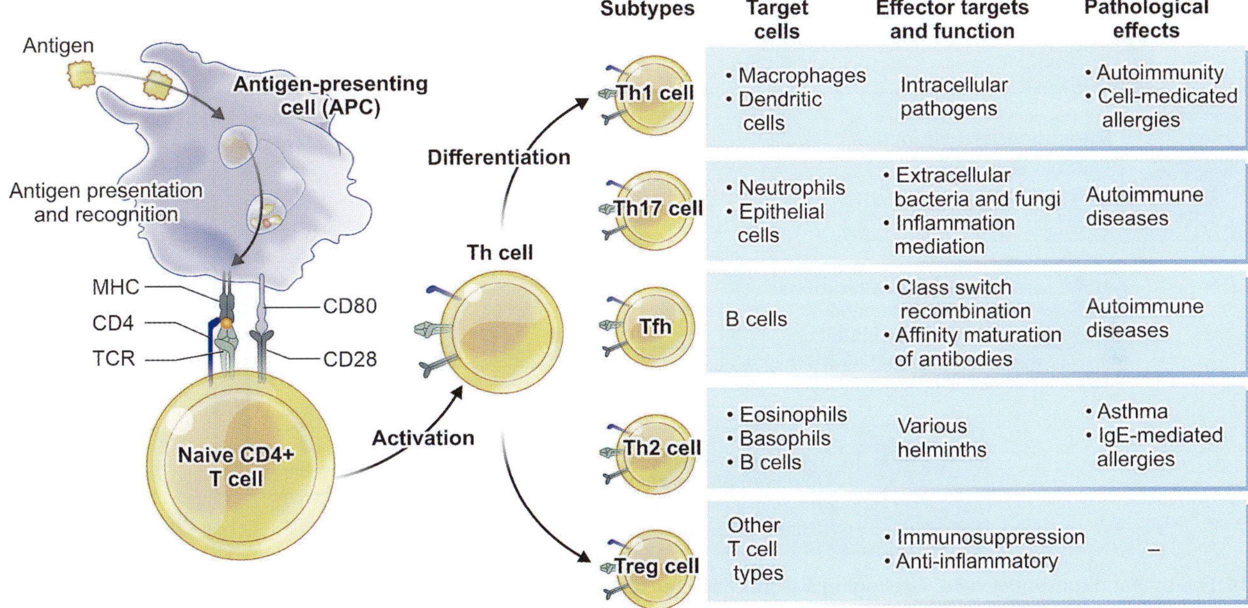

FIG. 15: T-helper cell differentiation.
Source: NEJM. Illustrated glossary. N Engl J Med [Internet]. 2002 [cited 2025 May]. Available from: https://illustrated-glossary.nejm.t/

survival. B-2 cells originate from lymphoid-biased HSCs and develop in a sequence from pro-B cells to pre-B cells and then to immature B cells in the bone marrow. Once mature, B cells exit the bone marrow and are found in two main peripheral pools: (1) Marginal zone (MZ) B cells and (2) follicular (FO) B cells. MZ B cells are primarily located in the MZ of the spleen and respond rapidly to blood-borne pathogens, particularly T-cell-independent (TI) antigens, producing large amounts of IgM antibodies and presenting antigens to CD4+ T cells to initiate adaptive responses. In contrast, FO B cells are primarily found in the follicles of secondary lymphoid organs and depend on T follicular helper (TFH) cells for their activation. FO B cells interact with antigen-specific T follicular helper (TFH) cells to become germinal center (GC) B cells, which express the enzyme *activation-induced cytidine deaminase (AID)*. Under the influence of signals from TFH cells, *AID* is activated, leading to *class switch recombination (CSR)* and *somatic hypermutation (SHM)*. Class switching can

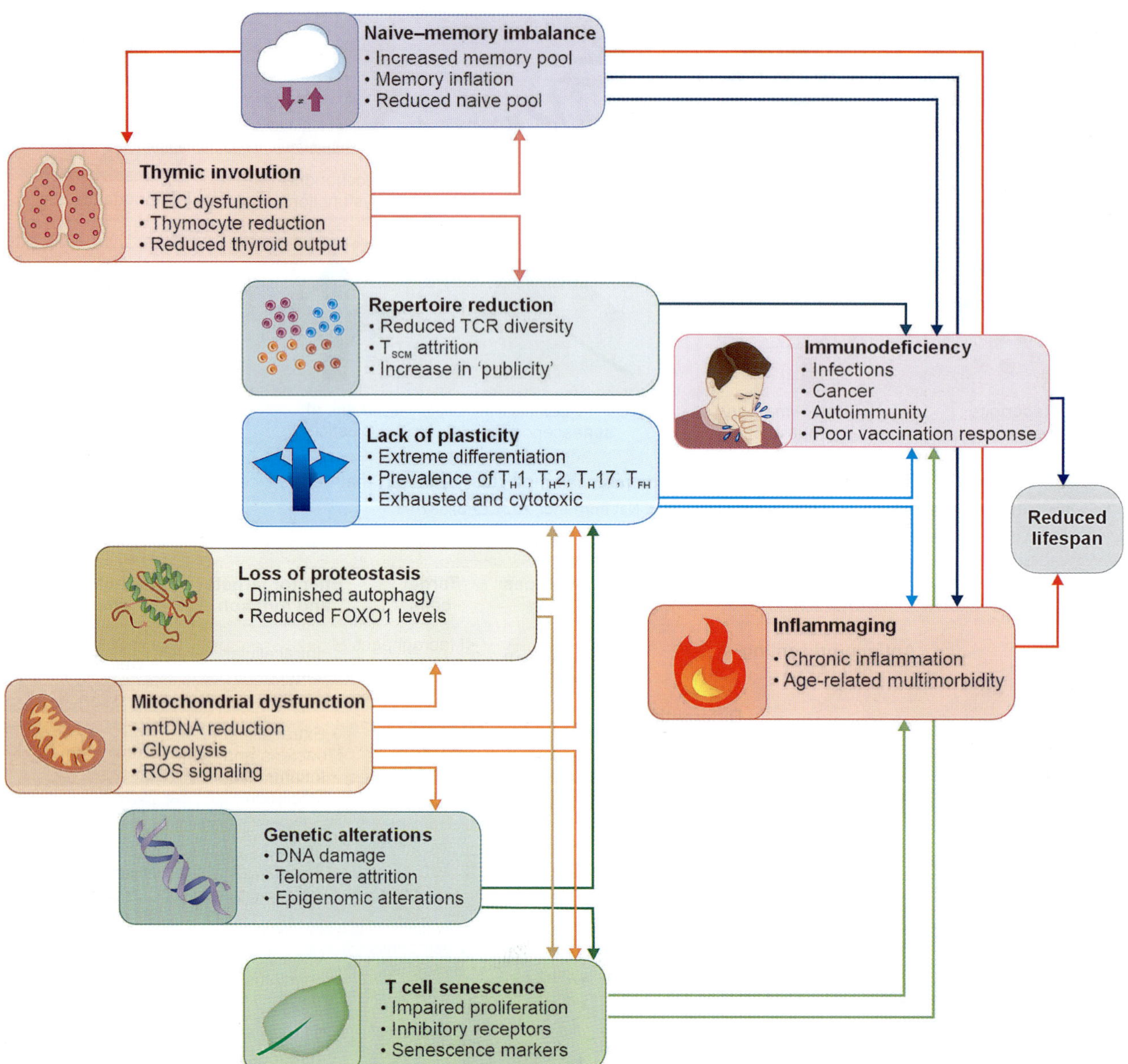

FIG. 16: Features and consequences of T-cell aging. Salient characteristics of each hallmark are listed, and the most important interconnections are indicated by arrows.

Source: Mittelbrunn M, Kroemer G. Hallmarks of T cell aging. Nat Immunol. 2021;22(6):687-98.

change the isotype of an antibody from IgM/IgD to IgG/IgA/IgE **(Fig. 17)**.

Mature B cells account for 5–10% of human peripheral blood lymphocytes, 20–30% of lymph node cells, 50% of splenic lymphocytes, and approximately 10% of bone marrow lymphocytes. These cells express intramembrane Ig molecules that serve as B-cell receptors (BCRs), functioning similar to T-cell receptors. Unlike T cells, which recognize processed peptide fragments presented by MHC class I and II molecules, B cells can recognize and respond to whole, unprocessed native antigens through their surface Ig (sIg) receptors. B cells also express surface receptors for the Fc region of IgG (CD32) and for activated complement components (C3d or CD21, C3b or CD35). Their primary role is antibody production, but they also act as efficient APCs, with their presentation abilities enhanced by various cytokines. B-cell development occurs in two phases: Antigen-independent phase, which takes place in primary lymphoid organs and includes all maturation stages up to the surface Ig-positive (sIg+) mature B cell, and antigen-dependent phase, initiated by antigen interaction with mature B-cell sIg, leading to

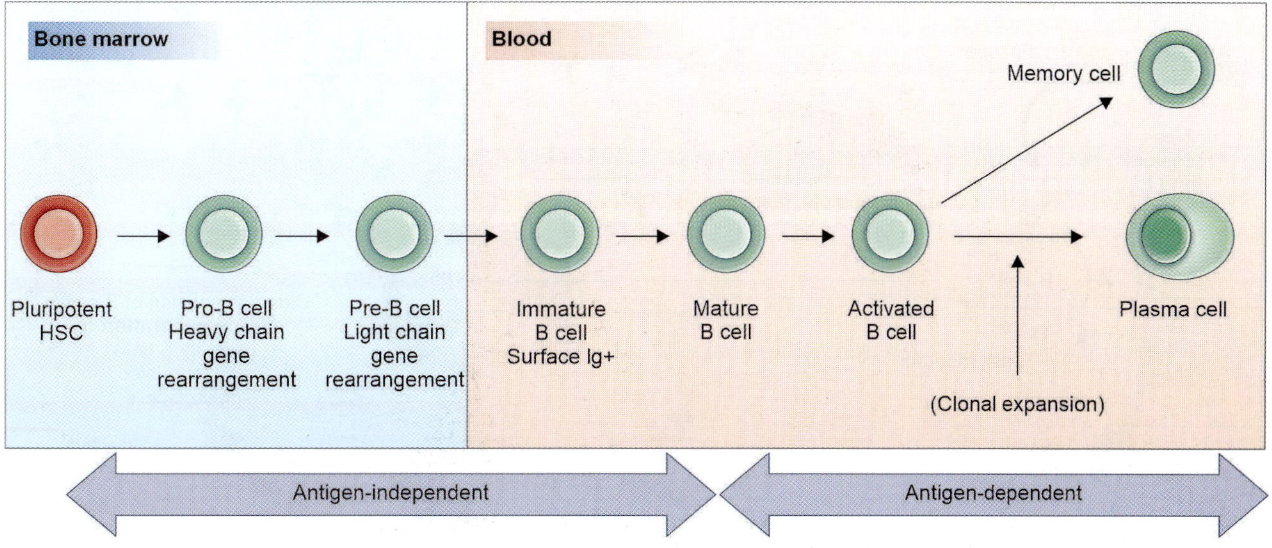

FIG. 17: Depiction of B-cell development. Immunoglobulin gene rearrangement (first of the heavy chain genes, followed by light chain gene rearrangement) is crucial to B lymphopoiesis, resulting in the generation of a library of mature B cells collectively expressing a highly diverse repertoire of surface immunoglobulin (the B-cell antigen receptor). Encounter with a specific antigen results in expansion of a clone of B cells recognizing that antigen and generation of memory B cells and plasma cells secreting immunoglobulin of the same specificity.

Source: Halter JB, Ouslander JG, Studenski S, High KP, Asthana S, Supiano MA, et al. Hazzard's Geriatric Medicine and Gerontology, 8th edition. New York: McGraw Hill; 2022.

memory B-cell induction, Ig class switching, and plasma cell formation. This latter phase occurs in secondary lymphoid organs such as lymph nodes, spleen, and gut Peyer's patches. Unlike T cells, which develop their repertoire intrathymically before encountering foreign antigens, B-cell diversity is shaped by somatic hypermutation that alters Ig genes following antigen stimulation in lymph node germinal centers **(Fig. 18)**.

During B-cell development, the antigen-binding variable region of immunoglobulins (Ig) achieves diversity through a series of ordered gene rearrangements, similar to those seen in T-cell receptors. The process begins with the heavy chain, where D segments rearrange to J segments, followed by the V gene segment joining the D-J sequence, ultimately aligning with a constant (C) segment to form a functional heavy chain gene (V-D-J-C). Subsequently, a κ or λ light chain gene is produced by rearranging a V segment to a J segment, resulting in a complete Ig molecule consisting of one heavy and one light chain. This rearrangement is tightly regulated to ensure that each B cell expresses a single antibody specificity through a mechanism known as *allelic exclusion*, wherein only one gene of each type is utilized. With around 300 Vκ genes and 5 Jκ genes, there are over 1,500 possible kappa light-chain combinations, while approximately 70 Vλ genes and 4 Jλ genes yield more than 280 lambda light-chain combinations. The diversity of these light chains is further augmented by somatic mutations within the V and J genes. In the case of heavy-chain rearrangement, the VH domain is constructed from the combination of VH, DH, and JH germline genes, resulting in even greater variability in the heavy chain's variable region compared to that of light chains.

Random rearrangements of immunoglobulin (Ig) genes can occasionally produce self-reactive antibodies, necessitating mechanisms to correct these errors. One such mechanism is B-cell receptor (BCR) editing, which mutates autoreactive BCRs to prevent interaction with self-antigens. If receptor editing fails, autoreactive B cells undergo negative selection in the bone marrow, leading to apoptosis upon BCR engagement with self-antigens. Once B cells exit the bone marrow, they populate peripheral sites such as lymph nodes and the spleen, where they await contact with foreign antigens that activate their clonotypic receptors. Antigen-driven activation triggers *somatic hypermutation*, introducing point mutations in the rearranged heavy- and light-chain genes, resulting in mutant sIg molecules with potentially improved antigen-binding capabilities. This process, known as affinity maturation, enables memory B cells in peripheral lymphoid organs to produce the highest-affinity antibodies. B lymphocytes that synthesize IgG, IgA, and IgE arise from mature sIgM+ and sIgD+ B cells through Ig class switching, which occurs in germinal centers of peripheral lymphoid tissues. This process is facilitated by the critical interaction between CD40 on B cells and CD40 ligand on T cells, along with T cell-produced cytokines such as IL-4 and TGF-β, and other cytokines such as IL-1, -2, -4, -5, and -6, which collectively stimulate mature B cells to proliferate and differentiate into antibody-secreting cells.

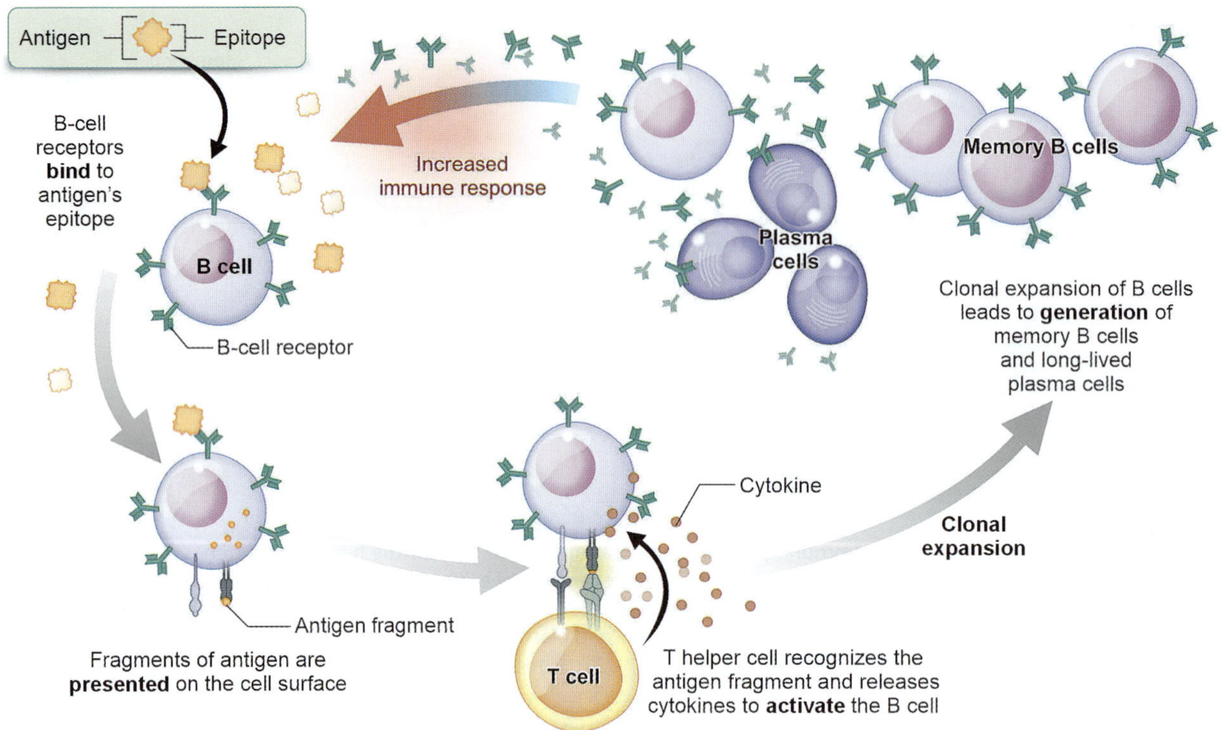

FIG. 18: Immunogenicity.
Source: NEJM. Illustrated glossary. N Engl J Med [Internet]. 2002 [cited 2025 May]. Available from: https://illustrated-glossary.nejm.t/

Aging and B-2 Cells

Recent studies indicate that aging significantly reduces the production of precursor B cells in the bone marrow of both mice and humans, likely due to changes in the bone marrow microenvironment, such as lower IL-7 levels and a shift in HSCs toward myeloid cell production. Aging reduces the B-cell antibody response to T cell-dependent antigens, primarily due to dysfunction in aged DCs and T cells, which show impaired expression of B cell-activation markers such as CD40L. This leads to fewer GC B cells and impaired isotype switching. Additionally, the number of regulatory T cells (TREGs), which can suppress B-cell function, increases with age, contributing to a defective antibody response. Isotype switching is impaired in aged B cells in both mice and humans, linked to reduced stability of E47 mRNA and lower transcription of *activation-induced cytidine deaminase (AID),* resulting in weaker and less durable immune memory.

While peripheral B-2 cell numbers remain stable in aged mice, the FO B-cell subset slightly declines, which may contribute to reduced GC numbers and affect naive and memory B-2 cells in aging humans. Aging also impacts the MZ B-cell subset; although the exact effects are unclear, some studies indicate an increase in autoreactive antibodies due to hypersensitivity to the prosurvival factor BAFF, while others report a reduction in MZ B cells attributed to declining MZ macrophages. Additionally, aged MZ B cells show defective antigen capture and antibody production, leading to diminished T cell-independent immune responses.

Additionally, aged MZ B cells show defective antigen capture and antibody production, leading to diminished T cell-independent immune responses **(Fig. 19)**.

Age-associated B Cells

Age-associated B cells (ABCs) have been identified in aged mice by researchers Hao et al. and Rubtsov et al. Hao et al. define them as CD43–CD21–/35–CD23– B cells, while Rubtsov et al. identify them as CD11b+CD11c+ B cells. Recent studies have shown that the transcription factor T-bet is significantly expressed in ABCs. The presence of T-bet in B cells is crucial for their ability to produce autoantibodies. There is a notable increase in the frequency and quantity of ABCs within the B-cell pool. Evidence shows that in the later stages of senescence, these cells can make up about 50% of the total splenic B-cell population. This rise is driven by the accumulation of genetic and epigenetic changes over time, suggesting that ABCs are a naturally occurring subset found in all animal species.

Evidence indicates a close relationship between ABCs and follicular (FO) B cells. Research has demonstrated that FO B cells can differentiate into ABCs in response to

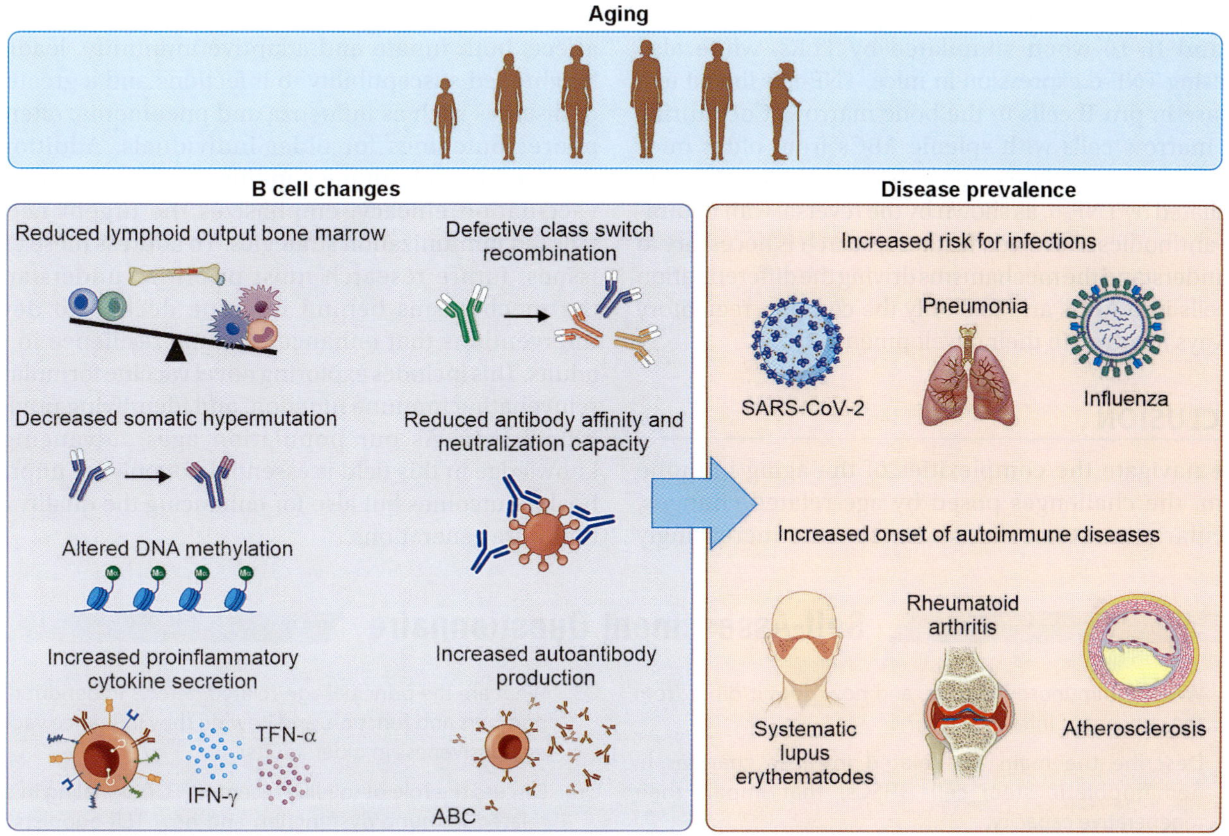

FIG. 19: Age-related effects on B cells and the impact on disease prevalence. Aging is associated with reduced lymphoid output in the bone marrow and intrinsic defects in B cells, including decreased CSR, SHM, and antibody affinity. The increase in ABCs also results in increased proinflammatory cytokine secretion and autoantibody reduction. Together, these age-related B-cell changes contribute to the increased risk for infections and autoimmune diseases upon aging.

(CSR: class switch recombination; SHM: somatic hypermutation)

Source: de Mol J, Kuiper J, Tsiantoulas D, Foks AC. The dynamics of B cell aging in health and disease. Front Immunol. 2021;12:733566.

stimulation via TLR 7 or 9, but not through BCR or CD40 signaling. This finding strongly suggests that FO B cells are a significant source of ABCs. Further studies have shown a positive correlation between T-bet levels and signals from IL-21 or IFN-γ via TLR7, indicating that TLR-mediated activation is crucial for the development of T-bet+ B cells. The differentiation of ABCs appears to require the costimulation of TLR7 alongside IL-21 or IFN-γ. While BCR signaling is not essential for ABC responses, a combination of TLR and BCR signals can enhance the proliferation and differentiation of ABCs. Notably, T-bet+ B cells cannot develop without MHC-II and CD40, suggesting that germinal center (GC) B cells may also be a potential origin for ABCs, although this has yet to be definitively proven. Additionally, T-bet is involved in the differentiation of CD11c+ B cells, which are significant precursors for producing IgG2a antibodies. This particular isotype is highly effective for antibody-dependent cellular cytotoxicity and plays a vital role in the antiviral immune response **(Flowchart 1)**.

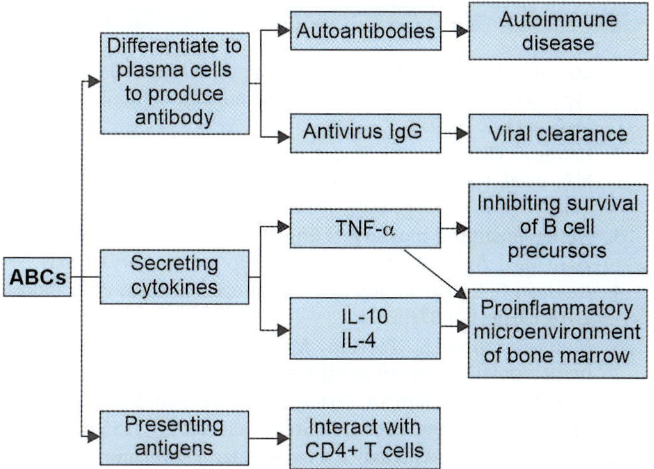

FLOWCHART 1: Functional properties of age-associated B cells (ABCs).

Source: Ma S, Wang C, Mao X, Hao Y. B cell dysfunction associated with aging and autoimmune diseases. Front Immunol. 2019;10:318.

In vitro studies show that ABCs preferentially produce IL-4 and IL-10 when stimulated by TLRs, while also increasing TNF-α expression in mice. TNF-α is linked to a decrease in pro-B cells in the bone marrow. Coculturing bone marrow cells with splenic ABCs from older mice inhibits the growth of B-cell precursors, and this inhibition is mediated by TNF-α, as shown by the reversal with neutralizing antibodies. However, further research is necessary to fully understand the mechanisms driving the differentiation of B cells into ABCs and to clarify the complex regulatory pathways involved in their development.

CONCLUSION

As we navigate the complexities of the aging immune system, the challenges posed by age-related changes, particularly immunosenescence, become increasingly evident. This gradual decline in immune function affects both innate and adaptive immunity, leading to heightened susceptibility to infections and a greater risk of diseases such as influenza and pneumonia, often with poorer outcomes for older individuals. Additionally, the rise in autoimmune conditions, alongside declining vaccination efficacy, emphasizes the urgent need for tailored immunization strategies. To address these critical issues, future research must prioritize understanding the mechanisms behind immune decline to develop interventions that enhance immune resilience in older adults. This includes exploring novel vaccine formulations, rejuvenating immune function, and identifying predictive biomarkers. As our population ages, advancing our knowledge in this field is essential not only for improving health outcomes but also for enhancing the quality of life for future generations.

Self-Assessment Questionnaire

Q1. What is immunosenescence, and how does it differ from the concept of inflammaging?

Q2. Describe the main age-related intrinsic changes in hematopoietic stem cells (HSCs) that impair their regenerative capacity.

Q3. How does aging affect myeloid and lymphoid lineage differentiation, and what are the consequences for immune function?

Q4. How do natural killer (NK) cells change in phenotype and function with advancing age?

Q5. What are the principal age-related defects in dendritic cell numbers and function, and how do they influence vaccine responsiveness in older adults?

Q6. Discuss the role of toll-like receptor (TLR) signaling in age-related immune dysfunction and how TLR agonists can enhance vaccine efficacy in older individuals.

Q7. Summarize the molecular hallmarks of T-cell aging and explain how thymic involution and mitochondrial dysfunction contribute to immunosenescence.

FURTHER READINGS

1. Loscalzo J, Fauci A, Kasper D, Hauser S, Longo D, Jameson JL. Harrison's Principles of Internal Medicine, 21st edition. New York: McGraw Hill; 2022.
2. Halter JB, Ouslander JG, Studenski S, High KP, Asthana S, Supiano MA, et al. Hazzard's Geriatric Medicine and Gerontology, 8th edition. New York: McGraw Hill; 2022.
3. NEJM. Illustrated glossary. N Engl J Med [Internet]. 2002 [cited 2025 May]. Available from: https://illustrated-glossary.nejm.t/
4. de Haan G, Lazare SS. Aging of hematopoietic stem cells. Blood. 2018;131(5):479-87.
5. Mejia-Ramirez E, Florian MC. Understanding intrinsic hematopoietic stem cell aging. Haematologica. 2020;105(1):22-37.
6. Kim MJ, Kim MH, Kim SA, Chang JS. Age-related deterioration of hematopoietic stem cells. Int J Stem Cells. 2008;1(1):55-63.
7. Li X, Li C, Zhang W, Wang Y, Qian P, Huang H. Inflammation and aging: signaling pathways and intervention therapies. Signal Transduct Target Ther. 2023;8(1):239.
8. Shaw AC, Goldstein DR, Montgomery RR. Age-dependent dysregulation of innate immunity. Nat Rev Immunol. 2013;13(12):875-87.
9. Han S, Georgiev P, Ringel AE, Sharpe AH, Haigis MC. Age-associated remodeling of T cell immunity and metabolism. Cell Metab. 2023;35(1):36-55.
10. Mittelbrunn M, Kroemer G. Hallmarks of T cell aging. Nat Immunol. 2021;22(6):687-98.
11. Zhang H, Weyand CM, Goronzy JJ. Hallmarks of the aging T-cell system. FEBS J. 2021;288(24):7123-42.
12. de Mol J, Kuiper J, Tsiantoulas D, Foks AC. The dynamics of B cell aging in health and disease. Front Immunol. 2021;12:733566.
13. Ma S, Wang C, Mao X, Hao Y. B cell dysfunction associated with aging and autoimmune diseases. Front Immunol. 2019;10:318.
14. Shaw AC, Joshi S, Greenwood H, Panda A, Lord JM. Aging of the innate immune system. Curr Opin Immunol. 2010;22(4):507-13.
15. Frasca D, Blomberg BB. Aging affects human B cell responses. J Clin Immunol. 2011;31(3):430-5.
16. Ruan P, Wang S, Yang M, Wu H. The ABC-associated immunosenescence and lifestyle interventions in autoimmune disease. Rheumatol Immunol Res. 2022;3(3):128-35.
17. Mogilenko DA, Shchukina I, Artyomov MN. Immune ageing at single-cell resolution. Nat Rev Immunol. 2022;22(8):484-98.

CHAPTER 5

Psychological Changes of Aging

Sweta Kedia, Lt Col Sumit Bhaskar

CASE VIGNETTE

Mrs Saraswati, a 76-year-old female, literate, unemployed, widow, living alone, presented with complaints of low mood and a decrease in daily functioning since 1 year. She reported feeling increasingly lonely and overwhelmed by a sense of purposelessness. She also complained of memory lapses, which made functioning difficult. Her interest in previously enjoyable activities had also gone down, and she would often be plagued with anxiety and negative thinking about life. A detailed psychological assessment revealed the following aspects:

- *Loneliness and social isolation*: She was staying alone. Though her neighborhood was cooperative, she often missed people at home. She had her brother's family nearby, but since the last few months, she had decreased her visits there due to a lack of motivation.
- *Anxiety*: She would often have anxious ruminations about falling ill and becoming dependent on others and also that people may not even come to know that she is no more as she stayed alone.
- *Cognitive changes*: An examination using Addenbrooke's Cognitive Examination-III (ACE-III), she obtained a score of 80 with a low score in the area of attention and concentration and recent memory.
- *Mood changes*: She appeared to have depressive symptoms and on Geriatric Depression Scale-30, she had a score of 15, indicating the presence of mild-to-moderate symptoms.
- *Physical health*: Her sugar was not controlled as she would not take her meals on time and would often skip medications.

Therapeutic Approach

- *Pharmacological management*: She was referred for medical management of her mood symptoms as well as to control her diabetes. She was also referred to a dietitian to ensure that her sugar levels did not fluctuate.
- *Psychoeducation*: She was educated about the relationship between mind and body, need for medication compliance, and dietary management.
- *Problem-solving techniques*: She was asked to give a key to her neighbors, who could check on her at least once in a day to ensure her well-being. She was also encouraged to visit her brother's house at least once in 2 weeks and them visiting her once in 2 weeks. This system ensured weekly visits with family.
- *Increasing social support*: She was encouraged to go to the park at least three times in a week and also visit the nearby temple, where she could meet like-minded people.
- *Memory support strategies*: She was provided with practical strategies to manage memory changes, such as using memory aids, creating routines, and engaging in mindful meditation.

INTRODUCTION

Aging is a complex, dynamic process that involves irreversible changes in living organisms over time. It encompasses a range of physiological transformations driven by genetic factors, as well as influenced by biological, environmental, and psychosocial elements. Although there is no universally accepted age that marks the onset of old age, the United Nations designates 60 years and older as the benchmark for considering individuals as older adults. In Asia, 57% of the population is aged 60 years or above, and this demographic is expected to double by 2050, reaching an estimated 2.1 billion people.

Biological aging refers to the natural, progressive alterations in metabolism and the physicochemical properties of cells that occur with age. These changes contribute to diminished self-regulation and regenerative abilities, resulting in structural and functional modifications in tissues and organs.

Psychosocial aging is often considered a secondary effect of biological aging. As individual organs and systems undergo age-related changes, these can impact mood, attitudes toward one's environment, physical health, and social engagement. Additionally, psychosocial aging influences an older person's role within their family and society. However, the extent of psychosocial aging is significantly influenced by how well a person prepares for and adapts to aging, and it evolves progressively over time.

As people age, they often face growing challenges in adapting to new situations. Bromley identifies five common approaches to adapting to old age:

1. *Constructive attitude*: Marked by acceptance of aging, internal harmony, and positive interactions with others
2. *Dependent attitude*: Characterized by increased dependency and passivity
3. *Defensive posture*: Involves rejecting help despite needing it, with a pessimistic view of aging and a tendency toward isolation
4. *Hostility toward the world*: Seen in individuals who are aggressive, suspicious, and dissatisfied, leading to social withdrawal
5. *Hostility toward oneself*: Involves self-criticism and a lack of belief in one's ability to influence their own life

This chapter delves into the psychological changes experienced during aging, explores common challenges, and discusses strategies for successful aging.

PSYCHOSOCIAL ASPECTS IN AGING

Adapting to Retirement

Retirement is viewed as an event, status, and process, with Atchley identifying six stages: (1) Preretirement, (2) retirement, (3) disenchantment, (4) reorientation, (5) retirement routine, and (6) termination of retirement. The initial "honeymoon" phase involves enjoying newfound leisure. Traditionally, retirement disrupts routines and can negatively impact health, as work is central to adult life. Successful adaptation to retirement is influenced by health, education, income, and social support.

Theories on retirement, aging, and productivity offer varied perspectives. Disengagement theory views retirement as a gradual withdrawal from societal interactions. In contrast, activity theory frames retirement as a crisis where the loss of work should be countered by engaging in other productive activities, which are crucial for self-worth and satisfaction. Continuity theory suggests that retirees maintain their preretirement roles and activities as much as possible. Research shows that retirement can relieve job-related stress, allowing for personal interests and improved health. Studies have found mixed results: Retirement often boosts mental health and life satisfaction in the short term, with some evidence of long-term benefits, but findings on its impact on depression and mental health vary. A recent study also indicated that positive reasons for retirement contributed to better outcomes with respect to psychological well-being.

Effects of Marital Status and Sexuality

Marriage significantly impacts elder health, with married individuals generally experiencing better health outcomes compared to those who are never married, widowed, or divorced. Studies have consistently shown a link between marriage and lower mortality rates. Several theories explain this association: Marriage may offer social and economic support (social causation theory), healthier individuals may be more likely to marry or stay married (selection theory), or married individuals may adopt healthier behaviors due to both the selection and direct effects of marriage. Additionally, the stress associated with bereavement or marital dissolution can affect health. A recent systematic review found an increased risk of psychological frailty in unmarried/single elderly men, while the opposite was true for elderly women. Another longitudinal study found the risk of dementia to be higher in any category of unmarried elderly, especially in the young-old age group. Gender differences were again observed in the study.

Sexuality remains a significant aspect of life for older adults, though many still hold the belief that older individuals should not engage in sexual activity. Physiological changes, health issues, and medication can negatively impact sexual function in the elderly. Psychological and social factors also play a role, such as the loss of a primary partner, diminished self-esteem, societal attitudes, body changes, fear of rejection, and performance anxiety, all of which can reduce sexual interest and activity. Research shows a decline in sexual activity with age, with and documenting this trend. A national study from the United States indicated a decrease in sexual activity from 73% among those aged 57–64 years to 26% among those aged 75–85 years. A study conducted on 477 Brazilian elderly found a significant positive relationship between sexuality and quality of life. Another study from India highlights that though sexuality decreased with age, 57% of individuals above 60 years were found to be sexually active. However, sociocultural factors such as religious/cultural prohibitions, interpersonal conflicts, and the presence of mental health issues negatively influenced the sexual activity in elderly women.

Coping with Bereavement and Loss

Aging often involves a heightened risk of experiencing multiple losses, such as the death of a spouse, siblings, peers, or even children as life expectancy increases. The likelihood of experiencing bereavement increases with age, and it is often believed that the elderly are naturally equipped to deal with the loss. On the other hand, a significant minority are at risk for developing prolonged grief disorder (9–25%), depression (about 15%), posttraumatic stress disorder (about 9–16%), existential distress, and loneliness. These mental health issues are also found to be associated with cognitive decline, vascular diseases, suicide, and overuse or underuse of healthcare services. Cultural practices affect how individuals express their grief and cope with the same.

To plan treatment, it is important to understand the various presentations of grief process given as follows **(Table 1)**:

- *Predeath grief/anticipatory grief*: A sense of grief while caring for a person whose death is impending
- *Acute grief*: Experienced when the loss happens
- *Integrated grief*: Dealing with grief and reorganizing life after loss. It usually lasts for 6–12 months. Some studies have shown that coping with the death of a child can take up to 10 years.
- *Complicated/prolonged grief*: It is a failure to adapt to the loss and persistent yearning for the person. The International Classification of Diseases 11th Revision (ICD-11) criteria for prolonged grief include:
    - Death of someone close at least 6 months ago
    - Either persistent and pervasive longing for the deceased or persistent and pervasive preoccupation with the deceased
    - Accompanied by more than or equal to one example of intense emotional pain, e.g., sadness, blame, guilt, anger, inability to experience positive emotions, emotional numbness, feeling one has lost a part of himself/herself
    - Substantial impairment in personal, family, social, educational, occupational, or other important areas of functioning
    - The grief response has persisted for an atypically long period (≥6 months) and clearly exceeds norms for the individual's social, cultural, or religious context.

Over the years, several models have been described to conceptualize grief, starting from Sigmund Freud to Elisabeth Kübler-Ross. One of the most studied models in the elderly has been the "dual-process model." As described in **Figure 1**, the model has three components:

1. *Loss orientation*: The stressful experiences linked directly to the death/loss, i.e., thinking about the deceased, remembering the events preceding or following the loss, and yearning.
2. *Restoration oriented*: The bereaved also has to deal with stressors secondary to the loss, i.e., alterations in daily routine or living arrangements, practical or legal issues, and navigating new roles and responsibilities.
3. *Oscillation*: Dealing with grief is not a linear process, and the bereaved dwindles between the two stressors to cope with the loss.

Normal grief is usually expected to become more tolerable after 6 months of the loss. If symptoms continue beyond that, then it is advised to seek professional help. Even within the first 6 months, if the aged person

TABLE 1: Grief, prolonged grief, and major depressive disorder (MDD).

Grief	Prolonged grief	MDD
Arise in response to a death	Arise in response to a death	Can arise spontaneously
Sadness, guilt, anxiety, and sleep/appetite changes	Sadness, guilt, anxiety, and sleep/appetite changes	Sadness, guilt, anxiety, and sleep/appetite changes
Intense yearning but usually starts improving within 2–3 weeks	Intense yearning and preoccupation with deceases that do not improve	Sadness as an expression of yearning
Nonsuicidal	May be suicidal	May be suicidal
Functionally less impaired	Functionally impaired	Functionally impaired
Typical period is 6 months to 2 years with gradual improvement	Symptoms are sustained; does not remit or improve without intervention	Minimum 2 weeks
Spontaneous remission	Needs targeted intervention	Usually needs intervention

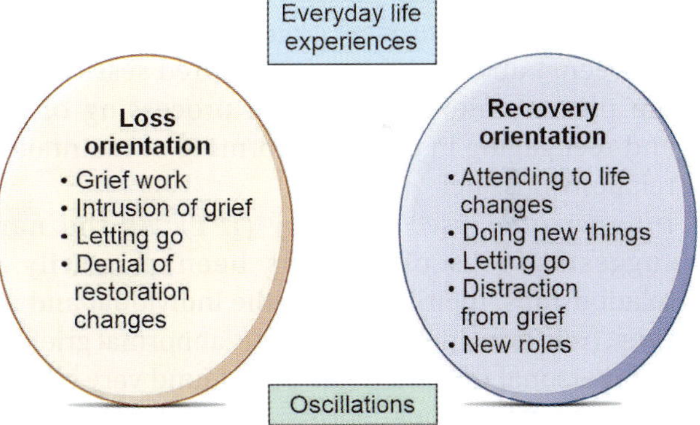

FIG. 1: Dual-process model of coping with bereavement.

shows symptoms of major depressive disorder, then pharmacological and psychosocial interventions are required. Despite elderly being more vulnerable to loss and bereavement, they have been a less studied population with respect to effective therapies. Some of the therapies that have small to some evidence base are:

- *Complicated grief therapy*: A 16-week program developed at Columbia University. The purpose is to help the bereaved person reinitiate their natural adaptive responses. The themes of the therapy are (1) sharing information, (2) self-regulation, and (3) rebuilding connections. These themes are covered through advancing aspirational goals, revisiting the story of the death, talking about how the world changed after the loss, and fostering continued bonds. In a randomized controlled trial (RCT), it was found to be significantly more effective compared to interpersonal therapy. A modified version includes sessions with family members.
- *Cognitive-behavior therapy (CBT)-modified for grief*: The focus is on psychoeducation about grief, cognitive restructuring of loss-related maladaptive thoughts, fostering adaptive thoughts, and behavior activation. A few studies have demonstrated promise of the intervention for older adults.
- *Dual-process bereavement group interventions*: Ranges between 4 and 14 weeks of structured sessions with the primary aim of emotional processing of grief and reengaging in activities, forming or maintaining relationships, etc.
- *Interpersonal psychotherapy (IPT)*: As the name suggests, focus of IPT has been primarily on relationships, their impact on the individual and vice versa (role transition, role dispute, abnormal grief, and interpersonal deficit). It has been found very effective in dealing with major depressive disorder. A couple of studies in elderly have found IPT to be effective when combined with other therapies such as peer support or psychoeducation.

Identified several key indicators of grief resolution:

- Capacity to remember both the positive and the negative qualities of the deceased
- Moving beyond the idealized memories of earlier stages
- Ability to offer support to others who are grieving
- Shifting focus from one's own loss
- Engagement in new relationships, rekindling old friendships, and pursuing new interests

Elderly Abuse

Elder abuse is a single or repeated act or lack of appropriate action, occurring within any relationship where there is an expectation of trust, which causes harm or distress to an older person. This type of violence amounts to a violation of human rights. Older adults are at risk of abuse, in its many forms, e.g.:

- Physical, verbal, psychological, financial, or sexual abuse
- Abandonment
- Neglect
- Serious losses of dignity and respect

Current evidence suggests that one in six older people experiences elder abuse. Elder abuse can have serious physical and mental health, financial, and social consequences, including, for instance, physical injuries, premature mortality, depression, cognitive decline, financial devastation, and placement in aged care facilities.

Life Satisfaction

Life satisfaction is a well-researched topic in studies of elderly populations and is often used as an indicator of successful aging, sometimes being equated with mental health. However, it is more accurately seen as a part of the broader concept of subjective well-being, which also includes measures of morale and mood. Defined life satisfaction as a comprehensive evaluation of life quality, based on comparing one's aspirations with their actual life conditions described it as a general measure of an individual's emotions and attitudes toward their life at a particular moment, ranging from negative to optimistic.

A recent review indicates that life satisfaction among older adults in Asia is influenced by various factors, including social functioning, health status, housing satisfaction, economic conditions, insurance coverage, quality and duration of sleep, social support, cognitive ability, marital status, preferred living arrangements, religiosity, education level, and daily life choices.

Changes in Cognitive Functions

Cognition plays a crucial role in maintaining functional independence as individuals age, affecting their ability to live alone, manage finances, follow medication regimens, and drive safely. Moreover, effective communication relies on intact cognitive functions, including processing sensory information and interacting appropriately with others. Cognitive abilities can be categorized into several domains, including attention, memory, executive function, language, and visuospatial skills. While cognitive abilities generally decline with age, distinguishing between typical age-related changes and those that might indicate the onset of a brain disease is essential for understanding and managing cognitive health, as shown in **Table 2**.

TABLE 2: Changes in cognitive functions with age.

Cognitive functions	Changes
Reaction time	• Progressively slows down from ages 30–70 years
Attention	• Decline in performance on complex tasks that require selective or divided attention • Simpler tasks, such as digit span, remain stable
Memory	• Historical, autobiographical, and procedural memory remain intact • Decline in the ability to learn new information and retrieval. Also, prospective memory declines
Executive functions	• Decreased performance on novel, complex, or timed tests • Decreased ability to inhibit certain responses, distinguish between relevant and irrelevant information, form concepts, abstract ideas, and exhibit mental flexibility
Speech and language	• Generally intact, including vocabulary, verbal reasoning, and comprehension • Older adults tend to be less verbose, more repetitive, and less precise in word choice during spontaneous speech compared to younger adults
Visuospatial functioning	• Visual recognition of objects, shapes, gestures, and conventional signs remains stable • Abilities related to visuoperceptual judgment and spatial orientation tend to decline
Intelligence	• Crystallized intelligence generally remains intact even up to the eighth decade of life • Progressive decline in fluid intelligence

Some of the nonpharmacological interventions used while dealing with cognitive impairments are given in the following text.

- *Cognitive rehabilitation*: It is a personalized approach, based on a problem-solving approach to help patients with dementia to improve their activities of daily living and enhance their functionality. The aim is not to remove the cognitive deficit but to help the patient to manage everyday challenges and the caregivers to develop effective strategies to support the patient. For example, keeping a to-do list, engaging the patient in day-to-day activities, and indulging in cue-controlled memory tasks.
- *Cognitive stimulation therapy (CST)*: It is a structured therapy of 14 group sessions that are held twice weekly. The themes include physical games, childhood memories, and current events to activities such as baking and word search. CST is one of the recommended therapies for dementia patients as per the National Institute for Health and Care Excellence (NICE) guidelines.
- *Reminiscence therapy*: It can be done in both individual and group settings. The aim is to improve long-term memory, build connectiveness, and improve the use of language. The therapist dwells into memories from childhood, adolescence, etc., using a multitude of objects such as photographs, toys, and leisure-time activities.

Other Mental Health Issues

Apart from dementia, one of the most common mental health issues faced by the elderly is depression. In the Longitudinal Aging Study in India-Diagnostic Assessment of Dementia (LASI-DAD) study, the self-reported prevalence of any psychiatric disorder in individuals over 60 years of age was found to be 0.4%, while that of depression in individuals was found to be 0.8%. Other common mental illnesses found in elderly are anxiety disorders, psychosis, and substance-use disorders, especially nicotine-dependence disorder.

A review of Indian studies in 2015 found that depression in Indian elderly ranged from 8.9 to 62.16% in the community, while clinic-based studies have reported the prevalence to be between 42 and 72%. In general, depression in elderly presents with anxiety or irritability, sleep and appetite disturbances, anhedonia, preoccupation with somatic symptoms, and significant cognitive complaints, especially forgetfulness and low energy levels. Some of the risk factors for developing depression include painful or disabling physical illness, loneliness, recent loss or other adverse life events, past or family history of depression, medications (e.g., steroids), and being a woman. Some of the commonly used assessment tools are Geriatric Depression Scale-15 and -30 items (validated in Hindi), Patient Health Questionnaire-9 and -15, and Hamilton Depression Rating Scale.

Anxiety disorders, in elderly, are significant causes of distress, disability, and mortality. In community samples, anxiety disorders range from 1.2 to 15%, with the most common being generalized anxiety disorder. The risk factors for developing anxiety disorders in elderly are female gender, recent stressful life events, chronic medical illnesses such as respiratory disorders, and the presence of mental illness such as depression. Childhood traumas such as poverty, parental loss, and mental illness in parents have also been found to be associated with the development of anxiety in later life. Presentation of anxiety in elderly may present differently compared to young adults. The anxiety may be more focused on health-related issues, may be more evident in terms of symptomatology, but not easily expressed in words and more often than not is associated with underlying depression.

Table 3 highlights various anxiety disorders found in elderly.

Quite a few scales have been developed to assess anxiety disorders:

- Abbreviated Penn State Worry Questionnaire
- Geriatric Anxiety Inventory-Short Form
- Adult Manifest Anxiety Scale-Elderly Version
- Geriatric Anxiety Scale
- State-Trait Anxiety Inventory
- Beck Anxiety Inventory
- State-Trait Inventory for Cognitive and Somatic Anxiety

Somatic symptom disorder is not a widely studied topic in the elderly, with prevalence ranging from 1.5 to 13%. It is understood as a tendency to experience and express somatic distress and then repeatedly seek medical help for the same. The scales used in young adults are also used in elderly but may overestimate the severity in older adults. Some of the scales include Patient Health Questionnaire-15, Somatization subscale of the Symptom Checklist 90-item version (SCL-90 SOM), Somatic Symptom Scale-8 items, and Somatization subscale of Brief Symptom Inventory.

The treatment of mental health issues may involve either pharmacotherapy, psychotherapy, or a combination of both. Prejudices such as ageism have always created therapeutic nihilism in clinicians dealing with the elderly. Freud believed that psychotherapy should not be attempted with elderly as they did not have the capacity to change. However, over the years, various reviews and systematic reviews have found psychotherapy to be as effective in medication. In a recent study of 100,000 elderly, it was found that they responded better to psychotherapy compared to working adults. However, the majority of the psychotherapy studies have taken place in Western societies, and evidence in low- and middle-income countries (LMICs) is very limited.

Various changes have been made in the psychotherapy modalities to match the needs of the elderly clients such as keeping the language simple, giving session summaries and homework in a written format, and including a caregiver and shorter therapy sessions unless the client needs to ventilate.

The following points elucidate the various evidence-based psychotherapies used with elderly population:

- *CBT*: It focuses on changing negative automatic thoughts, cognitive distortions, and dysfunctional behavior patterns, solve problems, and create realistic goals. It also involves use of relaxation techniques such as deep breathing or muscular relaxation. CBT has been found to be efficacious in major depressive disorder, fear of falling, and somatoform disorder. However, contradictory results are there with respect to anxiety.
- *Cognitive analytic therapy*: It combines cognitive therapy and object relation theory with an emphasis on "shared meaning" and "dialogue" as a source of catharsis.

TABLE 3: Commonly found anxiety disorders in elderly.

Disorders	Symptom summary
Generalized anxiety disorder	Diffuse and constant worry and negative ruminations
Obsessive–compulsive disorder	Intrusive thoughts, images, and impulses that may or may not be associated with repetitive behaviors and rituals
Panic disorder	Episodes of intense anxiety along with autonomic arousal (palpitations, shortness of breath, flushing, fear of dying, or losing control)
Agoraphobia	Fear of being trapped in a place from where escape appears difficult, leading to avoidance of such places
Social phobia	Intense anxiety in social situations
Specific phobia	Intense fear of specific objects, situations, or animals (e.g., claustrophobia, cynophobia, and hydrophobia)
Posttraumatic stress disorder	Reexperiencing of a traumatic event, such as the death of a loved one, accompanied by autonomic arousal, nightmares, and avoidance of everything associated with the trauma
Health anxiety	Fear of developing a chronic and debilitating illness or disability
Death anxiety	Fear of death of self or loved ones

- *Problem-solving therapy*: It is based on the premise that daily life's problems can precipitate and maintain depressive symptoms. The therapy involves both skill training (in solving problems) and cognitive restructuring. In some community settings, problem-solving therapy has been found to be an effective treatment as well as a prevention strategy for depression.
- *Behavior therapy*: It focuses on changing maladaptive behavior (e.g., lying on the bed whole day) and reinforcing adaptive behaviors such as following a daily routine or meeting with friends. It has been found effective in the treatment of depression and insomnia, even in elderly with dementia.

SUCCESSFUL AGING

For over 20 years, the notion of "successful aging" has been pivotal in both academic research and public discussions about aging. The nomenclature also includes terms such as, "healthy aging," "active aging," "productive aging," and "aging well."

The classic definition of successful aging involves high physical, psychological, and social functioning in elderly without any major disease.

A meta-analysis elucidated four main domains of healthy aging as: (1) avoiding disease and disability; (2) being actively engaged; (3) having high mental, physical, and cognitive functions; and (4) being psychologically well adapted. In definition of successful aging included six dimensions: (1) Autonomy, (2) control over one's environment, (3) self-acceptance, (4) purpose in life, (5) personal growth, and (6) positive relationship with others.

However, contemporary studies have also pointed out that individuals can age successfully even if they are suffering from a chronic disease and that successful aging is not an endpoint but a process as highlighted by the lifespan model of Selective Optimization with Compensation (SOC) model. As shown in **Flowchart 1**, successful aging is a multidimensional concept with interrelated aspects.

STRATEGIES FOR PROMOTING PSYCHOLOGICAL WELL-BEING IN AGING

Aging is not preventable; however, one can adopt certain strategies to increase the likelihood of enhanced physical and mental well-being, including:

- *Enhancing cognitive functions*: Engaging in intellectually stimulating activities such as puzzles, reading, and learning new skills
- *Adopting a healthy lifestyle*: Eating a well-balanced diet, engaging in regular physical exercise, and maintaining healthy sleep schedules
- *Mindfulness and relaxation*: Practicing yoga, mindfulness meditation, and other relaxation exercises such as *Pranayam* and deep breathing
- *Fostering social connection*: Participating in community activities, volunteer work, social groups, maintaining strong family connections, etc.
- *Addressing health concerns*: Going for regular health checkups and managing chronic conditions effectively

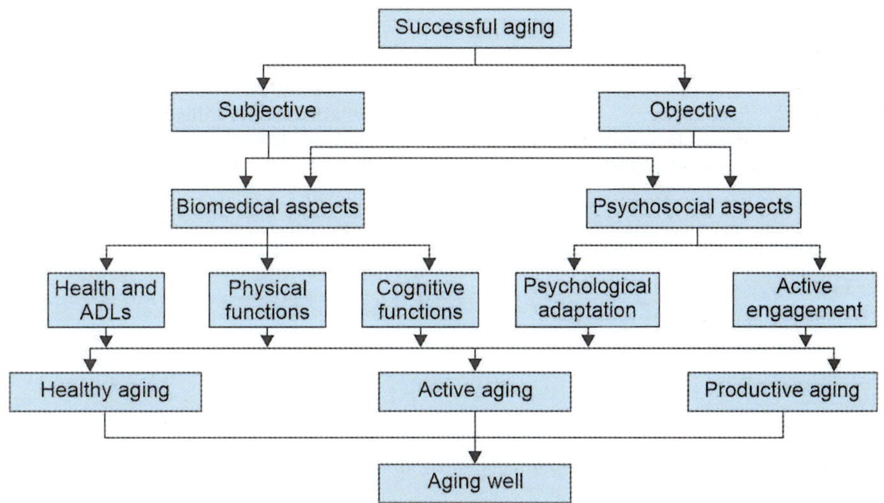

FLOWCHART 1: Dimensions of successful aging.
(ADLs: activities of daily living)
Source: Modified from Fernandez-Ballesteroz (2019) and Urtamo et al. (2019).

CONCLUSION

The psychological aspects of aging encompass a wide range of experiences, including cognitive changes, emotional adjustments, and social dynamics. Understanding these aspects and implementing strategies to support mental health can help older adults navigate the challenges of aging while maintaining a fulfilling and enriched life. By addressing the cognitive, emotional, and social needs of older adults, we can promote their well-being and enhance their quality of life in the later stages of life.

Self-Assessment Questionnaire

Q1. How does biological aging affect the body's metabolism and regenerative abilities?

Q2. What are the five common approaches to adapting to old age identified by Bromley, and how do they impact an older individual's quality of life?

Q3. How does marital status affect health outcomes in older adults, and what are some factors that influence these outcomes?

Q4. How does aging affect attention, and which types of attentional tasks are most impacted?

Q5. What are some common signs of anxiety disorders in elderly individuals, and how do these symptoms differ from anxiety in younger adults?

Q6. How has psychotherapy for elderly individuals been adapted to meet their specific needs, and which therapies have been found effective?

Q7. How has the concept of "successful aging" evolved over time, and what are the key components of this multidimensional approach?

Q8. What are some strategies that can enhance physical and mental well-being during aging?

Q9. What are the different types of grief that elderly individuals may experience, and how is complicated or prolonged grief identified?

Q10. What are some of the common mental health issues faced by the elderly, and which validated tools are available in India to assess these issues?

FURTHER READINGS

1. Bratt AS, Stenström U, Rennemark M. Effects on life satisfaction of older adults after child and spouse bereavement. Aging Ment Health. 2017;21(6):602-8.
2. Bülow MH, Söderqvist T. Successful ageing: a historical overview and critical analysis of a successful concept. J Aging Stud. 2014;31:139-49.
3. Dziechciaż M, Filip R. Biological psychological and social determinants of old age: bio-psycho-social aspects of human aging. Ann Agric Environ Med. 2014;21(4):835-8.
4. Harada CN, Love MCN, Triebel KL. Normal cognitive aging. Clin Geriatr Med. 2013;29(4):737-52.
5. Khodabakhsh S. Factors affecting life satisfaction of older adults in Asia: a systematic review. J Happiness Stud. 2022;23(3):1289-304.
6. Lee J, Meijer E, Langa KM, Ganguli M, Varghese M, Banerjee J, et al. Prevalence of dementia in India: national and state estimates from a nationwide study. Alzheimers Dement. 2023;19(7):2898-912.
7. McNicoll L. Issues of sexuality in the elderly. Med Health R I. 2008;91(10):321-2.
8. Morgan K. Psychological aspects of ageing. Psychiatry. 2007;6(12):484-7.
9. Roberts R. Knopman DS. Classification and epidemiology of MCI. Clin Geriatr Med. 2013;29(4):753-72.
10. Wilkinson RT, Allison S. Age and simple reaction time: decade differences for 5,325 subjects. J Gerontol. 1989;44(2):P29-35.

CHAPTER 6

Multimorbidity

Surekha Viggeswarpu, Madhulatha Alexander

CASE VIGNETTE

Patient information: A 65-year-old Ms Rukmini presented to the outpatient department for a regular checkup.

Presenting complaint: She is a known diabetic for the past 6 years and was recently diagnosed to have hypertension and osteoarthritis. Her daughter-in-law complained that she had become slower than usual and had some issues recalling recent events. Ms Rukmini had also become withdrawn of late and preferred to lie in her room, looking up at the ceiling. She had to be coaxed to eat and had lost her enthusiasm to do the things she was interested in, such as cooking and knitting. The daughter-in-law felt that she had lost some weight, and she occasionally had problems with constipation. She also noticed some urgency of urine, with occasional urinary incontinence, as she could not reach the restroom on time. There were no other lower urinary tract symptoms.

INTRODUCTION

After completing her final MBBS examination, she entered her internship expecting to see the "examination cases" buzzing around the outpatient department. To her astonishment, most of the cases she saw were for control of diabetes and its various complications, hypertension, osteoarthritis, and patients with numerous somatic complaints. The examination cases had vanished, and in their place were others with many medical problems that had to be tackled in parallel. There was no single diagnosis but a huge list!

This is multimorbidity in all its splendor—patients presenting with no specific chief complaint but a host of complaints that have affected their ability to perform their activities of daily living.

Aims

- To recognize and list all the problems a patient is burdened with
- To address each problem separately and in the totality of the patient as an individual
- To ensure that the management of the patient with multimorbidity is patient centered, focusing on the quality of life and promoting self-management toward agreed goals

MULTIMORBIDITY

Multimorbidity is the presence of multiple diseases and medical conditions—chronic or acute—in one person at one time.

These multiple diseases and conditions must be treated concurrently without a hierarchical order.

Certain conditions heighten the risk of developing other conditions; people with multimorbidity are likely to accumulate more diagnoses and experience escalating clinical complexity, increasing readmission rates and healthcare costs.

Multimorbidity is associated with poor treatment outcomes and longer hospital stays.

Interventions which focused on specific behavioral risk factors, medication management, or functional ability were more likely to improve health outcomes. This requires interprofessional collaboration. Sustainability was enhanced by integrating interventions into existing healthcare systems.

Conversely, comorbidity indicates a condition or conditions that coexist in the context of an index disease. Comorbidity, the conceptual predecessor of multimorbidity, was initially defined by Feinstein as "any distinct additional clinical entity that has existed or may occur during the course of a patient who has the index disease under study."

EPIDEMIOLOGY OF MULTIMORBIDITY

Around the world, advances in public health and changes in clinical interventions causing significant demographic shifts have resulted in increased life expectancy and greater longevity, escalating the burden of multimorbidity on individuals and the healthcare system. Therefore, there needs to be a radical shift from disease-specific care to a more holistic view of health, especially in the geriatric population. Geriatric patients carry a lot of baggage—both genetic and lifestyle—in the process of aging.

Multimorbidity has emerged as a significant public health issue worldwide as it increases the complexity of managing disease in patients. Considerable research has indicated a link between multimorbidity and health-service utilization, including hospitalization and total healthcare costs. Multimorbidity is associated with disability, poor functional status, poor quality of life, and adverse drug reactions due to multiple drugs prescribed for various ailments present in the individual. There is a higher mortality in patients with multimorbidity.

Bergman et al. described the central feature of frailty, which is commonly seen in the old, as "increased vulnerability to stressors due to impairments in multiple, interrelated systems that lead to a decline in homeostatic reserve and resiliency." The complex relationship between frailty and chronic disease is poorly understood, though some scales measuring frailty consider the "accumulation of multiple deficits" in their scoring matrix.

Risk factors for multimorbidity are as follows:

- Adults aged 65 years or older. However, younger persons also represent a large proportion of those with multimorbidity.
- Minimal physical activity, obesity, smoking, and alcohol abuse
- Childhood financial hardship
- Lower socioeconomic status—data is scarce.
- Lower educational level—primary school and below
- Widowhood
- Lifetime earnings were associated with multimorbidity. They exert a modest protective effect.

Bronfenbrenner, in 1977, proposed that health outcomes are affected by a range of variables, including the individual, behavioral, interpersonal, community, and policy environment. These are diagrammatically represented in the health ecology model of multimorbidity, as shown in **Figure 1**.

Leading chronic conditions causing death:

- Tobacco use
- Unhealthy dietary patterns
- Physical inactivity
- Alcohol consumption

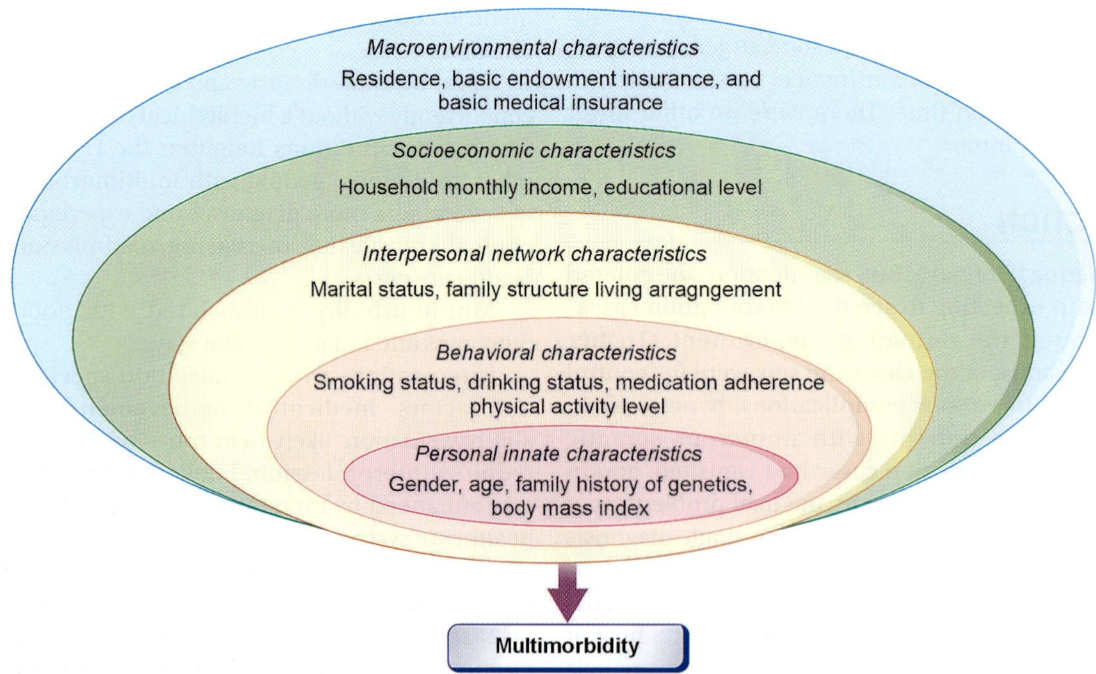

FIG. 1: Health ecology model of multimorbidity.

PREVALENCE AND GLOBAL PERSPECTIVE

The prevalence of multimorbidity among adults ranged from 4.0 to 92.8% in various studies. The results from 126 pooled studies estimated the prevalence of multimorbidity at 37.2% [95% confidence interval (CI) 34.9–39.4%, I^2 99.7%]. The pooled proportion of multimorbidity was the highest in South America with 45.7% (95% CI 39.0–52.5%, I^2 99.0%) and lowest in Africa with 28.2% (95% CI 15.6–40.8%, I^2 99.0%). In Asia, Europe, North America, and Oceania, the pooled prevalence of multimorbidity was estimated to be 35% (95% CI 31.4–38.5%, I^2 99.3%), 39.2% (95% CI 33.2–45.2%), and 43.1% (95% CI 32.3–53.8%), respectively.

In a large population-based administrative claims data study, 67% of the beneficiaries had multimorbidity, which increased in prevalence from 50% for those under the age of 65 years to 81.5% for those aged 85 years and above. Prevalence varied in various studies due to methodological biases. Hence, no two studies were comparable. Standardized methods for measuring multimorbidity are needed for more effective public health surveillance and prevention, especially in the geriatric population in the developing world.

MULTIMORBIDITY IN THE OLDER PERSON IN INDIA

According to the findings of the Longitudinal Aging Study in India (LASI) I study, the prevalence of single morbidity was 30.3% and that of multimorbidity was 32.1% among older people in India. Risk factors for the development of multimorbidity in India included being female, living in urban areas or alone, and being older. Hypertension, arthritis, and thyroid disorders were prevalent among females, and chronic lung diseases and stroke were prevalent among males.

The highest prevalence of multimorbidity was in Kerala—59.2%. It was highest as the population aged and in the western and southern parts of the state. Those who were living with a spouse were more likely to have multimorbidity. Disease-specific multimorbidity was high in chronic heart disease and low in angina. No specific reasons could be attributed to these findings.

Challenges in patients with multimorbidity include the following:

- *Fragmentation of healthcare*—due to patients visiting various "organ-specific specialists" for their various ailments. Overlapping treatments prescribed by these specialists can cause clinically relevant challenges. This leads to conflicts between the specialists, as they lack support and collaboration. On top of it all, different guidelines may offer conflicting recommendations.

  There is insufficient data regarding best practices in geriatric patients with multimorbidity due to inadequate published treatment guidelines and evidence-based medicine. Most treatments and practice guidelines target a single index condition, but patients with multimorbidity are complex and heterogeneous, especially in the geriatric age group.

  The traditional disease-focused approach to clinical medicine may render care, i.e., fragmented and poorly coordinated, and produce treatment plans that are inefficient, ineffective, or even harmful for patients with multimorbidity. Clinicians have limited guidance or evidence on which to base care decisions for such patients.

  It is important to remember that as age increases, heterogeneity between individuals continues to diverge.
- *Conflicts* also arise between treating physicians and patients, as patient priorities are not considered. There are numerous challenges in delivering patient-centered care, which believe in incorporating shared decision-making.
- The *cost of treatment* should also be considered. The mainstay of the treatment of most of these chronic diseases starts with lifestyle modification, which may not be palatable to some people. Also, individuals may change their minds regarding the treatment options.
- Data on the structural intervention directed at social determinants of chronic disease, including health systems, is scarce **(Fig. 2)**

CLINICAL PRESENTATION AND EVALUATION OF MULTIMORBIDITY IN OUTPATIENT SETTINGS

Clinical presentation: These patients often walk into the outpatient department for a medical checkup. A detailed listing of all the patient's problems—active, inactive, and those that have surfaced after eliciting a thorough history—is imperative. The "brown bag check" should be complete and well documented. Social, financial, and psychological aspects should be delved into.

A detailed physical examination should ensue, including a postural blood pressure estimation. This constitutes a comprehensive geriatric assessment. A problem list will then emerge.

Before proceeding, kindly list the patient's problem from the case vignette.

Specific Investigations in the Evaluation of Multimorbidity

Ordered investigations should be relevant, and their costs should be considered, as most of these patients belong to

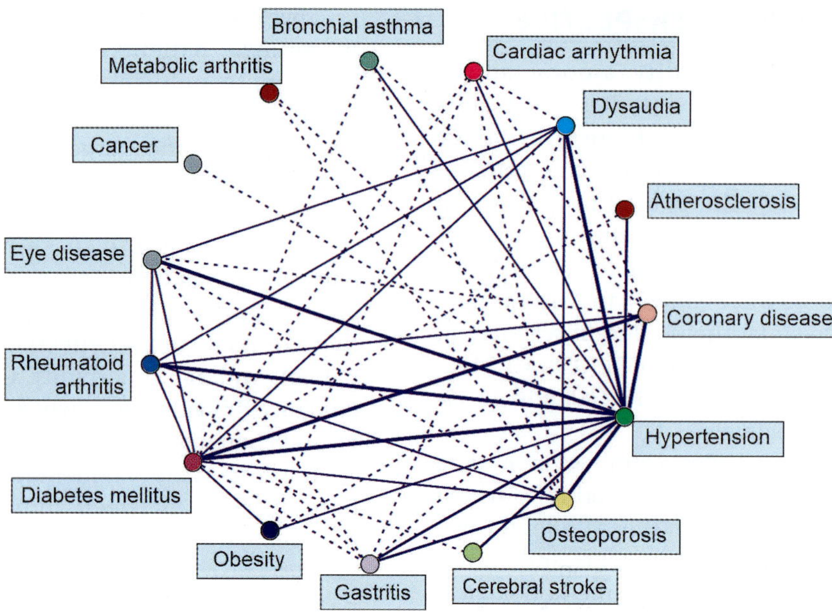

FIG. 2: Web graph of association between chronic diseases.

the unorganized sector in our country. This group lacks insurance or pension and has poor financial reserves.

- *Laboratory tests*: A complete blood count and other investigations are essential to assess the extent of each morbidity and its complications/target organ damage.
- *Imaging studies*: A chest X-ray is a must to assess cardiac size and to rule out tuberculosis and other chronic lung conditions.

  Other imaging modalities should be done on a case-by-case basis—such as ultrasound, MRI/CT of the brain, high-resolution computed tomography (HRCT) of the thorax, and positron emission tomography (PET) scans—depending upon the presentation, findings, and clinical judgment.
- *Invasive studies*: Biopsies from affected sites, bone marrow, cerebrospinal fluid (CSF) studies, scopies, etc., should be ordered at the discretion of the treating physician as per the patient's wishes.
- *Cardiac and neurological tests*:
  - A 12-lead ECG can pick up chamber hypertrophy and silent ischemia.
  - An ECHO may also have to be done.
  - A Holter, EEG, and EMG may be ordered depending on the clinician's comprehensive examination and judgment.

Systematic Evaluation and Development of a Care Plan

Depending on the problems, one may have to call in the services of a specialist or enlist the intervention by the multidisciplinary team, which involves nurses, physio and occupational therapists, dieticians, swallow therapists, social workers, etc. These are called upon on a need basis.

A physiotherapist's clinical assessment and training of the family members in addressing the patient's mobility and balance issues can go a long way in preventing falls. Vision and hearing impairment, ruling out peripheral neuropathy, and prescription of appropriate footwear are vital. The rationalization of medication, resistance training exercises, and vitamin D replacement may prevent further falls. An occupational therapist visits the home—virtually or physically—and suggests specific and low-cost modifications to aid in fall prevention. A dietitian can suggest a nutritious diet that does not pinch the pocket, is easy to prepare, and is palatable. A swallow therapist can reiterate safe swallow techniques, especially in patients with Parkinson's disease or following a stroke.

Based upon all their assessments, existing published guidelines, and availability of services in the community/family, an individualized plan of action in consultation with the patient and their carers is drawn up and executed. Along with your rational medical prescription, the treatment modalities offered by the multidisciplinary team should be added to the final treatment plan.

Regular follow-ups are encouraged, and progress is communicated to the patient and carer, thus upholding the tenet of shared responsibility in caring for the patient.

Now, add a list of investigations and interventions to your problem list.

Also, make a note of the specialists you would like to consult and which members of the multidisciplinary team you would call upon to make an impact on Ms Rukmini's quality of life.

MANAGEMENT OF MULTIMORBIDITY

Patients with multimorbidity typically experience a fluctuating health status, with particular ailments rotating into and out of the forefront and influencing the patient's overall well-being.

Control of symptoms and a conscious effort to reduce flares and complications to keep the symptoms of chronic illnesses at bay should be the mantra. However, the heterogeneous nature of multimorbidity makes it challenging to control the array of coexisting conditions that may have impacted therapeutic strategies.

"Therapeutic competition" (a medication prescribed for one condition is harmful or exacerbating for another condition) and the concept of "time horizon to benefit" (how long it will take until the benefits of interventions are achieved) should be considered before the introduction of other drugs/treatment modalities.

Clinicians should be advised to look at the patient holistically despite competing health objectives. Thus, the cry of the knee with osteoarthritis should not be lost in the control of diabetes. The treatment strategies should incorporate the patient's physical, psychological, spiritual, and financial needs. The key to prioritizing among recommendations from multiple guidelines is understanding what matters most to the patient and what outcomes are most important or bothersome to the patient.

Overall approach from expert group guidelines: The American Geriatrics Society (AGS) has developed an algorithm for the management of multimorbidity **(Flowchart 1)**.

The five principles to address multimorbidity, as advocated by the American Geriatric Society, are as follows:

1. Elicit and incorporate patient preferences into medical decision-making.
2. Recognize the limitations of the evidence base in interpreting and applying the medical literature to persons with multimorbidity.
3. Frame clinical management decisions within the context of risks, burdens, benefits, and prognosis.
4. Consider treatment complexity and feasibility when making clinical management decisions.
5. Choose therapies that optimize benefit, minimize harm, and enhance the quality of life.

Guidelines for the management of multimorbidity, as laid out by the National Institute for Health and Care Excellence (NICE) in the United Kingdom, also run along similar lines:

- Tailor care to meet personal goals and priorities.
- Identify people who may benefit from care.

Approach to the evaluation and management of the older adult with multimorbidity

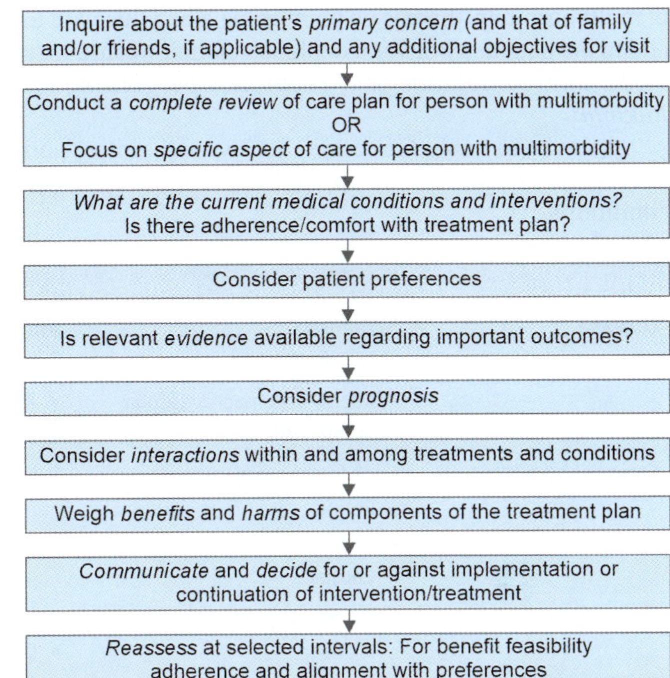

FLOWCHART 1: Evaluation of an older person with multimorbidity.

Note: Recognize that each person's health trajectory and priorities differ. Further interventions are based on the context of their overall health status, life expectancy, degree of functional impairment, and chronic disease burden.

Source: Uptodate.com.

- Identify the impact of disease and treatment burden on quality of life.
- *Review medications*: Consider nonpharmacologic approaches and stop all unnecessary medications.

Patients with multimorbidity experience frequent clinical encounters with multiple providers across many healthcare settings. Medical errors tend to occur at points where care is being transferred. Multidisciplinary forums, such as stroke teams and tumor boards, should be set up, wherein the voices of each person involved in the care of the individual, including the individuals themselves and their carers, are heard. Some carers give compelling insights into the lives of the patients they care for. Do not suppress their voice.

Polypharmacy: This is the result of addressing coexisting chronic conditions, resulting in a host of problems associated with drug dosage, drug–drug, and drug–food interactions.

"Start low, go slow" and "think before you ink" are strategies we must always use before prescribing any drug. Review the "brown bag" at every visit. It is well worth the time. Consolidate drug dosing schedules to minimize complexity and error.

Cancer screening: This is one of the main preventive strategies employed. Still, if life expectancy is poor in the face of multimorbidity, there is no point going along this path to add to the patient's woes and depletion of their wealth.

Finally, consolidate your problem list regarding Ms Rukmini.

As shown in **Table 1**, a comprehensive assessment and management plan can be applied to common geriatric conditions.

WHAT IS MULTIMORBIDITY?

Multimorbidity is the coexistence of two or more chronic medical conditions at the same time in one individual, which may or may not interact with one another.

The National Quality Forum defines multiple chronic conditions as "two or more chronic conditions that collectively have an adverse effect on health status, function, or quality of life and that require

TABLE 1: Comprehensive assessment and management plan for common geriatric conditions.

Disease	Screening	Management	Other inputs
Type 2 diabetes mellitus	• HbA1c • Micro- and macrovascular complications	• Lifestyle modification • Rationalize medication • Regular follow-up advised	Retinal evaluation to rule out retinopathy
Essential hypertension	Look for end-organ damage: • Retina • Renal • Cardiac	Rationalize medication	Look for other potential cardiovascular risk factors
Dyslipidemia	Chest and thyroid status	• Lifestyle changes • Drugs are to be added according to the ASCVD score	OT and PT input
Bilateral knee joint osteoarthritis		• Pain relief • PT input • Toilet modification—western toilet	PT input
Slow gait	Detailed neurological examination to exclude an extrapyramidal syndrome, peripheral neuropathy	• PT and OT input for gait and balance training and fall prevention	• Regular assessment of gait and balance at all visits • Would the patient benefit from a walking aid for offloading or improving balance? • Check vision and hearing • Supplement vitamin D is low
Functional urinary incontinence		Pain relief	Routine gynecological check
Pedal edema	Rule out: • Offending drugs • Liver/cardiac/renal cases for the same	Discontinue amlodipine, change to telmisartan	If not improving, look for other causes
Depression	Geriatric Depression Scale	• Involvement in social activities both at home and in the community • Look for suicidal risk • A trial of depressants may be needed	A psychiatrist may be consulted if symptoms persist
Mild cognitive impairment	• TSH and vitamin B12 estimation and replacement, if needed • Can review the patient at a later date and recheck memory	To be reassessed after a fair trial of involvement in social activities, and a trial of antidepressants may be given	• Address all vascular risk factors • Ask for a family history of dementia • Simple measures aid recall, making diary entries, calendar entries, etc.

(ASCVD: atherosclerotic cardiovascular disease; OT: occupational therapist; PT: physiotherapist; TSH: thyroid-stimulating hormone)

complex healthcare management, decision-making, or coordination."

There are so many ramifications and interactions between the illnesses and their treatments, and one should maintain a delicate balance between these to see that the patient is as good as they can get.

An individual suffers from multimorbidity due to multiple reasons ranging from comorbidities that may arise due to a common risk factor or due to the outcome of a particular disease leading to another disease, e.g., a particularly common chronic health problem, such as cardiovascular disease (CVD) or diabetes, may share various related risk factors. Treating the risk factor may alleviate the disease.

These complex patients are underrepresented in clinical research populations given their age and multimorbidity, which may mask or ruin the effect of the drug under investigation. Hence, no specific guidelines are present as to how to treat these older individuals with the latest drugs/interventions. It depends on the astute clinician to decide how they would individualize treatment for the patient, as they would have to look into drug–drug interaction, pharmacokinetics and pharmacodynamics, cost, and the patient's overall medical status.

IMPACT OF MULTIMORBIDITY

- Frailty
- Functional limitations and disability
- Diminished quality of life
- Financial burden
- Polypharmacy:
    - Adverse drug reactions
    - Treatment complications
- High health utilization:
    - Emergency department visits
    - Hospitalizations
    - Readmission
- Nursing home placement
- Death

PREVENTION OF MULTIMORBIDITY

Chronic disease prevention activities likely to have the most significant population impact include:

- Tobacco control
- Salt reduction
- Use of multidrug regimens for secondary prevention of CVDs.
  Healthy living is the cornerstone.

ROLE OF A GERIATRICIAN IN MULTIMORBIDITY

Identify and address issues that impact multiple conditions:

- *Nutrition*: Calorie intake and dietary restrictions due to multimorbidity should be addressed. Some concessions should be given to older individuals, and the regimen need not be too rigid.
- *Physical activity/exercise* should be incorporated into the treatment regimen.
- *Functional independence* in all activities of daily living (at least) should be encouraged.

Address:

- Sleep disturbances
- Mental health
- Safety of environment
- Adequacy of support at the current level of care
- Caregiver stress

Medically:

- Rationalize drug prescription—ensure that cost incurred does not cause a heavy financial burden
- Advise regular follow-up. The drugs the patient is on should be brought to the outpatient department whenever the patient sees the geriatrician.
- Spend time with the patient—do not be in a hurry to send them off.
- Patient and carer re-education is essential at every visit. Know Your Patient

Take Home Messages

- Encourage a healthy lifestyle.
- Make a proper problem list for each patient, which includes medical and social problems, to make a difference in their lives.
- There is a need for better interventions for older adults to avert a health crisis in later years of life.
- Proper policy measures and strengthening of the health system to ensure healthy aging in India are imperative to developing more sustainable and integrated models of care.
- Emphasis should be given to workforce training and quality improvement strategies to ensure better physical and functional health in older adults.
- Financial incentives may improve healthcare accessibility in cash-strapped households, especially in the unorganized sector

CONCLUSION

Multimorbidity pose an extraordinary challenge to modern geriatric practice.

It further stress the need holistic, personalized care in place of usual disease centric care

It also underscores the balanced approach by geriatrician between evidence-based medicine with individualized priorities, functional goals with rationalizing medications essential with minimum medication.

Strengthening health systems, workforce training, and policy measures is essential to ensure coordinated, and holistic care for older adults living with multimorbidity.

Self-Assessment Questionnaire

Q1. What is the difference between comorbidity and multimorbidity in older adults?

Q2. Based on the case vignette of Ms Rukmini, list at least five active medical and psychosocial problems she was facing.

Q3. Why is a comprehensive geriatric assessment (CGA) essential for patients with multimorbidity?

Q4. Describe at least three major risk factors contributing to multimorbidity in the Indian elderly population.

Q5. How does fragmentation of healthcare impact outcomes in patients with multimorbidity?

Q6. What are the key components of a patient-centered approach advocated by the American Geriatrics Society for multimorbidity management?

Q7. Discuss the role of the multidisciplinary team (MDT) in improving quality of life in multimorbid older adults.

Q8. Outline practical strategies to prevent or delay the onset of multimorbidity at the community and individual level.

Q9. How can a geriatrician balance medical, psychosocial, and financial priorities while managing complex multimorbid cases?

FURTHER READINGS

1. van den Akker M, Buntinx F, Knottnerus JA. Comorbidity or multimorbidity: what's in a name? A review of literature. Eur J Gen Pract. 1996;2(2):65-70.
2. van den Akker M, Buntinx F, Roos S, Knottnerus JA. Problems in determining occurrence rates of multimorbidity. J Clin Epidemiol. 2001;54(7):675-9.
3. Smith SM, Wallace E, O'Dowd T, Fortin M. Interventions for improving outcomes in patients with multimorbidity in primary care and community settings. Cochrane Database Syst Rev. 2016;2016(3):CD006560.
4. Feinstein AR. The pre-therapeutic classification of co-morbidity in chronic disease. J Chronic Dis. 1970;23(7):455-68.
5. Bergman H, Ferrucci L, Guralnik J, Hogan DB, Hummel S, Karunananthan S, et al. Frailty: an emerging research and clinical paradigm—issues and controversies. J Gerontol A Biol Sci Med Sci. 2007;62(7):731-7.
6. Pathirana TI, Jackson CA. Socioeconomic status and multimorbidity: a systematic review and meta-analysis. J Public Health. 2018;42:186-94.
7. Wolff JL, Starfield B, Anderson G. Prevalence, expenditures, and complications of multiple chronic conditions in the elderly. Arch Intern Med. 2002;162:2269-76.
8. Bronfenbrenner U. Toward an experimental ecology of human development. Am Psychol. 1977;32(7):513-31.
9. Chen Y, Shi L, Zheng X, Yang J, Xue Y, Xiao S, et al. Patterns and determinants of multimorbidity in older adults: study in health-ecological perspective. Int J Environ Res Public Health. 2022;19(24):16756.
10. Mokdad AH, Marks JS, Stroup DF, Gerberding JL. Actual causes of death in the United States, 2000. JAMA. 2004;291(10):1238-45.
11. Chowdhury SR, Das DC, Sunna TC, Beyene J, Hossain A. Global and regional prevalence of multimorbidity in the adult population in community settings: a systematic review and meta-analysis. eClinicalMedicine. 2023;57:101860.
12. Kudesia P, Salimarouny B, Stanley M, Fortin M, Stewart M, Terry A, et al. The incidence of multimorbidity and patterns in accumulation of chronic conditions: a systematic review. J Multimorb Comorb. 2021;11:26335565211032880.
13. Patel P, Muhammad T, Sahoo H. The burden of disease-specific multimorbidity among older adults in India and its states: evidence from LASI. BMC Geriatr. 2023;23(1):53.
14. Sinnott C, Hugh SM, Browne J, Bradley C. GPs' perspectives on the management of patients with multimorbidity: systematic review and synthesis of qualitative research. BMJ Open. 2013;3(9):e003610.
15. Fried TR, Tinetti ME, Iannone L. Primary care clinicians' experiences with treatment decision-making for older persons with multiple conditions. Arch Intern Med. 2011;171(1):75-80.
16. Gaziano TA, Galea G, Reddy KS. Scaling up interventions for chronic disease prevention: the evidence. The Lancet. 2007;370: 1939-46.
17. Uijen AA, van de Lisdonk EH. Multimorbidity in primary care: prevalence and trend over the last 20 years. Eur J Gen Pract. 2008;14(Suppl 1):28-32.
18. Khan MR, Malik MA, Akhtar SN, Yadav S, Patel R. Multimorbidity and its associated risk factors among older adults in India. BMC Public Health. 2022;22(1):746.
19. World Health Organization. (2024). Ageing and health. [online] Available from https://www.who.int/news-room/fact-sheets/detail/ageing-and-health. [Last accessed May, 2025].

CHAPTER 7

Longevity and Anti-aging

Prasun Chatterjee

CASE VIGNETTES

Case Vignette 1: Mr Ramesh Babu—A Life of Genetic Blessings

Profile

Mr Ramesh Babu, a 92-year-old man, is a noted businessman managing a successful multinational company. He is a social drinker and smoker who enjoys a carefree life, pursuing ambitious goals even in his advanced age. Despite his indulgent lifestyle, he exhibits remarkable longevity and vitality, often surprising his peers and healthcare professionals.

Family History

Mr Babu hails from a lineage of centenarians. His parents lived well past 100 years, enjoying robust health with minimal medical interventions. His father, a former industrialist, passed away at 104 years, while his mother, a homemaker with an active social life, lived to 92 years. This extraordinary genetic legacy has granted Mr Babu a resilience that defies the conventional consequences of his habits.

Lifestyle and Observations

Mr Babu has never adhered to a structured routine or strict health guidelines. His life reflects a mix of indulgence and optimism, thriving on his genetic "blessed gene," as he often refers to it. Despite his lack of regular exercise and his consistent consumption of tobacco, he has avoided significant health issues, a testament to the robust genetic foundation inherited from his parents.

Case Vignette 2: Mr SS Rudra—Discipline as the Key to Longevity

Profile

Mr SS Rudra, a 95-year-old man, is a living example of the benefits of discipline and perseverance. A lifelong disciplinarian, he has maintained a strict daily routine, including lifelong vegetarianism, small eating, and religiously exercising for over 40 years. His resilience has helped him navigate the ups and downs of life, and he continues to adapt and thrive despite the challenges of aging.

Family History

Unlike Mr Babu, Mr Rudra's family history does not feature notable longevity. His parents lived into their late 60s, with both succumbing to lifestyle-related conditions. This lack of genetic advantage makes his long life particularly remarkable, mainly attributed to his unwavering commitment to a healthy lifestyle.

Lifestyle and Observations

Mr Rudra's day begins with meditation and exercise, followed by a balanced diet rich in whole foods. He abstains from alcohol and smoking, practices mindfulness, and is known for his ability to remain calm in stressful situations. These habits have not only preserved his physical health but may also have induced favorable epigenetic modifications, altering gene expression to promote longevity and vitality.

These two contrasting case vignettes illustrate the interplay of nature and nurture in shaping health outcomes and longevity.

Both cases provide valuable insights into the dynamics of aging, demonstrating that while genetics may set the stage, lifestyle choices often determine the quality of the performance.

INTRODUCTION

Aging

With increasing global life expectancy, the aging population is growing rapidly. Understanding longevity and antiaging is critical for addressing age-related diseases, reduced productivity, and healthcare costs. Moreover, advancements in antiaging science provide hope for a future where aging may be more manageable and less debilitating.

The quest to know more about why people die started in 1900 with fungi *Candida albicans,* followed by further study in worms *Caenorhabditis elegans*, mice, and primates such as monkeys and human.

It took scientists more than a century to unravel the various pathways related to aging.

The first step in longevity science is to thoroughly understand aging pathways and hallmarks. This field aims to prognosticate aging patterns and potential antiaging interventions.

Let us understand a few terminologies related to longevity science.

Longevity

Longevity refers to the length of an individual's life, mainly focusing on extending the healthy years of life, often referred to as the "health span." It encompasses living longer and maintaining physical, mental, and emotional well-being throughout those extended years.

Lifespan is the total number of years we live, whereas health span is how many years we remain healthy and disease free.

Biological Age

Biological aging, also known as physiological or functional age, is the gradual decline of an organism's functional characteristics as it ages. It is different from chronological age because it considers other factors besides the day you were born.

The biological age is very different from the calendar or chronological age. Calendar aging is only a time-bound experience that vaguely describes the physiological well-being of an individual.

Calendar age poorly reflects internal biological processes and intraindividual variation of individuals; therefore, it is not an appropriate indicator of an individual's functional abilities.

Accelerated aging is when a person's biological age is more than their chronological age.

At the individual level, different cells, tissues, and organs exhibit different aging trajectories, so they have different biological ages.

The measurement of biological age is a complex phenomenon. Among various aging clocks (proteomic clock, transcriptomic clock, metabolomic clock, immune clock, and epigenetic clock) which tried to explain biological aging, epigenetic clock is considered as one of the best ways to measure biological age. Epigenetic changes are age-related changes in the methylation of CpG sites, thereby changing the activity of DNA and not its sequence.

The first-generation epigenetic clocks (Horvath clock, Hannum clock) show that epigenetic age can be estimated from DNA across multiple cell types, blood samples, tissues, and species. These clocks used machine-learning algorithms to estimate epigenetic age which could be compared with chronological age.

The second generation of clocks (PhenoAge, GrimAge) was trained on mortality and health indicators, i.e., to predict length of life and health rather than age.

The third generation of the epigenetic clock (DunedinPoAm38, Dunedin PACE—**Box 1**) measured

BOX 1 Dunedin PACE study.

Signs of aging:	*Health indicators*:
• Balance	• HbA1c
• Physical limitations	• Cardiorespiratory fitness
• Gait speed	• Waist–hip ratio
• Perceptual reasoning	• FEV_1/FVC
• Steps in place	• FEV_1
• Working memory	• Mean arterial pressure
• Chair stands	• BMI
• Processing speed	• Leukocyte telomere length
• Grip strength	• Creatinine clearance
• Self-rated health	• Urea nitrogen
• Motor coordination	• Lipoprotein
• Facial aging	• Triglyceride
	• Gum health
	• Total cholesterol
	• WBC
	• hsCRP
	• HDL cholesterol
	• ApoB100/ApoA1

(BMI: body mass index; FEV_1: forced expiratory volume in 1 second; FVC: forced vital capacity; HDL: high-density lipoprotein; WBC: white blood cell)

Source: Belsky DW, Caspi A, Corcoran DL, Sugden K, Poulton R, Arseneault L. DunedinPACE, a DNA methylation biomarker of the pace of aging. eLife. 2022;11:e73420.

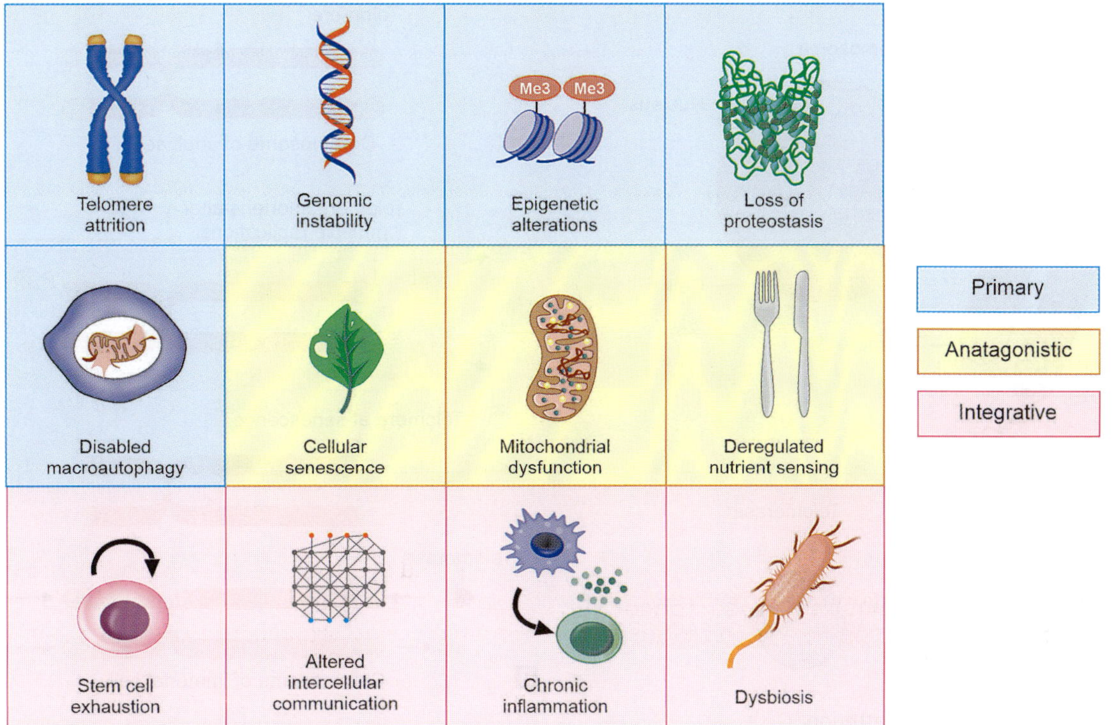

FIG. 1: Twelve hallmarks of aging.

Source: López–Otín C, Blasco MA, Partridge L, Serrano M, Kroemer G. Hallmarks of aging: an expanding universe. Cell. 2023;186:243-78.

the rate of change in epigenetic age. The pace or rate of aging was estimated over 20 years through 19 indicators reflecting health status and 12 aging signs.

HALLMARKS OF AGING

Aging researchers have proven the involvement of 12 hallmarks **(Fig. 1)**, such as (1) genomic instability, (2) telomere attrition, (3) epigenetic alterations, (4) loss of proteostasis, (5) deregulated nutrient sensing, (6) mitochondrial dysfunction, (7) cellular senescence, (8) stem cell exhaustion, (9) altered intercellular communication, (10) gut dysbiosis, (11) disabled macroautophagy, and (12) chronic inflammation in the process of aging.

1. *Genomic instability*: This is characterized by a tendency to undergo mutations, which are permanent, inheritable changes to the DNA sequence. It changes the gene expression and regulation, leading to age-related cellular degeneration and functional decay **(Flowchart 1)**.
2. *Telomere attrition*: Telomeres (TTAGGG) shorten with each cell division. Environmental factors can accelerate telomere shortening, impacting biological aging **(Figs. 2A and B)**.
3. *Epigenetic alterations*: These are changes in gene expression influenced without altering the DNA sequence. Changes include DNA methylation, histone modification, chromatin remodeling, noncoding RNA (ncRNA) regulation, and RNA modification. Most importantly, methylation patterns in DNA change with age, reflecting the impact of environment and lifestyle on the epigenome **(Fig. 3)**.

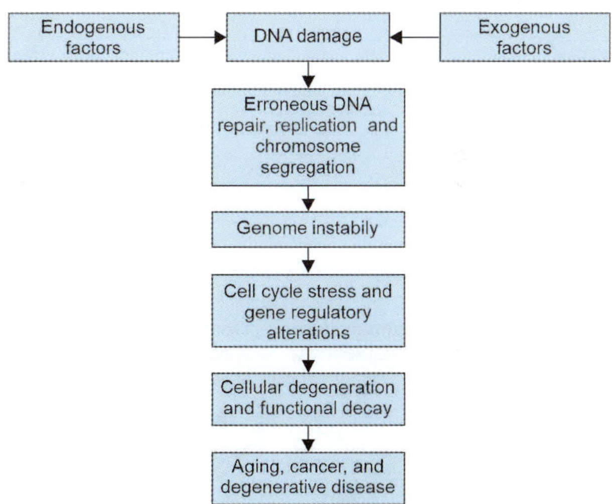

FLOWCHART 1: Genomic instability.

Source: Vijg J, Montagna C. Genome instability and aging: cause or effect? Transl Med Aging. 2017;1:5-11.

4. *Loss of proteostasis*: Proteostasis is the process through which cells maintain a balanced and functional

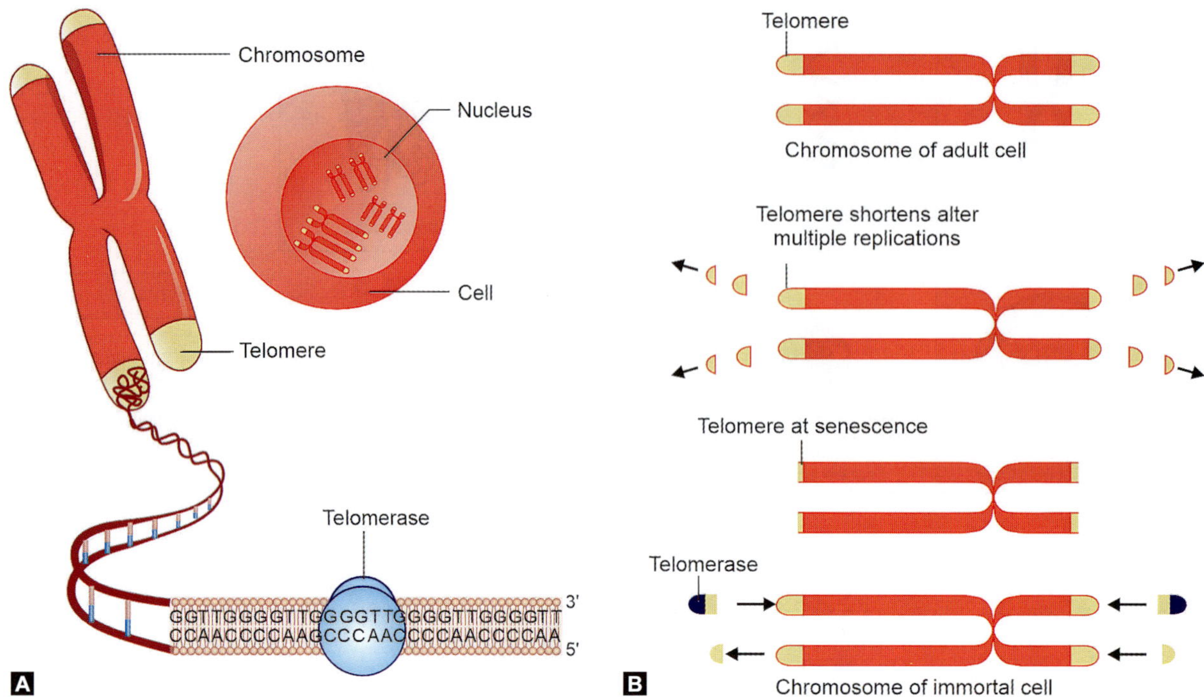

FIGS. 2A AND B: Telomere attrition.

Source: Vaiserman A, Krasnienkov D. Telomere length as a marker of biological age: state-of-the-art, open issues, and future perspectives. Front Genet. 2021;11:630186.

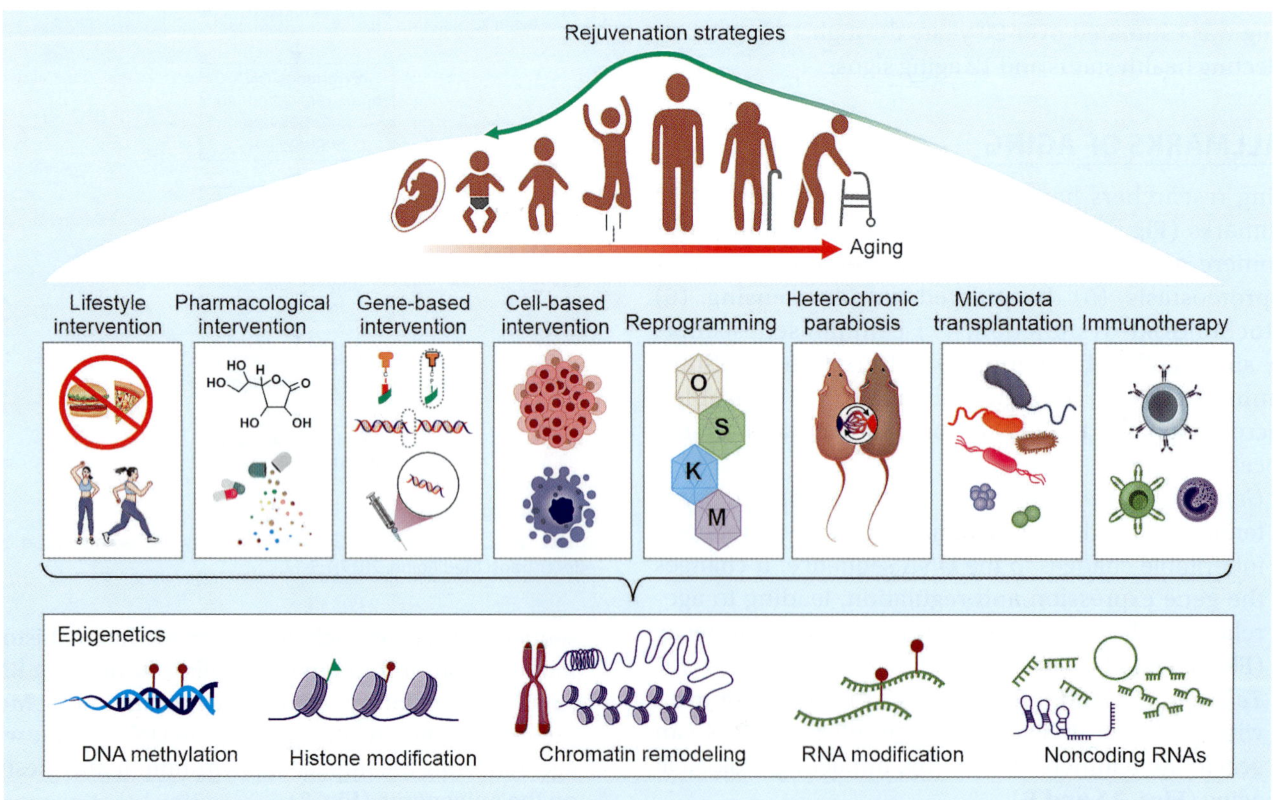

FIG. 3: Epigenetic alterations.

Source: Kong et al. Front Genet (2019).

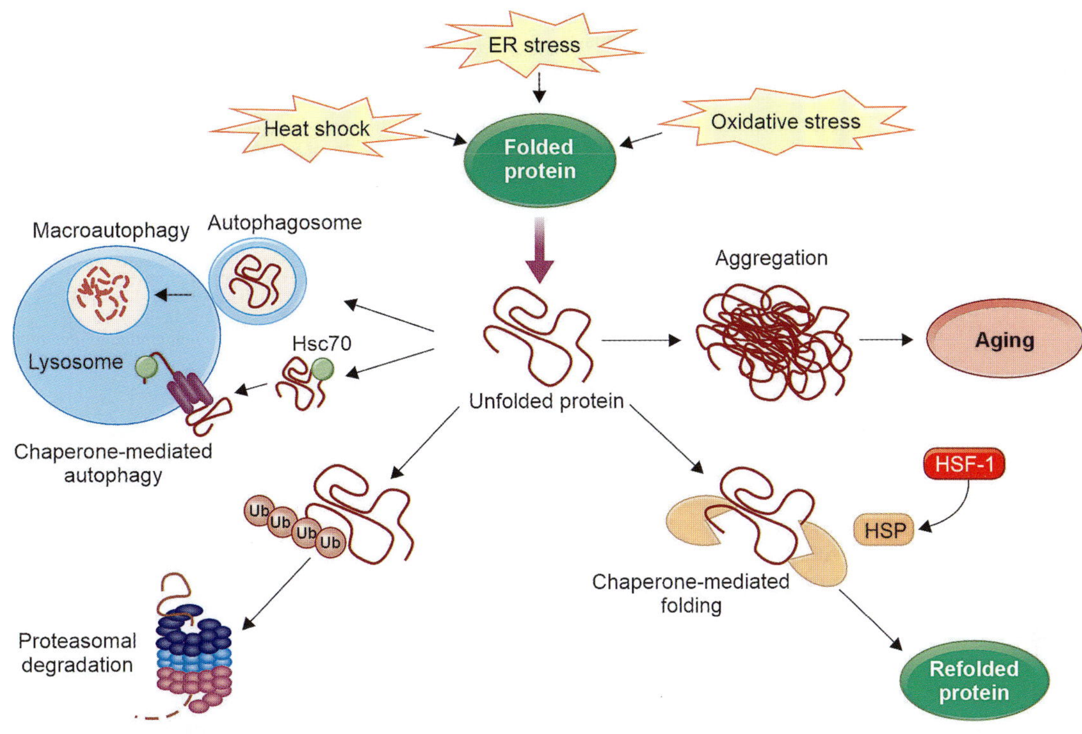

FLOWCHART 2: Folded protein.
(ER: endoplasmic reticulum)
Source: Khan S, et al. J Drug Deliv Sci Technol (2021).

proteome. Aging disrupts this balance, so misfolded and unfolded proteins are aggregated in the system **(Flowchart 2)**.

5. *Deregulated nutrient sensing*: Nutrient-sensing pathways regulate that the body takes in just the right amount of nutrition. The metabolic stress activities deregulate these nutrient-sensing molecules and downstream pathways, causing cells to age faster. Nutrient-sensing pathway is the basis for calorie restriction (CR) and antiaging interventions **(Flowchart 3)**.
6. *Mitochondrial dysfunction*: Accumulation of somatic mutations in mitochondrial DNA (mtDNA) occurs with age, affecting genes essential for the electron transport chain (ETC) and mitochondrial protein synthesis. Functional impairments in ETC activity contribute to aging and degenerative diseases **(Fig. 4)**.
7. *Cellular senescence*: This is an irreversible cell cycle arrest triggered by various insults such as DNA damage, metabolic stress, and telomere erosion. Senescent cells accumulate with age but are usually cleared by the immune system in younger individuals but not in older people. Senescent cells express senescence-associated secretory phenotype (SASP) which is the primary cause of the detrimental effects of senescent cells **(Flowchart 4)**.
8. *Stem cell exhaustion*: Stem cells are essential for tissue regeneration and homeostasis. Despite their resilience, our stem cells eventually lose their ability to divide as we age. The decrease in the renewal of stem cells leads to age-related disorders. Stem cell therapy is an innovative approach to replenishing decaying stem cells from undifferentiated ones **(Fig. 5)**.
9. *Altered intercellular communication*: Cell-to-cell communication is of particular importance for the proper development and function of the organism. Altered intercellular communication is a hallmark of aging when the body's cell-to-cell communication system breaks down through multiple pathways **(Fig. 6)**.

   Book Chapter: Aging, *From Fundamental Biology to Societal Impact, 2023, pages 257-274.*

10. *Gut dysbiosis*: This has recently emerged as an essential hallmark of aging. The human gut microbiota consists of trillions of microorganisms from four main bacterial phyla (Firmicutes, *Bacteroides*, Proteobacteria, and Actinobacteria), aiding digestion, nutrient absorption, vitamin production, and immune regulation. Aging alters gut microbiota, increasing proinflammatory microbes and reducing beneficial ones, leading to gut dysbiosis. The gut communicates with other organs in the body through gut–brain axis, gut–muscle axis, and gut–skin axes **(Fig. 7)**.

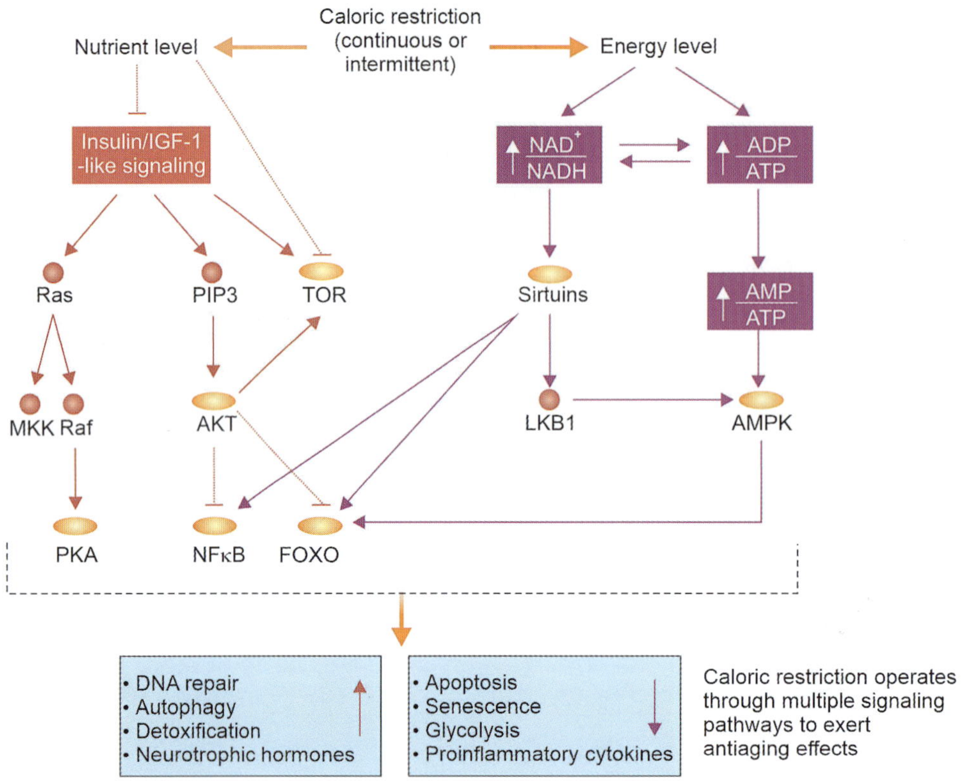

FLOWCHART 3: Nutrient-sensing pathway.

(ADP: adenosine diphosphate; ATP: adenosine triphosphate; IGF-1: insulin-like growth factor 1; NAD+: nicotinamide adenine dinucleotide; NADH: reduced nicotinamide adenine dinucleotide; NFκB: nuclear factor kappa B)

Source: Merck. (2025). Deregulated Nutrient Sensing. [online] Available from https://www.merckmillipore.com/IN/en/life-science-research/genomic-analysis/Epigenetics-and-Nuclear-Function/Deregulated-Nutrient-Sensing/FsCb.qB.u04AAAFQ6t52i0ib,nav?ReferrerURL=https%3A%2F%2Fwww.google.com%2F. [Last accessed May, 2025].

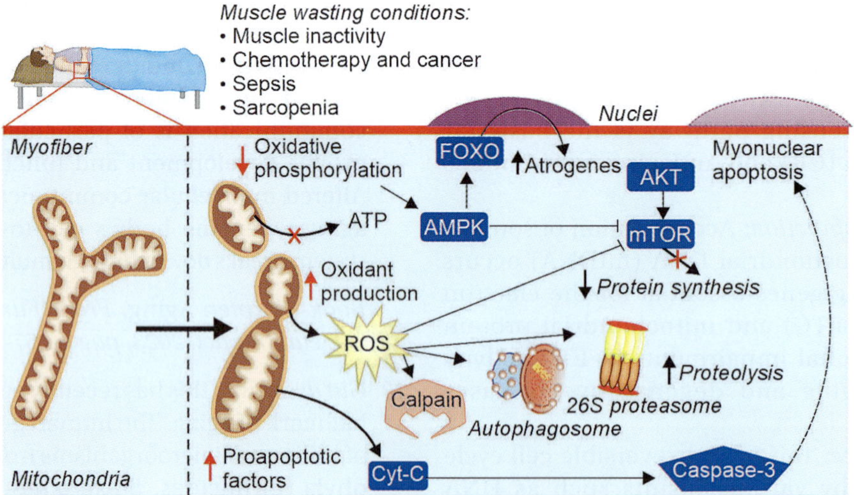

FIG. 4: Mitochondrial dysfunction.

(AMPK: AMP-activated protein kinase; ATP: adenosine triphosphate; mTOR: mammalian target of rapamycin; ROS: reactive oxygen species)

Source: Hyatt HW, Powers SK. Mitochondrial dysfunction is a common denominator linking skeletal muscle wasting due to disease, aging, and prolonged inactivity. Antioxidants (Basel). 2021;10(4):588.

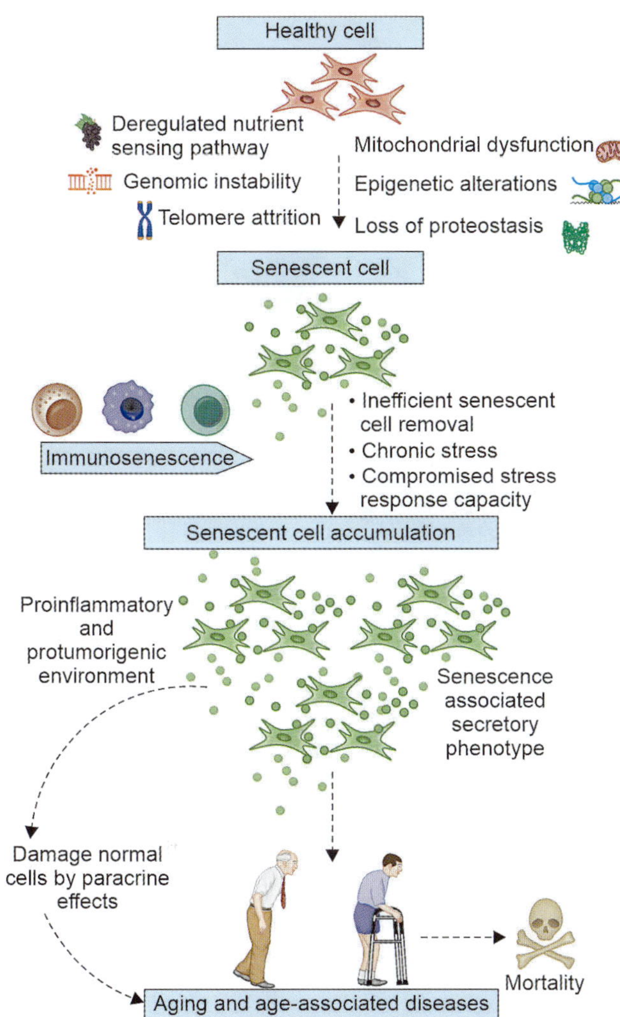

FLOWCHART 4: Cellular senescence.

Source: Diwan B, Sharma R. Nutritional components as mitigators of cellular senescence in organismal aging: a comprehensive review. Food Sci Biotechnol. 2022;31(9):1089-109.

11. *Disabled macroautophagy*: Autophagy removes damaged or dysfunctional cellular components. Dysregulation of autophagy is implicated in neurodegenerative disorders, diabetes, obesity, autoimmune disease, infections, and aging **(Fig. 8)**.
12. *Chronic inflammation*: Inflammaging is a chronic, low-grade inflammation that occurs with age and is a significant risk factor for morbidity and mortality in the elderly. Chronic inflammation can lead to excessive immune activity in the brain that shows up in many ways, such as cognitive decline, memory lapse, confusion, and sickness behavior **(Fig. 9)**.

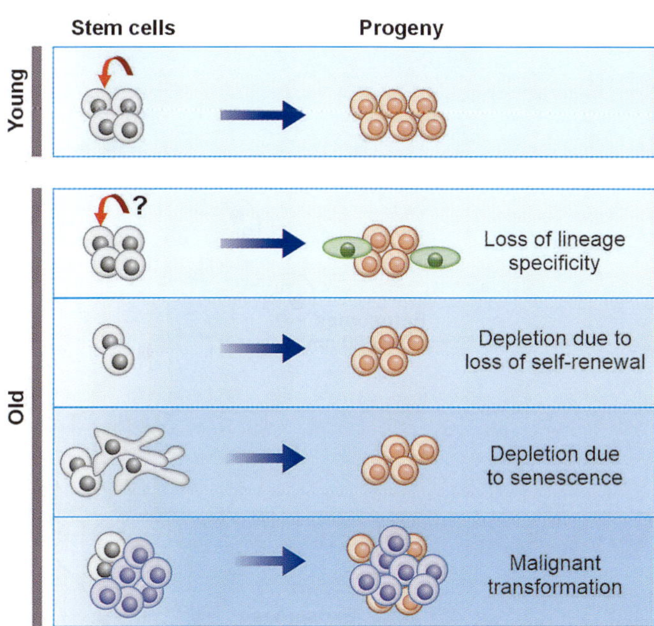

FIG. 5: Stem cell therapy.

Source: Liu L, Rando TA. Manifestations and mechanisms of stem cell aging. J Cell Biol. 2011;193:257-66.

FACTORS INFLUENCING LONGEVITY

There are a few essential molecules and pathways that play as intermediates among multiple hallmarks of aging, thereby influencing longevity.

Molecular Signaling Pathways

- Various signaling pathways specifically, the sirtuin 1 (SIRT1) and mammalian target of rapamycin (mTOR) pathways, adenosine monophosphate-activated kinase (AMPK) signaling is one of the central regulators of cellular and organism metabolism in eukaryotes. Specific AMPK activation protects against aging and extends the lifespan in *C. elegans* and rodents.
- SIRT1 is a well-known nicotinamide adenine dinucleotide (NAD^+)-dependent deacetylase that impacts several molecules to promote health. It is believed to increase the lifespan by the suppressing of cellular senescence through delaying age-related telomere attrition, sustaining genome integrity, and promoting DNA damage repair.
- The mTOR is a serine/threonine kinase. It exists as two distinct protein complexes: mTOR complexes 1 (mTORC1) and 2 (mTORC2). Inhibition of mTORC1 extends the lifespan and delays aging.

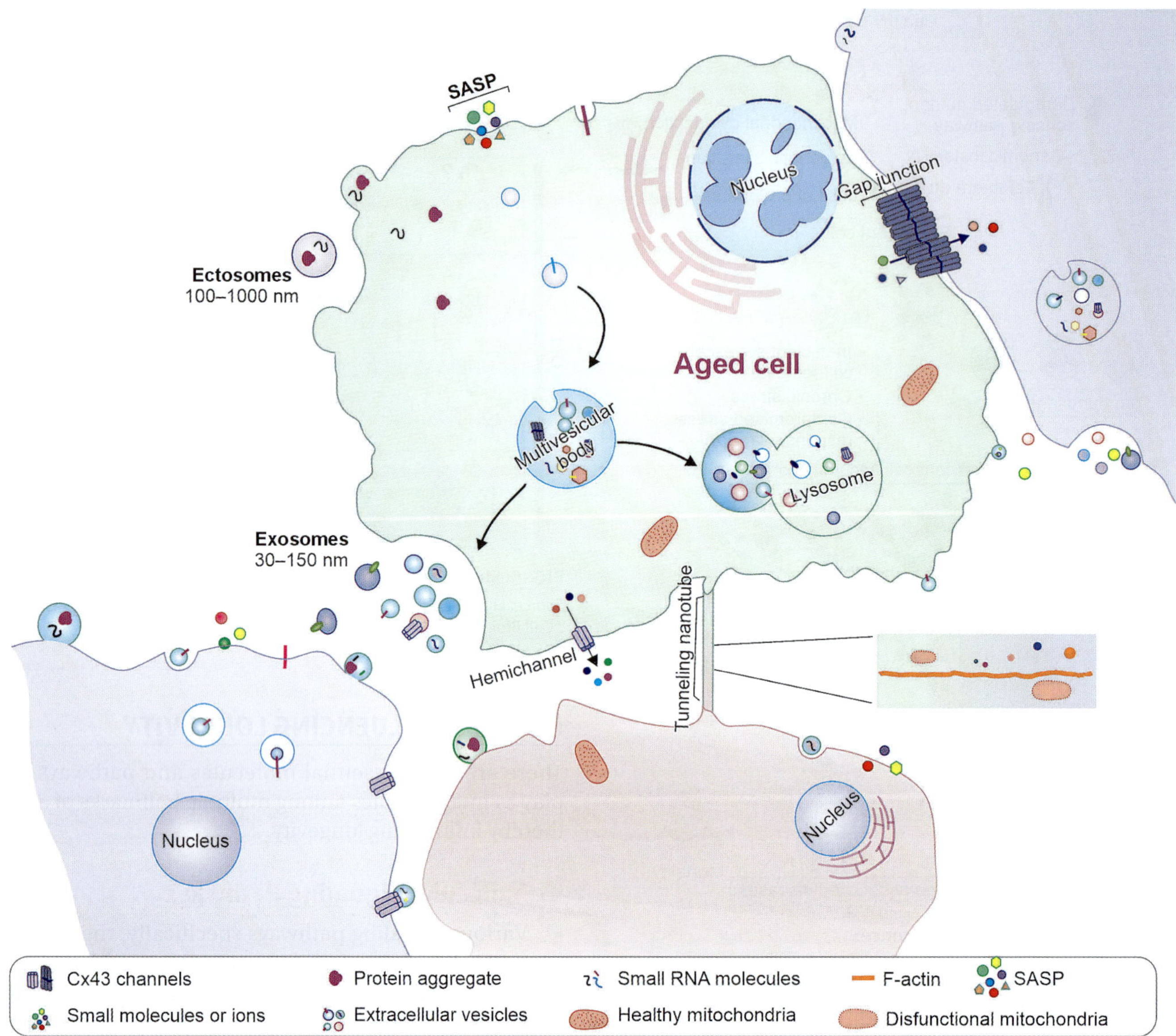

FIG. 6: Different types of intercellular communication. Connexins composed of hemichannels allow the exchange of small molecules between the cytoplasm and the extracellular milieu, or when in the form gap junctions facilitate communication between neighbor cells. Extracellular vesicles result either from the fusion of multivesicular bodies (MVBs) with the plasma membrane (PM), releasing small vesicles called exosomes, or from PM outward budding originating ectosomes. When in the extracellular space, these vesicles can fuse, dock, or be endocytosed by the recipient cell triggering a response. According to its properties, tunneling nanotubes (TNTs) ensure communication between connected cells by transference of organelles, protein aggregates, genetic material, and small molecules. Aged cells can be characterized by a particular secretory phenotype, senescence-associated secretory phenotype (SASP), whose components can propagate to other cells and throughout the organism potentially modulating younger cells' response.

- Insulin/insulin-like growth factor 1 (IGF-1) signaling accelerates the aging process later in the lifespan. It can control immunosuppression and cellular senescence through its several connections to STAT3 signaling.

Genetics

- Family history of longevity often indicates genetic predispositions to a longer life.
- In an Indian study published in NPJ Aging, genes involved in oxidative stress, apoptosis, DNA damage repair, glucose metabolism, and energy metabolism affected longevity significantly.

Lifestyle Factors

- *Diet*: Nutrient-dense, balanced diets are associated with longer lifespans. Caloric restriction has shown the potential to increase lifespan in animal studies.

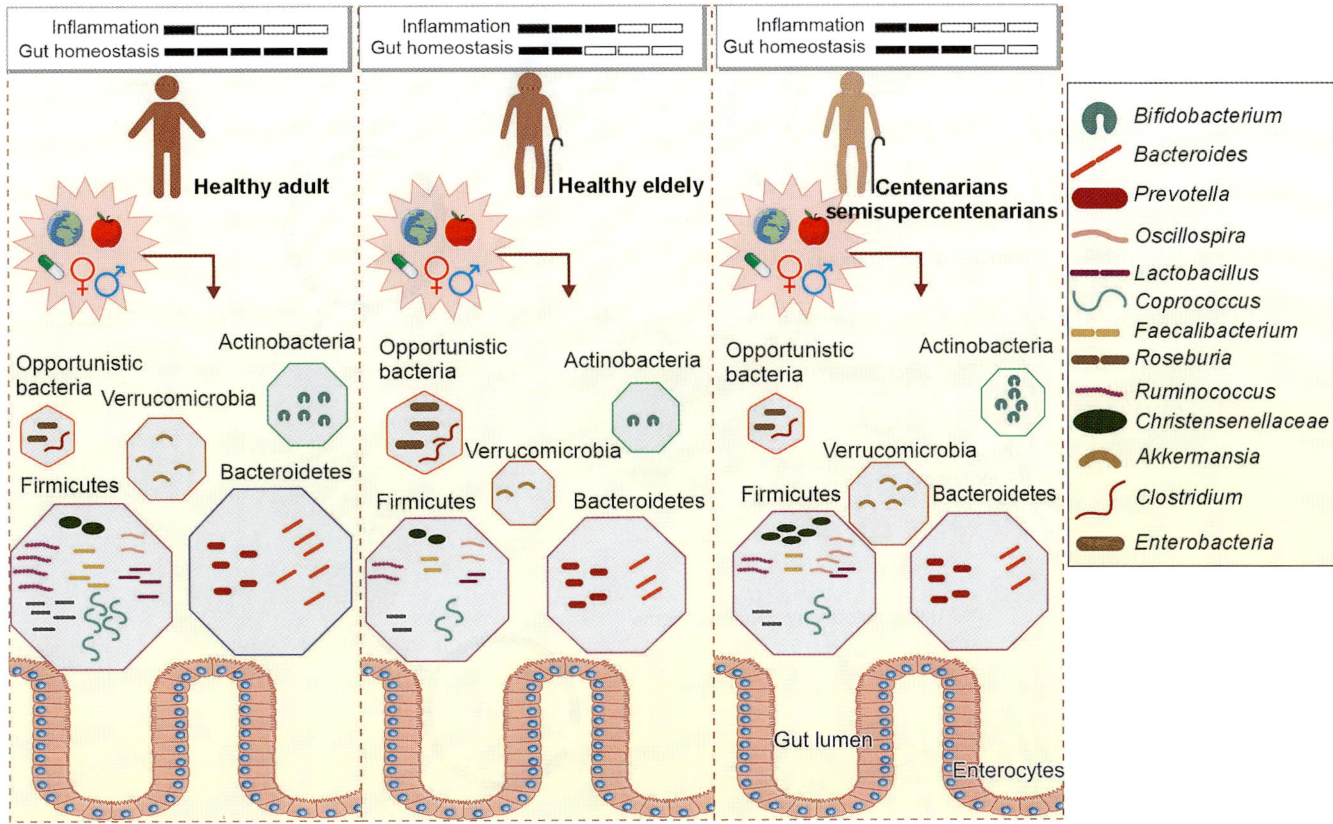

FIG. 7: Gut dysbiosis.
Source: Ragonnaud E, Biragyn A. Gut microbiota as the key controllers of "healthy" aging of elderly people. Immun Ageing. 2021;18(1):2.

- *Physical activity*: Regular exercise improves cardiovascular health, muscle mass, and metabolic functions.
- *Stress management*: Chronic stress accelerates aging processes.
- *Life circumstances*. Social support, socioeconomic status, and education levels can influence how long and well people live.

Environmental Factors

Pollution and exposure to toxins accelerated cellular aging.

SCIENCE OF ANTIAGING

Antiaging and its Importance

Antiaging is a multidisciplinary approach to slowing, halting, or reversing aging.

Antiaging measures include medical, nutritional, lifestyle, and technological interventions to improve quality of life and reduce the risks associated with aging-related diseases.

ANTIAGING PRACTICES AND LIFESTYLE

Dietary Approaches

- *Caloric restriction*: CR reduces calorie intake without malnutrition to delay the aging process. The CALERIE (Comprehensive Assessment of Long-term Effects of Reducing Intake of Energy) trial was conducted at three clinical centers in the United States and found that CR slowed the pace of aging in healthy adults. The different pathways regulated by CR include AMPK pathway, forkhead box (FOXO) pathway, mTOR signaling pathway, IGF-1 pathway, nuclear factor kappa B (NFκB) pathway, c-Jun N-terminal kinase (JNK) pathway, and p38 kinase pathway.
- *Specific diets*: There are some traditional healthy dietary patterns associated with longevity **(Box 2)**.

Exercise and Mobility

- *Resistance training (strength exercise)*: It helps preserve muscle mass and strength.
- *Aerobic exercise (endurance exercise)*: It improves cardiovascular and metabolic health.

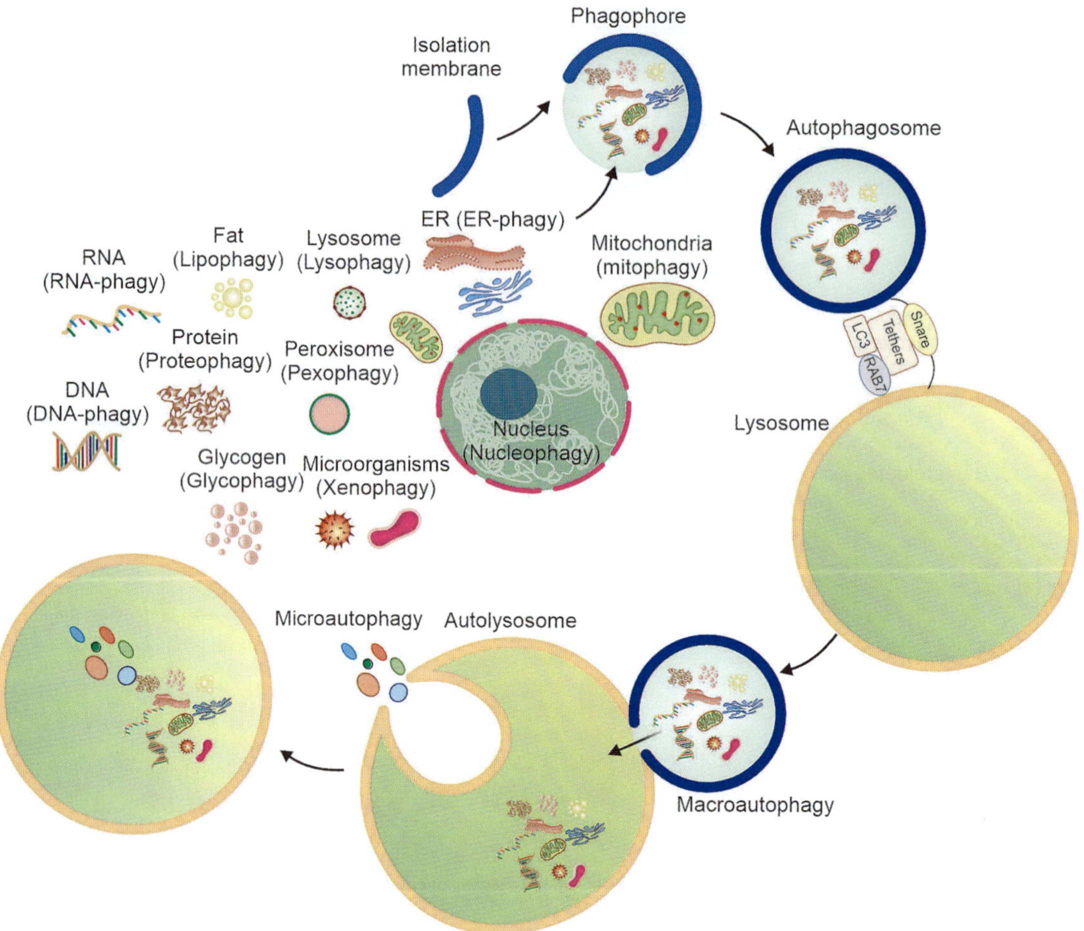

FIG. 8: Macrophagy and microautophagy.
Source: Tabibzadeh S. Role of autophagy in aging: the good, the bad, and the ugly. Aging Cell. 2023;22(1):e13753.

- *Flexibility training (stretching exercise)*: It improves the motion of joints, postural balance, and locomotion.
- *Balance training*: It builds stability, coordination, and strength to prevent falls in the elderly.
- Studies claim that higher moderate to vigorous exercise levels are associated with longer life expectancy.

Stress Reduction

- Stress can have a significant impact on aging and can accelerate the aging process.
- Practices such as yoga, meditation, and mindfulness reduce cortisol levels linked to aging.

Sleep Hygiene

- The circadian rhythm of sleep plays an essential role in the sleep-wake cycle, affecting the aging manifold.
- Aging is associated with advanced sleep timing, decreased nocturnal sleep time and efficiency, increased frequency of daytime naps, increased nocturnal awakenings, and decreased slow-wave sleep.
- Adequate and restorative sleep enhances cellular repair and reduces oxidative stress.

Cellular Interventions

Stem cell therapies: These replace damaged cells with healthy stem cells to regenerate tissues. Mesenchymal stem cells promise to slow or reverse the normal aging process. Mesenchymal stem cell preparations were in development for two main aging conditions: Physical frailty and facial skin aging. Approximately 16 clinical trials for both conditions are currently underway.

Molecular Approaches

- *Antioxidants*: Molecules such as vitamins C and E neutralize reactive oxygen species (ROS), reducing oxidative stress.

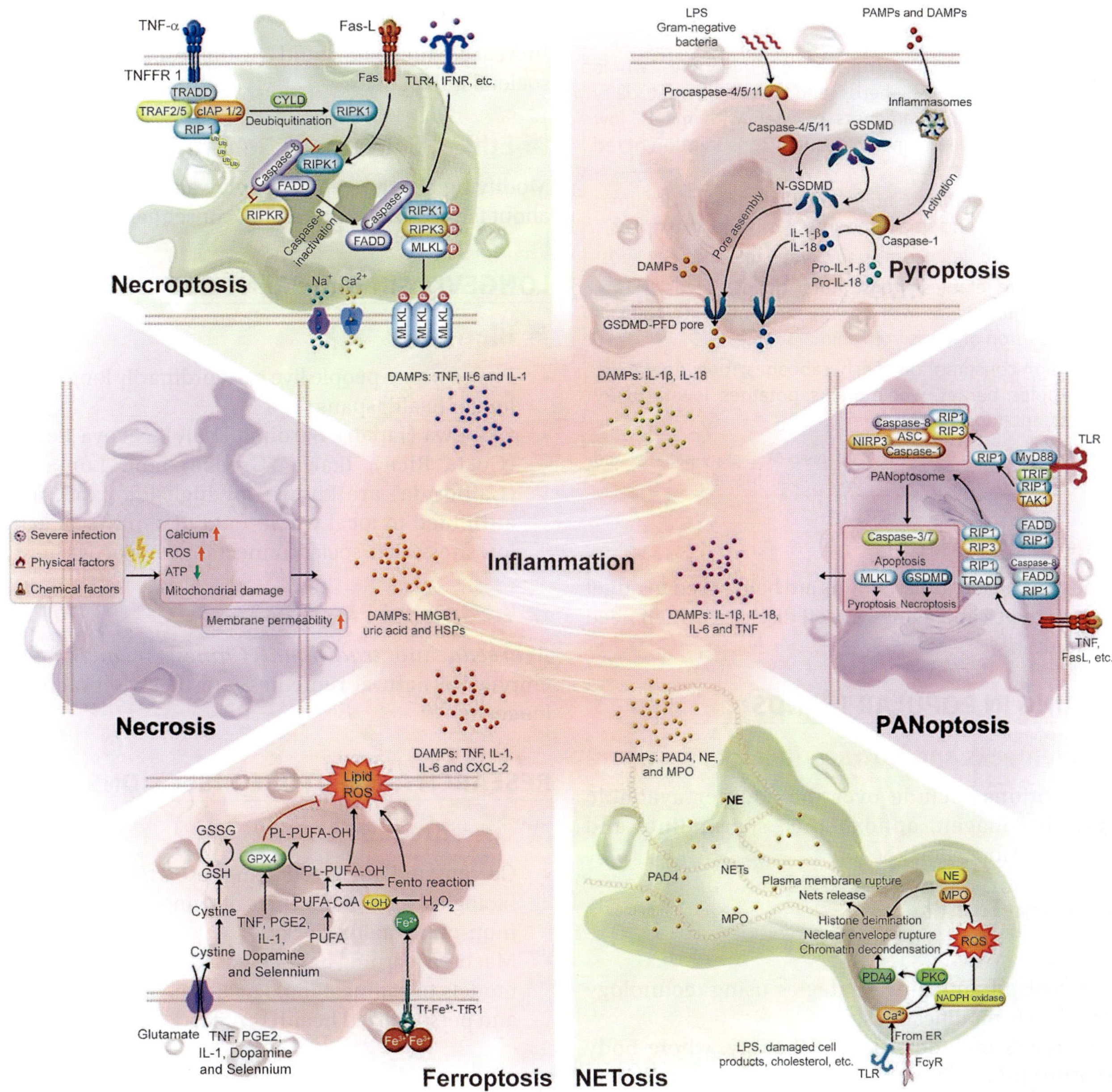

FIG. 9: Chronic inflammation.

Source: Zhang W, Xiao D, Mao Q, Xia H. Role of neuroinflammation in neurodegeneration development. Signal Transduct Target Ther. 2023;8(1):267.

- *Telomerase activators*: Drugs that lengthen telomeres, potentially delaying cellular senescence, e.g., TA-65.
- *Senolytics*: Drugs designed to eliminate senescent cells, reduce inflammation, and improve tissue function, e.g., dasatinib, quercetin, and fisetin.
- *NAD⁺ precursor supplementation*: Preservation of cognitive ability by increasing NAD⁺ levels through supplementation with NAD⁺ precursors, e.g., nicotinamide (NM) and nicotinamide riboside (NR).
- *mTOR inhibitors*: These emerge as potential antiaging therapeutics, e.g., rapamycin, RTB101, and everolimus.
- *Mitochondria-targeted supplementation*: MitoQ, Urolithin A, and elamipretide are promising drugs.

Most of these molecules are available over the counter for consumption. However, more randomized clinical trials are required to establish their efficacy.

Regenerative Medicine

Regenerative medicine indicates development of artificial organs and tissue engineering techniques to replace damaged or aging tissues.

BOX 2 Traditional healthy dietary patterns.

- *Mediterranean*: Vegetables, fruits, olive oil, legumes, whole grains, nuts, seeds, fish, herbs and spices, low-fat dairy and yogurt, moderate amounts of wine with meals, low consumption of sweets, and unfrequent consumption of red and processed meat
- *Okinawan*: Vegetables, fruits, whole grains, legumes (particularly soy), and small amounts of fish and lean meats
- *Japanese*: Vegetables, rice, fish, soy, green tea, and seaweeds
- *Vegetarian*: Vegetables, fruits, nuts, grains, seeds, herbs, spices, mushrooms, as well as vegetable oils with total or partial exclusion of foods from animal sources
- *Nordic*: High consumption of fish, cabbages, root vegetables, pears, apples, berries, whole grains, potatoes, low-fat dairy products, and rapeseed oil

Source: Dominguez LJ, Veronese N, Barbagallo M. Dietary patterns and healthy or unhealthy aging. Gerontology. 2024;70(1):15-36.

Genetic Engineering

Gene therapy-based interventions are being used to target aging phenotypes and aging-related diseases, which need further study.

ANTIAGING IN POPULAR TRENDS

Supplements and Nutraceuticals

Popular options include over-the-counter available resveratrol, collagen, antioxidants, spermidine, and coenzyme Q10 for cellular health

Emerging Trends

Biohacking

- Personalized antiaging strategies using technology and lifestyle modifications.
- New trends include red light therapy, whole-body cryotherapy, infrasound vibrations, hyperbaric chambers, and grounding.

Artificial Intelligence and Wearables

Artificial intelligence (AI)-powered digital health platforms generate exhaustive information about patient health for their personalized health profile. Wearables could provide real-time and continuous monitoring of patients' medical health information, helping physicians detect and monitor health indicators early.

ETHICAL CONSIDERATIONS AND CHALLENGES

Equity in Access

Antiaging treatments are often expensive and inaccessible to lower income populations, raising ethical concerns.

Social Implications

Increased lifespan could strain resources and create societal imbalances.

Ethical Concerns in Genetic Engineering

Modifying human genes to delay aging raises questions about fairness and unintended consequences.

LONGEVITY IN DIFFERENT CULTURES

Blue Zones

- Places where people live extraordinarily long lives with longer health spans.
- Okinawa (Japan), Sardinia (Italy), Nicoya Peninsula (Costa Rica), Ikaria (Greece), and Loma Linda (California) are known for high life expectancies, attributed to local whole-food diet, physical activity, low stress, rich, social connections, and active lifestyles.

Traditional Practices

Ayurveda and *traditional Chinese medicine (TCM)* emphasize natural remedies and lifestyle practices for longevity.

RESEARCH AND FUTURE DIRECTIONS

Current Studies

- Current and advanced aging research has focused on biological age, biomarkers of aging, and multidomain muti-omics aging clocks.
- Machine learning has been used to develop prediction models to estimate biological age, disease prediction, and personalized health profiles.

Promising Therapies (Fig. 10)

- Development of senolytics, gene therapies, and tissue regeneration technologies.
- Studies on drugs such as rapamycin and metformin for their antiaging effects.
- Precision medicine for longevity is being explored to provide tailor-made medical treatment and preventative care to an individual's health profile.

Aging as a Disease

- Emerging perspectives treat aging as a modifiable biological process rather than an inevitable decline.
- The notion that aging is a disease is poorly received within the scientific community, but the rebranding of aging would open new avenues in aging research.

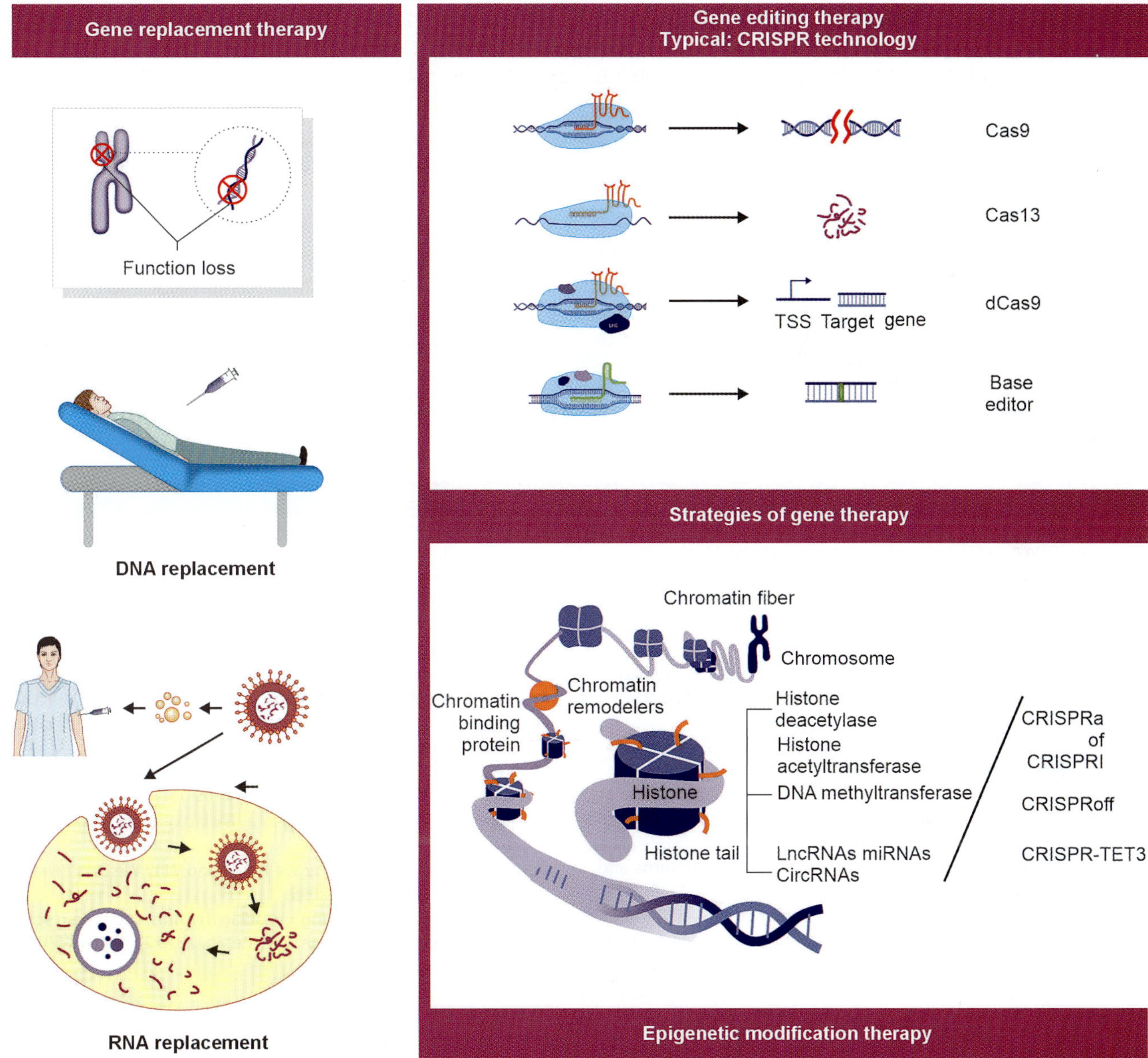

FIG. 10: Strategies of gene therapy.
(CRISPR: clustered regularly interspaced short palindromic repeats)
Source: Yu J, Li T, Zhu J. Gene therapy strategies targeting aging-related disease. Aging Dis. 2023;14(2):398-417.

- This idea is shifting aging research from basic to therapeutic and preventive science.

CONCLUSION

Summary

Longevity and antiaging are complex, multifaceted fields involving biology, lifestyle, medicine, and technology. While significant progress has been made, challenges remain in ensuring equitable access and addressing ethical concerns.

Future of Aging

With continued advancements, the possibility of significantly extending both lifespan and health span appears within reach, paving the way for a healthier, more vibrant aging process.

Self-Assessment Questionnaire

Q1. How do longevity and health span differ, and why is the latter increasingly emphasized in modern geriatric practice?

Q2. What is the significance of biological age over chronological age, and how do epigenetic clocks help estimate it?

Q3. Compare and contrast the longevity determinants in the two case vignettes—Mr Ramesh Babu and Mr SS Rudra.

Q4. Name the 12 hallmarks of aging and explain how mitochondrial dysfunction and cellular senescence contribute to age-related decline.

Q5. Describe the role of NAD^+, SIRT1, and mTOR pathways in regulating cellular aging and longevity.

Q6. Discuss the evidence and mechanisms behind caloric restriction and exercise as antiaging interventions.

Q7. What are senolytics and telomerase activators, and how do they aim to reverse cellular aging?

Q8. Explain how AI-powered wearables and biomarker-based aging clocks are transforming longevity science.

Q9. What are the major ethical and societal implications of antiaging research, particularly regarding gene therapy and equitable access?

FURTHER READINGS

1. López–Otín C, Blasco MA, Partridge L, Serrano M, Kroemer G. Hallmarks of aging: an expanding universe. Cell. 2023;186(3):243-78.
2. Belsky DW, Caspi A, Corcoran DL, Sugden K, Poulton R, Arseneault L. DunedinPACE, a DNA methylation biomarker of the pace of aging. eLife. 2022;11:e73420.
3. Vaiserman A, Krasnienkov D. Telomere length as a marker of biological age: state-of-the-art, open issues, and future perspectives. Front Genet. 2021;11:630186.
4. Tabibzadeh S. Role of autophagy in aging: the good, the bad, and the ugly. Aging Cell. 2023;22(1):e13753.
5. Zhang W, Xiao D, Mao Q, Xia H. Role of neuroinflammation in neurodegeneration development. Signal Transduct Target Ther. 2023;8(1):267.
6. Dominguez LJ, Veronese N, Barbagallo M. Dietary patterns and healthy or unhealthy aging. Gerontology. 2024;70(1):15-36.
7. Hyatt HW, Powers SK. Mitochondrial dysfunction is a common denominator linking skeletal muscle wasting due to disease, aging, and prolonged inactivity. Antioxidants (Basel). 2021;10(4):588.
8. Diwan B, Sharma R. Nutritional components as mitigators of cellular senescence in organismal aging: a comprehensive review. Food Sci Biotechnol. 2022;31(9):1089-109.
9. Yu J, Li T, Zhu J. Gene therapy strategies targeting aging-related disease. Aging Dis. 2023;14(2):398-417.
10. Ragonnaud E, Biragyn A. Gut microbiota as the key controllers of "healthy" aging of elderly people. Immun Ageing. 2021;18(1):2.
11. Barzilai N, Crandall JP, Kritchevsky SB, Espeland MA. Metformin as a tool to target aging. Cell Metab. 2016;23(6):1060-5.
12. Kennedy BK, Berger SL, Brunet A, et al. Geroscience: linking aging to chronic disease. Cell. 2014;159(4):709-13.
13. Niccoli T, Partridge L. Ageing as a risk factor for disease. Curr Biol. 2012;22(17):R741-52.
14. Sinclair DA. Lifespan: Why We Age—and Why We Don't Have To. New York: Atria Books; 2019.
15. Longo VD, Panda S. Fasting, circadian rhythms, and time-restricted feeding in healthy lifespan. Cell Metab. 2016;23(6):1048-59.

CHAPTER 8

Oral Health in Older Adults

Ritu Duggal, Bharathi Purohit

CASE VIGNETTE

Patient information: A 75-year-old male, Mr Virender Kothari, with a history of type 2 diabetes and hypertension, lives in an old age home with around 30 inmates.

Presenting complaint: Mr Kothari visits the nearby health center with concerns about masticatory discomfort due to the existing prosthesis. He is a healthy, independent person, demanding a new prosthesis with improved masticatory stability and better aesthetics.

History of present illness: Mr Kothari had difficulty in eating and swallowing food for 3–4 months, especially while chewing hard food. The partial denture in the lower left mandibular region becomes loose, and at times, he removes his lower denture while eating due to the discomfort caused by the denture. This has also affected his nutritional intake and his overall oral health and quality of life.

Medical history: Mr Kothari has a history of type 2 diabetes and hypertension, for which he has been taking antidiabetic and antihypertensive medications for the past 20 years. He has reported a history of visual disturbance for which he has undergone cataract surgery for both the eyes 3 years back. His last comprehensive oral examination was conducted 2 years back.

Social history: Mr Kothari lives in an old age home for the past 10 years after the death of his wife and receives necessary assistance and care in this facility. He actively engages in day-to-day tasks and physical and recreational activities with his inmates. He has a history of tobacco habit which he quit since his stay in the old age home. There was no history of past alcohol consumption.

Review of systems: There was no significant medical history reported by him, apart from few episodes of cold and fever in the past 3 months, for which he had self-medicated.

Physical examination: During the physical examination, his blood pressure was 138/85 mm Hg and heart rate was 82 beats/min.

Oral examination: He complains of mouth soreness and difficulty in eating anything hard. Dental history reveals that he had been wearing partial denture for the last 10 years and that his current denture was about 4 years old. He reported that he had a fear of choking, and history of strong gag reflex, especially when impressions were made. Oral examination showed mandibular extended edentulous areas and inappropriate prosthesis. The existing fixed prosthesis had aesthetic defects and incorrect peripheral fitting, leading to functional instability and extensive wear of the acrylic teeth. The patient had poor oral hygiene and generalized dental abrasions. The X-ray evaluation showed extreme resorption of the mandible on the left side.

INTRODUCTION

Changing demographics, including an increase in life expectancy and the growing number of elderly, has focused attention on the need for geriatric dental care. Oral health is often neglected in the elderly, and oral diseases associated with aging are complex, adversely affecting the quality of life. Among the most common diseases affecting older adults are chronic diseases of the oral cavity, including dental infections (e.g., caries, periodontitis), tooth loss, mucosal lesions, and oral cancer. These conditions can adversely affect nutrition, self-esteem, quality of life, and general health, and this highlights the importance of oral health for healthy aging.

Teeth loss is accelerated in the elderly population leading to functional disabilities. Masticatory function is compromised in these cases, affecting the nutritional status of the individual due to inappropriate food selection. On an average, every patient over 65 years has about five pathological conditions, and interdisciplinary collaboration is often necessary which also commonly requires consideration of the comorbidities, to improve the oral health.

In this chapter, we will explore the complexities of oral health in elderly population, with the primary objective of empowering geriatric healthcare providers with knowledge of epidemiology, required investigations, possible treatments, and rehabilitation of oral health status in the elderly. We will also explore other factors associated with this important issue including physiological, psychological, social, and cultural aspects that shape the experiences of the geriatric community.

ORAL DISEASE BURDEN IN THE ELDERLY

Oral health is often not the focus of attention when discussing health problems among the elderly, where numerous comorbidities occur that severely impact the quality of life of this population. However, the growing oral health needs of elderly have warranted considerable attention in the past few decades, with the changing demographics and at the same time remarkable progress in oral health awareness, research, and technology. Life expectancy at birth has increased, with an increasing number of the population retaining teeth for longer compared with previous generations. Therefore, understanding the epidemiology of oral diseases in elderly is important for healthcare providers to identify the multifactorial changes associated with aging that make oral health issues important and unique in this population.

Oral diseases, while largely preventable, pose a major health burden for many countries and affect people throughout their lifetime, causing pain, discomfort, disfigurement, and even death. The main conditions of interest when considering oral diseases among older people are tooth loss, dental caries, periodontitis, dry mouth, and oral precancer/cancer. Oral diseases are caused by a range of modifiable risk factors common to many noncommunicable diseases (NCDs), including sugar consumption, tobacco use, alcohol use, and poor hygiene, and their underlying social and commercial determinants.

EPIDEMIOLOGY AND GLOBAL PERSPECTIVE

It is estimated that oral diseases affect nearly 3.5 billion people in all age groups with untreated dental caries (tooth decay) in permanent teeth being the most common health condition according to the Global Burden of Disease 2019. According to this, edentulism (complete tooth loss), severe periodontitis (chronic gum disease), and untreated dental caries (tooth decay) account for 23.1 million disability-adjusted life years (DALYs) worldwide—a loss of approximately 284.6 years per 100,000 population. 28.02% of the increase in DALYs for oral conditions between 1990 and 2010 is solely attributed to population aging.

Most low- and middle-income countries do not have sufficient services available to prevent and treat oral health conditions. Treatment for oral health conditions is expensive and usually not part of universal health coverage (UHC). Without reforms in oral healthcare policies, the oral disease burden is likely to continue growing, amplified by the challenges of population aging.

Indian Scenario

In the billion-plus population of India, there are nearly 150 million elderly people (above 60 years of age), and it is expected to double to 20.8% by 2050. The proportion of elderly population in rural and urban India is almost similar, with approximately 7.7% in urban and 8.7% in rural areas, according to the 2011 census report of India. There also exists a trend in which more teeth are retained as age increases due to increased awareness and effective dental public health measures. This inevitably places an increased need for oral healthcare among the geriatric population.

Isolated cross-sectional studies have been conducted across India to assess the oral health status among elderly. Majority of the studies showed low oral hygiene scores among elderly with dental caries, periodontal disease, and lack of prosthesis being the most common diseases recorded. The overall prevalence of dental caries experience ranged from 31.5 to 91.9%; 16–85% had root caries and 22–73.2% had periodontal disease. Majority of the elderly had no prosthesis which ranged from 12 to 86.6%. The National Oral Health Survey in India (2002–2003) showed a prevalence of 85% dental caries, 80.2% periodontal disease among 65–74-year age group, and 29.3% of subjects were in need of full mouth prosthesis. The report of a multicentric study (2007) covering seven states across India reported 67.8% prevalence of dental caries in 65 years and older age group. Longitudinal Aging Study in India (LASI) Wave 1, 2017–2019, a nationally representative longitudinal survey, reported higher prevalence of common oral health problems (47%) among elderly aged 60 years and above.

Geriatric population is prone to root caries, periodontal disease, wearing of teeth, missing teeth, edentulism, poor quality of alveolar ridges, mucosal lesions, oral ulceration, dry mouth (xerostomia), oral cancers, etc. Many of these are the sequelae of neglect in the early years of life, for example, consumption of a cariogenic diet, lack of awareness regarding preventive aspects, and habits such as smoking and/or tobacco, pan, and betel nut chewing. Reduced immunity in old age and coexisting medical comorbidities further aggravate the existing oral diseases. Some of the unique challenges are as follows:

Age: Literature has reported that the two groups of 60–64 years (the new elderly) and 65–74 years (the transition group) had significantly more favorable attitudes toward dental care than the old elderly (>75 years) age group.

Socioeconomic status: Utilization of preventive health care is higher among higher social classes, as they can overcome any financial barrier to dental care, tend to be better educated, and are potentially more likely to be familiar with and to adopt favorable attitudes toward the maintenance of oral health.

Accessibility-related barriers: Access to dental services may present a barrier because of physical incapacity or disability, travel problems, lack of knowledge of dental services, or lack of dental services in a given area. Patients with problems of mobility, e.g., are less likely to visit dental clinics where stairs must be climbed.

Fear and anxiety: Most people experience some apprehension at the prospect of a dental visit, and sometimes, inherent fear and anxiety about routine dental procedures are an important barrier to the receipt of care in older people.

Psychosocial factors: Cultural and psychosocial aspects can also influence the utilization of dental services. Lack of family and social support can impact the oral health of elderly.

Professional Barriers: There is a need for improved awareness of dental care among health and allied health professionals to provide dental care guidance for this vulnerable population. Provision of basic oral hygiene education by healthcare providers is necessary whenever an elderly patient visits their clinic for any other health-related ailment.

Understanding the epidemiology of oral diseases in the Indian elderly is critical for tailoring preventive measures, clinical interventions, and developing healthcare policies to address this issue effectively. By recognizing the specific challenges and risk factors within the Indian context, healthcare professionals and policymakers can work toward reducing the oral disease burden and improve the oral and overall quality of life for the elderly population in India.

CLINICAL PRESENTATION AND EVALUATION OF ORAL DISEASES IN OUTPATIENT SETTINGS

In an outpatient setting, the assessment of oral diseases in elderly individuals and managing risk factors is important for improved masticatory abilities. This section provides an overview of the clinical presentation and the systematic evaluation of oral diseases in an outpatient context.

- *History of presenting illness*: A thorough dental and medical history is essential. Patients should be asked about their chief complaint, duration of symptoms, frequency of dental episodes, aggravating and relieving factors, and history of any self-medication should be recorded. If there are multiple dental problems, they need to be listed in the chronological order with their related symptoms.
- *History of adverse habits*: The most common adverse habits such as tobacco use (both smokeless form and smoked form of tobacco), duration, and frequency of use of each type of product should be recorded. Use of alcohol or any other addictive drugs should also be recorded.
- *Dental health behavior*: Patients should be asked about their routine oral hygiene measures. This is important because cultural factors and traditions influence the type of products used by them, which has an important influence on oral hygiene.
- *Coexisting medical conditions*: The presence of systemic diseases not only affects the patient's ability to maintain oral hygiene, but can also have a direct effect on the onset and progression of oral diseases. Though impairments are not life-threatening, they affect a person's quality of life. Identification and assessment of any coexisting medical conditions, such as diabetes, cardiovascular diseases, osteoporosis, or neurological disorders, play a critical role in the acceptance and success of the dental treatment plans.
- *Physical and mental conditions*: Physical and psychological conditions influence self-care capacity and the choice of treatment plan. For example, in institutionalized elders who are suffering from systemic diseases, the therapy of choice should be the least invasive one that is able to restore function at an acceptable level. Active healthy elders can be beneficiaries of complex prosthetic treatments.

Specific Investigations

To comprehensively evaluate dental condition of the patient in an outpatient setting, specific investigations are often necessary. These investigations help to tailor the effective treatment strategies. Some key investigations in routine practice are as follows:

- *Laboratory tests*: Blood glucose levels, blood pressure monitoring, and thyroid function tests are essential before planning any dental procedure. Other tests such as complete blood count (CBC), vitamin D levels, any history of surgical intervention, and history of any allergic/adverse reactions due to any medications should be thoroughly investigated. Comprehensive medication review is also essential to rule out possible drug interactions during dental treatment.
- *Radiographic investigations*: Dental X-rays are important for a comprehensive view of the oral cavity before planning the treatment. They help in assessing the condition of teeth and the roots, in addition to investigating the condition of facial and jaw bones.
    - *Intraoral periapical radiograph (IOPA)*: These X-rays cover the complete tooth/few teeth including some regions below teeth. They are helpful in day-to-day practice and are usually taken during most dental treatments.
    - *Orthopantograms (OPGs)* are a type of dental X-ray that produces a wide panoramic scanning of upper and lower jaws including temporomandibular joint (TMJ). OPGs are used regularly in routine check-ups to monitor and assess the health of jaws and teeth, fractures, or infections, such as periodontal disease, and TMJ disorders. OPG can detect bone loss due to periodontal disease, which can eventually lead to tooth loss.
    - *Dental cone beam computed tomography (CBCT)* is a special type of X-ray equipment used when regular dental or facial X-rays are not sufficient. By providing detailed three-dimensional (3D) images of a patient's teeth, jaw, and surrounding structures, CBCT machines have transformed the way dental professionals approach diagnosis and treatment planning.
- *Environmental safety evaluation*: The elderly are at a considerably higher risk of experiencing fall injuries compared to younger age groups, attributed to age-related physical and cognitive changes, comorbidities, and polypharmacy which increase their susceptibility. In certain cases, where there is a history of dental fracture due to a fall injury, a home safety evaluation may be needed to prevent future injuries and recommend modifications.

The selection of specific investigations should be guided by the patient's dental history and clinical findings. A thorough and systematic investigation allows dental care providers to identify the problem and develop an appropriate treatment plan.

MANAGEMENT OF ORAL DISEASES

The management of oral diseases in the elderly involves a multifaceted approach aimed at understanding the age-related changes in the oral cavity, addressing underlying causes, and promoting overall well-being. It often requires a collaborative effort among healthcare professionals, caregivers, and the patient. An overview of the age-associated oral health changes which need to be considered before planning the treatment is given in the following text.

Age-related Orofacial Changes

Nutrition in Old Age and Its Implications for Oral Care

Adequate nutrition is a vital factor in promoting the health and well-being of the aged. Missing dentition and ill-fitting dentures cause difficulty in chewing and altered perception of taste. A compromised nutritional status, in turn, can further undermine the integrity of the oral cavity. Maintaining dental health may help prevent or delay the onset of frailty and improve the quality of life in aging individuals. Therefore, diet and nutrition should be considered as an integral part of the oral health assessment and treatment planning.

Age Changes in Oral Mucous Membrane

The oral mucosa performs essential protective functions that profoundly affect the general health and well-being of the host. A decline in the protective barrier of the oral mucosa leads to increased susceptibility to various pathological conditions such as candidal infections and a decreased rate of wound healing. The tongue is reported to show marked clinical changes and become smoother with the loss of filiform papillae.

Salivary Glands and Salivary Secretion with Aging

The diminished function of salivary gland is commonly associated with aging. The presence of saliva protects the oral cavity, upper airway, and digestive tract and facilitates numerous sensorimotor phenomena. The absence of saliva thus has many deleterious consequences on the host. The main oral health problems of old age, i.e., xerostomia (mouth dryness) and dental caries, have been attributed to the reduced salivary flow.

Alveolar Bone

Resorption of maxillary and mandibular bones is common in elderly due to loss of teeth. The jaw bones may appear knife-edge in shape due to resorption.

Temporomandibular Joint

There may be partial or complete disc displacement and disc degeneration associated with aging.

Tooth Structure

Age changes in the morphology of teeth have important clinical implications as these changes may influence the outcomes of the restorative treatments and have a great bearing on the reparative responses. The changes in the dentin, enamel, cementum, and pulp and the prevalence of attrition and cervical abrasion affecting the form of the tooth are common in elderly.

Periodontal Tissue

Periodontal diseases are among the most prevalent chronic conditions in dentate older populations. Changes in structure and function during aging may affect the host response to plaque microorganisms, increasing the rate of periodontal destruction, coupled with inflamed gingiva and changes in salivary gland secretions.

Prosthetic Considerations

There is a high prevalence (~40% in some populations) of edentulism among elderly. The treatment plan and the prognosis are influenced by various systemic and local factors as well as a person's previous experience with dentures. The most important determinants are debilitating diseases, neurophysiological changes which limit the person's capacity for acquiring new muscle activity patterns, and atrophy of the masticatory muscles which may reduce chewing efficiency and cannot be sufficiently improved through prosthetic treatment. Instead, it is important to advise the person on how to attain an adequate diet, i.e., easy to chew. Reduced salivary secretion or xerostomia is frequently a complicating factor in diabetic patients and other debilitating diseases, which results in rampant caries, loss of denture retention, traumatic lesions, and infections of the oral mucosa. Meticulous oral hygiene supplemented by mouthwashes with chlorhexidine and use of artificial salivary substitutes are important means to reduce complications to denture wearing in xerostomia. The success of prosthetic management in geriatric dentistry is determined by several factors such as the patient's degree of cooperation, the financial resources available for care, and the technical quality of prosthetic materials.

Other Factors Influencing Utilization of Dental Care

General health-related factors, sociodemographic factors (age, gender, place of residence, and culture), service-related factors (accessibility, availability of dental services, attitude of the dentist, cost factor, and quality of service provided), and subjective factors (personal beliefs, perceived need, dental fear, and anxiety) also affect the dental care provision.

DENTAL CARE IN ELDERLY

Although the elderly are retaining their dentition longer than in the past, dental morbidity and prevalence of dental diseases continue to be high. Despite the high burden of dental diseases, preventive protocols present the dental profession with many challenges. This may be because most of the current elderly were not introduced to the concept of preventive dentistry at a young age or are of the opinion that tooth loss is a normal part of the aging and is not preventable. Others have adapted to a compromised oral health status and seek treatment only when an emergency arises. Another challenge in providing restorative as well as preventive care for elderly people is to develop an appreciation of the need for regular care.

Primary Prevention

Oral Prophylaxis

Oral prophylaxis involves professional cleaning of the accumulated plaque and calculus with the use of devices in the clinical setup. It is advisable to visit the dentist once in 6 months for maintaining good oral care. At the same time, patients are advised to follow oral care routine with the use of soft toothbrush, application of light pressure, and modification of the brushing method. Rotary electric toothbrushes are advised in case of reduced manual dexterity, impaired vision, or due to physical limitations associated with conditions such as stroke, Parkinson's disease, or severe arthritis.

Mouth Rinses

A therapeutic rinse such as chlorhexidine mouthwash can be an adjunct for controlling plaque and calculus. This is especially important for patients with physical and mental disabilities. It also reduces oral mucositis and candidiasis in immune-suppressed patients such as those on intensive chemotherapy. Remineralizing fluoride rinses as well as varnish application with antibacterial action and enhanced remineralization property can be used in elderly who continually experience new carious lesions because of severe xerostomia. Patients with xerostomia should be encouraged to hydrate frequently, avoid alcohol and foods and drinks that contain sugar, and use over-the-counter saliva substitutes as needed. Topical antifungal therapies are effective for treating denture stomatitis and angular cheilitis caused by candidiasis. Using reminders and prompts for oral hygiene care is also advisable.

Denture Care

The elderly who wear dentures should be educated about proper home care of both dentures and the supportive oral tissues as well as the need for continued professional care. Use of nonabrasive denture cleaners and soaking dentures overnight is important to prevent denture stomatitis, and the tissues can be prevented from harm by avoiding wearing the denture while retiring for the night.

Counseling and Education

Empowering the patients about the best dental practices for optimal oral health is an essential part of clinical care. Well-informed patients are more likely to comply with treatment plans, dispel misconceptions, implement new behaviors to adapt to medical conditions and physical limitations, and prevent further deterioration of the condition in the future.

Other Considerations

Offering psychosocial and community support to address the fear of dental treatment and enhance self-confidence are integral components of dental care. Regular monitoring and follow-up should be established to track improvements and address new concerns.

Secondary Prevention

Strategies include those that detect the disease early and intervene to prevent its progression. This may include various restorative procedures carried out to halt the progress of caries and periodontal therapies to improve gum health. Dentistry for the elderly should not be considered as the palliative treatment of terminal oral disease. We must recognize that there are a range of clinical entities and multiple levels of prevention as well as treatment.

Tertiary Prevention

Strategies include those that reduce morbidity by restoring function and reducing disease-related complications. Tertiary prevention includes all measures for oral rehabilitation. This includes the replacement of lost teeth (dentures, dental crowns or bridges, and implants) and the complex treatment of oral cancer. It aims to prevent further deterioration and restore oral health if significant dental tissue loss occurs.

Management of worn dentition using fixed or removable prostheses is a common method to rehabilitate those elderly patients who lose several teeth, which if left untreated might decrease the vertical dimension of occlusion, leading to reduced mastication and aesthetic efficiency.

Dental implants are medical devices surgically implanted into the jaw to restore masticatory ability and aesthetics, providing support for crowns, bridges, or dentures. Evidence from the literature has shown that age alone should not be a limiting factor for dental implant therapy and that old age does not seem to represent a factor of major prognostic significance in treatment with dental implants. Treatment with implants can be considered safe and predictable with minimal complications for older as well as for younger patients.

In the elderly, most patients have TMJ degeneration, where the symptoms are mild and self-limiting. However, if left untreated, TMJ problems in the elderly limit jaw mobility and cause lockjaw, chronic headaches, difficulty in biting and chewing, frequent tinnitus or ringing, and neck/shoulder pain. In the few patients who are refractory to conservative treatment, arthrocentesis and TMJ replacement are also available.

Therefore, an appropriate and efficient treatment plan is necessary to restore the patient's comfort, function, aesthetics, good speech, and health of the stomatognathic system. The management of oral health in the elderly is an ongoing process, and individualized care plans should be tailored to each patient's unique needs. Collaboration between healthcare providers, therapists, family members, and the elderly individuals themselves is essential to create a safe and supportive environment that reduces the oral disease burden and promotes healthy aging **(Fig. 1)**.

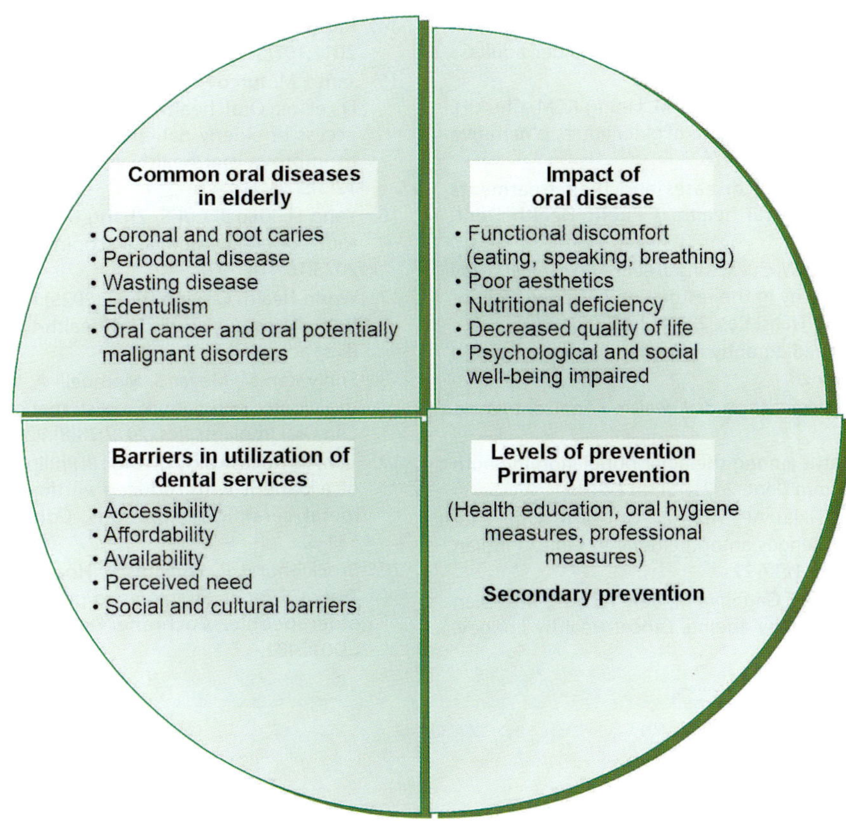

FIG. 1: Overview of oral health in elderly.
Source: https://edantseva.gov.in/

CONCLUSION

Oral health is an integral component of overall well-being in older adults, directly influencing nutrition, systemic health, and quality of life. The elderly face unique challenges due to age-related physiological changes, comorbidities, psychosocial barriers, and limited access to dental care. A comprehensive approach involving prevention, early diagnosis, and rehabilitation is essential for reducing the burden of oral diseases in this population. Strengthening awareness, integrating oral healthcare into general geriatric care, and adopting innovative service delivery models such as mobile clinics and teledentistry can help bridge existing gaps. Ultimately, collaborative efforts between healthcare providers, caregivers, policymakers, and the elderly themselves are crucial to promote healthy aging through improved oral health.

Self-Assessment Questionnaire

Q1. What is oral health?

Q2. What is geriatric dentistry?

Q3. How common are oral diseases in elderly?

Q4. What are the risk factors for oral diseases in elderly?

Q5. What are the oral health assessment tools?

Q6. Discuss oral health promotion in geriatric population.

FURTHER READINGS

1. Razak PA, Richard KM, Thankachan RP, Hafiz KA, Kumar KN, Sameer KM. Geriatric oral health: a review article. J Int Oral Health. 2014;6(6):110-6.
2. Batchelor P. The changing epidemiology of oral diseases in the elderly, their growing importance for care and how they can be managed. Age Ageing. 2015;44(6):1064-70.
3. Janto M, Iurcov R, Daina CM, Neculoiu DC, Venter AC, Badau D, et al. Oral health among elderly, impact on life quality, access of elderly patients to oral health services and methods to improve oral health: a narrative review. J Personal Med. 2022;12(3):372.
4. Murray Thomson W. Epidemiology of oral health conditions in older people. Gerodontology. 2014;31(Suppl 1):9-16.

5. Marchini L, Ettinger RL. The prevention, diagnosis, and treatment of rapid oral health deterioration (ROHD) among older adults. J Clin Med. 2023;12(7):2559.
6. Chan AKY, Tamrakar M, Jiang CM, Lo ECM, Leung KCM, Chu CH. Common medical and dental problems of older adults: a narrative review. Geriatrics (Basel). 2021;6(3):76.
7. Ghezzi EM, Ship JA. Systemic diseases and their treatments in the elderly: impact on oral health. J Public Health Dent. 2000;60(4):289-96.
8. Liu S, Wang S, Du Y, Zhang W, Cui X, Xing J, et al. The clinical study of CBCT imaging technology in the restoration of upper anterior teeth of the elderly. Am J Transl Res. 2021;13(6):7022-8.
9. Molander B. Panoramic radiography in dental diagnostics. Swed Dent J Suppl. 1996;119:1-26.
10. Ciancio SG. Medications' impact on oral health. J Am Dent Assoc. 2004;135(10):1440-8.
11. Salim R. Oral health status among the older population in South Kerala. J Oral Health Comm Dent. 2021;15(3):117-21.
12. Bharti R, Chandra A, Tikku AP, Arya D, Gupta R. Oral care needs, barriers and challenges among elderly in India. J Indian Prosthodont Soc. 2015;15(1):17-22.
13. Patel J, Wallace J, Doshi M, Gadanya M, Ben Yahya I, Roseman J, et al. Oral health for healthy ageing. Lancet Healthy Longev. 2021;2(8):e521-7.
14. Raphael C. Oral health and aging. Am J Public Health. 2017;107(S1):S44-5.
15. Janto M, Iurcov R, Daina CM, Neculoiu DC, Venter AC, Badau D, et al. Oral health among elderly, impact on life quality, access of elderly patients to oral health services and methods to improve oral health: a narrative review. J Pers Med. 2022; 12(3):372.
16. Yang H, Xiao J, Cui S, Zhang L, Chen L. Oral health assessment tools for elderly adults: a scoping review. J Multidiscip Healthc. 2023;16:4181-92.
17. World Health Organization. (2025). Oral health. [online] Available from: https://www.who.int/health-topics/oral-health#tab=tab_2. [Last accessed May, 2025].
18. Srinivasan M, Meyer S, Mombelli A, Müller F. Dental implants in the elderly population: a systematic review and meta-analysis. Clin Oral Implants Res. 2017;28(8):920-30.
19. Jain AR, Nallaswamy D, Ariga P, Philip JM. Full mouth rehabilitation of a patient with reduced vertical dimension using multiple metal ceramic restorations. Contemp Clin Dent. 2013;4(4): 531-5.
20. Brocklehurst P, Williams L, Hoare Z, Goodwin T, McKenna G, Tsakos G, et al. Strategies to prevent oral disease in dependent older people. Cochrane Database Syst Rev. 2019;2019(5): CD012402.

CHAPTER 9

Comprehensive Geriatric Assessment, Approach to Geriatric Patients

NN Prem, Anupa Pillai

CASE VIGNETTE

- An 85-year-old woman has uncontrolled hypertension on one blood pressure medication (185/80 mm Hg).
- Plan: Add a second blood pressure medication
- After 2 weeks, she had a fall.

INTRODUCTION

In 2010, 524 million individuals globally were aged 65 years or older. By the year 2050, the World Health Organization has predicted that 1.5 billion people will be 65 years or older. Nearly 80% of these older individuals will be living in low- and middle-income countries. In 2011, older persons constituted 8.6% of India's total population, equaling 103 million. This proportion is expected to increase exponentially and is projected to reach 19.5% in 2050, equaling 319 million people. This will have a tremendous impact on the global cancer burden. India is also witnessing a demographic transition.

"Geriatric syndrome" is a term that is often used to refer to common health conditions in older adults that do not fit into distinct organ-based disease categories and often have multifactorial causes. The list includes conditions such as cognitive impairment, delirium, incontinence, malnutrition, falls, gait disorders, pressure ulcers, sleep disorders, sensory deficits, fatigue, dizziness, and frailty. These conditions are common in older adults, and they may have a major impact on quality of life and disability. Geriatric syndromes can best be identified by a geriatric assessment.

ORIGIN OF COMPREHENSIVE GERIATRIC ASSESSMENT

- The emergence of a comprehensive geriatric assessment (CGA) as the best approach to the care of older persons was a critical milestone
- The idea that improving medical outcomes and quality of life in older persons requires a multidisciplinary approach
- The assessment cannot be limited to disease management that originated and developed in the UK healthcare system
- The operational idea that this complexity could be handled through a CGA was proposed by *Marjory Warren* in the late 1930s.

DEFINITION OF COMPREHENSIVE GERIATRIC ASSESSMENT

Comprehensive geriatric assessment is defined as a multidisciplinary diagnostic and treatment process that identifies medical, psychosocial, and functional limitations of a frail older person in order to develop a coordinated plan to maximize overall health with aging.

The healthcare of an older adult extends beyond the traditional medical management of illness. It requires evaluation of multiple issues, including physical, cognitive, affective, social, financial, environmental, and spiritual components that influence an older adult's health. CGA is based on the premise that a systematic evaluation of frail older persons by a team of health professionals may identify a variety of treatable medical and social problems and lead to better health outcomes.

The content of the assessment varies depending on different settings of care (e.g., home, clinic, hospital, and nursing home).

INDICATIONS FOR REFERRAL TO COMPREHENSIVE GERIATRIC ASSESSMENT

One must know whether the older adult is too fit or too sick to benefit from CGA.

The criteria could be:
- Age
- Medical comorbidities such as heart failure or cancer
- Psychosocial disorders such as depression or isolation
- Specific geriatric conditions such as dementia, falls, functional disability, or frailty
- Previous or predicted high healthcare utilization
- Consideration of change in living situation (e.g., from independent living to assisted living, nursing home, or in-home caregivers)

Multidisciplinary Team

The CGA multidisciplinary team may include:
- Medical, e.g., geriatrician, psychiatry of old age, palliative care specialist
- Nursing
- Medical social worker
- Physiotherapy
- Occupational therapy
- Speech and language therapy
- Dietetics
- Pharmacists
- Podiatry

Framework

The overall care rendered by CGA teams providing longitudinal assessment and care can be divided into six steps:
1. Data gathering
2. Discussion among the team increasingly including the patient and/or caregiver as a member of the team
3. Development, with the patient and/or caregiver, of a treatment plan
4. Implementation of the treatment plan
5. Monitoring response to the treatment plan
6. Revising the treatment plan

Each of these steps is essential if the process is to be successful at achieving maximal health and functional benefits. However, monitoring response and revising the treatment plan may be left to primary care providers if the model relies on a single consultation.

MODELS OF COMPREHENSIVE GERIATRIC ASSESSMENT

- Postdischarge assessment due to the pressure to decrease lengths of hospital stay and reduce readmissions.
- Early CGA programs focused on restorative or rehabilitative goals (tertiary prevention)
- Newer programs are aimed at primary and secondary prevention.

PRINCIPLES OF COMPREHENSIVE GERIATRIC ASSESSMENT

- *Goal*: Promote wellness, independence
- *Focus*: Function, performance (gait, balance, transfers)
- *Scope*: Physical, cognitive, psychological, social domains **(Table 1 and Fig. 1)**
- *Approach*: Multidisciplinary
- *Efficiency*: Ability to perform rapid screens to identify target areas
- *Success*: Maintaining or improving quality of life

TABLE 1: Domains and assessment tools used in comprehensive geriatric assessment.

Domain	Subdomain	Tests
Physical	• Functional status • Nutrition • Vision hearing	ADL, IADL, TUG, MNA
Cognition	Dementia, MCI	Mini-cog, HMSE
Psychological	Depression	GDS
Social	Support system	Caregiver, socioeconomic, advance directives

(ADL: activities of daily living; GDS: Geriatric Depression Scale; HMSE: Hindi Mental State Examination; IADL: instrumental activities of daily living; MCI: mild cognitive impairment; MNA: Mini Nutritional Assessment; TUG: timed up and go test)

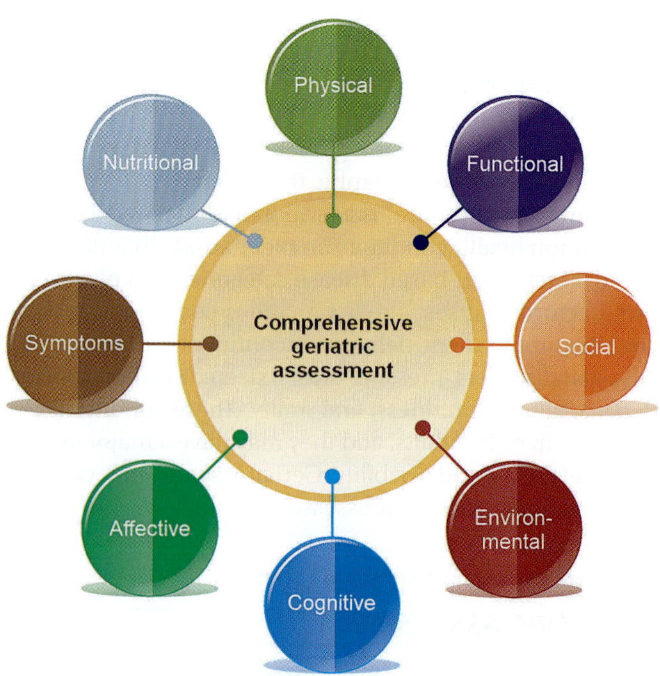

FIG. 1: Domains of comprehensive geriatric assessment.

DIMENSIONS OF GERIATRIC ASSESSMENT

The four main dimensions covered in a CGA should include: (1) physical, (2) functional, (3) psychological, and (4) social assessment, as given in **Box 1**.

BENEFITS OF COMPREHENSIVE GERIATRIC ASSESSMENT

The benefits of CGA, in comparison to less-structured multidisciplinary assessment, where each discipline approaches the patient's assessment and plan of care in isolation, include the following:
- Improves diagnostic accuracy
- Optimizes medical and rehabilitation treatment
- Enhances health and functional outcomes
- Informs the development of individualized care plans
- Assists in avoiding the potential complications of hospitalization
- Facilitates effective discharge planning

GOALS OF CARE

- *To improve process of care*:
  - Improve diagnostic accuracy
  - Improve medical treatment
  - Arrange for long-term case management
- *To improve outcomes of care*:
  - Improve functional status
  - Better quality of life

BOX 1 Four dimensions of geriatric assessment.

1. *Physical assessment*:
   - Presenting complaint
   - Past medical history
   - Medication reconciliation and review
   - Nutritional status
   - Alcohol
   - Immunization status
   - Advanced directives
2. *Psychological assessment*:
   - Cognition and mood
3. *Functional assessment*:
   - Activities of daily living
   - Balance
   - Mobility
4. *Social assessment*:
   - Living arrangements
   - Social support
   - Carer stress
   - Financial circumstances
   - Living environment

- *To contain costs of care*:
  - Reduce use of unnecessary formal services
  - Prolong tenure in the home/community

COMPREHENSIVE GERIATRIC ASSESSMENT IN DIFFERENT SETTINGS

Comprehensive Geriatric Assessment in Hospitals

- Comprehensive geriatric assessment is commonly divided into two types:
  i. *Geriatric evaluation and management units (GEMUs) or acute care for elders (ACE)*:
     a. Delivered by a team in a discrete ward
     b. With control over the delivery of the multidisciplinary team recommendations
  ii. *Inpatient geriatric consultation service (IGCS)*:
     a. A multidisciplinary team will assess patients.
     b. Deliver recommendations to the general physicians or internists
- The number of randomized controlled trials (RCTs) has shown GEMUs/ACEs associated with:
  - *Greater functional independence* at discharge
  - *Less frequent* institutionalization
  - Shorter and *less expensive hospitalization*
  - *Higher satisfaction* rate among patients, family members, physicians, and nurses

Mobile Acute Care of the Elderly

- Mobile services which incorporate the principles of CGA
- Deliver them to patients who are not on dedicated wards for older inpatients
- Similar to already existing inpatient geriatric consultation team
- But these teams attempt to overcome the key limitation of peripatetic geriatric assessment care:
  - Tendency not to implement the recommendations
- Delivering care directly on wards which do not normally provide such care

Comprehensive Geriatric Assessment in Emergency Department

- Emergency department (ED) will face increasingly high numbers of older people in the future with complex comorbidities.
- *The idea*:
  - Deliver CGA close to the point of presentation with acute illness
- *Achieved in a number of ways*:
  - Enhancing the ED team:
    - Placing specially trained nursing staff (advanced nurse practitioners)

    - Bringing the geriatric medicine team into the assessment process either during or after ED attendance and embedding CGA service
  - Creation of a dedicated physical environment for patents requiring CGA in the ED setting
- *ED-based CGA may*:
  - Reduce admissions to acute wards and the intensive care unit (ICU)
  - Increase referrals to palliative and hospice care
  - Increase patient satisfaction
  - Slow the decrease in functional status

Comprehensive Geriatric Assessment in Surgical Care

- Aging populations are at an increased risk of postoperative complications
- *CGA in surgical care has been described through*:
  - The use of *preoperative protocols*
  - Surgical patients in the ACE unit service
  - Delivering CGA for older patients requiring abdominal surgery
  - Multidisciplinary geriatric consultation team for older hip fracture patients
- *Reported effects*:
  - Improved function
  - Reduction in delirium
  - Reduction in falls and bed sores

Comprehensive Geriatric Assessment in Oncology

Comprehensive geriatric assessment is able to:

- Detect problems not found by routine examinations in the initial evaluation
- Assist in cancer treatment decisions
- *Predict complications and side effects from treatment*:
  - Chemotherapy-related toxicity
  - Tolerance of chemotherapy
  - Outcome in surgical oncology
  - Identification and treatment of new problems during follow-up care
- Estimate survival
- Improving functional status and quality of life (in primary care, medical and surgical clinics and wards, long-term care rehabilitation facilities and nursing homes, hospice, and palliative care networks)
- Improving the early identification of palliative care needs
- Reducing mortality (in outpatient care of surgical area, ED, and nursing homes)
- Reducing hospitalization (from nursing homes, hospice, and palliative care network)
- Reducing access rate to ED (in primary care setting and after discharge from the hospital medical wards)
- Reducing the length of hospital stay (in a surgical hospital setting)
- Optimizing postdischarge management pathways (in medical and surgical hospital setting)
- Improving medications appropriateness (in primary care, medical hospital setting, and nursing homes)
- Reducing postoperative complications (in surgical outpatient and hospital settings)
- Minimizing use of physical restraints (in medical hospital setting and nursing homes)

CASE AFTER COMPREHENSIVE GERIATRIC ASSESSMENT

An 85-year-old woman has uncontrolled hypertension on one blood pressure medication.

- Lives alone (daughter will help with medications)
- Gait and balance abnormality (home therapy)
- Osteoporosis (treated)
- Mild memory impairment (evaluated for dementia)
- Incontinent of urine (treated)
- Vision impairment (fix or find glasses, ophthalmology appointment)
- Over-the-counter (OTC) medications (discard)
- Difficulty with cleaning [home occupational therapy evaluation (OT-eval) for fall risk]

CONCLUSION

Caring for older adults is not just about treating illnesses , it is about understanding the whole person. Comprehensive Geriatric Assessment (CGA) recognizes that every older individual has unique physical, emotional, social, and functional needs. By bringing together different specialists and looking beyond diseases, CGA helps uncover hidden problems, prevents complications, and ensures that care plans are truly meaningful to the person's life. More than a checklist, it is a process that respects dignity, promotes independence, and supports families in their caregiving role. As populations age, especially in countries like India, the role of CGA will only become more vital. Its ultimate goal is to help older adults live healthier, safer, and more fulfilling lives.

Self-Assessment Questionnaire

Q1. What is meant by a comprehensive geriatric assessment (CGA), and how does it differ from a routine medical evaluation?

Q2. Which four major dimensions are included in a CGA, and what key elements are assessed in each?

Q3. Who are the essential members of a multidisciplinary CGA team, and what is the role of each in the assessment process?

Q4. What are the six key steps in the CGA framework, and why is it important to include the patient and caregiver in the process?

Q5. How does CGA improve diagnostic accuracy, treatment outcomes, and quality of life in older adults compared to standard care?

Q6. What are the common indications for referring an elderly person for CGA, and how can clinicians identify those who will benefit most?

Q7. How is CGA adapted for use in different healthcare settings such as hospitals, emergency departments, surgical care, and oncology?

Q8. Discuss the evidence supporting the benefits of GEMUs/ACE units compared to inpatient geriatric consultation services.

Q9. Reflect on the case vignette: How did applying CGA change the management plan for the 85-year-old woman with hypertension, and what lessons can be learned from this example?

FURTHER READINGS

1. Ellis G, Gardner M, Tsiachristas A, Langhorne P, Burke O, et al. Comprehensive geriatric assessment for older adults admitted to hospital. Cochrane Database Syst Rev. 2017;9(9):CD006211.
2. Pilotto A, Cella A, Pilotto A, Daragjati J, Veronese N, Musacchio C, et al. Comprehensive geriatric assessment in primary care settings: A case series. Eur Geriatr Med. 2017;8(5-6):395-400.
3. Rubenstein LZ, Stuck AE, Siu AL, Wieland D. Impacts of geriatric evaluation and management programs on defined outcomes: Overview of the evidence. J Am Geriatr Soc. 1991;39(9 Pt 2): 8S-16S.
4. Stuck AE, Siu AL, Wieland GD, Adams J, Rubenstein LZ. Comprehensive geriatric assessment: A meta-analysis of controlled trials. The Lancet. 1993;342(8878):1032-6.
5. The American Geriatrics Society. Comprehensive geriatric assessment toolkit for primary care physicians. New York: American Geriatrics Society. 2018.

CHAPTER 10

Government Schemes for Senior Citizens

Saumyarup Pal, Rashi Jain

INTRODUCTION

India, with its rich cultural heritage and demographic diversity, stands at the cusp of a significant transformation—the rapid aging of its population. As medical advancements extend life expectancies and fertility rates decline, the proportion of senior citizens is increasing at an unprecedented rate. This demographic shift presents both opportunities and challenges, particularly in ensuring the well-being and dignity of the elderly.

Recognizing the critical need to support this growing segment of the population, the Indian government has implemented a range of schemes and programs aimed at addressing the unique needs of senior citizens. These initiatives span various domains, including financial security, healthcare, social inclusion, and legal protection, reflecting a comprehensive approach to fostering a supportive environment for the elderly.

This chapter delves into the myriad government schemes designed for senior citizens in India, exploring their objectives, implementation mechanisms, and impact. By examining these initiatives, we gain insight into how the nation is preparing for its demographic future, ensuring that the aging population can lead fulfilling, independent, and secure lives. Through a detailed analysis, this chapter also highlights the successes and areas for improvement in the current frame.

TRENDS AND DIMENSIONS OF SENIOR CARE IN INDIA: POPULATION AGING AND SOCIETAL IMPACT

India is undergoing a profound demographic transition, with its elderly population projected to rise sharply in the coming decades. Currently, 12.8% of the population is above 60 years, and this share is expected to nearly double by 2050. The Longitudinal Ageing Study in India (LASI), a pioneering survey led by IIPS, Harvard, USC, and the Ministry of Health and Family Welfare, provides critical insights into the health, economic, and social dimensions of aging. The study shows that population aging is not only a healthcare challenge but also a societal shift with deep economic, cultural, and policy implications.

Health and Functional Challenges

Elderly health patterns are shifting from infectious diseases to noncommunicable diseases (NCDs) such as diabetes, hypertension, and cardiovascular illness. Nearly 75% of seniors suffer from at least one chronic condition, while 23% face multimorbidity, complicating care. Functional decline is widespread, with 24% reporting difficulties in daily living and over 48% struggling with instrumental tasks. Mobility restrictions affect more than half, but fewer than half use supportive devices, reflecting gaps in accessibility. Mental health burdens are equally significant—20% experience psychological issues, and one in three elders report depressive symptoms, often undiagnosed.

Nutrition and preventive care remain neglected. Over 27% of the elderly are underweight, while obesity is rising in urban areas. Adult immunization, though critical in preventing infectious diseases such as pneumonia and influenza, is largely absent from public health agendas. Additionally, climate change has intensified risks, with 31,000 heat-related elderly deaths recorded in 2018, underscoring seniors' vulnerability to environmental stressors.

Social Dimensions and Vulnerabilities

India's aging population is marked by strong gender and rural-urban divides. Women live longer but face higher rates of widowhood, poverty, and social isolation—54% of elderly women are widows, and many live alone with minimal support. Rural areas host 71% of the elderly, but infrastructure gaps, poor access to healthcare, and limited social security deepen inequalities. Social participation declines with age, and nearly 32% report low life satisfaction, exacerbated by financial dependency and family neglect. Elder abuse—reported by 5% of seniors, mostly at the hands of close relatives—remains an under-addressed issue.

Literacy and awareness gaps add to social exclusion. More than 55% of elderly Indians are illiterate, and knowledge of government schemes remains low, with only 28% aware of any entitlements. This lack of empowerment limits their ability to claim rights or access benefits.

Economic Implications

Population aging is reshaping India's economy, creating both challenges and opportunities. With 70% of seniors financially dependent on family and 78% lacking pension coverage, financial insecurity is widespread. Healthcare costs already consume a large share of elderly household expenditure, often pushing families into debt. At the same time, the "silver economy"—estimated at USD 7 billion and expanding rapidly—offers opportunities for innovation in health technology, home care, and insurance markets. However, elderly financial literacy is low, and risks of fraud and financial abuse are growing, particularly for socially isolated seniors.

Digital and Societal Transitions

The digital divide reinforces exclusion—85.8% of the elderly are digitally illiterate, with women and rural populations at greatest disadvantage. While health-tech and telemedicine are expanding, seniors often lack the skills or devices to benefit. Yet, digital healthcare, assistive devices, and teleconsultations could play a transformative role in senior care if access barriers are addressed.

SOCIETAL IMPACT AND WAY FORWARD

Population aging has wide societal implications. Rising dependency ratios will strain families and the working-age population. Changing family structures, with a shift to nuclear households, reduces traditional caregiving support, leaving many seniors vulnerable to isolation and neglect. Without robust social security, inclusive health systems, and age-friendly infrastructure, the burden of aging could intensify socioeconomic inequalities.

At the same time, seniors represent a vital social and economic resource. Harnessing the silver economy, strengthening community care models, expanding social security, and bridging digital divides can turn aging into an opportunity rather than a burden. Policies must emphasize integrated healthcare, social empowerment, financial inclusion, and digital literacy, alongside building resilience to climate and economic shocks.

In conclusion, aging in India is not merely a demographic phenomenon but a societal transition that will shape the country's future. Ensuring that seniors live healthy, dignified, and engaged lives require intersectoral collaboration, inclusive policies, and recognition of aging as a collective responsibility.

STRATEGIES OF INDIAN GOVERNMENT

Health Empowerment and Inclusion

- *Tailored service delivery*: A model for healthy and active aging in India should prioritize the independence and health of the elderly, requiring a customized service plan based on their needs and preferences.
- *Healthcare needs assessment*: Trained health workers should conduct standardized assessments covering basic health status, medical history, risk assessment, nutritional needs, functionality, continuity, personal goals, and expectations.
- *Integrated healthcare ecosystem*: The government should develop a comprehensive healthcare system focusing on health literacy, primary healthcare services, tele-consultations, healthcare infrastructure, skilled workforce, and accessibility of services. The geriatric healthcare structure in India consists of three National Centre for Ageing (NCA) at the central level, followed by various points of care at regional, district, community, primary, and subcenter levels. This hierarchy includes NCA (3), regional geriatric centers (18), district hospitals (718), community health centers (4869), primary health centers (18407), and sub-centers (90719). Under the Government of India's National Programme for the Health Care of the Elderly, there's a comprehensive healthcare package for the elderly encompassing several service areas. These areas include nutritional assessment, mental health assessment, management of NCDs such as hypertension and diabetes, oral assessment, ophthalmic assessment, and cardiovascular risk assessment. Nutritional assessment involves screening using a Geriatric Assessment Tool and

Mini-Nutritional Assessment Scale. Mental health assessment includes screening for mental health disorders. NCD management covers screening, management, and follow-up of hypertension and diabetes. Oral assessment includes oral care examination, screening for dental caries, and assisted oral care. Ophthalmic assessment involves visual acuity testing, near vision testing, and screening for cataracts. Cardiovascular risk assessment includes history taking regarding smoking and alcohol, along with health education to prevent cardiovascular diseases.

- *Promoting health literacy*: Initiatives to enhance understanding of geriatric health issues and available healthcare programs among seniors and caregivers, utilizing plain language and digital technology for education.
- *Strengthening primary healthcare*: Enhancing Ayushman Bharat centers to screen and manage age-specific disorders, with packages for fall prevention, women's health, and psychosocial support.
- *Expanding tele-consultation services*: Broadening telemedicine coverage for seniors through outreach efforts, home-based care, and accessible platforms.
- *Healthcare infrastructure enhancement*: Developing frameworks for senior care facilities, integrating geriatric healthcare into existing infrastructure, and ensuring specialized provisions for seniors.
- *Skilled workforce development*: Training healthcare professionals in geriatrics, incorporating geriatric competencies into curricula, and creating new workforce cadres for senior care. In India, the demand for skilled workers in elderly care is increasing, prompting the availability of various certification courses. Institutions such as All India Institute of Medical Sciences (AIIMS) New Delhi, Christian Medical College (CMC) Vellore, and others offer Doctor of Medicine (MD) in Geriatrics. Numerous institutions also offer postgraduate diplomas and fellowships in geriatrics, such as CMC Vellore and Indira Gandhi National Open University (IGNOU). The curriculum for these courses includes topics such as gerontology, public policy, clinical geriatrics, psychology, and counseling. Despite the availability of these specialized programs, geriatrics has limited representation in family medicine and public health courses. Undergraduate medical education includes minimal formal training in geriatrics, typically just 1–2 weeks.

  For nursing, the Graduate Nursing Bachelor of Science in Nursing (BSc Nursing) and Post Basic BSc Nursing curriculum includes medical-surgical nursing for adults and a 1-year postbasic diploma in Gerontological Nursing, as per the guidelines of the Indian Nursing Council (INC). CMC Vellore, AIIMS, and Manipal College of Nursing integrate medical-surgical nursing into their graduate nursing programs, focusing on adult and elderly care.

  The National Institute of Social Defence (NISD) offers a Certificate Course in Geriatric Care (6 months), which trains individuals to provide hands-on care for the elderly. HelpAge India provides short-term caregiver training programs focusing on elderly care in home or institutional settings, covering dementia care, hygiene, and nutrition. Annamalai University and other institutions offer distance education programs such as a Postgraduate Diploma in Gerontology or related fields. IGNOU offers a Certificate in Geriatric Health and Care (CGHC) starting from the July 2025 session.
- *Increasing service accessibility*: Strengthening home-based care with regulatory provisions, operationalizing Poshan Abhiyan for seniors, improving mental health services, and ensuring emergency response infrastructure.
- *Technology integration*: Leveraging technology for health services accessibility, including assistive devices, smart monitoring, and virtual assistants.
- *Rehabilitation services enhancement*: Improving rehabilitation infrastructure and capacity building for physiotherapy and palliative care.
- *Incentivizing preventive health*: Encouraging periodic screenings, elder immunizations, Ayush practices integration, and promoting healthy lifestyles.
- *Research strengthening*: Establishing a national senior care resource center, robust data repositories, and research institutions for geriatric healthcare knowledge enhancement.
- *Data repository establishment*: Creating repositories for age-specific health issues, NCDs screening, management, and out-of-pocket expenditure (OOPE) data.
- *Promoting healthy lifestyles*: Encouraging physical activities, yoga, ayurvedic diets, and nutritious eating habits for seniors.
- *Evidence-based policy formulation*: Utilizing research and data repositories to formulate evidence-based strategies and policies for senior care.
- *Continued education and training*: Implementing ongoing capacity building programs for healthcare providers and family caregivers on identifying early signs of geriatric health issues.
- *Community outreach programs*: Increasing awareness of mental health conditions and regular mental health check-ups among the elderly through community outreach initiatives.

- *Senior-specific vaccination programs*: Strengthening immunization programs for preventable diseases among the elderly, in line with recommendations from leading medical societies.
- *Integrating Ayush practices*: Integrating ayurvedic and other traditional Indian medical practices into conventional healthcare systems to promote wellness and disease prevention among seniors.

Efforts to be Made in Social Domain

- *Comprehensive social support system*: Government efforts should focus on creating an integrated system to socially include seniors, addressing socioeconomic barriers to welfare scheme utilization.
- *Social needs assessment*: Assessments should cover patient demographics, family and caregiver situations, daily living activities, social interactions, and awareness levels to tailor support strategies.
- *Awareness initiatives*: Sensitizing communities about elderly needs and legal safeguards through workshops, legal clinics, and online orientations can enhance social inclusion.
- *Peer support groups*: Establishing peer support groups and self-help models can provide emotional and social support for seniors, addressing various needs such as mental health, livelihoods, and advocacy.
- *Legal reforms*: Strengthening welfare acts and maintenance laws to protect seniors from abuse and abandonment, expedite case disposal, and ensure access to legal aid are crucial.
- *Elderly-friendly housing reforms*: Developing regulatory frameworks, quality standards, model by-laws, and care facilities accreditation can improve living conditions for seniors.
- *Community-based care services*: Supporting informal caregiving and enabling home-based services can facilitate "aging in place," ensuring seniors receive care within their communities.
- *Centralized portal for senior care*: A national portal can streamline access to services, provide information, training modules for caregivers, and offer grievance redressal mechanisms.
- *Promotion of care economy*: Recognizing and supporting care workers, particularly women, through rights protection, skilling programs, and regulatory oversight can enhance the senior care sector.
- *Enhancing awareness of legal safeguards*: Informing seniors about their rights and available welfare schemes can empower them to access necessary support services.
- *Peer support networks*: Establishing platforms for seniors to share experiences and support each other can foster a sense of community and mutual assistance.
- *Strengthening legal protections*: Improving laws and regulations to safeguard seniors from abuse, neglect, and financial exploitation is essential for their social inclusion and protection.
- *Improving housing accessibility*: Creating more elder-friendly housing options and ensuring accessibility standards are met can enhance seniors' quality of life.
- *Empowering community care*: Investing in community-based care programs and support services can help seniors remain independent and engaged within their communities.
- *Facilitating access to resources*: Developing centralized platforms and services can streamline access to information, resources, and support networks for seniors and their caregivers.
- *Advocating for care workers*: Supporting the rights and welfare of care workers is crucial for maintaining high-quality care standards and ensuring seniors receive adequate support.
- *Promoting social inclusion*: Implementing initiatives to combat social isolation and promote active participation in community life can improve seniors' overall well-being.
- *Creating supportive environments*: Designing public spaces and communities with seniors' needs in mind can enhance their mobility, safety, and sense of belonging.
- *Strengthening community networks*: Building strong community networks and partnerships can facilitate the delivery of comprehensive support services to seniors.
- *Promoting lifelong learning*: Providing opportunities for seniors to engage in lifelong learning activities can promote social inclusion and cognitive well-being.

Economic Domain

- *Financial needs assessment*: Evaluating work status, financial independence, and insurance penetration among seniors is crucial to understand their economic needs.
- *Reskilling initiatives*: Introducing age-friendly labor markets, incentivizing employment, and supporting reskilling in tech-based roles can enhance elderly employment opportunities.
- *Public funds and infrastructure*: Increasing coverage of schemes like PMJAY and extending pension support to the unorganized sector can improve financial security for seniors.
- *Mandatory savings plans*: Implementing regulatory mechanisms for viable interest rates on senior

citizen deposits can ensure sustainable income for retirees.

- *Geriatric health insurance*: Encouraging the private sector to develop comprehensive insurance products for seniors covering various health services can alleviate financial burdens.
- *Liquidity and capital allocation*: Reassessing the reverse mortgage mechanism and tax reforms can increase liquidity for seniors and support the senior care industry.
- *Protection from financial fraud*: Raising awareness about financial fraud and ensuring accessibility to safeguards and redressal mechanisms are essential to protect seniors from exploitation.
- *Incentives for senior-owned businesses*: Providing financial incentives and tax benefits to senior-owned businesses can promote economic independence among the elderly.
- *Enhanced pension schemes*: Reforming pension schemes to adapt to inflation and increasing coverage for nonmedical needs can improve financial stability for seniors.
- *Encouraging private sector engagement*: Engaging the private sector and leveraging corporate social responsibility (CSR) avenues are essential strategies for enhancing eldercare comprehensively and efficiently. This approach not only fosters economic development and job creation but also ensures the well-being of the elderly population. Private sector involvement can encompass adding new capacity, augmenting existing services, and addressing areas with limited public facilities. Incentivizing private sector participation through strengthened public-private partnerships (PPPs) and channeling CSR funds toward elderly care initiatives can significantly impact the senior care ecosystem. Opportunities for private sector engagement include establishing elder care homes, sponsoring mobile medical units, developing insurance products tailored for seniors, organizing health camps, deploying technology-enabled care solutions, sponsoring skill-building programs, and launching advocacy campaigns. Furthermore, fostering innovations through incubation support and seeking patient capital can further enhance the senior care landscape. Overall, embracing private sector collaboration and CSR initiatives is pivotal for achieving comprehensive eldercare solutions.

Digital Domain

Efforts to ensure digital empowerment and inclusion in the Indian senior care ecosystem involve providing digital devices, internet connectivity, and digital literacy training to seniors by governments, private companies, and nonprofit organizations. Interventions aim to address digital literacy levels and penetration among seniors, ensuring they are not left behind in the digital age. Priority areas include improving access to affordable digital devices, increasing digital literacy through targeted campaigns and workshops, and harnessing modern technology such as artificial intelligence and the internet of things to streamline routine procedures in senior care. Additionally, support for startups and entrepreneurship in the senior care space is crucial for creating a digital-ready workforce and promoting digital transformation in elderly care.

SCHEMES, PROGRAMS, AND ACTIVITIES OF MINISTRIES AND VARIOUS DEPARTMENTS OF THE GOVERNMENT OF INDIA FOR THE WELFARE OF THE SENIOR CITIZENS

Ministry of Social Justice and Empowerment

Atal Vayo Abhyudaya Yojana

The Atal Vayo Abhyudaya Yojana (AVYAY), formerly known as the National Action Plan for Senior Citizens (NAPSrC), stands as a testament to India's commitment to ensuring the well-being and dignity of its elderly population. AVYAY, serving as a comprehensive framework, has been operational since April 1, 2021, encompassing various schemes such as the Integrated Program for Senior Citizens (IPSrC), State Action Plan for Senior Citizens (SAPSrC), Rashtriya Vayoshri Yojana (RVY), National Helpline (Elderline), and Senior Care Ageing Growth Engine (SAGE) aimed at promoting the silver economy. The funding sources for these schemes vary, with some being supported by the Budget and others by the Senior Citizens' Welfare Fund (SCWF). With a rapidly aging demographic, it has become imperative for nations to formulate comprehensive plans to address the unique needs and challenges faced by seniors. AVYAY is structured to address the four fundamental pillars of senior citizens' well-being—financial security, access to food, healthcare facilities, and opportunities for social engagement and dignity. Recognizing the vulnerability of elderly individuals, especially those from economically disadvantaged backgrounds, AVYAY also extends its ambit to encompass matters related to seniors' safety, protection, and awareness generation within society.

Objectives and initiatives: The primary objective of AVYAY is to ensure that senior citizens lead fulfilling and dignified lives during their golden years. To achieve this, the scheme has delineated several key initiatives:

- *Financial security*: AVYAY aims to provide seniors with financial stability through various measures such as pensions, subsidies, and welfare programs. By alleviating financial burdens, the scheme enables seniors to meet their basic needs and maintain a decent standard of living.
- *Access to healthcare*: Under AVYAY, seniors are entitled to comprehensive healthcare services, including preventive care, treatment, and rehabilitation. The scheme emphasizes the importance of affordable and accessible healthcare, particularly for elderly individuals with chronic conditions or disabilities.
- *Social interaction and dignity*: AVYAY recognizes the significance of social engagement in enhancing seniors' overall well-being. It promotes initiatives that foster community participation, recreational activities, and intergenerational bonding. By facilitating opportunities for seniors to remain active and connected, AVYAY promotes a sense of dignity and belonging.
- *Safety and awareness*: AVYAY prioritizes the safety and protection of senior citizens by implementing measures to prevent abuse, exploitation, and neglect. Additionally, the scheme focuses on raising awareness about seniors' rights, entitlements, and available support services. Through education and outreach programs, AVYAY endeavors to create a society that values and respects its elderly population.

Scheme of Integrated Program for Senior Citizens

The IPSrC has its roots in the National Policy on Older Persons (NPOP) introduced by the Government of India in 1999. This policy aimed to address the various challenges faced by the aging population and ensure their well-being and social integration. Subsequently, the IPSrC was launched as a comprehensive program under the Ministry of Social Justice and Empowerment to implement the objectives outlined in the NPOP. The IPSrC focuses on providing essential services such as healthcare, financial assistance, social security, and recreational activities to senior citizens. Over the years, the scheme has undergone several revisions and expansions to adapt to the changing needs of the elderly population and improve its effectiveness in promoting their welfare. Today, the IPSrC continues to play a crucial role in supporting and empowering senior citizens.

The following projects are eligible for assistance under the IPSRC:

- Support for the maintenance of senior citizens homes (SrCHs) catering to 25 beneficiaries, providing essential services such as food, care, and shelter for at least 25 indigent Senior Citizens.
- Support for the maintenance of senior citizens' homes accommodating 50 beneficiaries, offering food, care, and shelter for a minimum of 50 indigent Senior Citizens, either male only or a combination of male and female residents.
- Support for the maintenance of SrCHs specifically for 50 elderly women, recognizing the heightened vulnerability of older single women to poverty and economic crises.
- Support for the maintenance of continuous care homes and homes for senior citizens suffering from Alzheimer's disease or dementia, catering to a minimum of 20 seriously ill senior citizens requiring continuous nursing care or those afflicted with Alzheimer's disease or dementia.
- Support for the maintenance of Regional Resource and Training Centres (RRTCs), which act as key agencies for aged care coordination and technical support under the oversight of the Department of Social Justice and Empowerment. Their responsibilities include mentoring SrCHs, advocacy, stakeholder training, database management, inspections, and liaison with relevant state governments.
- Support for the maintenance of mobile medicare units (MMU) and physiotherapy clinics for senior citizens, with ongoing projects being continued under the IPSRC. However, no new MMUs will receive support under the scheme.

Also, the Department of Social Justice and Empowerment has established norms concerning old age homes, covering aspects such as land, living space, facilities, and operational standards encompassing nutrition, medical care, recreation, security, clothing, accommodation, hygiene, and sanitation.

State Action Plan for Senior Citizens

Financial assistance is allocated to states/UTs for undertaking state-specific initiatives aimed at the well-being of senior citizens. This assistance is disbursed based on the requests submitted by the respective states/UTs along with the necessary documentation. SAPSrC, initiated in the fiscal year 2019–20, facilitates funding for various endeavors, including the following:

- *Operation of MMU for senior citizens*: These units deliver medical services to elderly individuals residing in remote, rural, and underserved areas lacking proper healthcare facilities. Grants are directed toward district-level hospitals in aspirational districts to enhance healthcare provisions in these underserved regions. The objective is to empower senior citizens to actively engage in maintaining and enhancing their health, with each unit expected to cater to a minimum of 400 seniors monthly, making at least 10 trips per month.

- *Establishment of physiotherapy clinics for senior citizens*: Financial support is extended to agencies with a credible track record in senior citizen welfare for running physiotherapy clinics, catering to a minimum of 50 seniors monthly, exclusively in government district hospitals.
- *Training of geriatric caregivers*: Grants are allocated to agencies with a strong history in healthcare, particularly geriatric care, to provide training for a pool of geriatric caregivers or offer bedside assistance to elderly individuals in need.
- *Special campaigns for cataract surgeries*: The senior citizens rural outreach program for cataract surgery aims to support the national program for control of blindness by organizing special drives for cataract surgeries, especially considering the increasing prevalence of cataract blindness among the senior population. These surgeries are conducted annually in all districts, ensuring that each district progresses toward becoming cataract-blindness free for seniors, with free surgeries provided to senior citizen below the poverty line (BPL) cardholders.
- *State-specific welfare initiatives*: States/UTs are encouraged to allocate approximately 20% of their funds for innovative programs catering to the welfare of indigent senior citizens within their jurisdiction.

Senior Care Aging Growth Engine—Advancing Silver Economy

To inspire young minds to address elderly issues and devise innovative solutions for elderly care, fostering their development into startups with equity support, not exceeding 49%, managed by Industrial Finance Corporation of India (IFCI) Venture Capital Ltd. on behalf of the Ministry. Each chosen startup receives a maximum equity share of 1 crore.

Utilizing CSR Funds for Elderly Care

This initiative aims to efficiently direct CSR funding toward projects related to elderly care, such as establishing old age homes, daycare centers, and similar facilities for senior citizens, in accordance with Schedule VII of Section 135 of the Companies Act.

Scheme for Awareness Generation and Capacity Building for Senior Citizens' Welfare

This scheme encompasses various components such as the national helpline for senior citizens, research endeavors, awareness campaigns, and sensitization programs aimed at educating both the youth and other segments of society about issues concerning the elderly.

National helpline: Launched on October 1, 2021, the National Helpline for Senior Citizens, accessible via toll-free number 14567, offers free information, guidance, emotional support, and field intervention in abuse cases, enhancing the overall well-being of senior citizens. Operational from 8 am to 8 pm every day, Elderline is managed by the NISD, serving as the Central Nodal Agency.

Rashtriya Vayoshri Yojana

This initiative aims to supply physical aids and assisted living devices to senior citizens who are BPL and experiencing age-related disabilities or infirmities, with the goal of restoring their bodily functions as much as possible. The SCWF is financing this scheme.

Starting from the financial year 2020–21, the scheme has undergone revisions. The updated criteria now include senior citizens with a monthly income of <15,000/-who suffer from age-related disabilities/infirmities, expanding the pool of eligible beneficiaries beyond just those classified as BPL.

The revised RVY scheme has increased the number of devices provided. Currently, the distribution includes the following items:

- *Generic items*: Walking sticks, elbow crutches, walkers/crutches, tripods/quad pods, hearing aids, artificial dentures, and spectacles
- *Special items*: Wheelchairs, wheelchairs with commode, chair/stool with commode, silicon foam cushion, knee brace, spinal support, cervical collar, lumbosacral belt (LS), walker/rollator with brakes, walking stick with seat, and foot care kit

The central government fully finances (100% funded) the scheme through the Citizens' Welfare Senior Fund. The level of assistance provided for the distribution of "Physical Aids and Assisted-Living Devices" corresponds to the severity of the disability/infirmity among eligible senior citizens. In cases of multiple disabilities/infirmities, assistive devices will be provided for each condition. The Implementing Agency will offer 1 year of free maintenance for the supplied aids and assisted living devices. The maximum cost per beneficiary for devices will not exceed 7,000/.

Senior Citizens' Welfare Fund

Established following the Budget Announcement 2015–16, this fund is designated for the advancement of senior citizens' welfare. Oversight of the fund is managed by an Inter-Ministerial Committee, comprising the Department of Financial Services, the Ministry of Health and Family Welfare, the Ministry of Rural Development, the Ministry of Housing and Urban Affairs, and the Ministry of Labour and Employment, with the Ministry of Social Justice and Empowerment as the Nodal Ministry for administration.

National Council of Senior Citizens

In line with the National Policy for Older Persons (NPOP), the National Council for Older Persons (NCOP) was formed in 1999 to supervise policy implementation and advise the Government on issues concerning the elderly. Renamed and reconstituted as the National Council of Senior Citizens (NCSrC) in 2012, its mandate encompasses advising both Central and State Governments on various welfare issues and improving the quality of life for senior citizens.

Vayoshrestha Samman

Recognizing outstanding contributions by senior citizens and institutions toward elderly welfare, the Ministry of Social Justice and Empowerment began commemorating the International Day of Older Persons (IDOP) from October 1, 2005. Evolving from the Vayoshrestha Samman, the initiative was elevated to a National Award through the Scheme of National Awards for Senior Citizens, officially notified in the Gazette of India on January 22, 2013. The awards span 13 categories and were first presented on October 1, 2013, coinciding with IDOP.

Accessible India Campaign (Sugamya Bharat Abhiyan, Department of Empowerment of Persons with Disabilities)

Launched in 2015, the Accessible India Campaign aims for universal accessibility for Persons with Disabilities (PwDs). This involves creating elder-friendly, barrier-free environments in various public spaces such as buildings, public toilets, buses, bus stands, airports, and other public areas to foster age-friendly cities.

e-Anudaan Portal

An initiative by the Ministry of Social Justice and Empowerment, the e-Anudaan portal facilitates online registration for nongovernment organizations (NGOs) to apply for grant-in-aid to support the implementation of various Ministry schemes.

Ministry of Finance

Pradhan Mantri Vaya Vandana Yojana

Pradhan Mantri Vaya Vandana Yojana (PMVVY) is a pension scheme launched by the Government of India aimed at providing financial security and stability to senior citizens. Launched in May 2017, PMVVY offers guaranteed returns and regular pension payments to individuals aged 60 years and above. Under this scheme, pensioners can opt for monthly, quarterly, half-yearly, or annual pension payouts, depending on their preference. PMVVY provides a fixed interest rate for a period of 10 years, ensuring a steady income stream for retirees. This scheme is particularly beneficial for elderly citizens who seek a reliable source of income during their postretirement years, thus promoting financial independence and well-being among the senior population.

Administered by the Life Insurance Corporation (LIC) of India, it guarantees an 8% annual return, disbursed monthly for a decade, with a loan option available after 3 policy years. Any variance between LIC's returns and the assured 8% will be subsidized annually by the Government of India. Initially open for subscription from May 4, 2017, to May 3, 2018, the scheme required a minimum family purchase price of ₹1.5 lakh for a minimum monthly pension of ₹1,000, extendable to ₹7.5 lakh for a maximum pension of ₹5,000. Following the 2018–19 budget announcement, the cabinet extended the scheme until March 31, 2020, and raised the maximum purchase price to ₹15 lakh per senior citizen. Subsequently, in May 2020, the Union Cabinet approved a further extension until March 31, 2023, with adjustments to interest rates and minimum investment requirements. However, the PMVVY scheme was officially closed for fresh investments on March 31, 2023. After this date, new enrollments into PMVVY were no longer permitted.

Ayushman Vay Vandana Card

The Ayushman Vay Vandana Card (AVVC), launched in October 2024, is a major step toward strengthening health security for India's senior citizens. Targeted at individuals aged 70 years and above, the card provides cashless health insurance coverage of up to ₹5 lakh per year under the Ayushman Bharat-Pradhan Mantri Jan Arogya Yojana (AB-PMJAY) framework. What makes this scheme particularly senior-friendly is that it covers nearly 2,000 medical procedures, including treatment for chronic and age-related conditions, and accepts preexisting illnesses from day 1, with no waiting period. By December 2024, over 25 lakh elderly citizens had enrolled, and thousands had already availed of its benefits. For older adults who face high healthcare costs and often depend on family support, the AVVC offers a sense of security, dignity, and independence by ensuring timely access to both public and empaneled private hospitals across the country.

Pradhan Mantri Suraksha Bima Yojana

Pradhan Mantri Suraksha Bima Yojana (PMSBY) is accessible to individuals aged 18–70 who possess a bank or post office account and consent to automatic debiting. The scheme provides coverage of ₹2 lakh for accidental death or total permanent disability and ₹1 lakh for partial permanent disability.

Atal Pension Yojana [Pension Fund Regulatory and Development Authority (PFRDA)]

Launched on May 9, 2015, Atal Pension Yojana (APY) aims to establish a comprehensive social security system for all Indians, particularly targeting the poor, underprivileged, and those in the unorganized sector. It is open to all Indian citizens aged 18–40 years with a bank or post office account. The scheme offers five pension plan options ranging from ₹1,000 to 5,000, guaranteed by the Government of India upon reaching 60 years of age.

Varishtha Pension Bima Yojana

The Varishtha Pension Bima Yojana (VPBY) provides subscribers with a guaranteed pension rate per annum, paid monthly upon a lumpsum payment. Any deficit in the guaranteed return compared to LIC's generated return is compensated by the Indian government through subsidy payments. Subscribers can withdraw deposit amounts after 15 years of policy purchase. The scheme is managed by the LIC of India.

Senior Citizens' Saving Scheme

The Senior Citizens' Saving Scheme (SCSS) is designed as a retirement benefit program. Individuals aged 60 years and above can participate in SCSS through individual or joint investments. Installment amounts range from ₹1,000 to 15 lakh, designated for retirement benefits. The scheme also offers tax benefits.

Senior Citizens Savings Account Interest Rates: Elderly individuals with savings accounts in banks and post offices receive preferential interest rates.

Doorstep Banking

Following Reserve Bank of India directives, banks are mandated to offer basic banking services such as doorstep banking, encompassing cash withdrawals, cash pickup for demand drafts, submission of KYC documents, and life certificate collection at the homes of senior citizens and PwDs.

Income Tax Benefits for Senior Citizens

The Ministry of Finance provides income tax rebates for senior citizens' income. This includes tax exemptions up to ₹3 lakh, a 5% levy on income between ₹3 lakh and ₹5 lakh, complete income tax exemption for seniors above 80 years up to ₹5 lakh, increased deductions under section 80DDB for specified diseases, and tax benefits under section 80TTB for interest income up to ₹50,000 from deposits with banking institutions, post offices, or cooperative societies. Moreover, section 207 of the Income Tax Act exempts resident senior citizens from advance tax payments if they have no income chargeable under the "profits and gains of business or profession" category.

Health Insurance Incentives

To encourage caregiving for parents' medical needs, section 80D of the Income Tax Act allows deductions for health insurance premiums paid for parents. Similar deductions are available for Hindu Undivided Families (HUFs) regarding health insurance premiums for any member.

Service Tax Exemptions

Entities registered under Section 12AA of the Income Tax Act are exempt from service tax for educational or skill development programs targeting individuals over 65 years residing in rural areas.

Reverse Mortgage Scheme

Introduced by the Ministry of Finance in 2007, this scheme enables senior citizens to mortgage their property with banks and receive loans up to 60% of the property's value. The mortgage tenure ranges from 10 to 20 years.

Health Insurance Guidelines

The Insurance Regulatory and Development Authority (IRDA) issued instructions in 2009 regarding health insurance for senior citizens. These directives include allowing entry into health insurance schemes until the age of 65 years, transparency in premium rates, recording reasons for proposal denials, and ensuring renewability without arbitrary refusals.

Ministry of Health and Family Welfare

The National Programme for Health Care of the Elderly

The National Programme for Health Care of the Elderly (NPHCE), launched in 2010–11, is a state-oriented initiative aimed at providing comprehensive healthcare services to individuals aged 60 years and above. The NPHCE is significant as it is India's first dedicated program for elderly health, ensuring comprehensive care from community to tertiary level. It addresses the rising burden of chronic and age-related diseases through preventive, promotive, curative, and rehabilitative services. By building specialized infrastructure and trained workforce, it lays the foundation for healthy and dignified aging in India. NPHCE operates across all levels of primary, secondary, and tertiary levels of public healthcare system.

Primary and secondary geriatric care services: Initially implemented in 100 districts during the 11th plan period, the program has expanded to cover 718 health districts. Services include outpatient departments (OPDs), 10-bedded geriatric wards, physiotherapy, and laboratory services.

Tertiary level activities: Renamed as "Rashtriya Varishth Jan Swasthya Yojana" in 2016–17, tertiary care services are provided through regional geriatric centers (RGCs) in selected medical colleges. These centers offer specialized OPDs, geriatric wards, specialized beds in various medical specialties, human resource development, and research activities. Currently, 18 RGCs offer OPD services, 16 provide inpatient services, 14 offer physiotherapy, and 13 provide laboratory services. Two NCAs have been established as centers of excellence for geriatric care, located at Madras Medical College, Chennai, and AIIMS, New Delhi, respectively. Under the expansion phase, a new geriatric center at IMS-BHU, Varanasi, has been established under NPHCE umbrella.

Training modules: Three sets of training modules have been developed for medical officers, nurses, and community-based workers to deliver comprehensive geriatric care. State-level training of trainers for medical officers has been conducted in various states to ensure the effective implementation of geriatric care services.

LASI: LASI is one of the most important initiatives to understand the needs of older adults in the country. Convened by the Ministry of Health and Family Welfare, Government of India, and supported by the International Institute for Population Sciences (IIPS), Harvard School of Public Health, and the University of Southern California, LASI is the first large-scale national study that looks not only at the health of people aged 45 years and above, but also at their family life, social support, finances, and overall well-being. Funded jointly by the Government of India, the US National Institute on Aging, and other global partners, the study covers more than 72,000 individuals across all states and union territories (UTs). Findings reveal that around 24% of older adults report multiple chronic conditions, nearly 30% experience symptoms of depression, and almost one in five seniors face difficulties in performing daily activities without assistance. The study also highlights social concerns, with nearly 20% of older adults reporting loneliness and many relying heavily on family for financial security. By following individuals over time, LASI helps track how health and social challenges evolve with age. For those working in senior care whether family members, caregivers, doctors, or policymakers; LASI provides evidence to design better health services, community programs, and support systems that make aging more comfortable and dignified.

Ayushman Bharat–Pradhan Mantri Jan Arogya Yojana

The AB-PMJAY was launched by the Government of India to extend healthcare coverage to over 10 crore impoverished and vulnerable families, approximately 50 crore beneficiaries. It offers coverage up to ₹5 lakh per family annually for secondary and tertiary hospitalization. With the introduction of PMJAY, the Rashtriya Swasthya Bima Yojana (RSBY) and the Senior Citizen Health Insurance Scheme (SCHIS) have been amalgamated into it, ensuring that all enrolled beneficiary families from RSBY and SCHIS receive benefits under PMJAY.

The PMJAY eliminates age restrictions, so even the oldest members of the family are eligible. Unlike RSBY and SCHIS, which had lower coverage and limited packages, PMJAY covers a wide range of treatments for chronic diseases common in older age, such as cardiac ailments, cancer, kidney disorders, joint replacements, and neurological conditions, which were previously unaffordable for many.

Health and Wellness Centers

Health and wellness centers (HWCs), formerly known as Ayushman Arogya Mandir, are being activated in excess of 150,000 locations. These centers include provisions for elderly care and palliative health services.

Senior Citizen Health Insurance Scheme

The SCHIS, initiated in 2016, provided top-up insurance coverage to senior citizens enrolled under RSBY. Offering an additional health cover of ₹30,000 beyond the existing RSBY coverage, it extended this benefit in multiples of ₹30,000 for families with multiple senior citizens. Treatment packages under SCHIS were expanded beyond the 1,516 packages covered under RSBY before being incorporated into PMJAY.

Central Government Health Scheme

The Central Government Health Scheme (CGHS) has been delivering comprehensive medical care to central government employees and pensioners for six decades. It stands out due to its vast beneficiary base and open-ended approach to healthcare provision. As of August 29, 2023, the scheme has benefitted a total of 1,768,717 pensioners.

Ministry of Rural Development

The National Social Assistance Program (NSAP) operates as a centrally sponsored scheme, extending financial aid to elderly individuals, widows, and PwDs falling under the BPL category and meeting the eligibility criteria outlined in the NSAP guidelines. The assistance provided ranges from ₹200 to 500 per month. Additionally, in the event of the breadwinner's demise, a lumpsum assistance of ₹20,000 is granted to the grieving family. The implementation of the scheme is carried out by states/UTs, with state governments/UT administrations offering additional top-up assistance beyond the central support. NSAP encompasses the following schemes targeting the elderly and differently-abled individuals, outlined as follows:

- *Indira Gandhi National Old Age Pension Scheme (IGNOAPS)*: This initiative extends a monthly pension of ₹200 to elderly individuals aged 60–79 years falling within the BPL category. Upon reaching 80 years of age, the pension amount escalates to ₹500 per month. The scheme benefits a total of 221 lakh beneficiaries.
- *Indira Gandhi National Disability Pension Scheme (IGNDPS)*: Targeting individuals aged 18–79 years with severe and multiple disabilities (80% disability level) from the BPL category, this scheme provides a monthly pension of ₹300. Upon reaching the age of 80, the pension amount increases to ₹500 per month. Currently, the scheme benefits 10.58 lakh beneficiaries.

Ministry of Ayush

- The Ministry provides various medical facilities for senior citizens, including free consultation and yoga therapy through Yoga and Naturopathy programs. Additionally, OPD services are available in government hospitals across several states, including Delhi, Haryana, Tripura, Kerala, Madhya Pradesh, Andhra Pradesh, and Jharkhand.
- Free yoga training is conducted at 50 Yoga Parks through NGOs in different states, promoting holistic wellness among the elderly. Various other programs such as Health Promotion Programs, Yoga Therapy Training Programs, Individual Yoga Therapy Sessions, Weekend Yoga Training Programs, and Monthly Clinical Yoga Therapy Workshops are also offered.

Ayurveda, Homoeopathy, and Siddha Research Councils, operating under the Ministry of Ayush, provide specialized health services to the elderly through dedicated geriatric clinics nationwide. The AYURSWASTHYA Yojana Ayush and Public Health (PHI) component aims to address common public health concerns related to communicable and NCDs, maternal and child health, mental health, and geriatric care. The recently approved Vayo Mitra program under the National Ayush Mission focuses on providing comprehensive Ayush Geriatric Healthcare Services to raise awareness about aging-related issues, reduce morbidity in old age, and emphasize the importance of maintaining a high quality of life among the elderly population.

Ministry of Consumer Affairs, Food, and Public Distribution

Annapurna Scheme

The Department of Food and Public Distribution collaborates with the Ministry of Rural Development to allocate food grains according to projected requirements under the Annapurna Scheme. This initiative targets indigent senior citizens who do not receive a pension under IGNOAPS, providing them with 10 kg of food grains per person per month, free of charge.

Antyodaya Anna Yojana

This scheme offers heavily subsidized rice and wheat to households headed by widows, terminally ill individuals, disabled persons, and senior citizens who lack assured means of maintenance or societal support. Through Antyodaya Anna Yojana (AAY), these vulnerable groups receive essential food items at affordable rates to alleviate their economic burden and ensure their nutritional needs are met.

Other Ministries and the Schemes Run by Them

Ministry of Textiles

The ministry provides financial assistance to handicrafts awardee artisans above 60 years of age, with an annual income below ₹50,000. Beneficiaries receive ₹3,500 per month to support their livelihood and sustain their craftwork.

Department of Pension and Pensioners Welfare

This department oversees the distribution of retirement benefits, including pensions, to Central Government employees upon their retirement. The scheme ensures that retirees can lead an active and dignified life post-retirement, providing them with financial security and stability.

Ministry of Home Affairs

The ministry has issued detailed advisories to all state and UT governments, urging them to take immediate measures to enhance the safety and security of elderly individuals. These initiatives include senior citizen identification, sensitization of police personnel, regular beat staff visits, establishment of toll-free helplines, setting up of senior citizen security cells, and verification of domestic helps and drivers. The goal is to prevent neglect, abuse, and violence against the elderly and ensure their well-being and protection in society.

Indian Railways

Computerized Passenger Reservation System (PRS) automatically allocates lower berths to senior citizens based on availability, even if no preference is given during booking.

A specific quota of lower berths is earmarked for senior citizens, female passengers over 45 years, and pregnant women in various classes of trains, including sleeper, AC 3 tier, and AC 2 tier classes, with different allocations for different train types.

Central and Western Railways allocate accommodation for senior citizens during specified hours on suburban sections.

Wheelchair provision at stations is mandated, with instructions for free-of-cost battery-operated vehicles and e-wheelchair booking available online through the IRCTC portal.

"Yatri Mitra Sewa" by IRCTC at major stations offers wheelchair and porter services for passengers needing assistance.

Onboard ticket-checking staff can allot vacant lower berths to disabled persons, senior citizens, or pregnant women if available after departure.

Separate counters at PRS centers are designated for reservations from physically disabled persons and senior citizens.

Electric multiple unit (EMU) local trains have compartments designated for differently-abled persons, with wheelchair-friendly doorways.

Special coaches designed for disabled passengers, such as SLRD (Second class cum Luggage cum Guard Van and Disabled Friendly Compartment) and LHB Second Luggage, Guard & Divyangs Compartment (LSLRD), are being manufactured and incorporated into trains.

Production units are instructed to provide wider doors in newly manufactured coaches for improved accessibility.

Integrated Braille Signage is installed in newly manufactured coaches, with ongoing retrofitting in existing coaches to assist visually impaired travelers.

Ministry of Civil Aviation

Airlines and airport operators are mandated to provide automated buggies free of charge for senior citizens at airports with annual aircraft movements of 50,000 or more, facilitating their access to boarding gates located beyond reasonable walking distance.

Airport operators must prominently display information about the availability of automated buggies and small trolleys in the terminal building and on their websites.

Physical barriers at airports and airlines should be removed to ease entry and exit for senior citizens.

Frisking booths in security hold areas should be redesigned to eliminate the need for elderly individuals to climb and descend during security checks.

Special assistance should be provided to senior citizens, especially after they alight from vehicles at airports and until they reach the check-in counters.

Attention should be given to the elderly and those needing assistance at airline booking offices, with dedicated check-in counters and departure gates/lanes for their convenience.

Priority should be given to senior citizens at pre-queuing areas and Pre-Embarkation Security Check (PESC) points to streamline their travel process.

The Ministry of Social Justice and Empowerment allocated budgetary support from the Senior Citizens Welfare Fund to the Ministry of Civil Aviation in 2018–19 for operating electric-operated golf carts at designated airports and facilitating senior citizens' movement. Additionally, funds were released to the Airports Authority of India (AAI) to enhance facilities for flyers with reduced mobility, with 20 AAI airports now equipped with Ambu lifts.

Ministry of Housing and Urban Affairs

This ministry has introduced several initiatives to create an elder-friendly environment in urban areas. One such initiative is the Model Building Bye-Laws, 2016, which prescribe standards for barrier-free infrastructure in buildings and toilets. Additionally, the Urban Bus Specification-II emphasizes the procurement of low-floor buses with ramps to facilitate easy access for disabled persons and senior citizens. Moreover, all metro rail projects across the country incorporate disabled and elder-friendly infrastructure, including proper ramps/lifts and reserved seats in metro coaches. Furthermore, the Housing for All Mission/Pradhan Mantri Awas Yojana Guidelines prioritize families with senior citizens for allotment on the ground floor or lower floors of housing units. Alongside, the ministry implements the Deendayal Antyodaya Yojana-National Urban Livelihoods Mission (DAY-NULM) to provide permanent shelter equipped with essential services to urban homeless individuals, regardless of age.

Ministry of Road Transport and Highways

This ministry has introduced amendments to the Central Motor Vehicles Rules aimed at creating a Divyang/elderly-friendly environment. These amendments include provisions for priority seats, signage, securing of mobility aids, and wheelchair accessibility in vehicles. Additionally, the Ministry of Road Transport and Highways (MoRTH) issued accessibility guidelines for bus terminals and bus stops to ensure ease of access for all individuals, including Divyangjan. These guidelines focus on planning and designing accessible infrastructure in bus terminals and stops, with the aim of seamless inclusion of Divyangjan.

Ministry of Culture

This ministry provides financial assistance to veteran artists aged 60 years and above through a monthly allowance scheme.

Ministry of Communications

This ministry offers concessions to senior citizens, including exemptions from registration charges for Landline Telephone Connection by Bharat Sanchar Nigam Limited (BSNL) and a 25% concession in installation/activation charges and monthly services/rental charges for Landline connections under Plan-250 by Mahanagar Telephone Nigam Limited. (MTNL).

Ministry of Women and Child Development

This ministry has constructed a Home for Widows in Vrindavan, Uttar Pradesh, providing a safe and secure environment along with health services and other amenities, designed to cater to the needs of senior citizens and individuals with special challenges.

Existing Gaps

Despite several government schemes and community initiatives, elderly care in India continues to face significant gaps. There is limited awareness of welfare and health programs, leading to underutilization, especially in rural and marginalized populations. Health services remain fragmented and disease-focused, with inadequate emphasis on preventive, palliative, and long-term care. A severe shortage of trained geriatric specialists and caregivers, coupled with weak integration of institutional and home-based care, further limits accessibility. Financial security schemes often exclude the poorest elderly or provide inadequate support in the face of rising healthcare and living costs. Additionally, social isolation, lack of age-friendly infrastructure, and weak monitoring mechanisms undermine the effectiveness of existing programs. These gaps highlight the need for a more integrated, inclusive, and holistic approach to ensure dignified and healthy aging in India.

REMEDIAL MEASURES

To bridge these gaps, India needs a comprehensive and integrated approach to elderly care. Strengthening the primary healthcare system with geriatric-friendly services, expanding the NPHCE to every district, and ensuring better linkage with PMJAY can provide continuity of care. Community-based interventions such as home-based care, caregiver training, and day-care centers should be scaled up to reduce dependence on hospitals. Financial support schemes must be made more inclusive and inflation-linked, so that even the poorest elderly benefit meaningfully. At the same time, digital and social innovations, such as telemedicine, mobile health units, and social participation platforms, can reduce isolation and improve access. Stronger policy convergence across ministries, effective monitoring, and active participation of civil society and private sector will be key to creating a holistic, sustainable, and age-friendly ecosystem for India's growing elderly population.

CONCLUSION

In conclusion, government schemes for senior citizens in India play a crucial role in addressing the diverse needs of this demographic segment. These schemes reflect the government's commitment to ensuring the well-being and social security of senior citizens across the country. Through a multitude of initiatives, the government aims to provide financial assistance, healthcare support, and social inclusion opportunities to elderly citizens. Schemes such as the NSAP provide financial assistance to senior citizens living below the poverty line, helping them meet their basic needs. Additionally, healthcare schemes such as the NPHCE focus on promoting geriatric healthcare services and preventive measures. Pension schemes like the IGNOAPS offer monetary benefits to destitute and vulnerable senior citizens. Moreover, schemes such as the Integrated Programme for Older Persons (IPOP) aim to enhance the quality of life for senior citizens by providing daycare, recreational activities, and other support services. The government also prioritizes housing schemes tailored to the needs of elderly citizens, ensuring accessibility and affordability. Furthermore, initiatives such as the RVY distribute assistive devices to senior citizens with disabilities, improving their mobility and independence. These schemes underscore the government's recognition of the invaluable contributions made by senior citizens to society and its commitment to ensuring their dignity and well-being in their golden years. Through continuous evaluation and enhancement of these schemes, the government strives to address emerging challenges and effectively cater to the evolving needs of senior citizens in India.

Self-Assessment Questionnaire

Q1. What are the fundamental pillars of senior citizens' well-being addressed under the Atal Vayo Abhyudaya Yojana (AVYAY)?

Q2. What are the main objectives of the State Action Plan for Senior Citizens (SAPSrC), and how does it differ from national-level programs?

Q3. Define "Silver Economy" and what its implications are.

Q4. Describe the eligibility criteria and benefits of the Rashtriya Vayoshri Yojana.

Q5. How does the National Programme for Health Care of the Elderly (NPHCE) integrate primary, secondary, and tertiary-level services for older adults?

Q6. What are the key financial protection mechanisms available for seniors from the Government of India?

Q7. Explain the role of the National Social Assistance Programme (NSAP) in ensuring social security for the elderly and other vulnerable populations.

Q8. What are the significant gaps and remedial measures identified in the chapter to improve implementation and awareness of elderly welfare schemes in India?

FURTHER READINGS

1. Age Well Foundation. (2022). Contribution of Older Women. [online] Available from https://www.agewellfoundation.org/wp-content/uploads/2024/04/STATUS-OF-ELDERLY-WOMEN-IN-INDIA-MAR-2024-for-site.pdf [Last accessed September, 2025].
2. NITI Aayog. (2024). Senior Care Reforms in India. [online] Available from https://www.niti.gov.in/sites/default/files/2024-02/Senior%20Care%20Reforms%20in%20India%20FINAL%20FOR%20WEBSITE_compressed.pdf [Last accessed September, 2025].
3. Ministry of Rural Development, Government of India. (n.d.). National Social Assistance Programme (NSAP). Retrieved October, 2025, from https://nsap.nic.in
4. Mundada PS, Sharma S, Gupta B, Padhi MM, Dey AB, Dhiman KS. Review of health-care services for older population in India and possibility of incorporating AYUSH in public health system for geriatric care. Ayu. 2020;41(1):3-11.
5. Tattari S, Gavaravarapu SM, Pullakhandam R, Bhatia N, Kaur S, Sarwal R, et al. Nutritional requirements for the elderly in India: A status paper. Indian J Med Res. 2022;156(3):411-20.
6. Sastry NB, Vempadapu M, Sivananjiah S. Toward adapting the UN's healthy aging agenda for India: tailoring to unique historical context and traditions. Front Public Health. 2024;11:1346962.
7. Department of Social Justice & Empowerment, Government of India. (2023). Atal Vayo Abhyuday Yojana (AVYAY): Empowering the Elderly for a Dignified Life. [online] available from https://socialjustice.gov.in/writereaddata/UploadFile/63491659437974.pdf [Last accessed September, 2025].
8. Department of Social Justice & Empowerment. Integrated Programme for Senior Citizens (IPSrC). Government of India. Press Information Bureau. [online] Available from https://www.pib.gov.in/PressReleasePage.aspx?PRID=2008128&utm_source=chatgpt.com"Press Release:Press Information Bureau
9. Department of Social Justice & Empowerment, Government of India. (2024). State Action Plan for Senior Citizens (SAPSrC). [online] Available from https://scw.dosje.gov.in/state-action-plan-senior-citizens?utm_source=chatgpt.com"State Action Plan for Senior Citizens (SAPSrC) | Ageing With Dignity Department of Social Justice & Empowerment - Government of India [Last accessed September, 2024].
10. Ministry of Social Justice & Empowerment, Government of India. (2021). Senior Care Ageing Growth Engine (SAGE). [online] Available from https://scw.dosje.gov.in/seniorcare-ageing-growth-engine?utm_source=chatgpt.com"SAGE | Ageing With Dignity Department of Social Justice & Empowerment - Government of India [Last accessed September, 2025].
11. Ministry of Social Justice & Empowerment, Government of India. (2025). Rashtriya Vayoshri Yojana (RVY). [online] Available from https://scw.dosje.gov.in/rashtriya-vayoshri-yojana?utm_source=chatgpt.com"Rashtriya Vayoshri Yojana (RVY) | Ageing With Dignity Department of Social Justice & Empowerment - Government of India [Last accessed September, 2025].
12. NITI Aayog, Government of India. (2024). Senior Care Reforms in India. [online] Available from https://www.niti.gov.in/sites/default/files/2024-02/Senior%20Care%20Reforms%20in%20India%20FINAL%20FOR%20WEBSITE_compressed.pdf [Last accessed September, 2025].
13. Ministry of Railways, Government of India. (n.d.). Yatri Mitra Sewa. Retrieved October, 2025, from https://indianrailways.gov.in
14. International Institute for Population Sciences (IIPS), Harvard T.H. Chan School of Public Health, University of Southern California. Longitudinal Ageing Study in India (LASI) Wave 1, 2017–18, India Report. Mumbai: IIPS; 2020.
15. Ministry of Rural Development, Government of India. Indira Gandhi National Old Age Pension Scheme (IGNOAPS)—Operational Guidelines. New Delhi: MoRD; 2007.

SECTION 2

Geriatric Specifics

CHAPTER 11

Healthy Aging and Intrinsic Capacity

Meenal Thakral

CASE VIGNETTES

Case 1: Healthy Aging through Preserved Intrinsic Capacity

Background

Mr Sharma, a 72-year-old retired government employee, lives with his wife in an urban setting. He has a history of controlled hypertension and hyperlipidemia but remains active in his daily life. He takes regular morning walks, volunteers at a local library, and participates in community yoga sessions.

Assessment of Intrinsic Capacity

- *Locomotion*: Despite his age, Mr Sharma continues his daily walks (30 minutes) and performs strength exercises twice a week, maintaining muscle strength and balance.
- *Cognition*: He reads newspapers daily and stays mentally active by playing chess and solving puzzles. His recent cognitive assessment [Mini-Mental State Examination (MMSE) score: 28/30] suggests excellent cognitive function for his age.
- *Vitality*: His weight and body mass index (BMI) are within normal limits, and he follows a balanced diet with adequate protein intake. Blood tests reveal normal vitamin D and hemoglobin levels.
- *Sensory function*: No hearing difficulties were noted, and he uses reading glasses for presbyopia but reports no vision issues.
- *Psychological well-being*: He reports no depressive symptoms and actively engages in social activities. His social network supports his emotional well-being.

Outcome

Mr Sharma demonstrates high intrinsic capacity, which contributes to his ability to age healthily. He experiences minimal functional limitations and remains independent in all activities of daily living (ADLs). His lifestyle and intrinsic capacity help him preserve resilience against age-related decline, ensuring a high quality of life.

Case 2: Diminished Intrinsic Capacity in Early Age-related Decline

Background

Mrs Lakshmi, an 82-year-old widow, lives with her daughter in a semirural area. She has multiple chronic conditions, including type 2 diabetes and mild osteoarthritis. In the past year, she has started experiencing episodes of fatigue and minor falls, leading to concerns about her overall function.

Assessment of Intrinsic Capacity

- *Locomotion*: She walks short distances within her home but complains of knee pain from osteoarthritis. A recent gait analysis showed mild unsteadiness, and she uses a cane for longer walks. Her muscle strength is borderline low (SARC-F score: 3).
- *Cognition*: She occasionally forgets names and appointments, though she remains independent in decision-making. Her cognitive assessment (MoCA score: 22/30) indicates mild cognitive decline.
- *Vitality*: Mrs Lakshmi has unintentionally lost 3 kg in the last 6 months. Her BMI is slightly below normal, and her appetite has reduced. Laboratory tests reveal low hemoglobin (9.8 g/dL), raising concerns about nutritional deficiencies.

- *Sensory function*: She has reduced hearing, especially in noisy environments, but does not use hearing aids. Her vision is also impaired due to cataracts, awaiting surgical intervention.
- *Psychological well-being*: Mrs Lakshmi expresses feelings of loneliness since the death of her husband and feels anxious about her health. A Geriatric Depression Scale (GDS) score of 7/15 suggests mild depressive symptoms.

Outcome

Mrs Lakshmi exhibits declining intrinsic capacity, particularly in locomotion, cognition, and vitality. Early interventions, including cataract surgery, nutritional support, physiotherapy for strength and balance, and social engagement activities, may help prevent further functional decline. Addressing intrinsic capacity holistically will support healthy aging and maintain her independence for as long as possible.

INTRODUCTION

Healthy aging is the process of developing and maintaining functional ability, enabling well-being in older age. Functional ability comprises the health-related attributes that enable people to be and to do what they have reason to value. It includes the individual's intrinsic capacity, relevant environmental characteristics, and the interactions between the individual and these characteristics. Intrinsic capacity is the composite of all the physical and mental capacities of an individual. Environments comprise all the factors in the extrinsic world that form an individual's life context. These include home, communities, and the broader society. Well-being is considered in the broadest sense and includes domains such as happiness, satisfaction, and fulfilment.

PROCESS OF HEALTHY AGING

Healthy aging starts at birth with our genetic inheritance. However, we are also born into a social milieu, so the environment also plays a huge role.

- *Personal characteristics*:
  - Fixed: Sex and ethnicity
  - Mobile: Occupation, educational attainment, and wealth

  These contribute to the social position within a particular context and time, which further shapes the exposure, opportunities, and barriers faced and the access to the resources.
- *Health characteristics*: There is a gradual accumulation of molecular and cellular damage with aging that results in a general decrease in physiological reserves. These physiological and homeostatic changes and a range of positive and negative environmental influences vary significantly among individuals at any chronological age. These changes influence the development of other health characteristics such as physiological risk factors (e.g., high blood pressure), diseases, injuries, and broader geriatric syndromes.

  The interaction between these health characteristics further determines the intrinsic capacity of the individuals, i.e., the composite of all the physical and mental capacities that an individual can draw on.

COMPONENTS OF HEALTHY AGING

The three components of healthy aging are: (1) functional capacity, (2) intrinsic capacity, and (3) environment.

Intrinsic Capacity

Intrinsic capacity is defined as the combination of the individual's physical and mental capacities, including psychological capacities. The key domains of intrinsic capacity are:

- Cognitive capacity
- Psychological capacity
- Locomotor capacity
- Vitality
- Visual capacity
- Hearing capacity

Domains of intrinsic capacity are interrelated. Older people who experience declines require an integrated person-centered approach to assessment and management. For example, hearing helps people to communicate, maintain autonomy, and sustain mental health and cognition.

Functional Ability

Functional ability consists of the intrinsic capacity of the individual, the environment of the individual, and the interactions between them. Functional ability enables people to be and to do what they have reason to value. The five key domains of functional capacity that are essential for older people are:

1. To meet their basic needs—such as being able to afford diet, clothing, housing, and healthcare services, including medications
2. Learn, grow, and make decisions—strengthening a person's autonomy, dignity, integrity, freedom, and independence
3. Be mobile—for completing daily tasks and participating in activities

4. Build and maintain relationships—with children, family, partners, neighbors, and others
5. Contribute to society—by assisting friends, mentoring younger people, caring for family members, volunteering, pursuing cultural activities, and working

Environments

Environments are where people live and conduct their lives. Environments shape what older people with a given level of intrinsic capacity can be and do. Environments include the home, community, broader society, and all the factors within them. Key domains relate to:

- Products, equipment, and technology that facilitate movement, sight, memory, and daily functioning
- The natural or built environment
- Emotional support, assistance, and relationships provided by other people and animals
- Attitudes (as these influence behavior both negatively and positively)
- Services, systems, and policies that may or may not contribute to enhanced functioning at older ages.

TRAJECTORIES OF HEALTHY AGING

Intrinsic capacity and functional ability decline with increasing age as a result of the aging process, as well as the underlying disease. **Figure 1** shows the typical pattern of intrinsic capacity and functional ability across adult life. This typical pattern can be divided into three common periods: (1) A period of high and stable capacity, (2) a period of declining capacity, and (3) a period of significant loss of capacity characterized by dependence on care. **Table 1** depicts the challenges for each period of intrinsic capacity and responses from the healthcare systems.

Variation in intrinsic capacity is greater across people in older age than across younger groups. One individual may have the age difference of 10 years or more compared with another person but a similar intrinsic capacity or functional ability. This is why chronological age is a poor marker of health status. Identifying conditions associated with losses in intrinsic capacity provides an opportunity to intervene to slow, stop, or reverse the declines.

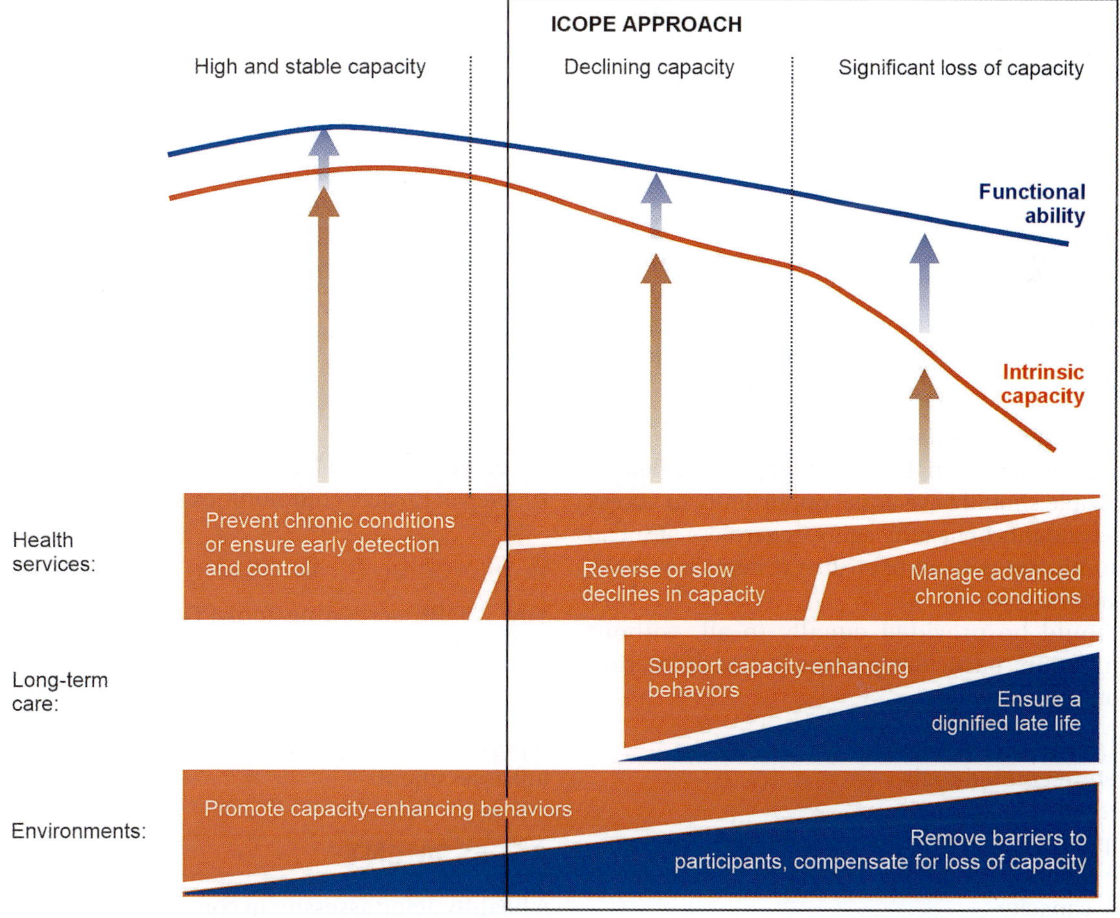

FIG. 1: A public health framework for healthy aging.
(ICOPE: integrated care for older people)

TABLE 1: The common periods of intrinsic capacity in older age and the key responses of a health system.

Period	High and stable capacity	Declining capacity	Significant loss of capacity
Risk and challenges	Risk behaviors, emerging NCDs	Falling mobility, sarcopenia, frailty, cognitive impairment, and sensory impairments	Difficulty performing basic tasks, pain, and suffering caused by advanced chronic conditions
Responses	• Reduce risk factors and encourage healthy behaviors • Early detection and management of chronic diseases	• Treat the underlying causes of declines in capacity • Maintain muscle mass and bone density through exercise and nutrition	• Interventions to recover and maintain intrinsic capacity • Care and support to compensate for losses in capacity • Rapid access to acute care • Palliative and end-of-life care

(NCDs: noncommunicable diseases)

Assessment and Management of Intrinsic Capacity

Declining intrinsic capacity is very frequently characterized by common problems in older age such as difficulties in hearing, seeing, remembering, moving, or performing daily social activities. Approaching older adults through the lens of intrinsic capacity and the environment in which they live helps to ensure that health services are oriented toward the outcomes that are most relevant to their daily lives. This approach can also help to avoid unnecessary treatment, polypharmacy, and side effects.

ICOPE Guidelines

In October 2017, the World Health Organization (WHO) published integrated care for older people (ICOPE) guidelines to manage declines in intrinsic capacity. The ICOPE approach embodies the focus on optimizing intrinsic capacity and functional ability as the key to healthy aging.

Principles of ICOPE. guidelines:

- Older people have the right to the best possible health.
- Older people should have equal opportunity to access the determinants of healthy aging, regardless of social or economic status, place of birth or residence or other social factors.
- Care should be provided equally to all, without discrimination, particularly without discrimination based on gender or age.

The ICOPE guidance describes how to:

- Set person-centered goals
- Support self-management
- Develop a care plan that includes multiple interventions to manage conditions associated with losses in intrinsic capacity
- Screen for losses in intrinsic capacity and assess health and social care needs
- Support caregivers
- Develop a personalized care plan

Person-centered Assessment and Pathway

Person-centered care addresses individual's health and social care needs rather than being driven by isolated health conditions or symptoms. The five steps of this pathway are:

- *Step 1*: *Screen* for declines in intrinsic capacity
- *Step 2*: Undertake a person-centered *assessment* in primary care c 2A: Understand the life of the older person
  - 2B: Assess in greater depth for conditions associated with loss in intrinsic capacity
  - 2C: Assess and manage underlying diseases
  - 2D: Assess social and physical environments and social care and support needs
- *Step 3*: Define the goal of care and develop a *personalized care plan*
  - 3A: Define with the older person the goal of care
  - 3B: Design a care plan
- *Step 4*: Ensure a *referral pathway and care plan monitoring* with links to specialized geriatric care
- *Step 5*: Engage communities and support *caregivers*

Screening for Decline in Intrinsic Capacity

The ICOPE screening tool **(Table 2)** can be used by trained healthcare workers to identify people with losses in intrinsic capacity in a community or at home. It is the first step in each car pathway. Those who show signs of or report losses in capacity at this first step should go on to a full assessment.

ASSESSMENT

A healthy aging assessment considers multiple domains of intrinsic capacity and the environments in which people live.

TABLE 2: ICOPE screening tool to screen for decline in intrinsic capacity.

Domain declines	Tests	Assess fully any domain with a checked square
Cognitive decline	• Remember three words: Flower, door, and rice (for example) • Orientation in time and space: What is the full date today? Where are you now (home, clinic, etc.)? • Recall the three words?	☐ Wrong to either question or does not know ☐ Cannot recall all three words
Limited mobility	Chair rise test: Rise from the chair five times without using arms. Did the person complete five chair rises within 14 seconds?	☐ No
Malnutrition	• Weight loss: Have you unintentionally lost >3 kg over the last 3 months? • Appetite loss: Have you experienced the loss of appetite?	☐ Yes ☐ Yes
Visual impairment	Do you have any problems with your eyes: Difficulties in seeing far, reading, eye diseases, or currently under medical treatment (e.g., diabetes, high blood pressure)?	☐ Yes
Hearing loss	Hears whispers (whisper test), screening audiometry result is 35 dB or less, or passes automated app-based digits-in-noise test	☐ Fail
Depressive symptoms	Over the past 2 weeks, have you been bothered by: • Feeling down, depressed, or hopeless? • Little interest or pleasure in doing things?	☐ Yes ☐ Yes

(ICOPE: integrated care for older people)

Care Pathways to Manage Cognitive Decline

Cognitive decline presents as increasing forgetfulness, loss of attention, and reduced ability to solve problems. This care pathway is intended to apply to older people with some degree of cognitive decline but who do not have dementia.

A person who fails the screening for cognitive decline undergoes the following pathway → Assessment of cognitive capacity → Assess and manage associated conditions → Prevent further declines in cognitive capacity → Assess and manage cardiovascular diseases and risk factors → Assess and manage social and physical environments.

Cognitive Assessment

The tools listed in **Table 3** can be used to assess cognition in older adults in primary care settings. Cognitive assessment can be limited if a person has <5 or 6 years of schooling or no schooling. Instead, it must rely on interviews and clinical judgment. A person with cognitive decline should be assessed for difficulty with activities of daily living (ADLs) or instrumental ADLs (IADLs) to plan for social care and support as a part of the personalized care plan. If the ADLs are affected, the person needs a specialized assessment to diagnose dementia:

TABLE 3: Examples of cognition assessment tools used in primary healthcare settings.

Cognitive assessment tool	Time taken (minutes)
Mini-Cog	2–4
Montreal Cognitive Assessment (MoCA)	10–15
Mini–Mental State Examination (MMSE)	7–10
General Practitioner Assessment of Cognition (GPCOG)	5–6

- *Assessment of associated conditions*: A full diagnostic workup is required to uncover the reversible conditions that can cause cognitive decline. The common reversible conditions are dehydration, malnutrition, infections, and medication problems. Assess the history of vascular disease in the brain (stroke/transient ischemic event) and prevent further events. Identify the cause (medical conditions, intoxication from substances, and use of drugs) and treat delirium. Assess depressive symptoms as per the depressive symptom's pathway.

- *Prevent further declines in cognitive capacity*: Provide multimodal exercises and cognitive stimulation.
- *Assess and manage cardiovascular diseases and risk factors*: Provide integrated management of diseases and reduce cardiovascular risk factors:
  - Suggest smoking cessation
  - Treat hypertension and diabetes
  - Provide dietary advice for weight control
- *Assess and manage social and physical environments*:
  - Assess the need for social care.
  - Provide personal care and support with ADLs.
  - Give advice to maintain independent toileting skills.
  - Assess for caregiver burden or strain and develop a social care and support plan, including support to caregivers.

Care Pathways to Improve Mobility

When a person fails the chair rise test in screening, mobility *assessment* using short physical performance battery (SPPB) **(Flowchart 1)** is done.

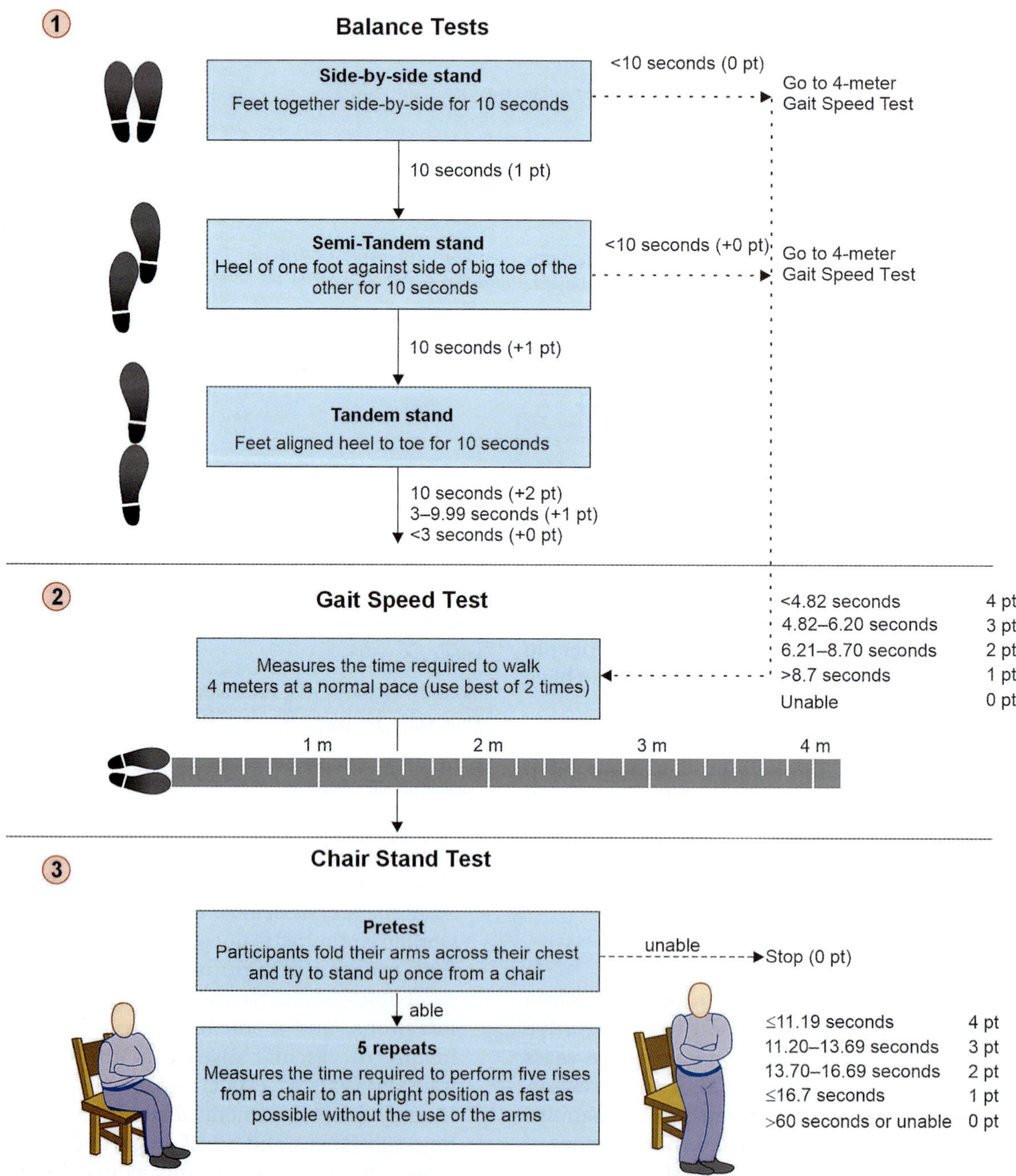

FLOWCHART 1: Short physical performance battery for mobility assessment.
(pt: points)

In case of normal mobility (score of 10–12 points), multimodal exercises are recommended at home.

In case of limited mobility (score of 0–9 points):

- Provide multimodal exercise with close supervision,
- Consider referral to rehabilitation,
- Consider increasing protein intake,
- Consider and provide assistive devices to aid mobility,

A multimodal exercise program for people with limited mobility is given in **Table 4**.

Limitations of multimodal exercises:

- *Pain*: Pacing physical activity in manageable chunks of time and slowly increasing physical task helps the body to build resilience and manage pain.
- *Severely reduced mobility*: Start with exercise training in bed or seated in a chair.
- *Cognitive impairment*: A simple and less structured exercise program is more suitable.

Assess and Manage Associated Conditions

- Polypharmacy: Review medication and aim to reduce.
- Osteoarthritis and osteoporosis: Integrated management of diseases
- Frailty and sarcopenia
- Pain: Consider pain management.

Assess and Manage Social and Physical Environment

- Assess the physical environment to reduce the risk of falls.
- Include fall prevention interventions such as home adaptations.
- Consider and provide assistive devices to aid mobility.
- Provide safe spaces for walking.

Care Pathways to Manage Malnutrition

When a person screens positive for malnutrition, nutritional assessment tools like Mini Nutritional Assessment (MNA) are used to categorize the extent of malnutrition **(Table 5)**.

Dietary advice:

- Help people to identify specific foods that are available locally and that provide adequate energy, protein, and micronutrients.
- Protein intake of 1–1.2 g/kg of body weight is recommended for healthy older adults. A person recovering from weight loss or acute illness may need up to 1.5 g/kg of body weight.
- Advise physical activity, which enables protein to be incorporated into the muscle and builds appetite.

TABLE 4: Multimodal exercise program for people with limited mobility.

Type of exercise	Benefits	Examples
Strength/resistance training	Requires muscles to work under load, using weights, resistance bands, or body weight	Squats, lunges, and sit-to-stand exercises
Aerobic/cardiovascular training	Increases heart rate until a person is slightly out of breath but can maintain a conversation	• Brisk walking • Cycling
Balance training	Challenges balance system, which includes static and dynamic exercises, can progress to different surfaces, and with eyes open and shut	• Standing on one leg at a time • Walking heel-to-toe in a straight line
Flexibility training	• Improves the extensibility of the tissues, such as muscle • Improves the range of joint movement	• Yoga • Pilates

TABLE 5: Mini Nutritional Assessment (MNA).

MNA score	Malnourished (MNA score: <17 points)	At risk of malnutrition (MNA score: 17–23.5 points)	Normal nutritional status (MNA score: 24–30 points)
Management	• Nutritional intervention is necessary • Give oral supplemental nutrition with increased protein intake (400–600 kcal/day) • Offer dietary advice • Monitor weight closely	• Offer dietary advice • Consider oral supplemental nutrition if unable to improve food intake • Monitor weight closely • Consider multimodal exercise	Reinforce generic health and lifestyle advice or usual care Reassess: • After an acute event or illness • Once a year for older people living in the community • Every 3 months for older people with social care needs

- Advise family-style meals and social dining, particularly for older people living alone or who are socially isolated.

Blood tests: These help one to personalize nutrition plan. The patient should be screened for common nutritional deficiencies of vitamins D and B12.

Oral supplemental nutrition (OSN) provides additional high-quality protein, calories, and adequate amounts of vitamins and minerals. OSN adds to food and should not replace food. It should be taken between meals and not with meals. People need continuing support and encouragement from family members to keep eating as well as possible. Ideally, the goal should be to stop OSN once the risk of malnutrition has passed and the diet provides adequate nutrition.

Assess and Manage Associated Conditions

Sarcopenia and frailty are conditions that can be associated with poor nutrition.

Assess and Manage Social and Physical Environments

Caregivers and communities can help to overcome barriers to older people's nutritional health.

- Organization of social dining events for older people
- Facilitating access to groceries
- Assistance to prepare food or receive food via a community-based catering service
- Access to help with managing finances

Care Pathways to Manage Vision

Ask the screening question → Test visual acuity → Assess visual impairment and eye diseases → Assess and manage associated conditions → Assess and manage social and physical environments.

Test the Visual Acuity

Both distant and near vision can be tested at primary care using the WHO simple eye charts. Simple screening for visual loss should be carried out at least once a year for people aged 50 years and older. If the vision is normal or the off-the-shelf simple reading glasses solve the problem, then reinforce eye care and provide vision hygiene advice, i.e., avoid lengthy electronic media watching, extensive time spent using near vision, use of better lighting and contrast, washing hands frequently, not rubbing the eyes, using only mild soap for eyelids, and refraining from eye cosmetics. Reassess yearly, even in the absence of visual impairment.

Assess Visual Impairment and Eye Diseases

- A primary care professional can examine the eyes for signs of common eye diseases.
- In case of sudden or rapidly progressing loss of vision in one or both eyes, secretions, scars, ongoing pain, and photophobia, specialist eye care is recommended.
- For people with irreversible low vision, assistive devices—desk or mobile magnifiers—can be useful.

Assess and Manage Associated Diseases

- *Hypertension*: It is an important risk factor for retinal diseases and glaucoma.
- *Diabetes*: A person with diabetes should have an eye examination by an eye care specialist each year to check for diabetic retinopathy.
- *Steroid use*: Long-term steroid therapy can cause raised intraocular pressure or lead to cataract. Patients receiving long-term steroid therapy need regular eye examinations.

Assess and Manage Social and Physical Environments

- *Introduce home adaptations*: Improve lighting, reduce glare, create contract like colored plate so that food comes out in contrast, use of black pen for writing.
- Use the most legible type of font on electronic media.
- Use vision assistive tools like devices with text-to-speech functions.
- Remove hazards from the usual walking path.

Care Pathways to Manage Hearing

Age-related hearing loss may be the most common sensory impairment in older people. Untreated hearing loss interferes with communication and can lead to social isolation. Limitations of other capacities, such as cognitive decline, can make these social consequences worse. Hearing loss is linked to many other health issues, including cognitive decline and risk of dementia, depression and anxiety, poor balance, falls, hospitalizations, and early death.

Test hearing → Assess hearing capacity → Assess and manage social and physical environments.

Test Hearing

Initial assessment is done by whisper voice test, screening audiometry (if the instrument is available), or an automated app-based digit-in-noise test which is available as a mobile app, e.g., hearWHO. If the person passes the screening, then give generic advice on caring for ears, i.e., do not put dirty fingers in ears or forget to wash hands before working with food, do not eat with dirty hands, always wash your hands after going to the toilet, do not swim or wash in dirty water, and do not put anything in your ears such as hot or cold oil, herbal remedies, or liquids such as kerosene.

Assess Hearing Capacity

Hearing assessment can involve three tests with specialized equipment: (1) A diagnostic audiometer for pure tone, (2) speech audiometry, and (3) tympanometry for middle ear assessment. These tests can help to identify the need for rehabilitation. These tests are done by an ENT specialist **(Table 6)**.

Assess and Manage Social and Physical Environments

- Provide emotional support and help with managing emotional distress.
- Provide auditory aids across the house (telephone, doorbells).
- Provide communication strategies for family members and caregivers:
  - Let the person see your face when you speak.
  - Make sure there is good light on your face to help the listener to see your lips.
  - Get the person's attention before you speak.
  - Speak clearly and more slowly. Do not shout.
  - Do not give up speaking to people who have difficulty hearing. This would isolate them and could lead to depression.

Care Pathways to Manage Depression

The term "depressive symptoms" (or low mood) applies to older adults who have two or more simultaneous symptoms of depression most of or all the time for at least 2 weeks, but who do not meet the criteria for a diagnosis of major depression. Depressive symptoms are more common in older people with long-term and disabling conditions, in social isolation, or who are caregivers with demanding care responsibilities. These issues should be considered as part of a comprehensive approach to managing depressive symptoms **(Table 7)**.

Screen for depressive symptoms → Assess mood → Assess and manage associated conditions → Assess and manage social and physical environments.

Assess Mood

If a person has at least one of the core symptoms and one or two additional symptoms, they may have depressive symptoms. If a person has more than two symptoms, they may qualify for a diagnosis of depressive disorder. It is important to distinguish depressive symptoms from depressive disorder because their treatments differ.

Assess and Manage Associated Conditions

- *Polypharmacy*: Review medications such as antidepressants, antihistamines, and antipsychotics.
- *Anemia and malnutrition*: These can lead to depressive symptoms because of deficiencies of iron and vitamins such as folate, vitamin B6, and vitamin B12. To manage depressive symptoms, it is crucial to manage anemia and improve nutritional status.
- *Hypothyroidism*: This is a common disorder in older people, especially women. The symptoms of hypothyroidism can be nonspecific and vary from

TABLE 7: Psychological and behavioral management of depression in older adults.

Depressive symptoms (0–2 additional symptoms)	Depression (≥3 additional symptoms)
• Offer brief, structured psychological interventions: ○ Cognitive behavioral therapy ○ Problem solving, counseling, or therapy ○ Behavioral activation ○ Life review therapy • Multimodal exercise • Mindfulness practice	• Treat depression: Refer to specialized care

TABLE 6: Hearing assessment test.

Deafness (audiometry ≥ 81 dB)	Moderate-to-severe hearing loss (audiometry 36–80 dB)	Normal hearing capacity (audiometry ≤ 35 dB)
• Refer to specialized hearing care • Evaluate and provide hearing devices (hearing aids or cochlear implants)	Ask about: • Risk factors (such as noise exposure and ototoxic medications) • Pain in the ear: History of active drainage of fluid from the ear(s), sudden or rapidly progressive hearing loss • Dizziness • Chronic otitis media • Unilateral hearing loss ○ If the answer is no to all the above, then provide hearing aids ○ If no hearing aids are available, inform about lip reading and signing as well as other communication strategies	• Reinforce generic advice on caring for ears or usual care • Reassess once every year

person to person, but they can include depressive symptoms. It should be managed by specialists.
- *Pain*: Assess and manage pain

The presence of the following conditions would suggest a different approach to the treatment of depression:
- Major loss in the last 6 months
- History of mania
- *Cognitive decline*: The cognitive functions affected in depression are attention, learning, and visual memory, as well as executive functions. Depression could be a psychological response to the individual's self-awareness of mild cognitive decline that has not yet begun to interfere with daily functioning.
- *Hearing loss and visual impairment*: Sensory losses in older individuals lead to social isolation, loneliness, and eventually depression.
- *Reaction to disability due to illness or injury*: Depression is a common secondary condition in people with disabilities. Older people with new disabilities are at risk of developing anxiety and depression.

Assess and Manage Social and Physical Environments

- Reduce stress and strengthen social support.
- Motivate older people to stay mobile and socially connected.
- Promote functioning in daily activities.
- Encourage participation in community-based exercise programs and skills development. Identify and tackle loneliness and social isolation (consider technology-assisted interventions).

Social Care and Support

For people with significant losses of intrinsic capacity, dignity is often possible only with others' care, support, and assistance. Social care and support include helping with activities of daily living, facilitating access to community facilities and public services, reducing isolation, helping with financial security, providing a suitable place to live, freedom from abuse, and participation in meaningful activities. Community health workers can screen for losses in functional abilities with a simple questionnaire. Interventions tailored to an older person's priorities can improve functional ability **(Table 8)**.

Caregiver Support

When declines in intrinsic capacity and functional ability make a person dependent on others for care, caregiving often falls on a spouse, another family member, or others in the household. Depending on the older person's needs, the burden of providing care can put the caregiver's well-being at risk. Every caregiver interviewed is asked about three areas **(Table 9)**.

TABLE 8: Questionnaire for loss in functional abilities.

Domain	Questions	Intervention
Personal assistant	• Do you have difficulty getting around indoors? • Do you have difficulty using the toilet or commode? • Do you have difficulty dressing yourself? • Do you have difficulty using the bath or shower? • Do you have difficulty keeping up your personal appearance? • Do you have difficulty feeding yourself?	• Assess and modify physical environment • Consider assistive technologies and aids • Assess support from family or caregivers
Accommodation	Do you have problems with the place where you live? If yes, ask: • Your safety and security where you live? • The condition of your house? • The location of your home? • The costs of housing? • The repair and maintenance of your home? • Managing to live independently where you are?	• Home adaptations • Alternative accommodation • Refer to the community housing program
Finances	Do you have problems with your finances? If yes, ask: • In general, how do your finances work out at the end of the month? • Are you able to manage your money and financial affairs? • Would you like advice about financial allowances or benefits?	• Referral for specialist financial advice • Advice on delegation of financial decision-making with protection against financial abuse

Continued

Continued

Domain	Questions	Intervention
Isolation	Do you feel lonely?	Review ways to enhance: • Close social connections (spouse, family, friends, and pets) • Use of local community resources (clubs, faith groups, day centers, sports, leisure, and education) • Opportunities to contribute (volunteering, employment) • Connectivity using communications technology
Meaningful activities	Are you able to pursue leisure interests, hobbies, work, volunteering, supporting your family, and educational or spiritual activities that are important to you?	• Provide a list of local community services • Encourage the older person to use these services
Elder abuse	• Observe for cues of possible elder abuse • Behavior of the older person • Behavior of the caregiver/relative • Signs and symptoms of physical abuse	Refer for specialist assessment through social work, adult protection, or law enforcement systems

TABLE 9: Areas of assessment.

Areas of assessment	Questions	Management
Burden of caregiving	• Does your role as a caregiver have a negative impact on your life? • Do you feel unsupported in your role as a caregiver?	Support for caregivers: • Training • Counseling • Coaching
Mood of caregiver	Over past 2 weeks, have you been bothered by: • Feeling down, depressed, or hopeless? • Little interest or pleasure in doing things?	• If yes: Assess the mood and manage depression • If no: Address the strain with support and psychoeducation • Provide problem-solving counseling • Provide cognitive behavioral therapy
Financial costs of caregiving	Ask: Are you facing loss of income and/or additional expenses because of the needs of care?	• If yes: explore local financial support options and strengthen links with formal long-term care systems and community support • If no: Reassess every 6 months

CONCLUSION

Aging is a natural journey, but how we age can make all the difference. Healthy aging is about much more than living longer it is about living well. When older adults maintain their physical strength, mental sharpness, and emotional well-being, they preserve their independence and sense of purpose. Intrinsic capacity reminds us that even small actions like staying active, eating well, keeping the mind engaged, and nurturing relationships can protect resilience and dignity in later years. With the right support from families, communities, and health systems, older adults can continue to contribute, connect, and thrive. In this way, healthy aging becomes not only an individual goal but also a collective responsibility, ensuring that growing older is a stage of life marked by fulfillment and meaning rather than decline.

Self-Assessment Questionnaire

Q1. Define "healthy aging" as per the World Health Organization (WHO). How does it differ from traditional concepts of successful aging, and what are the key determinants of healthy aging?

Q2. Explain the concept of "intrinsic capacity" and its components. How is intrinsic capacity measured, and why is it central to the WHO's approach to healthy aging?

Q3. Discuss the relationship between intrinsic capacity and functional ability. How can a decline in intrinsic capacity be prevented or managed in older adults?

Q4. Identify key clinical interventions or approaches to assess and enhance intrinsic capacity in older adults. How would these differ from conventional geriatric assessments?

Q5. How can healthcare systems support healthy aging by promoting intrinsic capacity at different stages of the life course? Provide examples of policy or community-based interventions.

FURTHER READINGS

1. World Health Organization. (2015). World report on aging and health. [online] Available from https://www.who.int/publications/i/item/9789241565042/. [Last accessed May, 2025].
2. World Health Organization. Integrated Care for Older People (ICOPE): A Manual for Primary Care Physicians (trainee's Handbook). India: World Health Organization, Regional Office for South-East Asia; 2020.
3. World Health Organization. Global Strategy and Action Plan on Aging and Health. Geneva: World Health Organization; 2017.
4. de Fátima Ribeiro Silva C, Ohara DG, Matos AP, Pinto ACPN, Pegorari MS. Short physical performance battery as a measure of physical performance and mortality predictor in older adults: a comprehensive literature review. !nt J Environ Res Public Health. 2021;18(20):10612.
5. World Health Organization. Decade of Healthy Aging: Baseline Report. Geneva: World Health Organization; 2020.

CHAPTER 12

Frailty

Laxmi Kant Goyal

CASE VIGNETTE

Patient information: Mrs Vandana Jain, a 77-year-old female with a history of coronary artery disease, hypertension, hearing impairment, and osteoarthritis of knee.

Presenting complaint: She has presented with progressive generalized fatigue for 4 years.

History of present illness: She has been having generalized fatigue progressing for the last 4 years, leading to recurrent hospitalizations. She is also having difficulty in performing her daily activities.

Medical history: She has a history of coronary artery disease and hypertension, managed with oral medication. She has severe osteoarthritis of the knee and a hearing impairment.

Social history: She is a homemaker and lives with her husband, son, daughter-in-law, and her one grandchild in a joint family setup. She has no history of alcohol or tobacco use.

Review of systems: Apart from the generalized fatigue, she has mild depression and urinary incontinence. She denies any other significant symptoms.

Physical examination: During the physical examination, her blood pressure is 150/90 mm Hg and her heart rate is 80 beats per minute. Examination of her musculoskeletal system reveals reduced joint mobility in her knees and a slightly curved spine. She also has a significant hearing impairment in both ears.

INTRODUCTION

Frailty is a multifaceted clinical syndrome that represents a heightened vulnerability to adverse health outcomes due to a significant decline in physiological reserve and resilience across multiple body systems. This syndrome is prevalent in the geriatric population and is characterized by decreased physical strength, reduced endurance, and diminished capacity to cope with stressors, leading to an increased likelihood of falls, disability, hospitalization, and mortality. Unlike specific chronic diseases, frailty encompasses a more generalized state of physiological decline that transcends individual health conditions, positioning it as a distinct and crucial entity in geriatric medicine.

As a public health challenge, frailty affects 10–15% of adults over the age of 65 years, with prevalence increasing with age and reaching approximately 25–50% in those over 85 years old. Frailty is more commonly observed in women, partly due to their longer life expectancy and differences in body composition, as well as hormonal and immune system variations. Importantly, frailty is not an inevitable consequence of aging but rather the result of complex interactions among biological, psychological, and social factors. Identifying and addressing frailty early in older adults is critical, as it enables healthcare providers to implement preventive and management strategies aimed at preserving function, independence, and quality of life.

Frailty is often associated with other geriatric syndromes, such as cognitive impairment, depression, and polypharmacy, which can interact synergistically to exacerbate overall decline. Social determinants of health, including isolation, financial instability, and limited access to resources, further compound frailty risk and underscore its complexity as a geriatric syndrome. Given this, frailty management requires a multidimensional approach, including physical, cognitive, emotional, and social interventions that collectively support resilience.

IMPACT OF FRAILTY ON GERIATRIC CARE

Frailty has profound implications for healthcare delivery, as frail older adults tend to have higher healthcare needs and incur greater costs due to frequent hospitalizations, prolonged recovery times, and increased use of long-term care facilities. Identifying frailty in older adults enables healthcare providers to tailor interventions that address specific deficits and minimize risks associated with common age-related conditions. Frailty assessments are especially valuable in predicting outcomes of surgical and nonsurgical treatments, as frail individuals often have poorer recovery and higher complication rates. Consequently, incorporating frailty assessment into routine geriatric care can lead to more targeted, personalized care plans that mitigate adverse outcomes and enhance patient quality of life.

In the broader context, frailty assessments contribute to public health strategies by identifying at-risk individuals in the community, facilitating early interventions, and optimizing resource allocation. The prevalence of frailty in aging populations highlights the importance of developing geriatric services that emphasize preventive care, timely diagnosis, and multidisciplinary interventions.

PATHOPHYSIOLOGY OF FRAILTY

The pathophysiology of frailty is complex and involves a dynamic interplay between biological, physiological, and psychosocial mechanisms that progressively reduce an individual's ability to withstand stress. Frailty is driven by chronic low-grade inflammation, sarcopenia (muscle loss and dysfunction), hormonal changes, oxidative stress, and psychosocial factors, each contributing to the decline in physiological reserve and overall resilience.

Chronic Inflammation ("Inflammaging")

Chronic low-grade inflammation, often termed "inflammaging," is a central component of frailty's pathophysiology. Aging disrupts immune function, leading to an ongoing inflammatory state characterized by elevated levels of inflammatory markers such as C-reactive protein (CRP) and interleukin 6 (IL-6). These markers are significantly higher in frail individuals and are implicated in the breakdown of muscle and tissue integrity. Persistent inflammation results in tissue damage and accelerates the aging process across multiple organ systems, impairing the body's ability to repair and regenerate.

Additionally, chronic inflammation exacerbates other pathophysiological mechanisms underlying frailty, such as muscle degradation and oxidative stress. This systemic inflammation often originates from cellular senescence, where aging cells lose their ability to divide and instead release proinflammatory cytokines. The presence of these senescent cells in tissues contributes to a continuous cycle of inflammation and cellular damage, leading to further physiological decline.

Oxidative Stress and Mitochondrial Dysfunction

Oxidative stress, which involves an imbalance between free radical production and antioxidant defenses, plays a significant role in frailty. As individuals age, the body's ability to neutralize free radicals diminishes, leading to an accumulation of oxidative damage in cells and tissues. This damage affects essential cellular components, including DNA, proteins, and lipids, compromising cell function and contributing to the physical decline observed in frail older adults. Mitochondria, the powerhouse of the cell, are particularly susceptible to oxidative damage, which impairs their capacity for efficient energy production. Mitochondrial dysfunction further exacerbates fatigue, weakness, and decreased endurance, the hallmark features of frailty.

In frail individuals, mitochondrial dysfunction disrupts cellular energy balance, leading to lower energy availability for physical activity, muscle contraction, and organ function. This dysfunction creates a cycle where cells struggle to meet energy demands, accelerating the loss of function and physiological reserve, particularly in muscle and cardiovascular tissues. The interaction between oxidative stress, mitochondrial dysfunction, and chronic inflammation creates a self-perpetuating feedback loop that drives the progression of frailty.

Sarcopenia: A Key Component of Frailty

Sarcopenia, defined as the loss of skeletal muscle mass, strength, and function, is both a hallmark and a key driver of frailty. Sarcopenia arises from a combination of reduced muscle protein synthesis, increased protein breakdown, and altered muscle composition. These changes are fueled by multiple factors, including reduced physical activity, hormonal imbalances, and poor nutrition.

Age-related hormonal declines in anabolic hormones, such as testosterone, growth hormone, and insulin-like growth factor-1 (IGF-1), contribute significantly to sarcopenia. These hormones are essential for muscle growth and repair, and their reduction leads to decreased muscle mass and strength. Concurrently, higher levels of catabolic cytokines, such as tumor necrosis factor-alpha (TNF-α), increase protein degradation within muscle tissues. Over time, this hormonal and cytokine imbalance promotes muscle wasting and decreases physical capacity, which are central to the physical manifestations of frailty.

Sarcopenia also involves neuromuscular changes that impair muscle activation and coordination. Age-related degeneration of motor neurons reduces the number and function of motor units, affecting muscle contraction and leading to weaker, slower movements. The resulting decline in physical capacity increases the risk of falls and restricts mobility, further exacerbating frailty. Sarcopenia and frailty share a reciprocal relationship, where declining muscle mass and function feed into other frailty-related deficits, creating a cycle of functional impairment.

Neuroendocrine Dysregulation

Frailty involves shifts in the neuroendocrine system, particularly involving hormones that regulate muscle, bone, and metabolic function. Aging reduces anabolic hormone levels—such as testosterone, dehydroepiandrosterone (DHEA), growth hormone, and IGF-1—which are critical for maintaining muscle mass and strength. Additionally, there is often an increase in cortisol, a catabolic hormone associated with muscle degradation and bone resorption. These hormonal shifts reduce the body's capacity for muscle maintenance, bone health, and energy metabolism, contributing to frailty's progression.

The hypothalamic–pituitary–adrenal (HPA) axis, which modulates stress response, also becomes dysregulated with age. Frail individuals often have an exaggerated or prolonged response to stress, further increasing cortisol levels and promoting catabolic processes. This hormonal imbalance decreases resilience and reduces the body's ability to recover from physiological and psychological stressors, thereby accelerating frailty.

Psychosocial Factors

Psychosocial factors, including social isolation, depression, and cognitive impairment, play a significant role in frailty's development and progression. Social isolation is particularly detrimental, as it is associated with reduced physical activity, poor nutritional intake, and increased stress. Loneliness and isolation create a feedback loop that exacerbates physical and cognitive decline, making older adults more vulnerable to frailty.

Depression, another common psychosocial factor, negatively affects motivation, energy, and self-care. Depressive symptoms decrease physical activity levels, further contributing to muscle wasting and decreased mobility. Cognitive impairment also plays a role in frailty by limiting the individual's ability to manage chronic conditions, adhere to treatments, and engage in health-promoting behaviors. Together, these psychosocial factors amplify frailty's physical manifestations and underscore the need for a holistic approach to frailty assessment and management.

Interaction with Chronic Diseases

Frailty frequently coexists with multiple chronic diseases, such as cardiovascular disease, diabetes, and chronic obstructive pulmonary disease (COPD), which further accelerate the decline in physiological reserves and resilience. Chronic conditions impose additional metabolic demands on the body, compounding the impact of frailty and increasing the risk of adverse health outcomes. For instance, cardiovascular disease reduces cardiac output, leading to fatigue and decreased physical endurance. Similarly, diabetes is associated with sarcopenia and neuropathy, impairing mobility and functional independence.

The presence of chronic disease exacerbates frailty through a cycle of reduced activity, decreased muscle mass, and diminished energy reserves, ultimately limiting the body's capacity to cope with stressors. As these conditions worsen over time, they contribute to frailty's progression, resulting in a cumulative impact on health and quality of life. Recognizing this interaction is essential in managing frail older adults, as it requires addressing not only the primary disease but also the multifactorial deficits associated with frailty.

SCREENING AND ASSESSMENT OF FRAILTY

The screening and assessment of frailty in older adults are critical steps in identifying individuals at high risk for adverse health outcomes and guiding personalized care plans. Various validated tools are used to detect frailty, assess its severity, and guide clinical decisions. These tools often evaluate physical, cognitive, and social domains, as frailty is a multidimensional syndrome involving multiple body systems.

Purpose of Screening and Early Detection

Early identification of frailty allows for timely interventions that can prevent further decline and improve quality of life. Screening for frailty is particularly important because many individuals may not present with overt symptoms until they experience a significant event, such as a fall or hospitalization. Identifying frailty early enables healthcare providers to apply interventions that preserve physical function, reduce hospital admissions, and lower mortality rates.

Routine screening for frailty is recommended in primary care settings and in any clinical context where older adults frequently present, such as outpatient clinics, emergency departments, and rehabilitation centers. By incorporating frailty screening into routine evaluations, healthcare providers can recognize individuals who may benefit from comprehensive geriatric assessment (CGA) and multidisciplinary management.

Key Screening and Assessment Tools

Multiple tools exist for frailty assessment, each with distinct criteria, advantages, and limitations. Some widely used tools are given as follows:

- *Fried frailty phenotype*: Developed by Dr Linda Fried and her colleagues, this phenotype model classifies frailty based on five criteria: (1) Unintentional weight loss, (2) exhaustion, (3) weakness (grip strength), (4) slow walking speed, and (5) low physical activity. Individuals meeting three or more criteria are considered frail, while those meeting one or two are classified as prefrail. The Fried frailty phenotype focuses on physical aspects, making it useful in both clinical and research settings. This straightforward approach is suitable for primary care and allows for easy identification of physically frail individuals.
- *Rockwood Clinical Frailty Scale (CFS)*: The CFS is a judgment-based tool that assesses frailty across multiple domains, including cognitive and functional status. It categorizes individuals on a scale from 1 (very fit) to 9 (terminally ill), offering a comprehensive view of frailty. The Rockwood scale is particularly valuable for assessing individuals with complex health conditions, as it captures the broader context of frailty by including social and psychological factors. It is commonly used in hospitals and long-term care settings.
- *Frailty index (FI)*: The FI, based on the cumulative deficit model, assesses frailty by calculating the ratio of deficits present (such as symptoms, diseases, or functional impairments) to the total number of deficits considered. The FI provides a nuanced assessment that reflects an individual's accumulated health challenges, allowing for personalized risk stratification. While comprehensive, it may require more time and detail, making it most suitable for comprehensive assessments rather than quick screenings.
- *Short Physical Performance Battery (SPPB)*: The SPPB evaluates lower extremity function by testing balance, gait speed, and chair stand abilities. Lower scores on the SPPB indicate reduced physical performance and are predictive of frailty. This tool is practical for assessing physical function and can be quickly administered in clinical settings, particularly for patients with limited mobility.
- *Timed Up and Go test*: The TUG test measures the time it takes for an individual to stand up from a seated position, walk a short distance, turn, return, and sit down again. A longer completion time indicates impaired mobility and higher frailty levels. The TUG test is a simple, effective way to assess mobility and fall risk, and it can be used alongside other assessments in primary care and hospital settings.

Comprehensive Geriatric Assessment

In frail older adults, a positive frailty screening should prompt a CGA, a multidimensional diagnostic process that evaluates medical, psychological, functional, and social domains. CGA identifies deficits that may benefit from intervention and guides the development of individualized care plans. CGA typically involves a multidisciplinary team, including geriatricians, nurses, social workers, physiotherapists, and dietitians, to address all aspects of frailty comprehensively.

Through CGA, healthcare providers can identify specific needs, such as nutritional supplementation, physical therapy, social support, or medication adjustments, which are integral to effective frailty management. Studies show that CGA improves outcomes in frail older adults by reducing hospitalizations, enhancing functional independence, and improving quality of life.

Predictive Value and Outcomes of Frailty Assessments

Frailty assessment tools are instrumental in predicting adverse outcomes, such as falls, disability, hospitalization, and mortality. Identifying frail individuals allows providers to implement preventive measures and guide decision-making in acute and long-term care settings. For instance:

- *Surgical outcomes*: Frailty is a predictor of poor outcomes in surgical patients, including increased rates of postoperative complications, longer hospital stays, and higher mortality rates. Recognizing frailty preoperatively enables providers to tailor perioperative care, such as prehabilitation programs and enhanced recovery protocols, to improve outcomes.
- *Emergency care*: In emergency settings, frailty assessments can inform decisions about hospitalization, discharge planning, and the need for follow-up care. Frail individuals discharged from the emergency department may benefit from additional support or monitoring to prevent readmission.
- *Chronic disease management*: Frailty is associated with poorer outcomes in chronic conditions such as cardiovascular disease and COPD. Recognizing frailty allows for adjustments in disease management strategies, such as medication optimization, lifestyle interventions, and closer monitoring to reduce exacerbations and improve long-term outcomes.

MANAGEMENT OF FRAILTY

The management of frailty involves a comprehensive, individualized approach that addresses biological, physical, and psychosocial domains. Effective frailty management aims to improve physical resilience, reduce risks of adverse events, and enhance quality of life.

Nutritional Interventions

Nutrition is a cornerstone of frailty management, as malnutrition and muscle wasting are common in frail older adults. Nutritional interventions focus on the following:

- *Protein intake*: Adequate protein intake is essential for maintaining muscle mass and function. Protein requirements may be higher for frail older adults to counteract muscle loss, and foods rich in essential amino acids, especially leucine, help stimulate muscle protein synthesis. Protein-rich foods, including lean meats, eggs, dairy, and legumes, are recommended, and protein supplements may be used in cases of poor dietary intake.
- *Micronutrient support*: Vitamin D and calcium are vital for bone health and muscle function. Vitamin D supplementation is particularly important in frail older adults at risk of falls and fractures, as deficiency is linked to muscle weakness and osteoporosis. Omega-3 fatty acids, antioxidants, and B vitamins also support muscle and bone health and may reduce inflammation.
- *Individualized nutritional plans*: Frail older adults often face challenges such as reduced appetite, dental issues, and taste changes, which may impair food intake. Working with dietitians to create personalized meal plans that are nutrient-dense, easy to prepare, and palatable is key to addressing specific nutritional needs and promoting overall well-being.

Physical Activity and Exercise

Physical activity is crucial for preventing and managing frailty, as it can improve muscle strength, balance, and endurance. Exercise interventions should include the following:

- *Resistance training*: Resistance exercises, such as weightlifting or resistance band exercises, help build muscle strength and counteract sarcopenia. Progressive resistance training has been shown to improve physical performance and reduce frailty severity in older adults.
- *Aerobic exercises*: Low-impact aerobic activities, such as walking, swimming, or cycling, improve cardiovascular health and endurance. Regular aerobic exercise enhances oxygenation and reduces fatigue, improving overall functional capacity.
- *Balance and flexibility training*: Exercises such as tai chi, yoga, and specific balance routines reduce fall risk by improving stability and flexibility. These activities are beneficial for frail individuals, as they help maintain mobility and reduce the risk of injury.
- *Individualized exercise programs*: Exercise regimens should be tailored to each individual's functional status, comorbidities, and preferences to ensure safety and adherence. Physiotherapists play a crucial role in developing and supervising these programs, especially for those with mobility limitations.

Pharmacological Interventions

Although no medications are currently approved specifically for frailty, pharmacological strategies may target symptoms or underlying conditions that exacerbate frailty:

- *Hormone replacement therapy*: Testosterone replacement may benefit older men with low testosterone and significant muscle loss, while growth hormone supplements may improve muscle mass, though their use must be balanced against potential risks.
- *Angiotensin-converting enzyme (ACE) inhibitors*: Evidence suggests that ACE inhibitors may improve muscle strength and physical performance in older adults with hypertension or heart failure. The exact mechanism is unclear, but it may involve modulation of muscle metabolism and reduction of inflammation.
- *Deprescribing*: Frail individuals often take multiple medications, increasing the risk of polypharmacy and adverse drug events. Regular medication reviews to deprescribe unnecessary medications reduce polypharmacy risks, improving physical and cognitive function in frail patients.

Multidisciplinary Care

A multidisciplinary approach to frailty management involves a team of healthcare professionals, including geriatricians, dietitians, physiotherapists, occupational therapists, social workers, and nurses. Each professional addresses different aspects of frailty:

- *Geriatricians* provide medical oversight, coordinate care, and adjust treatments to accommodate frailty.
- *Dietitians* offer nutritional guidance, ensuring adequate intake of essential nutrients.
- *Physiotherapists* develop exercise programs to improve physical function, balance, and endurance.
- *Occupational therapists* assist with activities of daily living (ADLs) and recommend assistive devices for safety.
- *Social workers* connect individuals with community resources and support systems to combat isolation and access

CHALLENGES AND FUTURE DIRECTIONS IN FRAILTY

Barriers in Diagnosis and Management

Diagnosing and managing frailty presents several challenges due to its inherently multifaceted nature. One of the primary barriers is the variability in definitions and assessment tools used to identify frailty. Various criteria and scales, such as the Fried frailty phenotype, the CFS, and others, may yield inconsistent results when applied in different clinical settings. This lack of standardization makes it difficult to uniformly identify frailty across healthcare systems and can result in significant discrepancies in patient management. Inconsistent identification can lead to both underdiagnosis, where patients do not receive necessary interventions, and overdiagnosis, where individuals may be subjected to unnecessary treatments.

Furthermore, frailty often coexists with other geriatric syndromes, including cognitive impairment, depression, and chronic diseases, complicating the diagnostic process. The overlapping nature of these conditions can obscure the recognition of frailty, leading to delays in appropriate management and a missed opportunity for early interventions that could improve patient outcomes. For example, cognitive decline may hinder an individual's ability to participate in physical activities or adhere to treatment plans, further exacerbating frailty.

The lack of awareness and training among healthcare providers regarding frailty assessment and management remains a significant obstacle. Many practitioners may not fully understand the implications of frailty or how to conduct effective assessments. This gap in knowledge can lead to insufficient attention being paid to frailty in clinical evaluations and treatment planning.

Healthcare systems also face logistical challenges in addressing frailty effectively. Limited resources, including insufficient time during consultations and fragmented care models, can hinder the implementation of comprehensive frailty management programs. Coordinating multidisciplinary care, which is essential for addressing the diverse needs of frail older adults, requires a robust infrastructure and collaboration among various healthcare professionals, including geriatricians, primary care providers, physical therapists, and social workers. The absence of integrated care pathways can lead to gaps in service delivery and fragmented patient experiences.

Emerging Therapies and Research

Advancements in our understanding of the pathophysiology of frailty have opened new avenues for developing targeted therapies. One promising area of research involves the use of anti-inflammatory agents to counteract the chronic inflammation commonly associated with frailty. Inflammation is recognized as a significant contributor to the decline in physical function and health status in older adults. Clinical trials are currently exploring the potential of these agents to improve physical function, reduce frailty-related complications, and enhance overall quality of life for frail individuals.

Senolytics, a class of drugs designed to target and eliminate senescent cells, represent another emerging therapy in frailty management. The accumulation of senescent cells is linked to various age-related conditions, including frailty, as they promote inflammation and tissue damage. Preclinical studies have shown that senolytics can improve physical function and extend health span in animal models, raising hopes for their application in human frailty management. Ongoing research aims to evaluate the safety and efficacy of these drugs in frail older adults, with the goal of translating these findings into clinical practice.

Additionally, mitochondrial enhancers that improve mitochondrial function and energy production are being investigated as potential therapies for frailty. These agents may help mitigate fatigue and muscle weakness, two common manifestations of frailty, thereby enhancing overall physical performance. Nutraceuticals, including supplements such as omega-3 fatty acids and antioxidants, are also being studied for their role in frailty prevention and management. The potential for these agents to positively influence health outcomes underscores the importance of a comprehensive approach to frailty that includes both pharmacological and lifestyle interventions.

Personalized Interventions

Personalized interventions tailored to individual frailty profiles hold great promise for improving outcomes among older adults. Biomarkers, such as inflammatory markers and genetic factors, can assist in identifying individuals at risk of frailty and guiding personalized treatment strategies. Precision medicine approaches that incorporate genetic, epigenetic, and environmental factors can optimize interventions, enhancing their effectiveness and relevance for each patient.

Developing predictive models to assess the risk of frailty and its progression is another crucial research direction. These models can integrate clinical, biological, and lifestyle data to provide a comprehensive risk assessment for frailty. Early identification of at-risk individuals allows healthcare providers to implement timely interventions aimed at preventing or delaying the onset of frailty. Such proactive approaches are essential in promoting healthier aging and improving the overall quality of life for older adults.

Technology and Innovation

Technological innovations offer exciting opportunities to enhance frailty management. Telemedicine and digital health platforms can facilitate remote monitoring, consultations, and intervention delivery, particularly for older adults with mobility issues or those living in rural areas with limited access to healthcare facilities. This approach can help bridge the gap in care delivery and ensure that frail individuals receive the support they need, regardless of their location.

Wearable devices, such as fitness trackers and smartwatches, are gaining traction in monitoring physical activity, heart rate, and other vital signs, providing real-time data that can be invaluable for assessing and managing frailty. These devices can help individuals track their physical activity levels and adherence to prescribed exercise regimens, promoting engagement in health-enhancing behaviors.

Furthermore, artificial intelligence (AI) and machine learning (ML) algorithms hold great potential for analyzing large datasets to identify patterns and predict frailty risk. These technologies can support clinical decision-making by providing personalized recommendations and identifying individuals who may benefit from specific interventions. By integrating AI and ML into electronic health records (EHRs), healthcare systems can streamline frailty assessment and management, making it easier for providers to deliver tailored care.

CONCLUSION

Frailty is a multifaceted syndrome with profound implications for older adults, influencing their health status, functional abilities, and overall quality of life. Early identification and comprehensive management are key to mitigating its impact and enhancing well-being in this vulnerable population. By addressing the biological, physical, and psychosocial aspects of frailty, healthcare providers can create more effective care strategies that support the aging population. Continued research and innovation are essential to developing effective interventions, optimizing personalized care approaches, and improving outcomes for frail individuals.

Through collaboration among researchers, healthcare providers, and policymakers, the goal of achieving healthier aging and improved quality of life for older adults can be realized.

Self-Assessment Questionnaire

Q1. What is frailty and why is it important in geriatric care?

Q2. Describe the role of sarcopenia in the pathophysiology of frailty.

Q3. What are the key clinical tools used to assess frailty?

Q4. How do nutritional interventions help in managing frailty?

Q5. What challenges exist in diagnosing and managing frailty?

Q6. What is the Fried frailty phenotype, and how is it used to assess frailty?

Q7. Why is a multidisciplinary approach important in managing frailty?

Q8. How does chronic inflammation contribute to the development of frailty?

Q9. What role do physical activity and exercise play in preventing and managing frailty?

Q10. What are some of the emerging therapies being investigated for frailty?

CHAPTER 13

Sarcopenia

Shakti Kruti

CASE VIGNETTE

Mrs S, an 80-year-old woman, with no prior comorbidities presents to her primary care physician with complaints of weakness and difficulty in performing daily activities such as climbing stairs and lifting groceries. She reports a recent unintentional weight loss of 5 kg over the past 6 months. Mrs S also mentions feeling fatigued easily and notices that her arms and legs seem thinner.

INTRODUCTION

Sarcopenia is a disease of the muscles, characterized by progressive loss of muscle mass and muscle function. Sarcopenia stands as a global health challenge, particularly affecting the geriatric population. The Asian Working Group for Sarcopenia (AWGS) in 2019 defined sarcopenia as the age-related loss of skeletal muscle mass combined with decreased muscle strength and/or reduced physical performance. The prevalence of sarcopenia varies depending upon the definition used to define sarcopenia. The pooled prevalence of sarcopenia for all definitions was found to be 10%. In a meta-analysis of 58,402 community-dwelling older adults, aged 60 years and above, the overall global prevalence of sarcopenia was found to be 10%. However, in a cross-sectional study, the prevalence of sarcopenia in the rural south Indian population was found to be 14.2%. Clinicians frequently encounter cases of sarcopenia in their daily practice. Therefore, understanding sarcopenia is crucial for the effective prevention, diagnosis, and treatment of this condition in the aging population.

Although sarcopenia is commonly associated with aging, its origins can be traced back earlier in life. This realization underscores the importance of early detection and proactive interventions. Sarcopenia is associated with several adverse health outcomes such as falls and fractures, impaired ability to perform activities of daily living (ADL), increased risk of cardiac disease and respiratory disease, and mobility disorders.

Trivia

The term *sarcopenia* is derived from a Greek words "sarx" meaning flesh and "penia" meaning poverty of flesh.

RISK FACTORS

Sarcopenia is not an unavoidable consequence of aging; it is influenced by various risk factors, some of which are modifiable. Recognizing these factors can aid in their prevention. Age is a significant risk factor for sarcopenia. Lifestyle factors, including less physical activity, inadequate nutrition, dental health, shorter and longer sleep durations, and smoking, are associated with increased risk. Additionally, cardiometabolic factors such as diabetes and its complications, hypertension, dyslipidemia, and osteoporosis contribute to the risk.

TYPES

Primary and secondary sarcopenia represent two categories of sarcopenia: Primary and secondary sarcopenia. Primary sarcopenia, is age-related, which occurs without an identifiable underlying cause. It is considered as a complex geriatric syndrome with multifactorial pathogenesis seen in older adults. Secondary sarcopenia, conversely, can manifest in any age group and is linked to an underlying cause. The list of causes for secondary sarcopenia is extensive and can be broadly categorized as medical, endocrinological, and metabolic **(Box 1)**. In most cases, the etiology of sarcopenia tends to be multifactorial. Thus, characterizing individuals as having solely primary or secondary sarcopenia is challenging due to significant overlap between the two categories.

Trivia

In 1989, Rosenberg proposed the term "sarcopenia."

BOX 1 Causes of secondary sarcopenia.

Medical conditions:
- Renal disease: Chronic kidney disease (CKD), end-stage renal disease (ESRD)
- Cardiac disease: Chronic heart failure (CHF)
- Liver disease: Liver cirrhosis
- Respiratory disease: COPD
- Neurological diseases: Stroke, primary muscular disease
- Malignancy
- Trauma, burns
- Arthritis: Osteoarthritis, rheumatoid arthritis

Endocrinological conditions:
- Hypothyroidism and hyperthyroidism
- Diabetes
- Osteoporosis
- Hypogonadism and menopause
- Obesity

Metabolic conditions:
- Fatty liver/NAFLD

Other conditions:
- Dementia
- Polypharmacy
- Psychiatric/psychological conditions: Dementia and anorexia nervosa
- Sepsis
- HIV and AIDS, etc.

(AIDS: acquired immunodeficiency syndrome; COPD: chronic obstructive pulmonary disease; HIV: human immunodeficiency virus; NAFLD: nonalcoholic fatty liver disease)

Source: Dhar M, Kapoor N, Suastika K, Khamseh ME, Selim S, Kumar V, et al. South Asian Working Action Group on SARCOpenia (SWAG-SARCO)—a consensus document. Osteoporos Sarcopenia. 2022;8(2):35-57.

PATHOPHYSIOLOGY AND PATHOGENESIS

Multiple factors can contribute to the development of sarcopenia. Aging disrupts the balance between muscle protein breakdown and synthesis, leading to a loss of skeletal muscle. Muscle regeneration depends on the activation of the mammalian target of rapamycin (mTOR) by serine-threonine kinases, which promote muscle protein synthesis. Factors such as insulin-like growth factor-1 (IGF-1), testosterone, and exercise stimulate this process. However, with aging, levels of IGF-1 and testosterone decline, and due to a sedentary lifestyle, there is reduced muscle protein synthesis. Additionally, the activation of the ubiquitin-proteasome pathway increases muscle breakdown.

In addition to the pathogenic mechanisms mentioned above, cellular changes such as decrease in the size and number of myofibers, transition of type 2 to type 1

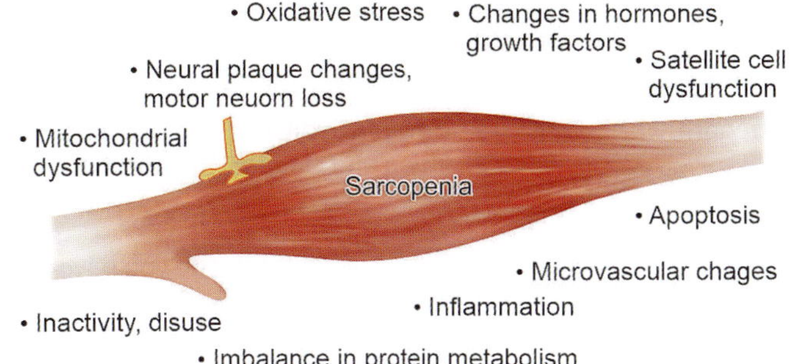

FIG. 1: Pathophysiology of sarcopenia.

Source: Cruz-Jentoft AJ, Sayer AA. Sarcopenia. Lancet. 2019;393(10191):2636-46.

myofibers, an increase in inter- and intramuscular fat infiltration, a decrease in the number of type 2 satellite cells, mitochondrial dysfunction in myocytes, and oxidative stress can all contribute to the development of sarcopenia **(Fig. 1)**.

DIAGNOSIS

The diagnosis of sarcopenia requires measurement of muscle mass, strength, and physical performance. While all definitions of sarcopenia require at least two parameters for diagnosis, each guideline employs different cutoff points. Let us look into the AWGS 2019 recommendations for diagnosing sarcopenia.

- *Case finding*: The initial step in diagnosing sarcopenia involves case finding. Tools such as calf circumference (CC), SARC-F **(Table 1)**, and SARC-CalF are recommended by AWGS 2019 for this purpose. In acute to chronic healthcare or clinical research settings, case finding can be accomplished by identifying conditions such as functional limitations, unintentional weight loss, depressive mood, cognitive impairment, repeated falls, malnutrition, or chronic illnesses such as heart failure and chronic obstructive pulmonary disease (COPD). In settings where these clinical indicators are absent, the case-finding tools mentioned above can be utilized. Case-finding tools of sarcopenia have been summarized in **Table 2**.
SARC-CalF score is calculated by adding 10 points to the SARC-F score if the CC is <34 cm in men and <33 cm in women.
- *Measurement of muscle strength*: According to AWGS 2019, handgrip strength is recommended as an indicator of muscle strength, and dynamometers are used to measure it. Two types of dynamometers are commonly used: (1) Spring-type (Smedley) dynamometer **(Fig. 2)** and (2) hydraulic-type (Jamar) dynamometer **(Fig. 3)**. When using the Smedley dynamometer, it is advised to stand with full elbow extension, while for the Jamar dynamometer, sitting with a 90° elbow flexion is recommended. If older adults are unable

TABLE 1: SARC-F questionnaire.

Component	Question	Scoring	Score
Strength	How much difficulty do you have in lifting and carrying 10 pounds?	• None = 0 • Some = 1 • A lot or unable = 2	
Assistance in walking	How much difficulty do you have walking across a room?	• None = 0 • Some = 1 • A lot, use aids, or unable = 2	
Rise from a chair	How much difficulty do you have transferring from a chair or bed?	• None = 0 • Some = 1 • A lot or unable without help = 2	
Climb stairs	How much difficulty do you have climbing a flight of 10 stairs?	• None = 0 • Some = 1 • A lot or unable = 2	
Falls	How many times have you fallen in the past year?	• None = 0 • One to three falls = 1 • Four or more falls = 2	

TABLE 2: Case-finding tools for sarcopenia.

Case-finding tools	Measurement	Cutoff	
Calf circumference (CC)	Measured using a nonelastic tape as maximum value in both calves	Men < 34 cm Women < 33 cm	Moderate-to-high sensitivity and specificity for predicting sarcopenia
SARC-F	It is a questionnaire which has five components, which are strength, assistance in walking, rising from a chair, climbing stairs, and fall	SARC-F score ≥ 4	Low sensitivity and high specificity
SARC-CalF	It involves adding CC to SARC-F score	SARC-CalF score ≥ 11	It has better sensitivity than SARC-F

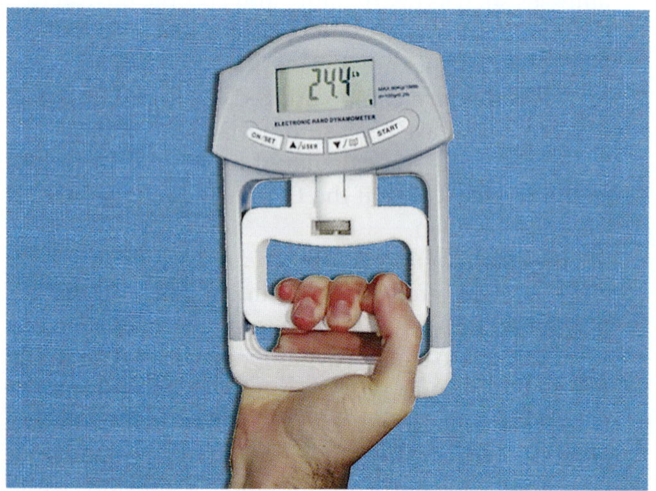

FIG. 2: Spring-type (Smedley) dynamometer.

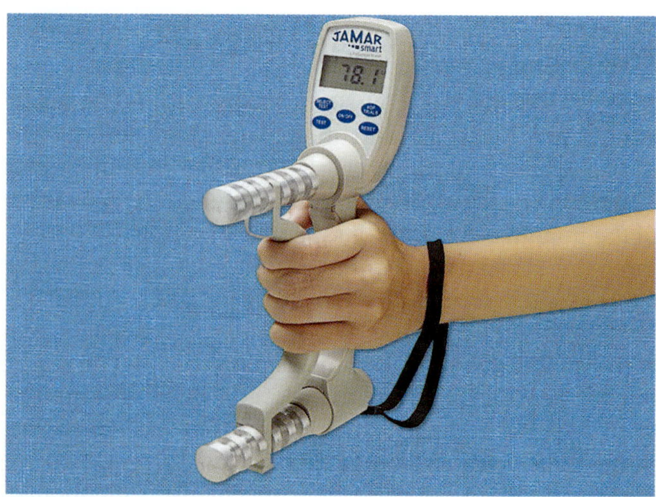

FIG. 3: Hydraulic-type (Jamar) dynamometer.

to stand unassisted, measurements can be taken in a seated position. AWGS 2019 recommends obtaining the maximum reading from at least two trials, either using both hands or the dominant hand, during a maximum-effort isometric contraction. The cutoff point for handgrip strength is <28 kg for men and <18 kg for women.

- *Measurement of skeletal muscle mass*: Skeletal muscle mass can be estimated through various methods such as MRI, CT, dual-energy X-ray absorptiometry (DXA), and bioelectrical impedance analysis (BIA). AWGS 2019 recommends using height-adjusted DXA or multifrequency BIA to measure muscle mass for diagnosing sarcopenia. The cutoff for low skeletal muscle mass is <7 kg/m^2 in men and <6.7 kg/m^2 in women by DXA, and <7 kg/m^2 in men and <5.4 kg/m^2 in women using BIA. BMI-adjusted muscle mass measured by DXA can also be utilized. According to the National Institutes of Health criteria, <0.789 kg/BMI for men and <0.512 kg/BMI for women, measured by DXA, are recommended cutoffs for low skeletal muscle mass.
- *Assessment of physical performance:* Various tests can assess physical performance, including the short physical performance battery (SPPB) **(Fig. 4)**, 6-minute walk test, stair climb power test, and five-time chair stand test. However, according to the AWGS 2019 recommendations, defining low physical performance should primarily rely on the SPPB, 6-minute walk test, or five-time chair stand test. The cutoff values are ≤9 for the SPPB, <1 m/s for the 6-minute walk test, and >12 seconds for the five-time chair stand test. A description of these tests has been summarized in **Table 3**.

After evaluating muscle strength, mass, and physical performance, a diagnosis of possible sarcopenia, sarcopenia, or severe sarcopenia can be determined. In primary healthcare or community preventive settings, if a diagnosis of possible sarcopenia is established, appropriate lifestyle interventions and health education are provided, and patients are referred to hospitals for confirmation of the diagnosis. **Flowchart 1** illustrates the AWGS 2019 recommended algorithm for diagnosing sarcopenia.

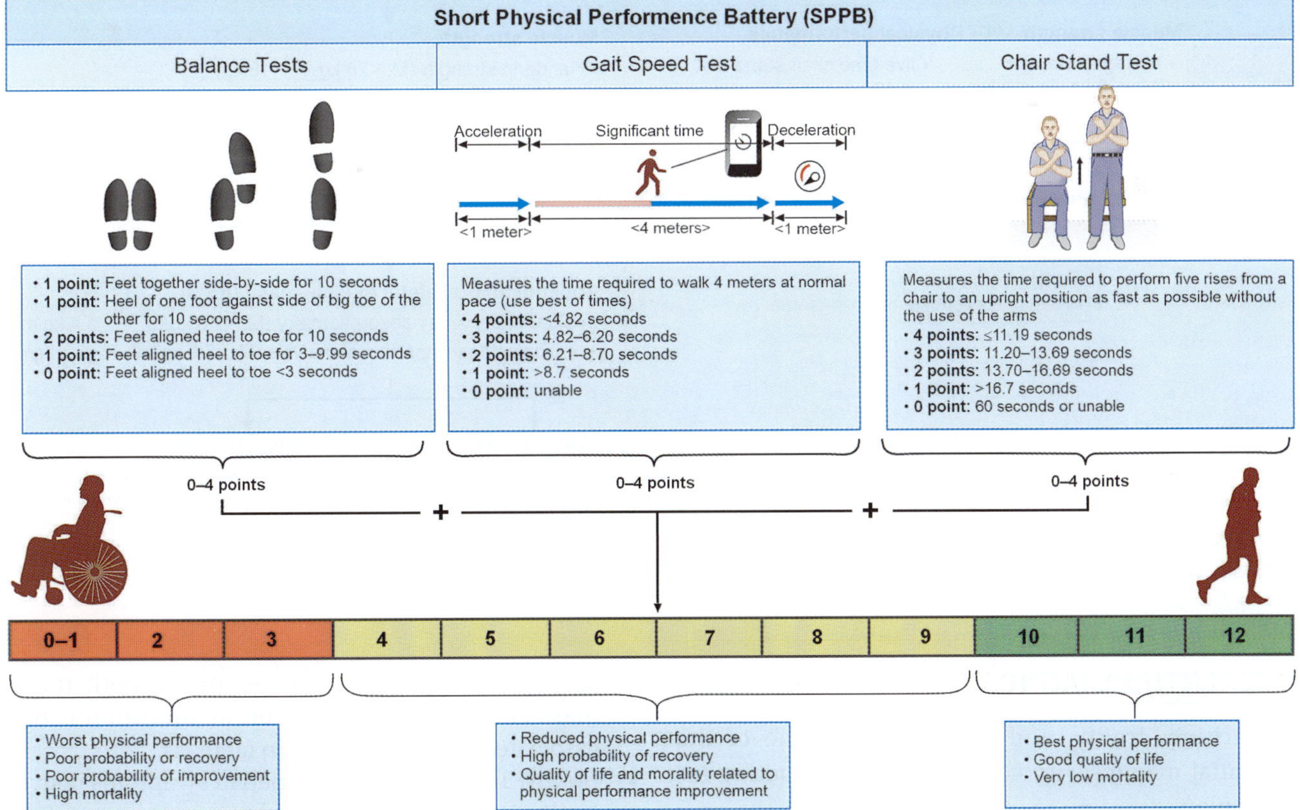

FIG. 4: Short physical performance battery (SPPB).

Source: Tonet E, Raisi A, Zagnoni S, Chiaranda G, Pavasini R, Vitali F, et al. Multidomain lifestyle intervention in older adults after myocardial infarction: rationale and design of the PIpELINe randomized clinical trial. Aging Clin Exp Res. 2023;35(5):1107-15.

TABLE 3: Tests for assessment of physical performance in sarcopenia.		
Test	**Description**	**Cutoff**
Short physical performance battery	• Balance test • Gait speed test • Chair stand test	≤9
6-minute walk test	• The participant is instructed to walk as far as possible for 6 minutes on a flat, measured course. The total distance covered is recorded	<1 m/s
Five-time chair stand test	• The participant sits in a chair with their arms folded across their chest and feet flat on the floor • They are instructed to rise to a full standing position and sit back down five times consecutively, as fast as possible, without using their arms for assistance • The time taken to complete all five repetitions is recorded	>12 seconds

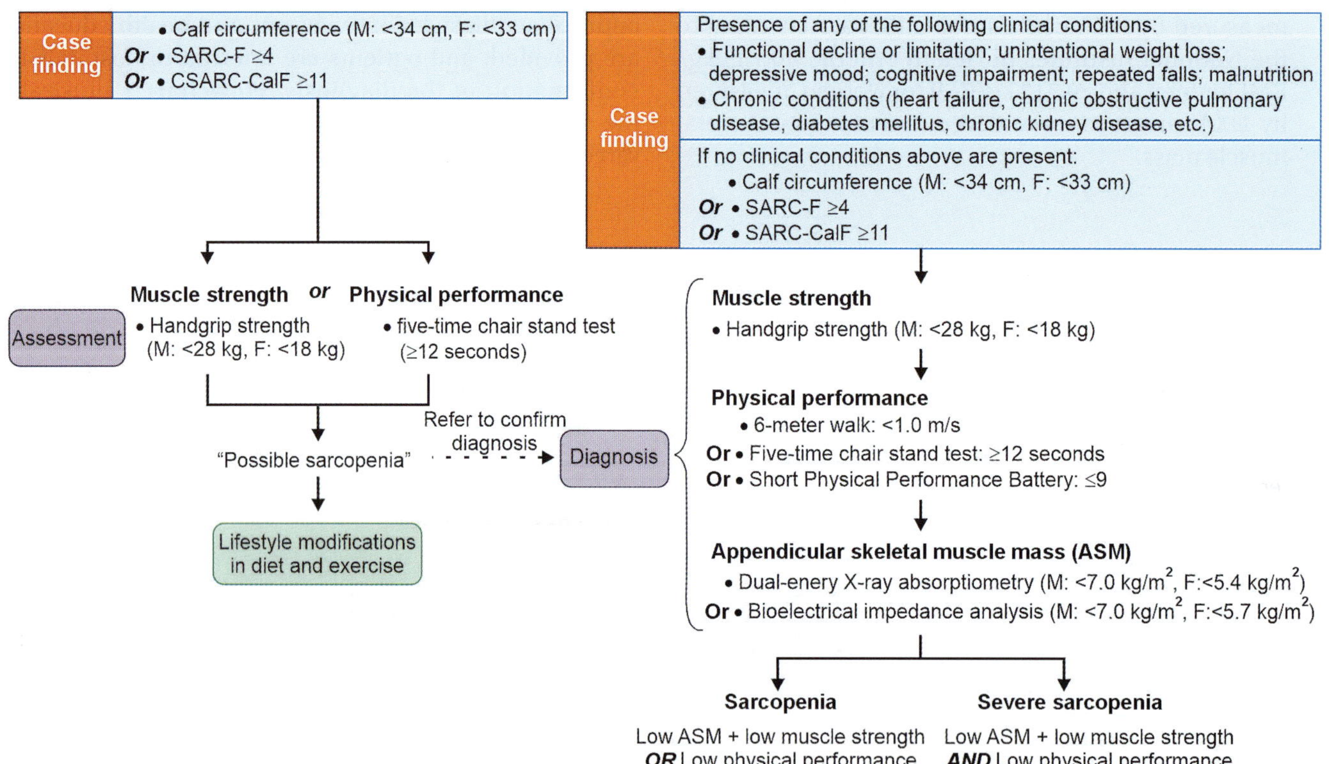

FLOWCHART 1: Algorithm for diagnosis of sarcopenia, AWGS 2019.
(AWGS: Asian Working Group for Sarcopenia)

DIFFERENTIAL DIAGNOSIS

Malnutrition, frailty, and cachexia are some of the differential diagnoses to consider when evaluating for sarcopenia.

- *Malnutrition*: Low muscle mass combined with normal muscle function suggests malnutrition, as sarcopenia typically involves loss of both muscle mass and function. Moreover, malnutrition is often associated with a reduction in fat mass.
- *Frailty*: There can be an overlap in symptoms between frailty and sarcopenia, and they often coexist in the elderly. Frailty represents a state of increased vulnerability to poor resolution of homeostasis

following a stressor event due to cumulative decline across various physiological systems. Frailty is a multisystem impairment and manifests through symptoms such as unintentional weight loss, weakness (evidenced by low grip strength), self-reported exhaustion, slow walking speed, and reduced physical activity. In contrast, sarcopenia primarily affects the musculoskeletal system.

- *Cachexia*: This is a condition characterized by severe weight loss and muscle wasting, frequently linked to underlying conditions such as cancer, human immunodeficiency virus-acquired immunodeficiency syndrome (HIV-AIDS), or end-stage organ failure. Both cachexia and sarcopenia can coexist, and the Glasgow Prognostic Score can aid in distinguishing between the two conditions, often severe muscle wasting with underlying disease goes in favor of cachexia.
- *Hand osteoarthritis (OA)*: This can lead to false-positive low grip strength measurements. Therefore, in patients suspected of severe hand OA, assessing muscle strength in the lower limbs may provide a more accurate evaluation. Lower limb strength can be assessed through functional tests such as the sit-to-stand test or timed up and go test, which provides a more accurate evaluation than relying on grip strength alone.

MANAGEMENT

The primary goal of treating patients with sarcopenia is to prevent further decline in muscle mass and strength, thereby reducing the risk of falls and disability. Treatment also aims to prevent or reduce hospitalizations and ultimately decrease mortality rates among affected patients.

- *Nonpharmacological management*:
    - Exercise and physical activity: A combination of various exercises, including resistance, aerobic, balance, and flexibility exercises, can be employed to manage sarcopenia.
        - Resistance exercises, such as weightlifting, using resistance bands, or performing bodyweight exercises against gravity, are beneficial for improving muscle mass, function, and performance, as well as enhancing gait and balance. These exercises are effective for both primary and secondary sarcopenia.
        - Aerobic exercises, such as jogging, cycling, or brisk walking, contribute to muscle protein synthesis, decrease muscle catabolism, and induce positive cellular changes, thereby promoting increases in muscle mass, strength, and aerobic capacity. In cases where patients with sarcopenia are unable to perform traditional aerobic exercises, low-impact alternatives are preferable, particularly in patients with osteoporosis.
        - Flexibility exercises, such as stretches, can be incorporated as either pre-exercise warm-ups or postexercise cool-downs. Additionally, activities such as tai chi and yoga serve as effective flexibility exercises. They enhance joint mobility across all ranges of motion.
        - Balance exercises, including standing on heels or toes, tandem walking, and walking on various surfaces, aim to stabilize the osteo-arthro-muscular triad, thereby reducing the risk of falls. It is essential for all prescribed exercises to be performed regularly, at least three times per week, considering the patient's exercise capacity. Balance, flexibility, and strength-training exercises must be done before aerobic exercises to ensure stability and to prevent fall.
    - *Nutritional optimization*: This can be achieved through dietary counseling and/or nutritional supplementation. It is recommended that daily protein intake be between 1 and 1.2 g/kg of body weight, as it plays a crucial role in maintaining and building muscle mass. Essential amino acid (EAA) supplementation has been shown to enhance muscle mass and protein synthesis, but it does not seem to impact muscle strength or physical performance. In a systematic review and meta-analysis of 35 randomized controlled trials (RCTs) conducted in sarcopenic older adults, branched-chain amino acid (BCAA)-rich supplementation showed beneficial effects on muscle strength and mass. Another systematic review and meta-analysis of six RCTs found that leucine supplementation improved muscle strength in sarcopenic older adults. However, in a double-blind, placebo-controlled RCT conducted in cirrhotic patients with sarcopenia, the addition of BCAA to exercise, dietary counseling, and standard medical therapy did not result in an improvement in muscle mass. Omega-3 fatty acid supplementation has demonstrated benefits in improving muscle mass, strength, and physical performance, particularly when combined with resistance training and/or protein supplementation. However, supplementation with beta-hydroxy beta-methyl butyric acid has yielded inconsistent results across studies regarding its effectiveness in enhancing muscle mass, strength, and physical performance.

- *Holistic care strategies*: Optimizing medical comorbidities that contribute to secondary sarcopenia through nonpharmacological and pharmacological management is crucial, alongside exercise and nutritional enhancements. Environmental modifications, such as installing grab rails and ramps, can enhance home safety for patients with sarcopenia. Additionally, providing assistive devices to sarcopenic patients facilitates their mobility and ADL. Psychological support is essential for these patients, and consulting with a clinical psychologist is advisable. Patients and caregivers must acknowledge the presence of sarcopenia in the patient and recognize the necessity for rehabilitation. Since nonpharmacological interventions such as exercise and nutritional optimization are paramount in managing sarcopenia, understanding and adhering to the rehabilitation program are essential.

- *Pharmacological management*: None of the medications for treating sarcopenia has been approved by the Food and Drug Administration (FDA). Let us take a brief look at pharmacotherapy options for sarcopenia.
  - *Vitamin D and calcium*: Vitamin D has been shown to improve muscle strength and physical performance, especially in women with low baseline levels. However, the optimal dose and duration of vitamin D supplementation for treating sarcopenia are still under investigation.

    Calcium supplementation has been shown to have positive regulation of muscle health in calcium-deficient patients.
  - *Myostatin inhibitors*: Myostatin is a negative regulator of muscle growth, and myostatin inhibitors are a class of drugs which target this protein. By binding to and neutralizing myostatin, these drugs have been shown to increase muscle protein synthesis, leading to an increase in muscle mass and function. They also offer additional benefits such as enhancing satellite cell activation and differentiation, improving mitochondrial function, and reducing inflammation. However, these drugs are still in the experimental stage and have not yet been approved for clinical use.

    MYO-029, the first myostatin (MSTN) inhibitor developed by Pfizer, showed no significant improvements in muscle size, strength, or function in clinical trials, leading to its discontinuation. Landogrozumab, another myostatin inhibitor, showed modest gains in appendicular lean mass and functional improvements in elderly patients, but subsequent trials in OA and cancer cachexia were largely unsuccessful. Bimagrumab is an antibody targeting MSTN/activin receptor ActRIIB and ActRIIA. This monoclonal antibody showed an increase in thigh muscle volume and improvements in gait speed and walking distance in sarcopenia patients, especially slower walkers. However, no functional benefits were seen in studies with chronic obstructive pulmonary disease (COPD) patients or older adults recovering from hip fractures, despite gains in muscle mass. Clinical trials are still underway.
  - *Testosterone and anabolic steroids*: Testosterone increases muscle mass and reduces muscle fat mass. However, it is associated with side effects such as fluid retention, gynecomastia, and cardiovascular effects. Additionally, there is inconclusive evidence regarding whether the increase in muscle mass correlates with an increase in muscle strength and physical performance. Anabolic steroids increase the fat-free mass, handgrip strength, and muscle mRNA level for several growth factors; however, they are associated with steroid-induced side effects.
  - *Hormonal replacement therapy*: It has been shown to increase the muscle mass; however, this effect is not seen in women >65 years and obese women.
  - *Selective androgen receptor modulators (SARMS)*: They selectively target and activate androgen receptor in muscle and bone tissue and promote muscle growth, while minimizing the activation of androgen receptor in other tissues such as prostate gland. They have not yet been approved by the FDA for clinical use in sarcopenia.
  - *Growth hormone (GH)*: While GH increases the lean muscle mass and reduces the muscle fat mass, it is expensive and associated with side effects such as fluid retention and orthostatic hypotension.

CONCLUSION

Sarcopenia represents a significant health concern, particularly among the elderly population, with its prevalence rising as life expectancy increases globally. While non-pharmacological interventions such as exercise and nutritional optimization play a pivotal role in its management, the exploration of pharmacotherapy options holds promise, albeit with ongoing research required to determine optimal dosages and efficacy.

Self-Assessment Questionnaire

Let us go back to the case of Mrs S.

Q1. What diagnostic criteria would you use to confirm sarcopenia in Mrs S?

Q2. How does sarcopenia impact Mrs S's ability to perform daily activities, and what are the implications for her quality of life?

Q3. Which nonpharmacological interventions, such as exercise and nutrition, are most effective in managing sarcopenia in elderly patients?

Q4. What are the potential long-term consequences if sarcopenia is left untreated in Mrs S's case?

Q5. How can primary care physicians incorporate screening for sarcopenia into routine evaluations of elderly patients?

FURTHER READINGS

1. Carvalho do Nascimento PR, Bilodeau M, Poitras S. How do we define and measure sarcopenia? A meta-analysis of observational studies. Age Ageing. 2021;50(6):1906-13.
2. Shafiee G, Keshtkar A, Soltani A, Ahadi Z, Larijani B, Heshmat R. Prevalence of sarcopenia in the world: a systematic review and meta-analysis of general population studies. J Diabetes Metab Disord. 2017;16:21.
3. Shaikh N, Harshitha R, Bhargava M. Prevalence of sarcopenia in an elderly population in rural South India: a cross-sectional study. F1000Res. 2020;9:75.
4. Schneider SM, Al-Jaouni R, Filippi J, Wiroth JB, Zeanandin G, Arab K, et al. Sarcopenia is prevalent in patients with Crohn's disease in clinical remission. Inflamm Bowel Dis. 2008;14(11):1562-8.
5. Chen LK, Woo J, Assantachai P, Auyeung TW, Chou MY, Iijima K, et al. Asian Working Group for Sarcopenia: 2019 consensus update on sarcopenia diagnosis and treatment. J Am Med Dir Assoc. 2020;21(3):300-7.e2.
6. Yuan S, Larsson SC. Epidemiology of sarcopenia: prevalence, risk factors, and consequences. Metabolism. 2023;144:155533.
7. Santilli V, Bernetti A, Mangone M, Paoloni M. Clinical definition of sarcopenia. Clin Cases Miner Bone Metab. 2014;11(3):177-80.
8. Dhar M, Kapoor N, Suastika K, Khamseh ME, Selim S, Kumar V, et al. South Asian Working Action Group on SARCOpenia (SWAG-SARCO)—a consensus document. Osteoporos Sarcopenia. 2022;8(2):35-57.
9. Cruz-Jentoft AJ, Sayer AA. Sarcopenia. Lancet. 2019;393(10191):2636-46.
10. Jang JY, Kim D, Kim ND. Pathogenesis, intervention, and current status of drug development for sarcopenia: a review. Biomedicines. 2023;11(6):1635.
11. Cesari M, Landi F, Vellas B, Bernabei R, Marzetti E. Sarcopenia and physical frailty: two sides of the same coin. Front Aging Neurosci. 2014;6:192.
12. Dodds R, Sayer AA. Sarcopenia and frailty: new challenges for clinical practice. Clin Med (Lond). 2016;16(5):455-8.
13. Douglas E, McMillan DC. Towards a simple objective framework for the investigation and treatment of cancer cachexia: the Glasgow Prognostic Score. Cancer Treat Rev. 2014;40(6):685-91.
14. Park WT, Shon OJ, Kim GB. Multidisciplinary approach to sarcopenia: a narrative review. J Yeungnam Med Sci. 2023;40(4):352-63.
15. Wetzlich B, Nyakundi BB, Yang J. Therapeutic applications and challenges in myostatin inhibition for enhanced skeletal muscle mass and functions. Mol Cell Biochem. 2025;480(3):1535-53.
16. Bai GH, Tsai MC, Tsai HW, Chang CC, Hou WH. Effects of branched-chain amino acid-rich supplementation on EWGSOP2 criteria for sarcopenia in older adults: a systematic review and meta-analysis. Eur J Nutr. 2022;61(2):637-51.
17. Lee SY, Lee HJ, Lim JY. Effects of leucine-rich protein supplements in older adults with sarcopenia: a systematic review and meta-analysis of randomized controlled trials. Arch Gerontol Geriatr. 2022;102:104758.
18. Mohta S, Anand A, Sharma S, Qamar S, Agarwal S, Gunjan D, et al. Randomised clinical trial: effect of adding branched chain amino acids to exercise and standard-of-care on muscle mass in cirrhotic patients with sarcopenia. Hepatol Int. 2022;16(3):680-90.

CHAPTER 14

Fall

Abhijith Rajaram Rao

CASE VIGNETTE

Patient information: Mrs Saroj Gupta, a 72-year-old female with a history of type 2 diabetes, hypertension, and osteoporosis.

Living situation: Lives with her son and daughter-in-law in a joint family.

Primary care physician: Dr Ananya Sharma.

Presenting complaint: Mrs Saroj Gupta, a 72-year-old retired school principal, visits the local healthcare clinic with concerns about multiple falls she has experienced over the past year. She reports having fallen three times, with the most recent fall occurring last week when she tripped on her way to the kitchen. She expresses worry about her frequent falls and their potential impact on her independence.

History of present illness: Mrs Gupta describes her falls as often happening when she is navigating uneven surfaces or attempting to perform daily activities. She says that the falls have led to minor injuries, such as sprained wrists and minor abrasions, but she has not suffered any major fractures or injuries. She attributes her unsteadiness to the pain in her arthritic knees and osteoporotic bone health. She expresses concerns about falling when her family is not around to assist her and is afraid of being a burden to her son and daughter-in-law.

Medical history: Mrs Gupta has a history of type 2 diabetes, managed with oral medication, and hypertension, for which she takes antihypertensive medications. She was diagnosed with osteoporosis and is prescribed calcium and vitamin D supplements, as well as alendronate. She has not experienced any recent changes in medication or dosages. Her last comprehensive physical examination was conducted 6 months ago.

Social history: Mrs Gupta lives with her son, his wife, and their two children in a joint family setup. She plays an active role in household activities, including helping to care for her grandchildren. She does not have a history of alcohol or tobacco use.

Review of systems: Apart from the falls and associated musculoskeletal pain, Mrs Gupta denies any other significant symptoms, such as dizziness, chest pain, visual disturbances, or urinary incontinence.

Physical examination: During the physical examination, her blood pressure is 138/82 mm Hg and heart rate is 78 beats per minute. Examination of her musculoskeletal system reveals reduced joint mobility in her knees and a slightly curved spine. Neurological examination does not reveal any focal deficits, and gait assessment shows a mildly unsteady gait.

INTRODUCTION

Within the realm of geriatric medicine, few challenges are as pervasive and consequential as the issue of falls among the elderly. As India undergoes a demographic transformation characterized by a rapidly growing aging population, the prevalence of falls among older individuals has become an increasingly significant concern.

Falls represent a critical concern, not just in India but across the globe. In the context of an aging society, understanding the causes, consequences, and prevention of falls in the elderly has become a paramount focus of healthcare and research. Within this chapter, we will explore the intricacies of falls in elderly individuals.

Our primary objective is to equip future geriatric healthcare professionals with an extensive comprehension of the epidemiology, etiology, and management of falls in the elderly. We will embark on an evidence-based journey, examining the multifaceted aspects of this issue, from the physiological and psychological factors to the societal and cultural influences that shape the experiences of elderly individuals.

Within the realm of geriatric medicine, few challenges are as pervasive and consequential as the issue of falls among the elderly. As India's aging population grows, falls among older individuals are becoming a major national and global concern. In an aging society, understanding the causes, consequences, and prevention of falls in the elderly is a key focus of healthcare and research. This chapter will delve into the complexities of falls in the elderly, aiming to equip future geriatric healthcare professionals with an extensive comprehension of the epidemiology, causes, and management of falls. We will take an evidence-based approach, exploring the physiological, psychological, societal, and cultural factors influencing this issue.

EPIDEMIOLOGY OF FALLS IN THE ELDERLY

Understanding the epidemiology of falls in the elderly is crucial for healthcare practitioners and researchers in the field of geriatric medicine. Falls among older individuals are a significant public health concern both globally and in India, and a comprehensive overview of their epidemiological factors helps us better comprehend the scope of the issue. We explore the key aspects of falls in the elderly, with a focus on the Indian context.

Prevalence and Global Perspective

Falls are alarmingly common among the elderly population worldwide. According to the World Health Organization (WHO), an estimated 646,000 individuals die each year due to falls, making them the second leading cause of unintentional injury-related deaths globally. For every fatal fall, many more result in nonfatal injuries, such as fractures, head injuries, and soft-tissue injuries. Every second of every day, an older adult (age 65+ years) suffers a fall in the United States, with 36 million falls resulting in 32,000 deaths each year. In India, the prevalence of falls among older adults ranges from 14 to 53%.

In the context of the aging global population, the prevalence of falls is expected to rise. The elderly, often defined as individuals aged 65 years and older, are at a considerably higher risk of experiencing falls compared to younger age groups. Factors such as age-related physical and cognitive changes, comorbidities, and polypharmacy contribute to this increased susceptibility.

Falls in the Indian Elderly

India's aging population is rapidly expanding, and the country is expected to become one of the world's most aged nations by 2050. In this context, the epidemiology of falls among the elderly in India presents unique characteristics:

- *Higher proportion of falls*: In India, falls constitute a substantial portion of injuries and hospitalizations among the elderly. This can be attributed to factors such as inadequate infrastructure, poor accessibility, and the prevalence of chronic diseases.
- *Gender disparities*: Studies have shown that elderly women in India are at a higher risk of falling compared to men. Sociocultural factors, including a higher prevalence of osteoporosis and lower physical activity levels among elderly women, contribute to this gender disparity.
- *Urban versus rural variances*: Epidemiological data indicate variations in fall rates between urban and rural areas. Factors such as uneven terrain and limited access to healthcare facilities can contribute to an increased risk of falls in rural regions.
- *Chronic health conditions*: The burden of chronic conditions such as diabetes, hypertension, and arthritis is high among the elderly in India. These conditions can lead to complications, polypharmacy, and impaired mobility, all of which elevate the risk of falls.
- *Malnutrition*: This is a prevalent issue among elderly individuals in India. Inadequate nutrition can lead to muscle weakness and frailty, increasing the likelihood of falls.
- *Psychosocial factors*: Cultural and psychosocial aspects can also influence the epidemiology of falls. Stigma around aging, mental health issues, and lack of social support can impact an individual's risk of falling.

CLINICAL PRESENTATION AND EVALUATION OF FALLS IN OUTPATIENT SETTINGS

In an outpatient setting, assessing and evaluating falls in elderly individuals are paramount for determining the underlying causes, managing risk factors, and preventing future episodes. This section provides an overview of the clinical presentation and the systematic evaluation of falls in an outpatient context.

Clinical Presentation

- *History of falls*: A thorough medical history is essential. Patients should be asked about their history of falls, including details of the most recent incident. Information about the frequency, circumstances, and any resultant injuries should be documented.
- *Prefall symptoms*: These symptoms are not a widely recognized medical or psychological term, but they

could refer to a range of potential symptoms or experiences leading up to a fall or accident. Some common signs or prefall symptoms to watch out for include:

- *Balance problems*: Difficulty maintaining balance or unsteadiness when walking
- *Muscle weakness*: Reduced strength in the legs, which can affect stability
- *Gait changes*: Alterations in the way a person walks, such as shuffling or taking shorter steps.
- *Dizziness or lightheadedness*: Feeling dizzy or faint can lead to falls.
- *Vision problems*: Poor vision or issues with depth perception can contribute to falls.
- *Medication side effects*: Some medications can cause drowsiness, dizziness, or impaired coordination.
- *Foot problems*: Wearing improper footwear or experiencing foot pain can increase the risk of falls.
- *Cognitive impairment*: Conditions such as dementia can affect judgment and decision-making, increasing the risk of falls.
- *Environmental hazards*: Clutter, slippery floors, poor lighting, and uneven surfaces at home can lead to falls.
- *Fear of falling*: Anxiety about falling can make a person more cautious, which can paradoxically lead to instability and an increased risk of falling.

- *Fall-related injuries*: Assess any injuries sustained during the fall, such as fractures, bruises, or head injuries. Document the location of the injuries and their severity.
- *Symptoms and complaints*: Inquire about any symptoms or complaints that the patient may be experiencing as a result of the fall. This may include pain, dizziness, nausea, or changes in physical or cognitive function.
- *Medication review*: Review the patient's medication list. Polypharmacy, medication interactions, and certain medications, such as sedatives, antihypertensives, and psychotropics, can increase the risk of falls.
- *Coexisting medical conditions*: Identify and assess any coexisting medical conditions, such as diabetes, cardiovascular diseases, osteoporosis, or neurological disorders, which can contribute to falls.
- *Functional assessment*: Evaluate the patient's functional status, including mobility, balance, and activities of daily living (ADLs). Impairments in these areas can increase the risk of falls.
- *Environmental factors*: Consider the patient's living environment. Identify any hazards in the home that may contribute to falls, such as loose rugs, inadequate lighting, or slippery surfaces.

Systematic Evaluation

- *Physical examination*: A comprehensive physical examination should be conducted. This includes a neurological assessment, musculoskeletal evaluation, and assessment of gait and balance.
- *Cognitive assessment*: Evaluate cognitive function, as cognitive impairment can be a risk factor for falls. The Mini-Mental State Examination (MMSE) or other cognitive screening tools can be useful.
- *Medication review*: Reassess the patient's medication regimen to identify any inappropriate medications or drug interactions. Adjustments may be necessary to mitigate fall risk.
- *Orthostatic hypotension*: Assess for orthostatic hypotension, a common cause of falls in the elderly. This can be done by measuring blood pressure in the supine and standing positions.
- *Vision and hearing assessment*: Impaired vision and hearing can contribute to falls. Evaluate visual acuity and hearing status and address any deficits accordingly.
- *Balance and mobility testing:* Utilize validated tests such as the timed up and go (TUG) test or the Berg Balance Scale to assess balance and mobility. These assessments help identify impairments and establish a baseline for measuring improvement.
- *Home environment evaluation*: If indicated, consider a home visit or refer to an occupational therapist for a thorough assessment of the patient's living environment to identify and rectify safety hazards.
- *Bone health assessment*: Assess bone health and risk of osteoporosis-related fractures. Dual-energy X-ray absorptiometry (DEXA) scans can help identify patients at risk of fractures.
- *Home environment assessment:* Factors such as adequate lighting, floor surfaces (loose rungs, carpets, slippery floor), furniture arrangements, bathroom safety, stairs and steps (handrails, free from clutter), and medication organization need to be evaluated to identify and avoid future risk of falls.

In the outpatient setting, a comprehensive evaluation of falls is a multidisciplinary effort involving physicians, nurses, physiotherapists, and occupational therapists. This collaborative approach ensures a holistic understanding of the patient's fall risk factors and allows for the development of tailored interventions to mitigate the risk of future falls.

Specific Investigations in the Evaluation of Falls

To comprehensively evaluate falls in an outpatient setting, specific investigations are often necessary. These investigations help identify underlying causes and contribute to tailored management strategies. Some key investigations commonly utilized are as follows:

- *Laboratory tests*:
  - *Complete blood count (CBC)*: A CBC can help identify anemia, which can contribute to weakness and falls.
  - *Basic metabolic panel (BMP) or comprehensive metabolic panel (CMP)*: These tests assess electrolyte levels, kidney function, and blood glucose, which may reveal metabolic imbalances that could lead to falls.
  - *Thyroid function tests*: Thyroid dysfunction, particularly hypothyroidism, can lead to muscle weakness, fatigue, and increased fall risk.
  - *Vitamin D levels*: Low vitamin D levels are associated with decreased bone density and increased fall risk. Assessing vitamin D status can guide supplementation.
- *Imaging studies*:
  - *X-rays*: X-rays are commonly used to evaluate for fractures or joint problems that may result from a fall. They are especially important if the patient presents with pain or localized symptoms after a fall.
  - *DEXA*: This scan measures bone mineral density and is essential for assessing osteoporosis and the risk of osteoporotic fractures.
  - *Magnetic resonance imaging (MRI) and magnetic resonance angiography (MRA)*: An MRI may be recommended when investigating neurological causes of falls, such as stroke, brain tumors, or structural abnormalities.
  - *Computed tomography (CT) scan*: CT scans are useful for assessing head injuries and intracranial bleeding that may result from a fall.
- *Cardiac evaluation*:
  - *Electrocardiogram (ECG or EKG)*: An ECG is performed to assess the heart's electrical activity and rhythm, which can reveal arrhythmias or conduction disorders that may cause syncope (fainting) and falls.
  - *Holter monitor*: For individuals with unexplained falls, a Holter monitor, which records the heart's electrical activity continuously, may be used to detect intermittent arrhythmias.
- *Neurological tests*:
  - *Electromyography (EMG) and nerve conduction studies (NCS)*: These tests evaluate peripheral neuropathy, which can lead to balance and gait problems.
- Gait and balance assessments:
  - *Computerized dynamic posturography:* This test objectively assesses a patient's balance and postural control and can help identify deficits.
  - *Functional gait and balance assessments*: Utilizing standardized tests such as the Tinetti Performance-oriented Mobility Assessment or the Berg Balance Scale helps gauge functional mobility and balance.
  - *Medication review*: Comprehensive medication review to identify potentially inappropriate medications or drug interactions that may contribute to falls.
  - *Home safety evaluation*: In certain cases, a home safety evaluation by an occupational therapist may be needed to identify environmental factors contributing to falls and recommend modifications.

The selection of specific investigations should be guided by the patient's clinical presentation, medical history, and physical examination findings. A thorough and systematic approach to these investigations allows healthcare providers to identify the root causes of falls and develop a personalized plan for fall prevention and management in the outpatient setting **(Flowchart 1)**.

MANAGEMENT OF FALLS

The management of falls in the elderly involves a multifaceted approach aimed at reducing the risk of future falls, addressing underlying causes, and promoting overall well-being. It often requires a collaborative effort among healthcare professionals, caregivers, and the patient. An overview of the key components of fall management is given in the following text:

- *Identification and management of underlying medical conditions*: Address underlying medical conditions that may have contributed to the fall, such as hypertension, diabetes, or heart disease, through appropriate medical treatment and management.
- *Medication review and optimization*: Review the patient's medications and consider discontinuing or adjusting medications that may increase fall risk or cause dizziness, sedation, or orthostatic hypotension.
- *Balance and strength training*:
  - Initiate or refer the patient to physical therapy for balance and strength training exercises. These programs can significantly improve gait, balance, and overall functional mobility, reducing the risk of falls.
  - Implementing targeted exercises to improve balance and strength can be highly effective in reducing this risk. A more detailed look at this aspect of fall prevention is as follows:
    - *Balance exercises*:
      - *Tai Chi*: This ancient Chinese martial art involves slow and controlled movements, promoting balance, flexibility, and muscle strength.

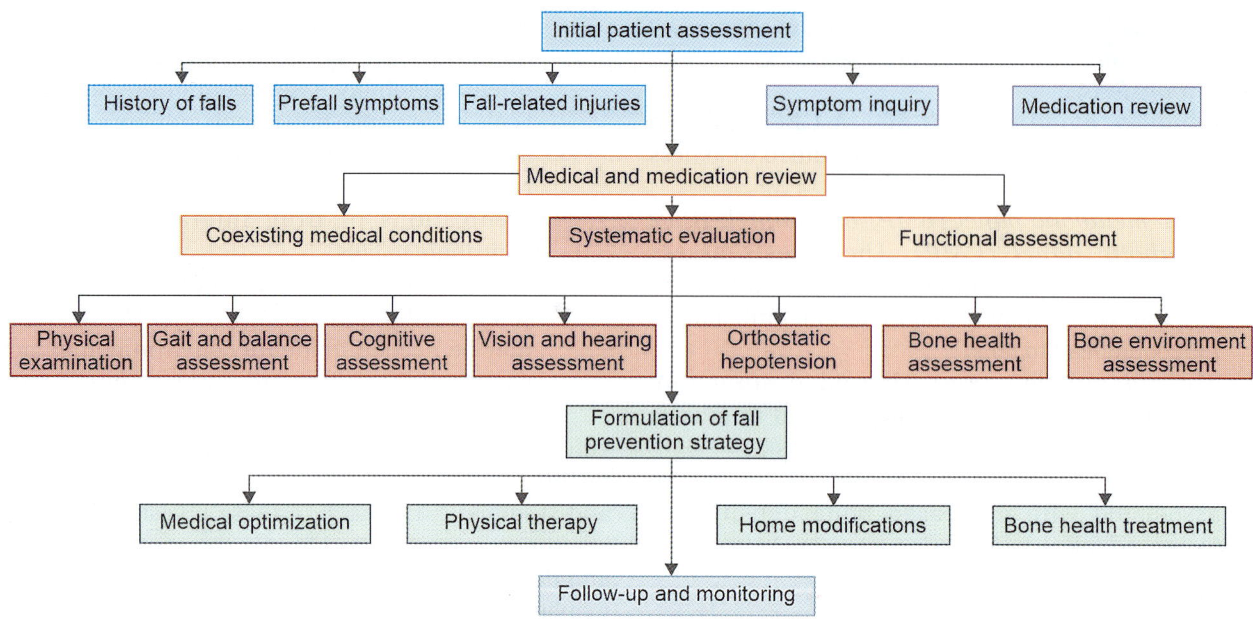

FLOWCHART 1: Outpatient evaluation of elderly patients with falls: Step-by-step approach.

- *Single-leg stands*: Standing on one leg for short durations helps improve balance. This can be done with support initially and then progressed to unsupported standing.
- *Heel-to-toe walk*: Walking in a straight line, placing the heel of one foot directly in front of the toes of the other, challenges balance.

– *Strength training*:
- *Resistance training*: Using resistance bands or weights can help strengthen muscles, particularly those in the legs and core.
- *Bodyweight exercises*: Squats, lunges, and leg lifts are effective exercises that can be performed using one's body weight.
- *Functional movements*: Focus on exercises that mimic daily activities, such as getting up from a chair or climbing stairs.

– *Specific muscle groups*:
- *Leg muscles*: Strengthening the quadriceps, hamstrings, and calf muscles is essential for stability and mobility.
- *Core muscles*: A strong core provides better support for the spine and improves overall stability.

– *Progressive challenge*:
- *Gradual increase*: Begin with exercises that match the individual's current fitness level and gradually increase the difficulty as strength and balance improve.
- *Dynamic movements*: Include dynamic movements that challenge the body's ability to adjust and maintain balance.

– *Frequency and consistency*:
- *Regular routine*: Establish a consistent exercise routine, aiming for at least 150 minutes of moderate-intensity exercise per week, as recommended by health guidelines.
- *Incorporate into daily life*: Encourage incorporating balance and strength exercises into daily activities, making them a natural part of the person's routine.

– *Supervised programs*:
- *Physical therapy*: A physical therapist can create a personalized program addressing specific weaknesses and challenges.
- *Group classes*: Joining group exercise classes designed for older adults can provide social support and motivation.

– *Fall prevention education*:
- *Awareness*: Educate older adults about the importance of balance and strength training in preventing falls.
- *Home exercises*: Provide simple exercises that can be performed at home to maintain progress.

• *Home safety assessment and modification*: Conduct a home safety evaluation and make necessary modifications to reduce fall hazards. This may include removing clutter, ensuring proper lighting, installing grab bars, and securing loose rugs.

- *Orthotic devices*: Consider the use of assistive devices such as canes, walkers, or orthotic devices, as appropriate, to enhance mobility and stability.
- *Footwear assessment:* Evaluate the patient's footwear and recommend appropriate shoes that provide good support, stability, and nonslip soles.
- *Vision and hearing correction*: Address visual and hearing impairments with appropriate corrective measures, such as glasses or hearing aids
- *Nutritional assessment*: Assess the patient's nutritional status and address malnutrition or vitamin deficiencies that may contribute to falls. Adequate protein and calcium intake are crucial for bone health.
- *Bone health management*: If indicated, initiate or optimize treatments for osteoporosis, such as calcium and vitamin D supplementation or prescription medications.
- *Fall prevention education*: Provide the patient and their caregivers with education on fall prevention strategies, including how to get up safely after a fall, the importance of proper nutrition, and environmental safety.
- *Psychosocial support*: Offer psychosocial support for individuals who have experienced a fall, as the emotional impact can be significant. Addressing fear of falling and enhancing self-confidence are integral components of fall management.
- *Monitoring and follow-up*: Regularly assess and monitor the patient's progress and adjust the management plan as needed. Scheduled follow-up appointments should be established to track improvements and address new concerns.
- *Fall alarms and alert systems*: In certain cases, fall alarms and alert systems may be recommended to notify caregivers or medical professionals in the event of a fall.
- *Community resources*: Explore community resources and support groups that can assist both elderly individuals and their caregivers in managing and preventing falls.

The management of falls in the elderly is an ongoing process, and individualized care plans should be tailored to each patient's unique needs. Collaboration between healthcare providers, therapists, family members, and the elderly individuals themselves is essential to create a safe and supportive environment that reduces the risk of falls and promotes healthy aging.

CONCLUSION

Falls in older adults are a major public health concern, often leading to serious morbidity, functional decline, and increased mortality. A fall is rarely a result of a single cause and should always prompt a multifactorial assessment, including evaluation of gait, balance, medications, vision, cognition, and home environment. Early identification of risk factors and a personalized, multidisciplinary intervention plan can significantly reduce the incidence of falls. Ultimately, fall prevention is not just about avoiding injury, but about preserving independence and quality of life in older adults.

Self-Assessment Questionnaire

Q1. What is fall?

Q2. How common is a fall in older people?

Q3. What are the risk factors of fall in older people?

Q4. How can it be known that older people may develop a fall in the future?

Q5. What are the consequences of a fall?

Q6. What are the steps that can be taken for the prevention of falls?

Q7. Explain the role of a geriatrician in fall prevention.

Q8. Discuss fall—a geriatric syndrome.

Q9. What is postfall evaluation?

FURTHER READINGS

1. Carter ND, Khan KM, McKay HA, Petit MA, Waterman C, Heinonen A, et al. Community-based exercise program reduces risk factors for falls in 65- to 75-year-old women with osteoporosis: randomized controlled trial. CMAJ. 2002;167(9): 997-1004.
2. World Health Organization. WHO Global Report on Falls Prevention in Older Age. Geneva: World Health Organization; 2008. p. 47.
3. Joseph A, Kumar D, Bagavandas M. A review of epidemiology of fall among elderly in India. Indian J Community Med. 2019;44(2):166-8.
4. Sasidharan DK, Vijayakumar P, Raj M, Soman S, Antony L, Sudhakar A, et al. Incidence and risk factors for falls among community-dwelling elderly subjects on a 1-year follow-up: a prospective cohort study from Ernakulam, Kerala, India. BMJ Open. 2020;10(7):e033691.

5. Vikaspedia Domains. (2021). Senior Citizens—Status in India. [online] Available from https://vikaspedia.in/social-welfare/senior-citizens-welfare/senior-citizens-status-in-india. [Last accessed May, 2025].
6. De Witt JK, Hagan RD, Cromwell RL. The effect of increasing inertia upon vertical ground reaction forces and temporal kinematics during locomotion. J Exp Biol. 2008;211(Pt 7):1087-92.
7. Pitchai P, Dedhia HB, Bhandari N, Krishnan D, D'Souza NRJ, Bellara JM. Prevalence, risk factors, circumstances for falls and level of functional independence among geriatric population - A descriptive study. Indian J Public Health. 2019;63(1):21.
8. Carpintero P, Caeiro JR, Carpintero R, Morales A, Silva S, Mesa M. Complications of hip fractures: a review. World J Orthop. 2014;5(4):402-11.
9. Devons CAJ. Comprehensive geriatric assessment: making the most of the aging years: Curr Opin Clin Nutr Metab Care. 2002;5(1):19-24.
10. Tinetti ME, Inouye SK, Gill TM, Doucette JT. Shared risk factors for falls, incontinence, and functional dependence. Unifying the approach to geriatric syndromes. JAMA. 1995;273(17):1348-53.
11. Chittrakul J, Siviroj P, Sungkarat S, Sapbamrer R. Physical frailty and fall risk in community-dwelling older adults: a cross-sectional study. J Aging Res. 2020;2020:e3964973.
12. Inouye SK, Studenski S, Tinetti ME, Kuchel GA. Geriatric syndromes: clinical, research and policy implications of a core geriatric concept. J Am Geriatr Soc. 2007;55(5):780-91.

CHAPTER 15

Syncope in Elderly

Raj Kumar Tata, Sunil Jyani

CASE VIGNETTE

Case Presentation

A 78-year-old male presents to the emergency department after experiencing a transient loss of consciousness while walking to the bathroom. His wife reports that he was unresponsive for approximately 30 seconds and recovered spontaneously without confusion or focal neurological deficits. There was no seizure activity or tongue biting.

The patient describes feeling lightheaded moments before the event and denies chest pain, palpitations, or dyspnea. His medical history includes hypertension, type 2 diabetes mellitus, and chronic kidney disease (stage 3). Medications include amlodipine, metformin, and aspirin.

Physical Examination

- *Vital signs*: Blood pressure 135/85 mm Hg (supine), 95/60 mm Hg (standing after 3 minutes), heart rate 82 bpm (supine) to 96 bpm (standing)
- *Cardiovascular*: Regular rate and rhythm, no murmurs or gallops
- *Neurological*: Normal cognitive function, no focal deficits
- *Other systems*: Unremarkable

Investigations

- *Electrocardiogram (ECG)*: Normal sinus rhythm, no ischemic changes, or conduction abnormalities
- *Complete blood count and metabolic panel*: Hemoglobin 11.5 g/dL, glucose 112 mg/dL, normal electrolytes, and creatinine 1.6 mg/dL
- *Echocardiography*: Preserved ejection fraction, no valvular abnormalities
- *Tilt table test*: Reproduction of symptoms with significant blood pressure drop and no compensatory tachycardia

Diagnosis

The patient is diagnosed with *orthostatic hypotension-related syncope* secondary to autonomic dysfunction, likely exacerbated by aging and comorbid conditions (diabetes mellitus and chronic kidney disease).

INTRODUCTION

Syncope is a transient, self-limited loss of consciousness due to acute global impairment of cerebral blood flow, which is rapid in onset, of brief duration, and recovery is spontaneous and complete. Transient loss of consciousness (TLOC) must be differentiated from syncope; key causes include seizures (aura, tonic–clonic movements, and postictal confusion), vertebrobasilar ischemia (focal neurological signs), hypoxemia (dyspnea, cyanosis), and hypoglycemia (autonomic symptoms, rapid recovery with glucose). Accurate diagnosis relies on history, examination, and targeted tests.

EPIDEMIOLOGY

Syncope is a common presenting symptom in the emergency department (ED), accounting for 1–2% of all ED visits and hospital admissions in the United States. Lifetime prevalence rates range from 10.5 to 19%.

In India, syncope is a prevalent medical issue, with lifetime incidence rates ranging from 15 to 39% in the general population. In the elderly Indian population, the incidence of unexplained syncope ranges from 6 to 11%. Neurocardiogenic syncope is identified as the most common cause, accounting for approximately 63.3% of cases.

The occurrence of syncope with aging shows bimodal variation, with a peak in late adolescence to early adulthood (mostly vasovagal in origin) and a second peak later in older age, with a sharp rise after the age of 70 years. In younger patients, reflex syncope (particularly vasovagal faints) overwhelmingly predominates as a cause. While reflex faints remain common as patients age, in older adult patients, disease-related abnormalities may not only predispose to transient hypotensive events (e.g., arrhythmias, orthostatic hypotension) but may also impair the ability to respond to physiologic stresses that would ordinarily not cause syncope.

ETIOLOGY

Etiology of syncope is given in **Table 1**.

History

Proper history is most important in making etiological diagnosis of syncope and, hence, in management.

- *Age*: Older adult patients are at a greater risk for adverse outcomes following syncope. Falls and associated fractures can occur. Aortic stenosis is of particular concern as patients get older, and it is the most common obstructive cardiac lesion. Older adult patients are more likely to have autonomic dysfunction, OH, and multiple medications, increasing the risk for syncope. Progression of diabetes can cause autonomic dysfunction and orthostasis, as can some other conditions such as Parkinson's disease.
- *Associated symptoms and triggers*: Concomitant symptoms can provide important diagnostic clues. As an example, chest pain may indicate an acute coronary syndrome or pulmonary embolism. Palpitations suggest an arrhythmia. Dyspnea raises concern for pulmonary embolism or heart failure. Abdominal or low back pain associated with syncope raises the

TABLE 1: Etiology of syncope.

Neurally mediated syncope	Orthostatic hypotension	Cardiac syncope
Vasovagal syncope: Provoked fear, pain, anxiety, intense emotion, sight of blood, unpleasant sight or odor, and prolonged standing	Primary autonomic failure—synucleinopathies	*Arrhythmias:* • Sinus node dysfunction • AV dysfunction • Supraventricular tachyarrhythmias
Situational reflex syncope	*Lewy body diseases*: • Parkinson's disease • Lewy body dementia • Pure autonomic failure • Multiple system atrophy	• Ventricular tachycardia • Inherited channelopathies
Pulmonary: Cough syncope, wind instrument player's syncope, weightlifter's syncope, "mess trick" and "fainting lark," and sneeze syncope	Secondary autonomic failure due to autonomic peripheral neuropathy	*Cardiac structural disease*: • Valvular disease • Myocardial ischemia • Obstructive cardiomyopathy
Urogenital: Postmicturition syncope, urogenital tract instrumentation, and prostatic massage	• Diabetes • Hereditary amyloidosis (familial amyloid polyneuropathy) • Primary amyloidosis	• Atrial myxoma • Pericardial effusion and tamponades
Gastrointestinal: Swallow syncope, glossopharyngeal neuralgia, esophageal instrumentation, rectal examination, and defecation syncope	Hereditary sensory and autonomic neuropathies (especially type III familial dysautonomia)	
Cardiac: Bezold–Jarisch reflex, cardiac outflow obstruction	• Autoimmune autonomic ganglionopathy • Sjögren's syndrome	
Carotid sinus: Carotid sinus sensitivity, carotid sinus massage	• Paraneoplastic autonomic neuropathy • HIV neuropathy	
Ocular: Ocular massage, ocular surgery, and ocular examination	Postprandial hypotension	
	Iatrogenic (drug-induced)	

(HIV: human immunodeficiency virus)

possibility of a ruptured abdominal aortic aneurysm. Headache raises the possibility of subarachnoid hemorrhage. Symptoms such as headache, paresthesias, or weakness may suggest a neurologic cause. The geriatrician should seek a history consistent with vasovagal syncope because this diagnosis carries a low risk for patient. A gradual prodrome generally precedes vasovagal syncope and often includes a sense of warmth, nausea and vomiting, diaphoresis, changes in vision, and pallor, either just prior to or shortly after the event. Inquiring about potential vasovagal triggers is also helpful. Triggers commonly associated with vasovagal syncope include visual stressors (e.g., seeing blood during phlebotomy or watching a childbirth), strong physical or emotional stress, micturition, defecation, coughing, swallowing, and prolonged standing in a warm environment.

- *Position*: Patients who lose consciousness with prolonged standing (i.e., minimum of 15–20 minutes) are more likely to have vasovagal syncope. Patients who lose consciousness while moving from a lying to a standing position are more likely to have orthostasis. Syncope while sitting or supine is suspicious for arrhythmia.
- *Onset*: Sudden loss of consciousness without warning or prodrome suggests arrhythmia. A prospective observational study of patients with recurrent syncope found that 64% of patients sustained an arrhythmia at the time of their sudden loss of consciousness when studied with a loop recorder. Injury from falls associated with an abrupt loss of consciousness can occur. Patients with prodromes are more likely to have vasovagal syncope and have repeatedly been shown to be low risk.
- *Duration of symptoms*: The duration of a syncopal event is difficult to quantify. Patients are generally unaware of the duration of their loss of unconsciousness, and events are often unwitnessed or poorly quantified if they are witnessed. As a rough guide, an "event" or loss of consciousness persisting for >4 or 5 minutes should raise concerns for seizure or other causes of altered mental status.
- *Exertional syncope*: Syncope with exertion raises the possibility of arrhythmia or cardiac outflow obstruction (e.g., aortic stenosis, hypertrophic cardiomyopathy, or pericardial tamponade).
- *Seizure versus syncope*: Differences between seizure and syncope are given in **Table 2**.
- *Medications*: A review of the patient's medications may reveal the cause of syncope. This is particularly important with older adult patients. Medications often implicated include calcium channel blockers, beta-blockers, alpha-blockers, nitrates, antiarrhythmics, diuretics (affecting volume status and electrolyte concentrations), and medications affecting the QTc interval (e.g., antipsychotics and antiemetics).

DIAGNOSTIC EVALUATION

- *Electrocardiogram (ECG)*:
  - Practice guidelines suggest that all patients presenting with syncope should receive an ECG even though the diagnostic yield is low.
  - Assess for arrhythmias, ischemia, conduction abnormalities (e.g., prolonged QT interval, bundle branch blocks), or signs of prior myocardial infarction
- *Laboratory tests*:
  - *Basic metabolic panel*: Electrolyte imbalances (e.g., hyponatremia, hyperkalemia)
  - *Blood glucose*: Rule out hypoglycemia.
  - Complete blood count (CBC), liver and kidney function tests
  - *Cardiac enzymes*: Suspected acute coronary syndrome and B-type natriuretic peptide (BNP)
- *Echocardiography*: Evaluate for structural heart disease, such as valvular dysfunction or left ventricular outflow obstruction
- *Holter monitoring or continuous cardiac monitoring*: For patients with suspected arrhythmias not detected on initial ECG
- *Tilt table testing*: Useful for diagnosing neurocardiogenic syncope or orthostatic hypotension
- *Neurological evaluation*: Consider brain imaging (MRI or CT) or EEG if seizures or vertebrobasilar insufficiency is suspected.
- *Carotid sinus massage*: Performed in monitored settings to diagnose carotid sinus hypersensitivity
- *Additional tests*:
  - *Stress testing*: If exertional syncope is reported
  - *CT pulmonary angiography*: If pulmonary embolism is suspected

TREATMENT

Treatment is based upon the underlying cause of syncope.

Neurally Mediated Syncope

- Reassurance, education, avoidance of provocative stimuli, and plasma volume expansion with fluid and salt are the cornerstones of the management of neurally mediated syncope.
- Isometric counterpressure maneuvers of the limbs (tensing of the abdominal and leg muscles, handgrip and arm tensing, and leg crossing) may raise blood

TABLE 2: Differences between seizure and syncope.		
Characteristics	**Generalized tonic–clonic seizure**	**Syncope**
Circumstances		
Situation	Awake or asleep	Usually upright, any position if cardiogenic
Precipitating factors	Sleep loss, alcohol withdrawal, flashing light	Emotion, injury, heat, crowds, none if cardiogenic
Motor phenomenon		
Vocalization	At onset (if any)	None
Location of motor component (if present)	Proximal limb	None
Generalized motor	Tonic, then clonic	Usually a tonic; if syncope lasts > 20 seconds, tonic and then clonic
Tonic posture	Partial flexion or straight	-
Head movements	To one side or none	-
Clonus/limb jerks	Bilateral (B/L) synchronous	B/L synchronous
Purposeful movement	Absent	Absent
Biting	Tongue, inside the mouth	Tongue biting rare
Babinski's sign	Present	Absent
Autonomic features		
Micturition	Frequent	Occasional
Eyes	Open	Open
Pupils	Dilated or hippus during attack	Dilated
Color	Cyanotic or gray	Pale
Pulse	Rapid and strong	Slow if vasovagal, weak if vasodepressor, or that of arrhythmias
Timing		
Usual duration	1–5 minutes	1–2 minutes
Onset	Sudden	Gradual, sudden if cardiogenic
Sequence of symptoms	Stereotypical	Stereotypical
Termination	Spontaneous	Rapid
Sequel		
Injury	Frequent, mild; scalp, face common	If a sudden onset
Postictal	Tired, confused, sleepy	Regains consciousness in 2–3 minutes, alert but tired

pressure by increasing central blood volume and cardiac output. Of these, abdominal muscle tensing is the most effective.

- *Approach to refractory recurrent syncope*: For patients with recurrent syncope despite the general measures described above, treatment is based upon the results of tilt testing and other clinical characteristics.
- For patients ≥ 40 years of age with recurrent syncope despite general measures, bradycardic or asystolic episodes (≥3 seconds if with syncope; ≥6 seconds if asymptomatic) documented by electrocardiographic monitoring, and *no* major vasodepressor component on tilt testing, permanent cardiac pacing may be an option.
- For patients with recurrent syncope despite general measures who do not have an indication for permanent cardiac pacing, we suggest treatment with fludrocortisone or midodrine. Based on limited

evidence, fludrocortisone may be preferred for patients with baseline systolic blood pressure < 120 mm Hg.

- *Fludrocortisone*: The drug is typically administered as 0.1–0.2 mg daily and is well tolerated. It may, however, cause loss of potassium from the body, and this effect should be monitored, with dietary replacement provided as needed. Fludrocortisone should generally be avoided in patients with hypertension or heart failure and also aggravate migraine susceptibility. In terms of dose, 0.2 mg daily is often needed, but over time (and especially if hypertension evolves), the dose can be reduced to 0.1 mg daily or even lower to 0.1 mg two to four times weekly.
- *Midodrine*: This is a prodrug; the active metabolite is an alpha-1-adrenergic agonist. Contraindications to midodrine therapy include hypertension and urinary retention. The usual starting dose for midodrine is 5 mg three times daily (morning, noon, and late afternoon). The dose range is 2.5 mg, twice daily, 4 hours apart, to 10 mg, three times daily, 4 hours apart. The maximum recommended total daily dose is 45 mg. Dosing within 3–4 hours of bedtime should be avoided due to the potential detrimental impact on sleep. In some patients, 5 mg twice daily is adequate if the patient has had a more positive response to lifestyle-based therapies.
- Cardioneural ablation is a potential approach for refractory cases, but indications for the procedure and optimal methodologies are still evolving.

Orthostatic Hypotension

- The first step is to remove reversible causes—usually vasoactive medications.
- *Nonpharmacologic interventions*: These include patient education regarding staged moves from supine to upright, warnings about the hypotensive effects of large meals, instructions about the isometric counterpressure maneuvers that increase intravascular pressure, and raising the head of the bed to reduce supine hypertension and nocturnal diuresis.
- Patients with nonneurogenic OH (nOH) should increase dietary salt and water intake to increase intravascular volume. Rapid intake of water induces an osmopressor reflex in the hour after ingestion due to the reduction of osmolarity in the portal vein. In addition to drinking water during meals and before exercise, patients are advised keeping a pitcher of water at the bedside and drinking rapidly before getting out of bed in the morning. Ingesting 500 mL of water upon awakening and reaching 1.5–3 L/day is a reasonable target. High sodium-containing foods or salt tablets also may be beneficial. While the optimal dose will vary among patients, typically a target dose of 6–10 g/day of sodium or a target urinary sodium level of 150–200 mEq is recommended.
- *Use compression stockings and abdominal binders*: The use of custom-fitted elastic compression stockings permits the application of graded pressure to the lower extremities and lower abdomen, thereby minimizing peripheral blood pooling. Such stockings should extend to the waist since most peripheral pooling occurs in the splanchnic circulation.
- *Pharmacotherapy*: Two drugs are approved by the US Food and Drug Administration (FDA) for the treatment of symptomatic nOH: (1) Alpha-adrenergic agonist midodrine, and (2) norepinephrine precursor droxidopa. Fludrocortisone, a synthetic mineralocorticoid, which is not specifically approved by the FDA for the treatment of nOH, is widely used but can lead to sustained hypertension in the supine position and other adverse effects.
- *Stepwise approach and monitoring*: Nonpharmacologic measures should be maximized before starting and must be continued after initiating pharmacotherapy.
- Pharmacologic approaches are based on two complementary strategies: (1) Expanding intravascular volume (typically with fludrocortisone) and (2) increasing peripheral vascular resistance with other medications.
- The selection of one strategy, the other, or both depends on the specific features and needs of each patient as well as the degree of peripheral sympathetic denervation, as determined by plasma norepinephrine levels.
- For patients with persistent nOH symptoms in whom nonpharmacologic measures such as volume augmentation with salt and water intake are insufficient to replenish intravascular volume, a regimen with fludrocortisone to augment volume and provide symptom relief is started. However, this approach may not be sufficient for some patients and is not ideal for those whose symptoms did not improve temporarily with volume augmentation.
- For patients with symptoms of nOH unresponsive to nonpharmacologic measures such as volume augmentation, a short-acting vasoconstrictor agent (such as a sympathomimetic) or atomoxetine as initial pharmacotherapy after nonpharmacologic measures is implemented. Measuring plasma norepinephrine levels can aid in the selection of therapy. Typically, a sympathomimetic agent (e.g., midodrine or droxidopa) for patients with a supine norepinephrine level <220 pg/mL, and atomoxetine, a norepinephrine transporter (NET) inhibitor, for other patients, is recommended.

- For the rare patient with nOH and severe anemia who has low serum erythropoietin concentrations, a trial of erythropoietin should be offered as a first line of treatment.
- *Fludrocortisone*: For patients with nOH symptoms that improve modestly or temporarily with nonpharmacologic measures to replete intravascular volume such as increased salt and water intake, fludrocortisone may provide symptom relief. Such patients are likely to have persistent volume depletion.
- Fludrocortisone is started at a dose of 0.05 mg/day and administered in the morning. If needed, it can eventually be increased up to 0.2 mg/day; little benefit is obtained by further dose increase, but the risk of adverse effects increases significantly. Fludrocortisone requires at least 5–7 days of treatment to exert significant clinical effects. Increments should not occur more rapidly than weekly.
- Short-term adverse effects of fludrocortisone are frequent and include hypokalemia, ankle edema, and supine hypertension. While fludrocortisone is well tolerated by most patients with chronic autonomic failure, many patients with nOH discontinue the drug due to adverse effects.
- Patients receiving fludrocortisone are advised to eat potassium-rich foods or take potassium supplements (potassium chloride 20 mEq/day) to reduce the risk of hypokalemia.
- Dependent edema may be managed with compression stockings when mild but may be worsened in many older patients with autonomic dysfunction who have concurrent conditions that promote edema.
- Supine hypertension is a frequent side effect that causes drug discontinuation in many patients.
- Long-term use of fludrocortisone exacerbates hypertension and organ damage, including left ventricular hypertrophy, congestive heart failure, and kidney failure, and is associated with a higher risk of all-cause hospitalization in patients with nOH.
- *Sympathomimetic agents*: For patients with nOH symptoms that do not improve with nonpharmacologic measures to replete intravascular volume such as increased salt and water intake and who have a serum norepinephrine level <220 pg/mL, a sympathomimetic agent is recommended as initial pharmacotherapy. Two sympathomimetic pressor agents are approved by the FDA for the treatment of nOH: Alpha-1-adrenergic agonist midodrine and norepinephrine precursor droxidopa.
- *Midodrine*: It should be titrated from 2.5 to 10 mg two to three times a day, owing to variable patient sensitivity to this agent. The maximum dose should not exceed 40 mg/day. Midodrine exerts an initial symptomatic benefit in most patients with nOH, although tachyphylaxis may occur. Patients should not take midodrine within 3–4 hours of bedtime to limit supine hypertension.
- Midodrine should not be used for patients with severe heart disease, uncontrolled supine hypertension, or urinary retention. Other potential adverse effects include pilomotor reactions (goose flesh), pruritus, gastrointestinal complaints, and urinary retention. Midodrine has no direct effect on heart rate as it does not stimulate cardiac beta-adrenergic receptors.
- *Droxidopa*: It is started at 100 mg three times daily. The target dose is from 100 to 600 mg up to three times a day, depending on individual circumstances. For example, for a patient with a movement disorder and nOH who is active for only a few hours in the morning (e.g., showering, preparing breakfast), it is reasonable to use a single morning droxidopa dose and skip the afternoon and evening doses. Other patients with different needs may receive droxidopa only twice daily or take a higher dose in the morning with lower doses in the afternoon and evening.
- The most common adverse effects of droxidopa are supine hypertension, headache, and nausea. Patients should not take droxidopa within 3–4 hours of bedtime to limit supine hypertension.
- *NET inhibitors*: For patients with nOH symptoms that do not improve with nonpharmacologic measures to replete intravascular volume such as increased salt and water intake and who have a serum norepinephrine level > 220 pg/mL, the recommendation is to start with atomoxetine, a NET inhibitor, as initial pharmacotherapy.
- Atomoxetine is a short-acting NET inhibitor that increases standing blood pressure and reduces the burden of symptoms for patients with nOH. The initial dose is typically 10 mg two times a day, which can be increased to 18 mg two times a day, depending on symptom relief and blood pressure response.
- NET inhibition enhances vasoconstriction at the sympathetic neurovascular junction and vasodilation at alpha-2 adrenergic receptors in the central nervous system. For patients with nOH and central autonomic dysfunction (e.g., multiple system atrophy), however, only peripheral vasoconstriction is apparent, making NET inhibitors particularly appealing for these patients. The higher the plasma norepinephrine level, the greater the pressor effect and expected symptomatic improvement.
- *Second-line combination therapy*: For patients with a suboptimal response to initial monotherapy, we

typically add a medication that may exert a synergistic benefit. As an example, a sympathomimetic agent may be used in combination with fludrocortisone or alone as the first pharmacotherapy for those unable or unwilling to tolerate fludrocortisone's adverse effects. Combining fludrocortisone with an alpha agonist can have synergistic effects and allow for a lower dose of both agents.

Cardiac Syncope

Treatment of cardiac disease depends on the underlying disorder. Therapies for arrhythmias include cardiac pacing for sinus node disease and AV block, ablation, antiarrhythmic drugs, and cardioverter defibrillators for atrial and ventricular tachyarrhythmias. These disorders are best managed by physicians with specialized skills in this area.

CONCLUSION

In summary, syncope in the elderly is a multifactorial and often complex clinical problem, with causes ranging from benign to potentially life-threatening. Its evaluation requires a careful, systematic approach that considers age-related physiological changes, comorbidities, and medication effects. Early identification of underlying causes, appropriate risk stratification, and targeted management are key to reducing morbidity and improving quality of life. Continued vigilance and a holistic, patient-centered approach remain essential in addressing syncope in the aging population.

Self-Assessment Questionnaire

Q1. What are the key differentiating features between syncope and other causes of transient loss of consciousness, such as seizure or vertebrobasilar ischemia?

Q2. Why are older people more prone to develop syncope compared to younger adults?

Q3. What are the most common neurally mediated triggers of syncope in older adults?

Q4. How does vasovagal syncope differ in its prodrome, onset, and recovery from arrhythmic syncope?

Q5. What are the nonpharmacological interventions recommended for patients with orthostatic hypotension?

Q6. How to treat recurrent syncope?

Q7. Outline a stepwise diagnostic approach for evaluating an elderly patient presenting with unexplained syncope in the emergency department.

FURTHER READINGS

1. Brignole M, Moya A, de Lange FJ, Deharo JC, Elliott PM, Fanciulli A, et al. 2018 ESC Guidelines for the diagnosis and management of syncope. Eur Heart J. 2018;39(21):1883-948.
2. Goldberger AL, Libby P. Syncope and orthostatic intolerance. In: Braunwald's Heart Disease: A Textbook of Cardiovascular Medicine, 12th edition. Philadelphia: Elsevier; 2022.
3. Shen WK, Sheldon RS, Benditt DG, Cohen MI, Forman DE, Goldberger ZD, et al. 2017 ACC/AHA/HRS guideline for the evaluation and management of patients with syncope: a report of the American College of Cardiology/American Heart Association task force on clinical practice guidelines and the Heart Rhythm Society. J Am Coll Cardiol. 2017;70(5):e39-110.
4. Kapoor WN. Evaluation and outcome of patients with syncope. Medicine. 2000;79(3):160-75.
5. Ungar A, Mussi C, Ceccofiglio A, Bellelli G, Nicosia F, Bo M, et al. Etiology of syncope and unexplained falls in elderly adults with dementia: syncope and dementia (SYD) study. J Am Geriat Soc. 2006;54(3):400-6.

CHAPTER 16

Incontinence

Ambica Singh

CASE VIGNETTE

Patient information: Mrs Dimple, a 70-year-old female with a history of diabetes.

Living situation: She resides with her both sons and daughters-in-law in residential quarters in Delhi.

Primary care physician: Dr A Singh.

Presenting complaint: She visited her primary care physician/geriatrician with complaints of a strong urge to urinate and leaks on the way to bathroom which she has been experiencing for the past 2 months. She also leaks a little when she coughs or sneezes hard, which she complains from past 1 year.

History of present illness: Patient was apparently well until 1 year back when she started facing issues of involuntary passage of urine leading to wetting of her underwear garment while coughing. She also noticed that the same complaint occurred whenever she sneezed. She could not reach out to any doctor due to embarrassment. She became more anxious while going out of the house and therefore reduced outings for only essential tasks.

For the past 2 months, she has been experiencing a strong urge to urinate, with increased frequency, which could not be deferred. Urine start to leak on the way to bathroom, due to which she stopped moving out of her room for embarrassment in front of family members.

Medical history: Mrs Dimple has a history of type 2 diabetes, which is managed with oral medications. She has not experienced any recent changes in medication or dosages. Her last comprehensive physical examination was conducted 1 year ago.

Social history: She lives with her sons, their wives, and their children in a joint family setup.

She plays an active role in household activities, including helping to care for her grandchildren. She does not have a history of alcohol or tobacco use.

Occupational history: She is a retired government clerk (retired 4 years back).

Review of systems: Apart from the falls and associated musculoskeletal pain, Mrs Dimple denies any other significant symptoms, such as dizziness, chest pain, visual disturbances, or urinary incontinence.

Physical examination: The patient was conscious, cooperative, and well oriented to time, place, and person. Glasgow Coma Scale (GCS) score is E4V5M6. Vitals were stable. Oral hygiene was satisfactory. General examination revealed no pallor/icterus/cyanosis/clubbing/lymphadenopathy/edema. Jugular venous pressure (JVP) was not raised. Patient had restricted mobility, with the support of a cane. Lumbar spine was found to have kyphoscoliosis. Respiratory examination revealed a few basal crepts apart from normal vesicular breath sounds all over. Cardiovascular and per abdominal examination were within normal limits. Neurological examination did not reveal any focal neurological deficits.

INTRODUCTION

The International Continence Society (ICS) and the International Urogynecological Association (IUGA) have defined the symptom of urinary incontinence (UI) as "the complaint of involuntary loss/leakage of urine." UI is a common and yet undertreated condition in elderly individuals. It is a stressful health issue which has socioeconomic impact. It results in deteriorated health-related quality of life. From a clinician's viewpoint, UI can be regarded as a specific diagnosis, while geriatricians consider it as a geriatric syndrome.

The severity of UI could range from occasional episodes of dribbling of urine to continuous urine leakage with concomitant fecal incontinence. Patients may be reluctant to initiate discussions about their incontinence and urinary symptoms due to embarrassment, lack of knowledge about treatment options, and/or fear of surgery.

The incidence and prevalence of UI increase with age. However, as against the general conception, UI should not be considered as a part of the normal aging process.

PREVALENCE AND GLOBAL PERSPECTIVE

The estimated global prevalence of UI in older men is 11–34% and 17–55% in older women. Studies from India show the prevalence of UI in women in their sixth and seventh decade, around 34% and 39%, respectively. There is a lack of sufficient data on the prevalence of incontinence among elderly men in India.

BLADDER PHYSIOLOGY

Urination is a dynamic process. At the basic level, urination is controlled by a reflex through the sacral micturition center. During normal bladder filling, afferent pathways via somatic and autonomic nerves carry information on bladder volume to the spinal cord. Motor output is adjusted according to the afferent information. Sympathetic tone contracts the bladder neck and inhibits parasympathetic tone, therefore relaxing the bladder musculature. Somatic innervation maintains tone in the pelvic floor musculature including striated muscle around the urethra. Voluntary pelvic floor muscle contracture also leads to inhibition of parasympathetic tone. For bladder emptying, sympathetic and somatic tones decrease, and parasympathetic, cholinergically mediated impulses increase for the bladder to contract **(Fig. 1)**.

Age-related Changes in Bladder Physiology

Refer to **Figures 2A and B**.

IMPACT OF URINARY INCONTINENCE ON HEALTH

Substantial negative health outcomes are associated with UI in older adults. The common effects of UI on the elderly are social isolation, depression, stigmatization, and embarrassment for many affected patients. UI affects overall levels of happiness and general and health-related quality of life (HRQoL) in older adults adversely **(Box 1)**.

RISK FACTORS

The risk factors for UI are outlined in **Table 1**.

TYPES OF INCONTINENCE

Transient versus Established

- *Acute/transient/reversible*: Situations in which the incontinence is of sudden onset, usually related to an acute illness or an iatrogenic problem, and subsides once the illness or problem has been resolved.
- *Chronic/persistent/established*: Incontinence that is unrelated to an acute illness and endures over time.

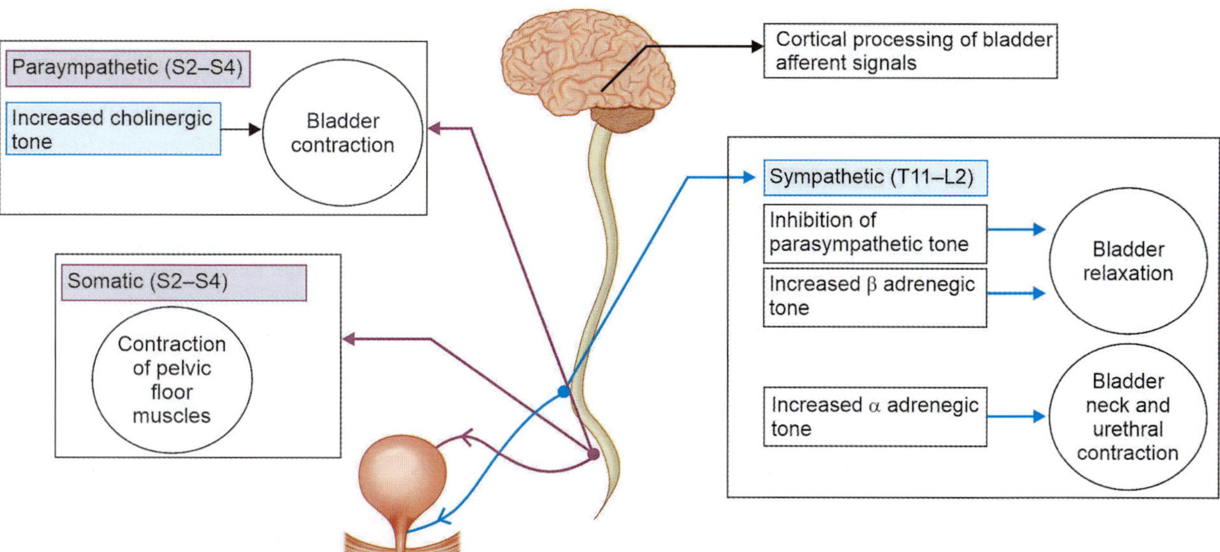

FIG. 1: Central and peripheral nervous system involved in micturition.

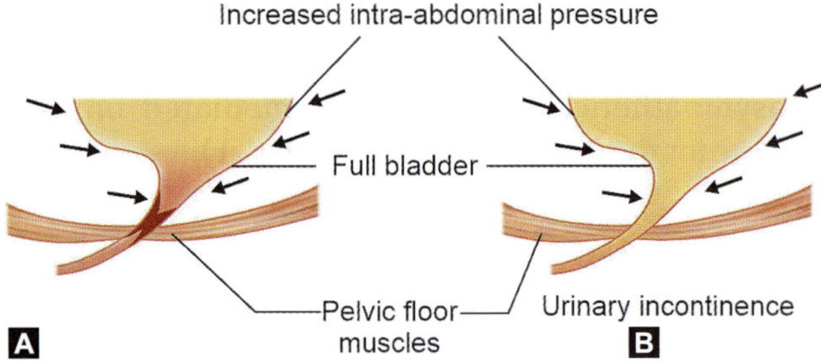

FIGS. 2A AND B: Schematic diagram showing age-associated changes in bladder, urethra-vesical position, and pelvic floor musculature predisposing to stress incontinence. (A) Normal anatomy leading to bladder outlet closure with a rise in intra-abdominal pressure; and (B) Age-associated changes such as estrogen deficiency, childbirth, and surgeries causing weakening of structures maintaining bladder positions, leading to urinary incontinence upon rise in intra-abdominal pressure.

BOX 1 **Impact of urinary incontinence on the health of a geriatric patient.**

- Overall quality of life
- Morbidity
- Sexual dysfunction
- Increased caregiver burden

However, the distinction between acute and chronic causes is although not always distinct. Reversible conditions that cause or contribute to UI in older persons are mentioned in **Box 2**.

Persistent UI is further subdivided, as described in **Table 3 and Box 3**.

Some authors also describe some other types of incontinence, which have been described below:

- *Neuropathic incontinence*: Incontinence due to neurological disease or conditions involving the brain, spinal cord, and peripheral nerve affecting the function and structure of the bladder and sphincter, as well as the synergic action of the two structures.
- *Continuous UI*: Complaint of continuous urine loss, day and night
- *Insensible UI*: Complaint of urine loss without knowledge of what precipitated the event or when it occurred

EVALUATION

The initial evaluation of UI includes characterizing and classifying the type of incontinence, identifying underlying conditions (e.g., neurologic disorder or malignancy)

TABLE 1: Risk factors for urinary incontinence.

Predisposing factor	Description	Promoting factor	Description
Gender	Female > Male	Smoking	Causes chronic cough and raised intra-abdominal pressure, damages blood vessels and nerves
Ethnicity	Caucasian > Afro-Caribbean	Obesity	Increased pressure on the bladder and pelvic floor muscles, hormonal imbalances
Family history	Identified for urgency urinary incontinence (UUI) but not stress urinary incontinence (SUI)	Infection (UTI)	Can irritate the bladder and lead to frequent urination
Neurological disorders	Spinal cord injury (SCI), stroke, multiple sclerosis (MS), Parkinson's disease (PD), dementia	Increased fluid intake	May not be a direct cause but it can exacerbate incontinence in some cases
Anatomical disorders	Vesicovaginal fistula (VVF), ectopic ureter in girls, urethral diverticulum, urethral fistula, bladder exstrophy, epispadias, urethral stricture, cystocele, rectocele	Medications	Diuretics, alpha-blockers, anticholinergics, sedatives, antidepressants (see **Table 2**)
Childbirth and pregnancy	Assisted vaginal delivery, increasing parity, pelvic floor muscle damage, perineal tears	Poor nutrition	Can contribute to overall health and bladder function
Pelvic, perineal, and prostate surgery	Radical hysterectomy, prostatectomy, transurethral resection of the prostate (TURP), pelvic floor repair surgery, pelvic radiation therapy	Aging	Weakening of pelvic floor muscles, decreased bladder capacity, and cognitive decline
Radical pelvic radiotherapy	Can damage pelvic nerves and muscles, leading to urinary incontinence	Cognitive deficits	Difficulty recognizing the urge to urinate, inability to hold urine
Diabetes	Can cause nerve damage (neuropathy) and bladder dysfunction	Poor mobility	Difficulty getting to the bathroom in time, especially for those with mobility impairments
		Estrogen deficiency	Can lead to decreased pelvic floor muscle tone and bladder support

TABLE 2: Medications for anatomical disorders.

Type of medication	Potential effects on continence	Specific examples
Diuretics	Polyuria, frequency, urgency	Loop diuretics (furosemide, torsemide), thiazide diuretics (hydrochlorothiazide, chlorthalidone)
Anticholinergics	Urinary retention, overflow incontinence, stool impaction	Oxybutynin, tolterodine, darifenacin, solifenacin
Psychotropics	Anticholinergic actions, sedation	Tricyclic antidepressants (amitriptyline, nortriptyline), antipsychotics (chlorpromazine, risperidone)
Antidepressants	Anticholinergic actions, sedation, immobility	Selective serotonin reuptake inhibitors (SSRIs) (fluoxetine, sertraline), serotonin-norepinephrine reuptake inhibitors (SNRIs) (venlafaxine, duloxetine)
Antipsychotics	Anticholinergic actions, sedation, immobility	First-generation antipsychotics (haloperidol, chlorpromazine), second-generation antipsychotics (olanzapine, risperidone)
Sedative–hypnotics	Sedation, delirium, immobility, urethral relaxation	Benzodiazepines (diazepam, lorazepam), z-drugs (zolpidem, eszopiclone)
Narcotic analgesics	Urinary retention, fecal impaction, sedation, and delirium	Morphine, hydromorphone, fentanyl
Alpha-adrenergic blockers	Urethral relaxation	Doxazosin, terazosin, tamsulosin
Alpha-adrenergic agonists	Urinary retention	Midodrine, pseudoephedrine
Angiotensin-converting enzyme inhibitors	Cough precipitating stress incontinence	Lisinopril, ramipril, enalapril
Beta-adrenergic agonists	Rarely may contribute to urinary retention	Albuterol, salmeterol, levalbuterol
Calcium channel blockers	May contribute to urinary retention	Diltiazem, verapamil, nifedipine
Alcohol	Polyuria, frequency, urgency, sedation, delirium, immobility	Ethanol
Caffeine	Polyuria, bladder irritation	Coffee, tea, soda, energy drinks

BOX 2 Reversible conditions that cause urinary incontinence in older persons.

- Conditions affecting the lower urinary tract:
  - Urinary tract infection (symptomatic with frequency, urgency, dysuria, etc.)
  - Atrophic vaginitis/urethritis
  - Postprostatectomy (incontinence will often resolve during first year)
  - Stool impaction
- Stool impaction
- Increased urine production:
  - Metabolic (hyperglycemia, hypercalcemia)
  - Excess fluid intake
  - Volume overload
  - Venous insufficiency with edema
- Congestive heart failure
- Impaired ability or willingness to reach a toilet
- Delirium
- Chronic illness, injury, or restraint that interferes with mobility
- Psychological

that may manifest as UI, and identifying potentially reversible causes of incontinence. Additional evaluation is warranted in the presence of complex medical conditions or concerning findings on history and/or physical examination **(Table 4)**.

TREATMENT

General Principles

- Treatments of UI must be carefully tailored to the individual geriatric patient.
- Patient education—available in booklets and on websites
- Treatment of predisposing conditions such as constipation, obesity, and heart failure
- Acute incontinence is generally transient if managed effectively.
- Environmental manipulation, appropriate use of toilet substitutes, avoidance of iatrogenic contributions to incontinence, modifications of diuretic and fluid intake patterns, and good skin care are all important.

TABLE 3: Types of persistent urinary incontinence.

Type	Description	Causes
Stress	Involuntary loss of urine with increased intra-abdominal pressure (e.g., coughing, laughing, exercising)	Weakness of pelvic floor musculature and urethral sphincter
Urgency	Leakage of urine because of an urgent need to void, often after sensation of bladder fullness	Detrusor hyperactivity, isolated or associated with one or more of the following: Local genitourinary condition, central nervous system disorders
Mixed	Combination of stress and urgency incontinence	Detrusor hyperactivity, isolated or associated with one or more of the following: Local genitourinary condition, central nervous system disorders
Functional	Urinary accidents associated with inability to toilet because of impairment of cognitive and/or physical functioning, psychological unwillingness, or environmental barriers	Severe dementia and other neurologic conditions, depression, and hostility
High postvoid residual (overflow)	Leakage of urine resulting from urethral obstruction or overdistended bladder, often contributing to urge leakage	• Anatomic obstruction by prostate, urethral stricture, severe cystocele • A contractile bladder associated with diabetes mellitus or spinal cord injury • Neurogenic (detrusor sphincter dyssynergy), associated with multiple sclerosis and other suprasacral spinal cord lesions • Medication effect

BOX 3 **Detrusor hyperactivity with impaired contractility (DHIC)—a special diagnosis in geriatric population.**

- Form of bladder dysfunction that is unique to the geriatric population
- During the bladder filling phase, the patient experiences typical symptoms of urinary urgency, frequency, potentially associated with urge UI
- During the voiding phase, the bladder does not contract efficiently to completely empty
- Functional combination of overactive and underactive bladder
- Monotherapy with antimuscarinic medications or other bladder relaxants can worsen urinary retention and promote development of chronic urinary retention with associated incontinence
- Treatment: Multimodal therapy, including behavioral interventions and medications, to inhibit detrusor overactivity and clean intermittent catheterization (CIC) to empty the bladder

TABLE 4: Evaluation of urinary incontinence.

All patients	Purpose
Focused history	Characterize the type of incontinence [three incontinence questionnaires (3IQ, *Brown JS et al., 2006*) can help], identify underlying medical conditions, assess medication history, and evaluate quality of life
Targeted physical examination	Assess pelvic floor muscle function, pelvic organ prolapse, and neurological symptoms
Urinalysis	Identify infections (UTI) or hematuria
Postvoid residual determination	Measure the amount of urine remaining in the bladder after voiding
Selected patients	**Purpose**
Laboratory studies	Assess for infections, kidney function, and blood sugar levels
Renal and/or bladder ultrasound	Evaluate the structure and function of the kidneys and bladder
Gynecologic evaluation	Assess for pelvic organ prolapse or other gynecological issues
Urologic evaluation	Assess the urethra, bladder, and prostate
Cystourethroscopy	Visualize the inside of the urethra and bladder
Urodynamic tests (considered in suspected overflow incontinence, history of diabetes, or neurological conditions)	Assess bladder function, bladder capacity, and urethral function

Behavioral therapies are a mainstay of the treatment of UI in geriatrics, although medications and surgeries can also be used successfully in this population.

Treatment of Stress Urinary Incontinence

- *Conservative management*:
  - Lifestyle modifications include weight loss, fluid intake optimization, restriction of alcohol and caffeine intake
  - Pelvic floor muscle training: Kegel's exercises
  - Electrical stimulation
  - Bladder training (maintaining a diary)
- *Pharmacotherapy*:
  - Duloxetine (serotonin and norepinephrine reuptake inhibitor)—acts by increasing α-adrenergic tone to the urethra
  - Pseudoephedrine—acts by stimulating contraction of urethral smooth muscle; adverse effects—headache, tachycardia, and elevation of blood pressure
- *Surgery*: The principal goal of surgery is to provide proper support of the vesicourethral segment. In patients with bothersome symptoms after attempts at nonsurgical treatment and in women with a significant degree of pelvic prolapse or intrinsic sphincter deficiency (ISD):
  - Bladder neck suspension
  - Midurethral tapes
  - Intraurethral injection of bulking agents
  - Artificial urinary sphincter

Treatment of Urge Urinary Incontinence

- Lifestyle modifications include weight loss, fluid intake optimization, restriction of alcohol and caffeine intake
- Behavioral techniques (bladder training)
- *Pharmacotherapy*:
  - Anticholinergic/antimuscarinic drugs:
    - Mechanism of action: Increasing bladder capacity and diminishing involuntary bladder contractions.
    - Potential adverse effects include dry mouth, constipation, blurry vision, elevated intraocular pressure, cognitive impairment, delirium.
    - For example, darifenacin, fesoterodine, imidafenacin, propiverine, solifenacin, tolterodine, trospium, oxybutynin
  - α-Adrenergic antagonists:
    - Mechanism of action: Relax smooth muscle of urethra and prostatic capsule
    - Useful in urge incontinence and related irritative symptoms associated with benign prostatic enlargement
    - Potential adverse effect includes postural hypotension
  - β3-agonist (mirabegron)—acts by increasing bladder capacity and diminishing involuntary bladder contractions.

Because of serious concerns about anticholinergics causing dementia and impaired cognition, mirabegron may be a better choice for treating overactive bladder (OAB) in the elderly.

  - Topical estrogen cream—helps strengthen periurethral tissue; side effect—local irritation.
- Options for nonresponders to drug therapy may include onabotulinumtoxinA (BOTOX) bladder injection or implanted sacral nerve stimulation such as InterStim therapy.
- More invasive surgical procedures, including bladder augmentation or urinary diversion for persistent severe UI, are rarely indicated.

Treatment of Overflow Incontinence

- Surgical removal of obstruction
- Bladder retraining—progressive lengthening or shortening of intervoiding interval, with intermittent catheterization used in patients recovering from overdistention injuries with persistent retention
- Catheterization—intermittent/indwelling

Treatment of Functional Incontinence

- Behavioral interventions which are dependent on the caregiver and include scheduled toileting, habit training, and prompted voiding
- Environmental manipulations
- Incontinence undergarments and pants

Role of Catheters in Managing Incontinence

- Catheters should be avoided in managing incontinence, unless specifically indicated.
- *There are three types of catheters*: (1) External, (2) intermittent straight, and (3) chronic indwelling.
  - External catheters, consisting of a condom attached to the drainage system, should be used only to manage intractable incontinence in male patients who do not have urinary retention and who are extremely physically dependent.
  - Intermittent catheterization can be used in patients with incontinence associated with urinary retention. Ideally, the bladder volumes should be kept <400 mL. However, in a nursing home setting, it carries the risk of nosocomial infections and anatomic abnormalities predisposing to the risk of injury.

- It is not advised to use incontinence undergarments and paddings on a convenience basis, since it fosters dependency.
- Chronic indwelling catheterization use should be limited to only specific settings such as persistent UI (that cannot be managed otherwise), skin wounds/bed sores, and care of critically ill to avoid complications such as chronic bacteriuria, bladder stones, periurethral abscesses, and even bladder cancer.

Prevention of urinary incontinence:
- Pelvic floor muscle training (PFMT), a group behavior modification program and an educational program to control UI and OAB, has shown some improvement in older women in some studies while others deliver comparable results.
- In men, postoperative UI is almost universal immediately after prostatectomy. There is some evidence showing the possibility of speed of recovery of continence using behavioral interventions such as PFMT initiated before surgery or immediately after surgery, with inconsistent results while both combined with promising results.

Treatment

- Treatment of constipation involves proper diet, including adequate fluid intake and bulk, improving mobility, positioning of the body during toileting, and the timing and setting of toileting.
- Pharmacologic therapy includes stool softeners, bulk forming agents such as bran, psyllium, osmotic cathartics, enemas, and suppositories.
- Specially designed incontinence undergarments are sometimes helpful.

CONCLUSION

Urinary incontinence is a highly prevalent 35–55% geriatric syndrome in elderly, with substantial negative effects on their health-related quality of life, including social isolation, depression, and embarrassment. UI should not be considered as a normal part of aging, but look for treatable causes and contributing factors such as neurological disorders, infection, diabetes, and medication usage etc.

Geriatrician should be proactive in case findings in their clinical practice to diagnose UI.

Effective treatment of UI in geriatrics demands an individualized, multimodal approach including behavioural therapies, lifestyle modifications, targeted pharmacotherapy, and surgical interventions when necessary.

Self-Assessment Questionnaire

Q1. How does the International Continence Society (ICS) define urinary incontinence (UI)?

Q2. List at least five risk factors associated with urinary incontinence in older adults.

Q3. Describe the impact of UI on the health and quality of life of elderly patients.

Q4. What are the major types of persistent urinary incontinence, and how can each be differentiated clinically?

Q5. What are the behavioral and lifestyle interventions recommended for managing stress and urge incontinence?

Q6. Why should catheter use be limited in managing incontinence, and what are the specific indications for its use?

Q7. Explain the condition detrusor hyperactivity with impaired contractility (DHIC) and its treatment approach.

FURTHER READINGS

1. Abrams P, Cardozo L, Fall M, Griffiths D, Rosier P, Ulmsten U, et al. The standardisation of terminology in lower urinary tract function: report from the standardisation sub-committee of the International Continence Society. Urology. 2003;61(1):37-49.
2. Thom D. Variation in estimates of urinary incontinence prevalence in the community: effects of differences in definition, population characteristics, and study type. J Am Geriatr Soc. 1998;46(4):473-80.
3. Sinha S, Agarwal MM, Vasudeva P, Khattar N, Madduri VKS, Yande S, et al. The Urological Society of India guidelines for the evaluation and management of nonneurogenic urinary incontinence in adults (executive summary). Indian J Urol. 2019;35(3):185.
4. Dugan E, Cohen SJ, Bland DR, Preisser JS, Davis CC, Suggs PK, et al. The association of depressive symptoms and urinary incontinence among older adults. J Am Geriatr Soc. 2000;48(4):413-6.
5. Lim YM, Lee SR, Choi EJ, Jeong K, Chung HW. Urinary incontinence is strongly associated with depression in middle-aged and older Korean women: data from the Korean longitudinal study of ageing. Eur J Obstet Gynecol Reprod Biol. 2018;220:69-73.

CHAPTER 17

Polypharmacy and Potentially Inappropriate Medications

Minakshi Dhar, Sudeep Mathew George

"The greatest medicine of all is to teach people how not to need it."

—Hippocrates

CASE VIGNETTE

An 88-year-old male, known case of hypertension, diabetes mellitus, and coronary artery disease, presented to his geriatrician for a regular follow-up. He reported that his dyspnea had worsened recently. He had mild symmetrical lower limb swelling. He had been visiting a few other clinics before the current visit for his complaints. His medications included tablet telmisartan (40 mg), tablet cilnidipine (20 mg), tablet metformin + vildagliptin (500/50 mg), tablet dapagliflozin (10 mg), tablet metoprolol succinate (50 mg), tablet torsemide + spironolactone (40/100 mg), tablet valsartan + sacubitril (24/26 mg), tablet aspirin + clopidogrel + atorvastatin (75/75/40 mg), tablet pantoprazole 40 mg, tablet clonazepam 0.25 mg, tablet calcium carbonate 500 mg, capsule coenzyme Q, and few other supplements.

INTRODUCTION

Drug prescribing in older adults poses a great challenge owing to the multiple comorbidities. There are specific pharmacokinetic (PK) and pharmacodynamic parameters that change with aging, leading to adverse reactions and consequences. Due to decreased renal and hepatic function, reduced lean body mass, and impaired hearing, vision, cognition, and mobility, older individuals are considerably more vulnerable to negative effects. This chapter focuses on the principles of pharmacotherapy and the challenges of drug prescribing in older adults.

AGE-ASSOCIATED CHANGES IN THE PHARMACOKINETICS AND PHARMACODYNAMICS

The changes in PKs and pharmacodynamics that occur as a part of normal aging account for the variability of drug response in older people. It is prudent to understand the physiological changes with aging to provide appropriate pharmaceutical care for them.

Pharmacokinetics

Pharmacokinetics describes the way how our body deals with the drug. Absorption, distribution, metabolism, and elimination of drugs are modified in older patients at different levels.

Absorption

Drug absorption is largely unaltered with aging. In the gastrointestinal tract, the majority of drugs undergo passive diffusion, which causes a delay in absorption but no overall change in the amount of absorption. Despite the delay in the time to attain maximum concentration after the first dose, no clinically significant change is seen once the steady state has been reached.

Reduction in gastric acid secretion, delayed stomach emptying, slowed transit time, and decreased blood flow are some age-related alterations in the gastrointestinal tract which may impact drug absorption. Concurrent use of several drugs also affects the drug absorption. Gastric pH also plays an important role in optimal drug

TABLE 1: Common drugs whose absorption is affected by achlorhydria.

Absorption effect	Generic name	Methods to minimize the problems
Increased rate	Enteric-coated tablets	Take on empty stomach
Increased extent	Alendronate	Take on empty stomach in an upright position with one full glass of water
Decreased extent	• Iron • Calcium carbonate	• Administer with citrus juice on an empty stomach • Take with meals

absorption. **Table 1** lists the common drugs whose absorption is affected by achlorhydria.

Distribution

Determining the appropriate dosage of a medication requires considering the possibility that the volume of distribution of the medicine may change in an older patient. Volume of distribution (V_d) is calculated as the amount of drug in the body divided by the concentration of drug measured in a biological fluid:

$$\text{Volume of apparent drug distribution } (L) = \text{Amount (mg)/concentration (mg/L)}.$$

The V_d is influenced by the body composition and the lipid or water solubility of a drug. The total body water content reduces with age. As people age, their percentage of body fat increases by 25–30%, but their muscle mass decreases by the same amount. These changes can affect the distribution of drugs, leading to a wider dispersion of fat-soluble drugs compared to water-soluble medications.

If volume of distribution of a drug is decreased, the loading dose required to reach the target concentration is also decreased and the half-life $t_{1/2}$ of the drug may be changed. Drugs that primarily distribute into muscle or body water will have a reduced volume of distribution, requiring lower doses to prevent the risk of toxicity.

Due to enlarged volume of distribution of lipid-soluble drugs, a prolonged duration of action will be problematic, when an adverse reaction occurs. **Table 2** lists the volume of distribution of commonly used drugs.

TABLE 2: Volume of distribution of commonly used drugs.

Increased volume	Decreased volume
• Prazosin • Acetaminophen • Salicylates • Diazepam • Oxazepam	• Phenytoin • Cimetidine • Theophylline • Gentamicin • Digoxin

Metabolism

Liver is the primary organ involved in the metabolism of drugs, although certain pharmaceuticals may also be metabolized by the kidney and the gastrointestinal system. The liver mass in an older adult can reduce in size by 20–40% with a 35% reduction in hepatic blood flow. As a consequence, the drugs with high first-pass metabolism can have high bioavailability in older adults.

Hepatic metabolism of drugs is categorized into phase I and phase II reactions. Phase I reactions include oxidations, reductions, and hydrolyses, whereas in phase II, drug molecules are conjugated to glucuronides, sulfates, or acetates. Phase I reactions involve cytochrome P45 monooxygenase (CYP450) enzymes which are majorly located in the smooth endoplasmic reticulum of hepatocytes. Numerous drugs that are frequently prescribed act as substrates for this enzyme system. Drugs that are metabolized through phase I mechanisms have a prolonged half-life owing to the substantial decrease in enzyme activity in older patients because of illness or drug interactions. In contrast, the drugs undergoing phase II metabolism by conjugation have not shown a change associated with advanced age.

Although this is primarily based on convention rather than concrete scientific data, it is advisable to decrease the dosage requirements for drugs that have phase I metabolism in older patients.

Elimination

Elimination of drugs from the body occurs primarily via the kidney. Physiological changes with aging such as reduction in blood flow and number of functioning nephrons can affect the elimination process of drugs. Altered renal clearance leads to prolonged half-lives of renally excreted drugs and increase in their serum concentration. Depending on the circumstances, one can either decrease the dosage, increase the time between doses, or do both to avoid an excessive buildup of a drug when its clearance is decreased.

Pharmacodynamics

Pharmacodynamics is the study of the relationship between the concentration of drug at the site of action and the biochemical and physiological effects. The physiological changes associated with aging include alterations in receptor number and affinity, signal transduction, and homeostatic mechanisms. The sensitivity to drug effects may either increase or decrease with advancing age. For instance, older persons may have enhanced sensitivity to the sedative effects of benzodiazepines but decreased sensitivity to the effect of drugs mediated by β-adrenergic receptors.

It should be highlighted that the majority of medications used in clinical practice have never had their PK and pharmacodynamics investigated in the elderly, particularly in those over 75 years or in those with concomitant comorbidities. Medication should be used cautiously to accomplish the goal of limiting hazards because older patients' responses to various drugs vary. A general dictum of "START SLOW AND GO SLOW" can be practiced while initiating drug therapy for older adults. **Table 3** summarizes the age-associated changes in PK and pharmacodynamics.

POLYPHARMACY

Although there is no standard definition, polypharmacy is often defined as the routine use of five or more medications. This includes over-the-counter, prescription, and/or traditional and complementary medicines used by a patient **(Flowchart 1)**.

With advancing age and multiple chronic ailments, the probability of polypharmacy increases dramatically. Polypharmacy poses a significant public health challenge. Various adverse health outcomes associated with polypharmacy include susceptibility to events such as drug–drug interactions, higher risk of falls, adverse drug reactions (ADRs), cognitive impairment, nonadherence, poor nutritional status, increased hospital stay, and mortality risk.

There is a lack of clinical guidelines for the management of older adults with multimorbidity. Currently, the majority of prescribing decisions are made using evidence-based guidelines specific to individual conditions. As a result, patients frequently receive multiple prescriptions from different specialists based on criteria relevant to their particular ailment. This can be a challenge to managing a single disease and potentially cause harm to the patient.

Both appropriate and undesirable cases of polypharmacy exist. When patients' clinical circumstances, comorbidities, allergy profiles, possible drug–drug and drug–disease interactions, and prescriptions are written based on the best available research, appropriate polypharmacy acknowledges that individuals may

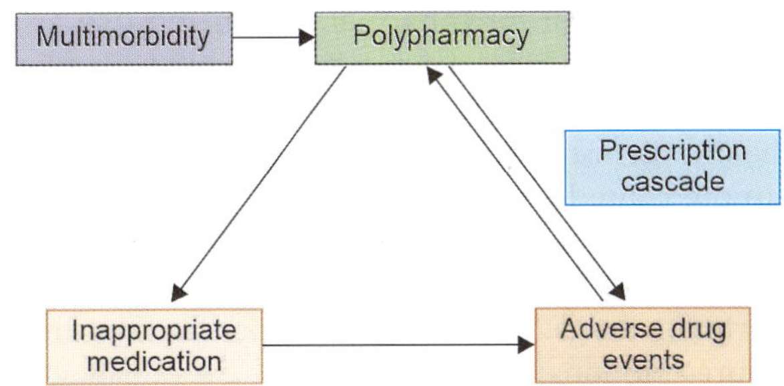

FLOWCHART 1: Polypharmacy and potentially inappropriate prescribing.

TABLE 3: Age-associated changes in pharmacokinetics and pharmacodynamics.

Pharmacological parameter	Age effect	Disease/factor effect	Clinical implication
Absorption	*Decrease in*: • Splanchnic blood flow • Gastrointestinal motility • Absorptive surface	Concurrent medications, tube feedings, and changes in pH	• Rate and extent are usually unaffected • Drug–drug and drug–food interactions can affect absorption
Distribution	*Decrease in*: • Total body water • Serum albumin • Lean body mass • Increased fat	Heart failure, ascites, and other conditions increase body water	• Fat-soluble drugs have a larger volume of distribution • Highly protein-bound drugs have a greater free concentration
Metabolism	Decreased liver blood flow and enzyme activity	Smoking, genotype, alcohol, and concurrent drug intake	Lower dosages may be therapeutic
Elimination	Decreased renal perfusion, glomerular filtration rate, and tubular secretion	Kidney impairment with acute and chronic diseases	Decreased renal elimination of drugs—dosage adjustments
Pharmacodynamics	Less predictable and often altered drug response at usual or lower concentrations	Drug–drug and drug–disease interactions may alter responses	Prolonged pain relief with opioids at lower dosages, altered sensitivity to beta-blockers

benefit from taking numerous medications. For example, four distinct pharmacological classes—beta-blockers, statins, antiplatelet agents, and angiotensin-converting enzyme (ACE) inhibitors—are utilized in the secondary prevention of myocardial infarction, where polypharmacy is considered both appropriate and required.

When one or more medications are prescribed that are not needed or are no longer evidence-based, this is known as inappropriate polypharmacy. This can occur for a number of reasons: (1) No evidence-based indication, an expired indication, or an excessively high dose; (2) one or more medications not meeting the intended therapeutic goals; (3) one or more medications causing ADRs or placing the patient at a high risk of developing ADRs; or (4) the patient is unwilling or unable to take one or more medications as prescribed.

Prevalence

The magnitude of polypharmacy is on the rise as the global population faces a demographic shift with a larger proportion of older people, along with a marked increase in the prevalence of multimorbidity.

In the United States, 70% of nursing home residents receive more than nine prescription pharmaceuticals, while over 80% of elders who live in the community use prescription drugs. The average older person uses three to eight prescriptions.

A systematic review found that 49% of older Indian adults (aged 60 years and above) were experiencing polypharmacy.

POTENTIALLY INAPPROPRIATE PRESCRIBING

Potentially inappropriate prescribing (PIP) is the misprescribing, overprescribing, or underprescribing of medication for older adults that may cause significant harm. PIP should always be assessed in conjunction with the multimorbidity, treatment goals, cognitive and functional status, and life expectancy of the older adults.

The screening criteria for PIP can be implicit (judgment-based) tools, explicit (criterion-based) tools, and tools showing a combination of both approaches. Implicit tools depend on the clinician's knowledge and attitude. These are usually time-consuming and have low reliability. However, these tools are patient-specific and take into consideration the entire drug regimen of the patient and shared decision-making. Examples of implicit tools include Medication Appropriateness Index (MAI) and Assessment of Underutilization (AOU) of Medication.

Explicit tools are developed after an extensive review of literature and consensus among experts, which comprise lists of medications that cause harmful effects in older adults. These can be easily applied to prescriptions and are less time-consuming. However, the patient preference or comorbidity burden is not addressed adequately. Commonly used explicit tools are illustrated in **Table 4**.

Beers Criteria

The American Geriatrics Society (AGS) Beers Criteria® (AGS Beers Criteria®) is one of the most widely used criteria to assess inappropriate drug prescribing. Beers et al. in 1991 were the first group to publish explicit criteria for PIP in older adults. The first iteration was focused on the frail nursing home resident population in the United States. The AGS issued the seventh iteration of Beers criteria in 2023, which is the most current update to the original set. With the exception of hospice and end-of-life care, the criterion is meant to be applied to persons 65 years of age and older in ambulatory, acute care, and institutionalized settings. The goals of the AGS Beers Criteria® are to (1) lessen the

TABLE 4: Commonly used explicit tools for PIP.

Criteria	Intended population	Specific advantages
Beers' criteria	≥65 years (excluding people with palliative care needs)	• Concise, robust grading methodology • Extensive evidence-based review
STOPP/START	Older people ≥ 65 years	Concise explanation of inappropriateness; organized by physiological system; includes underprescribing
EURO Fit foR The Aged (FORTA) list	Older people ≥ 65 years	Prescriber is directed to use the safest/most effective medications for common clinical scenarios
Australian Prescribing Indicators tool	Older people ≥ 65 years	Includes drug duplication and underprescribing
Norwegian General Practice (NORGEP) criteria	Elderly patients aged ≥ 70 years in general practice	Can be applied to medication list with no clinical information

(PIP: potentially inappropriate prescribing; START: Screening Tool to Alert doctors to the Right Treatment; STOPP: Screening Tool of Older Persons' Prescriptions)

amount of potentially inappropriate medications (PIMs) that older adults are exposed to through better medication selection, (2) inform patients and clinicians, and (3) act as a tool for assessing the cost, quality, and drug-use patterns of older adults.

The medications are grouped into five categories:
1. Medications that are potentially inappropriate in most older adults
2. Those that should typically be avoided in older adults with certain conditions
3. Drugs to use with caution
4. Drug-drug interactions
5. Drug-dose adjustment based on kidney function

STOPP/START Criteria

A set of explicit criteria known as STOPP (Screening Tool of Older Persons' Prescriptions)/START (Screening Tool to Alert Doctors to the Right Treatment) is based on physiological systems and aims to identify clinically significant prescribing issues with PIMs-STOPP criteria and possible prescribing omissions (PPOs-START criteria). The STOPP/START criteria were first released in two versions in 2008 and 2015. STOPP/START version 3 in 2023 includes 133 PIM criteria and 57 START PPO criteria.

PRESCRIPTION CASCADE

A prescription cascade starts when following administration of a drug, in case of any adverse event it is misinterpreted as a new medical problem; and this leads to the prescription of another medication to treat the adverse event caused by the previous one. As a consequence, the patient is put at risk for adverse reactions from the new drugs prescribed, leading to a vicious cycle of adverse reactions and prescribing **(Flowchart 2)**.

A few examples of prescription cascade are summarized in **Table 5**.

The prescription cascade leads to an increase in the pill burden and healthcare expenditure and causes preventable drug interactions and adverse reactions. Using clinical process maps is a workable way to locate and stop prescription cascades. It illustrates how a process moves along and serves to give documentation, promote communication, highlight areas that have gone wrong and can be fixed, and offer insight into the process.

Clinical process maps illustrate the temporal relationship between onset of symptoms and prescription cascade. It is always prudent to ask: "*Could my patient's new symptom be caused by a drug they are taking rather than a new medical condition*?", before doing further evaluation.

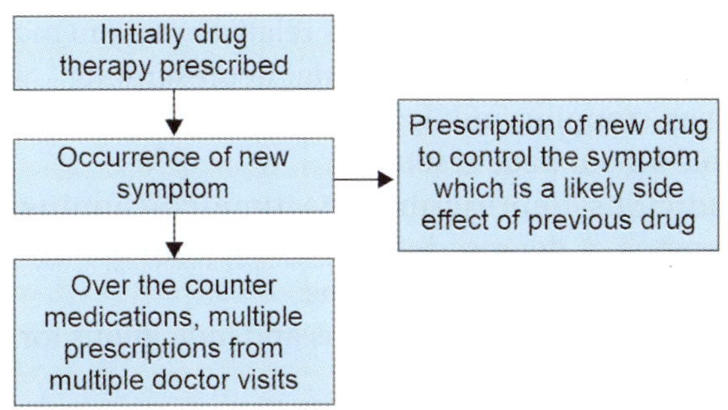

FLOWCHART 2: Prescribing cascade.

TABLE 5: Examples of prescription cascades.

Medicine	ADR	Second medicine prescribed to counter ADR
NSAIDs	Hypertension	Antihypertensives
Thiazide diuretics	Hyperuricemia, gout	Allopurinol
Metoclopramide	Movement disorder	Levodopa
Antipsychotic (typical and atypical)	Parkinsonism	Levodopa
ACE inhibitor	Cough	Cough suppressant/ antibiotics
Cholinesterase inhibitor	Incontinence	Anticholinergics
Calcium channel blockers	Edema	Diuretic
Vasodilators, diuretics	Dizziness	Prochlorperazine
Gabapentin	Peripheral edema	Diuretic

(ACE: angiotensin-converting enzyme; ADR: adverse drug reaction; NSAIDs: nonsteroidal anti-inflammatory drugs)

DEPRESCRIBING

In the context of a patient's care objectives, function, values, and preferences, deprescribing is the act of identifying and stopping drugs whose current or projected risks outweigh their potential benefits. The major goals of deprescribing include the risk reduction of geriatric syndromes such as delirium and falls and reduction in overall medication burden, thereby improving quality of life and drug adherence.

The evidence of deprescribing is still emerging. The clinical scenario may direct the deprescribing procedure. "Poly-deprescribing," which involves stopping several medications at once, may be more suitable for patients admitted to hospitals where it is relatively easy to monitor for withdrawal symptoms. "Serial deprescribing," which involves stopping medications one at a time, is more suitable for our patient settings.

Judicious deprescribing is time-consuming and challenging. A deprescribing protocol proposed by Scott et al. in 2015 comprises five steps:

1. List the ongoing medications and indications for their use
2. Assessment of the overall risk of drug-induced side effects in patients in determining the required deprescribing intervention
3. Evaluate every medication based on its potential for present or future benefits in comparison to its potential for current or future harm or burden
4. Prioritize stopping the medications that have the lowest benefit–harm ratio and likelihood of withdrawal reactions
5. Implementation of a deprescribing regimen and close monitoring for improvement in outcomes or onset of any adverse effects

Other deprescribing tools include:

- *Deprescribing.org*: Algorithms and guidelines
- *Medstopper.com*: Risk stratification and tapering tool
- *AGS Choosing Wisely*: https://www.choosingwisely.org/societies/american-geriatrics-society/
- Problem-based deprescribing (Molnar, Canadian Geriatrics Society, 2018)
- The Good Palliative–Geriatric Practice algorithm
- CEASE (current medicines, elevated risk, assess, sort, and eliminate) algorithm

STOPPFrail (Screening Tool of Older Persons' Prescriptions in Frail Adults with Limited Life Expectancy) (Table 6)

Both natural physiological aging and chronic illnesses can negatively affect cognitive function and functional abilities. Reevaluating treatment goals is necessary for these patients because their final months are often marked by frailty and increased dependency. This is especially true for medications with long-term preventative effects such

TABLE 6: Final STOPPFrail criteria 2021.

STOPPFrail version 2	
STOPPFrail is a list of potentially inappropriate prescribing indicators designed to assist physicians with deprescribing decisions. It is intended for older people with limited life expectancy for whom the goal of care is to optimize quality of life and minimize the risk of drug-related morbidity. Goals of care should be clearly defined, and, where possible, medication changes should be discussed and agreed with patient and/or family. Appropriate candidates for STOPPFrail-guided deprescribing typically meet all of the following criteria: • Activities of daily living dependency (i.e., assistance with dressing, washing, transferring, and walking) and/or severe chronic disease and/or terminal illness • Severe irreversible frailty, i.e., high risk of acute medical complications and clinical deterioration • Physician overseeing care of patient would not be surprised if the patient died in the next 12 months	
Section A: General	• Any drug that the patient persistently fails to take or tolerate despite adequate education and consideration of all appropriate formulations • Any drug without a clear clinical indication • Any drug for symptoms which have now resolved (e.g., pain, nausea, vertigo, and pruritus)
Section B: Cardiology system	• *Lipid-lowering therapies* (statins, ezetimibe, bile acid sequestrants, fibrates, nicotinic acid, lomitapide, and acipimox) • *Antihypertensive therapies*: Carefully reduce or discontinue these drugs in patients with systolic blood pressure (SBP) persistently < 130 mm Hg. An appropriate SBP target in frail older people is 130–160 mm Hg. Before stopping, consider whether the drug is treating additional conditions (e.g., beta-blocker for rate control in atrial fibrillation, diuretics for symptomatic heart failure) • *Antianginal therapy (specifically nitrates, nicorandil, and ranolazine)*: None of these antianginal drugs has been proven to reduce cardiovascular mortality or the rate of myocardial infarction. The aim is to carefully reduce and discontinue these drugs in patients who have had no reported anginal symptoms in the previous 12 months and who have no proven or objective evidence of coronary artery disease
Section C: Coagulation system	• *Antiplatelets*: No evidence of benefit for primary (as distinct from secondary) cardiovascular prevention • *Aspirin for stroke prevention in atrial fibrillation*: Aspirin has little or no role for stroke prevention in frail older people who are not candidates for anticoagulation therapy and may significantly increase bleeding risk

Continued

Continued

Section D: Central nervous system	• *Neuroleptic antipsychotics in patients with dementia*: Aim to reduce dose and discontinue these drugs in patients taking them for longer than 12 weeks if there are no current clinical features of behavioral and psychiatric symptoms of dementia (BPSD) • *Memantine*: Discontinue and monitor in patients with moderate-to-severe dementia, unless memantine has clearly improved BPSD
Section E: Gastrointestinal system	• *Proton-pump inhibitors*: Reduce dose of proton-pump inhibitors when used at full therapeutic dose >8 weeks unless persistent dyspeptic symptoms at lower maintenance dose • *112 receptor antagonists*: Reduce the dose of H_2 receptor antagonists when used at full therapeutic dose for >8 weeks, unless persistent dyspeptic symptoms at lower maintenance dose
Section F: Respiratory system	• *Theophylline and aminophylline*: These drugs have a narrow therapeutic index, have doubtful therapeutic benefit, require monitoring of serum levels, and interact with other commonly prescribed drugs putting patients at an increased risk of ADEs • *Leukotriene antagonists (montelukast, zafirlukast)*: These drugs have no proven role in chronic obstructive pulmonary disease; they are indicated only in asthma
Section G: Musculoskeletal system	• *Calcium supplements*: Unlikely to be of any benefit in short term unless proven, symptomatic hypocalcemia • *Vitamin D (ergocalciferol and cholecalciferol)*: Lack of clear evidence to support the use of vitamin D to prevent falls and fractures, cardiovascular events, or cancers • Antiresorptive/bone anabolic drugs *for osteoporosis* (bisphosphonates, strontium, teriparatide, and denosumab) • *Long-term oral nonsteroidal anti-inflammatory drugs*: Increased risk of side effects (e.g., peptic ulcer disease, bleeding, and worsening heart failure) when taken regularly for ≥2 months • *Long-term oral corticosteroids*: Increased risk of major side effects (e.g., fragility fractures, proximal myopathy, and peptic ulcer disease) when taken regularly for ≥2 months. Consider careful dose reduction and discontinuation
Section H: Urogenital system	• *Drugs for benign prostatic hyperplasia (five-alpha reductase inhibitors and alpha-blockers) in catheterized male patients*: No benefit with long-term bladder catheterization • *Drugs for overactive bladder (muscarinic antagonists and mirabegron)*: No benefit in patients with persistent, irreversible urinary incontinence unless clear history of painful detrusor hyperactivity
Section I: Endocrine system	• *Antidiabetic drugs*: Deintensify therapy. Avoid HbA1c targets [HbA1c < 7.5% (58 mmol/mol) associated with net harm in this population]. The goal of care is to minimize symptoms related to hyperglycemia (e.g., excessive thirst, polyuria)
Section J: Miscellaneous	• *Multivitamin combination supplements*: Discontinue when prescribed for prophylaxis rather than treatment of hypovitaminosis • *Folic acid*: Discontinue when the treatment course is completed. The usual treatment duration is 1–4 months unless malabsorption, malnutrition, or concomitant methotrexate use • *Nutritional supplements*: Discontinue when prescribed for prophylaxis rather than treatment or malnutrition

Disclaimer (STOPPFrail): While every effort has been made to ensure that the potentially inappropriate deprescribing criteria listed in STOPPFrail are accurate and evidence-based, it is emphasized that the final decision to deprescribe any drug referred to in these criteria rests entirely with the prescriber. It is also to be noted that the evidence base underlying certain criteria in STOPPFrail may change after the time of publication of these criteria. Therefore, it is advisable that deprescribing decisions should take account of current published evidence in support of or against the use of drugs or drug classes described in STOPPFrail.

(ADEs: adverse drug events; STOPPFrail: Screening Tool of Older Persons' Prescriptions in Frail Adults with Limited Life Expectancy)

as lipid-lowering, antidiabetic, and cognitive-enhancing drugs.

The tool was first published in 2017 and the second iteration was published in 2021. If an older adult meets all of the following criteria as listed, this tool offers a list of possibly inappropriate medication therapies that should be stopped:

- Activities of daily living dependency and/or chronic disease/terminal illness
- Severe irreversible frailty
- Patients who are likely to pass away in the next 12 months

PRACTICAL APPROACH TO OPTIMIZE PHARMACOTHERAPY IN OLDER ADULTS

An international group of eight geriatricians from six different nations produced the DRUGS guide to optimize

TABLE 7: DRUGS guide to optimizing medication safety for older adults.

	DRUGS guide to optimizing medication safety for older adults	Sex and gender considerations
D	*DISCUSS goals of care and what matters most to the patient*: • Include patients and caregivers in deprescribing discussions to ensure decisions focus on the goals of care	Women are more likely than men to be caregivers and might not have a caregiver to advocate for them

R	*REVIEW medications*:
	• Encourage patients to bring all prescribed and over-the-counter medications to their appointment
	• Review medications on an ongoing basis and when clinical conditions or goals of care change:
	  ○ Discontinue potentially unnecessary drugs
	  ○ Consider drug side effects as a potential cause for a new symptom
	  ○ Consider nonpharmacological options
	  ○ Change for safer alternatives
	  ○ Lower the dose
	• To identify possible prescribing cascades, determine when the medication was started and why
		Women use more prescribed and over-the-counter medications than men

U	*USE tools and frameworks*:
	• Identify drugs from the inappropriate prescribing tools, including Beers criteria or STOPP criteria
	• Use the STOPPFrail list when the individual is extremely frail and approaching the end of life
	• Consider whether the new or existing medical condition could be the result of a prescribing cascade and ask:
	  ○ Is a new drug being prescribed to manage a side effect from another prescribed drug?
	  ○ Could the initial drug be replaced with a safer drug or could the dose be reduced?
	  ○ Does the patient need the first drug or could this drug be stopped?
	• Pay attention to older people who are receiving the so-called good drugs with narrow therapeutic windows that might no longer be needed or for whom dose reduction might be beneficial
		Women are more often prescribed psychoactive drugs, whereas men are more often prescribed secondary prevention drugs; women might require lower doses; and men receive more aggressive medical therapy

G	*GERIATRIC medicine approach*: • Geriatricians carefully consider how multiple medical problems, frailty, cognitive impairment, and limited life expectancy reduce medication benefit, increase adverse events, or interfere with medication adherence	Women are more likely than men to have multiple medical problems, frailty, and adverse drug events; men are more likely than women to adhere to drug therapies; women might be less able than men to pay for medicines, decreasing adherence
S	*STOP the medications*: • Consider the algorithm created by Scott or the Good Palliative–Geriatric Practice algorithm to guide deprescribing	Women are more likely to discuss deprescribing with providers than men

medication safety for older persons. This manual provides instructions for prescribers on how to best prescribe medications to elderly patients. It stands for DISCUSS goals of care and what matters most, REVIEW medications, USE tools and frameworks, GERIATRIC medicine approach, and STOP the medications where appropriate. The detailed algorithm is explained in **Table 7**.

CONCLUSION

Polypharmacy in older adults presents a complex challenge in geriatric practice, requiring careful consideration and management. As highlighted in this chapter, understanding the nuances of medication interactions, side effects, and individual patient factors is crucial for optimizing therapeutic outcomes and minimizing harm.

By fostering interdisciplinary collaboration, implementing evidence-based prescribing practices, and prioritizing patient-centered care, healthcare providers can effectively address polypharmacy and promote healthier aging for older adults. Moving forward, continued research and education are essential for navigating the complexities of polypharmacy and enhancing the quality of care for this vulnerable population.

Self-Assessment Questionnaire

Q1. What are the significant age-related physiological changes that influence pharmacokinetics in older adults?

Q2. Define polypharmacy and differentiate between appropriate and inappropriate polypharmacy with suitable examples.

Q3. What are the common clinical consequences of polypharmacy in older adults?

Q4. Describe the main categories of drugs listed under the 2023 American Geriatrics Society (AGS) Beers Criteria®.

Q5. What is a prescription cascade? Give two examples and suggest strategies to prevent it.

Q6. What are the key indications for using the STOPPFrail criteria, and how does it guide deprescribing decisions in frail older adults?

Q7. Summarise the DRUGS guide for optimising medication safety in older adults and explain how it integrates a geriatric approach to pharmacotherapy.

FURTHER READINGS

1. Bushardt RL, Massey EB, Simpson TW, Ariail JC, Simpson KN. Polypharmacy: misleading, but manageable. Clin Interv Aging. 2008;3(2):383-9.
2. Hammerlein A, Derendorf H, Lowenthal DT. Pharmacokinetic and pharmacodynamic changes in the elderly. Clinical implications. Clin Pharmacokinet. 1998;35:49-64.
3. Lindblad CI, Gray SL, Guay DRP, Hajjar ER, McCarthy TC, Hanlon JT. Geriatrics. In: DiPiro JT, Talbert RL, Yee GC, Matzke GR, Wells BG, Posey LM (Eds). Pharmacotherapy: A Physiologic Approach, 6th edition. New York: McGraw-Hill Companies; 2005. pp. 103-13.
4. McLean AJ, Le Couteur DG. Aging biology and geriatric clinical pharmacology. Pharmacol Rev. 2004;56:163-84.
5. Hallworth M. Therapeutic drug monitoring. In: Marshall WJ, Lapsley M, Day AP, Ayling RM (Eds). Clinical Biochemistry: Metabolic and Clinical Aspects, 3rd edition. London: Churchill Livingstone; 2014. pp. 767-86.
6. Masnoon N, Shakib S, Kalisch-Ellett L, Caughey GE. What is polypharmacy? A systematic review of definitions. BMC Geriatr. 2017;17:230.
7. Molokhia M, Majeed A. Current and future perspectives on the management of polypharmacy. BMC Fam Pract. 2017;18:70.
8. Barnett K, Mercer SW, Norbury M, Watt G, Wyke S, Guthrie B. Epidemiology of multimorbidity and implications for healthcare, research, and medical education: a cross-sectional study. Lancet. 2012;380(9836):37-43.
9. Cadogan CA, Ryan C, Hughes CM. Appropriate polypharmacy and medicine safety: when many is not too many. Drug Saf. 2016;39:109-16.
10. Scottish Government Model of Care Polypharmacy Working Group. Polypharmacy Guidance, 2nd edition. Edinburgh: Scottish Government; 2015.
11. Morley JE. Polypharmacy in the nursing home. J Am Med Dir Assoc. 2010;11:289-91.
12. Bhagavathula AS, Vidyasagar K, Chhabra M, Rashid M, Sharma R, Bandari DK, et al. Prevalence of polypharmacy, hyperpolypharmacy and potentially inappropriate medication use in older adults in India: a systematic review and meta-analysis. Front Pharmacol. 2021;12:685518.
13. O'Connor MN, Gallagher P, O'Mahony D. Inappropriate prescribing: criteria, detection and prevention. Drugs Aging. 2012;29(6):437-52.
14. Beers MH, Ouslander JG, Rollingher I, Reuben DB, Brooks J, Beck JC. Explicit criteria for determining inappropriate medication use in nursing home residents. UCLA Division of Geriatric Medicine. Arch Intern Med. 1991;151:1825-32.
15. By the 2023 American Geriatrics Society Beers Criteria® Update Expert Panel. American Geriatrics Society 2023 updated AGS Beers Criteria® for potentially inappropriate medication use in older adults. J Am Geriatr Soc. 2023;71(7):2052-81.
16. O'Mahony D, Cherubini A, Guiteras AR, Denkinger M, Beuscart J-B, Onder G, et al. STOPP/START criteria for potentially inappropriate prescribing in older people: version 3. Eur Geriatr Med. 2023;14,625-32.
17. Rochon PA, Gurwitz JH. The prescribing cascade revisited. Lancet. 2017;389(10081):1778-80.
18. Graham-Rowe E, Lorencatto F, Lawrenson JG, Burr JM, Grimshaw JM, Ivers NM et al. Barriers to and enablers of diabetic retinopathy screening attendance: a systematic review of published and grey literature. Diabet Med. 2018;35:1308-19.
19. Scott IA, Hilmer SN, Reeve E, Potter K, Le Couteur D, Rigby D, et al. Reducing inappropriate polypharmacy: the process of deprescribing. JAMA Intern Med. 2015;175(5):827-34.
20. Woodford HJ, Fisher J. New horizons in deprescribing for older people. Age Ageing. 2019;48(6):768-75.
21. Anderson K, Stowasser D, Freeman C, Scott I. Prescriber barriers and enablers to minimising potentially inappropriate medications in adults: a systematic review and thematic synthesis. BMJ Open. 2014;4:e006544.
22. Lavan AH, Gallagher P, Parsons C, O'Mahony D. STOPPFrail (Screening Tool of Older Persons Prescriptions in Frail adults with limited life expectancy): consensus validation. Age Ageing. 2017;46:600-7.
23. Curtin D, Gallagher P, O'Mahony D. Deprescribing in older people approaching end-of-life: development and validation of STOPPFrail version 2. Age Ageing. 2021;50(2):465-71.
24. Rochon PA, Petrovic M, Cherubini A, Onder G, O'Mahony D, Sternberg SA, et al. Polypharmacy, inappropriate prescribing, and deprescribing in older people: through a sex and gender lens. Lancet Healthy Longev. 2021;2(5):e290-300.

CHAPTER 18

Pressure Ulcer

Mamta Saini

Pressure injuries are painful and costly but preventable.

INTRODUCTION

A pressure injury (PI) is a global "public health problem" among older adults. A pressure ulcer is a type of injury that causes the destruction of skin and underlying tissue due to constant pressure on the skin area for a specific time. This continuous pressure causes tissue ischemia and cessation of blood and nutrition supply to the tissue and leads to tissue necrosis.

Pressure sore is also known as bedsores or decubitus ulcers. The most common sites for pressure sores include the area covering bony prominence such as the sacrum, trochanters, heels, occiput, ischial tuberosities, and malleoli. PI causes increased hospital stay, readmission, financial cost for care, and mortality in older people. The personal burden includes pain related to PI, stress, anxiety, decreased autonomy, and social well-being.

EPIDEMIOLOGY

Pressure injuries occur in all healthcare settings and incidence differs in all clinical settings. The incidence rate ranges from 4 to 38% in hospitalization wards and the mortality rate is approximately 68% due to PI complications. About 70% of PIs occur in people aged > 65 years and in nursing home residents their prevalence is 6–22%.

In the United States, approximately 3 million adults are affected by PIs annually, and 60,000 die due to complications of the PI annually. The overall prevalence rates of pressure ulcers in a tertiary care hospital in India were 7.8% and 24.3% in the ICU. This PI management is also a source of economic burden. In the US, the estimated cost is $1.6 billion annually, and in the UK, the total cost is 4% of the total healthcare cost for PI management.

PATHOPHYSIOLOGY

A PI is the combined result of including intrinsic and extrinsic factors and leads to ischemia and necrosis. The external pressure must exceed the arterial capillary pressure of 32 mm Hg and venous capillary closing pressure of 8–12 mm Hg to impede blood flow and impair venous blood return. The external pressure above these values leads to tissue ischemia and necrosis **(Table 1)**.

Extrinsic Factors

- *Pressure*: It is a perpendicular force that is exerted on the specific skin area. The mechanisms causing PI due to pressure include the following:
  - *Ischemia caused by capillary occlusion*: Capillary occlusion due to applied pressure leads to ischemia and further interruption of cellular metabolism leading to accumulation of waste products. These cause increased capillary permeability, edema, and infiltration.

TABLE 1: Intrinsic and extrinsic factors of pressure injury.

Extrinsic factors	Intrinsic factors
• Pressure • Shear • Friction • Moisture	• Age • Malnutrition • Urinary incontinence • Neurological disease (stroke, degenerative neurologic disease, and spinal cord injury) • Peripheral vascular disease • Impaired sensation (diabetic neuropathy and medication-induced sedation)

- *Reperfusion injury*: During reperfusion, sudden entry of oxygen into previous ischemic tissue liberates free oxygen radicals including superoxide anions, hydroxyl radicals, and hydrogen peroxide leading to further endothelial damage.
- *Lymphatic flow obstruction*: Pressure over time occludes lymphatic circulation causing interruption of nutrition and accumulation of cellular waste products.
- *Deformation of tissue*: The constant high-magnitude pressure leads to the destruction of the cell membrane of the muscle. The pressure gradient at the vascular network increases when soft tissue available for pressure decreases causing pressure ulcers more on bony prominence. The characteristics of the involved tissue (type, size, and shape of involved tissue), mechanical properties stiffness, and tissue strength determine the degree of the deformation. Skin (epidermis and dermis) can withstand ischemic injury more prolonged than muscles, that's why PI starts first in muscles and subcutaneous tissue and visible skin changes occur later.

- *Shear*: Shear stress in comparison to pressure is a parallel force applied to the area of the body. It is the force against a surface as it is moved in the opposite but parallel direction that causes the deformation of tissue. Deeper structures such as muscles and subcutaneous tissue are more prone to shear than skin as the skin contains collagen and elastic fibers.
- *Friction*: In comparison to pressure and shear, friction mainly affects the superficial layer of skin rather than the deeper tissue. These are generally developed when the subject moves from one surface to another.
- *Moisture*: It can macerate the skin and make it more susceptible to breakdown by other forces.

Intrinsic Factors

- *Age*: Loss of fat and muscle and increased fragility of blood vessels and connective tissue lead to increased risk of PI.
- *Malnutrition*: Undernourished subjects have decreased adipose tissue at bony prominences which causes delayed wound healing. Obesity is also associated with an increased risk of PI as there is a chance of tissue-on-tissue injury, as soft tissue is difficult to offload.
- Urinary incontinence causes an increased risk of PI by creating moisture and skin maceration.
- Neurological diseases such as stroke and others leading to insensibility cause skin thinning and increased susceptibility to friction and shear forces.
- Peripheral vascular disease is responsible for negative wound healing by impaired perfusion to injured tissue.
- Impaired sensation leads to decreased protective phenomena like moving the body part to restore the blood flow when there is a pressure effect.
- Atrial fibrillation, myocardial infarction, and chronic obstructive disease all lead to decreased oxygen tension and increased PI.
- The coexistence of geriatric syndromes in older adults such as frailty, sarcopenia, urinary incontinence, cognitive impairment, and depression all contribute to PI formation via lack of self-care and increased sensitivity to pressure change as muscle mass decreases.

HISTORY AND EXAMINATION

For PI evaluation, a detailed history and physical examination are needed. People with normal sensation, mental status, and mobility develop discomfort and pain on continued pressure so they change their position to relieve pressure. Persons with any impairment in those have an increased risk of PI. A patient's relative reports PI mostly.

History regarding PI should include the following points:

- Duration of bedridden/immobility/restricted mobility
- Any history of hospitalization, and use of any medical device
- Site of PI (examine sacrum, greater trochanter, ischial tuberosity, lateral malleolus, and the heel of the foot)
- Total duration of PI
- Any change in size
- Associated symptoms such as pain (type, severity, frequency, and aggravating or alleviating factors)
- Any discharge and odor
- Any precipitating cause of immobility/bedridden such as stroke, fall, fractures, any road traffic accidents, encephalopathy, postsurgery, exacerbations of any other medical cause causing acute exacerbations of chronic obstructive pulmonary disease (AECOPD), and decompensated heart failure
- History regarding any comorbidities such as diabetes mellitus, neuropathy, peripheral vascular disease, any other immunocompromised condition, malignancy, and impaired nutritional status

Examination

- Total number of pressure ulcers
- Location of each PI
- Length (head-to-toe), width (side-to side), depth, and sinus tract, tunnels, undermining
- Wound characteristics such as appearance, any discharge or necrotic tissue, odor, and periwound skin condition

- Signs of infection—erythema, induration, warmth, tenderness or pain with palpation, and drainage (also noting amount, type, odor, and color)
- Staging of pressure ulcer
- Need to examine other systemic examination including cardiovascular, neurological, any sensory impairment, and motor weakness

Laboratory Studies

These studies include the following investigations:

- Complete blood counts with differentials
- Comprehensive metabolic panel
- Albumin and pre-albumin (for nutritional status)
- Glycated hemoglobin (HbA1c)
- Swab culture is needed in case of infected wound.

PRESSURE INJURY RISK ASSESSMENT

Pressure ulcer risk screening (PURS) should be done for all patients admitted to the healthcare facility to prevent pressure ulcers. The three most commonly used risk assessment tools are the (1) Norton Scale, (2) Waterlow Score, and (3) Braden Scale for predicting pressure ulcer risk.

Braden Scale: It is the most commonly used and accepted scale. It contains five sections with one to four points except one with one to three points.

1. *Sensory perception*: It is ability to respond to pressure-related discomfort or pain.
   a. *Completely limited*:
      i. Unresponsive to painful stimuli due to diminished level of consciousness or sedation (does not moan) or
      ii. Limited ability to feel pain all over the body
   b. *Very limited*:
      i. Responds only to painful stimuli, and
      ii. Unable to communicate discomfort except by moaning or
      iii. Due to sensory impairment, limited ability to feel pain, or discomfort over half of the body
   c. *Slightly limited*:
      i. Responds to verbal commands but not able to communicate discomfort always or
      ii. Has some sensory impairment which limits the ability to feel pain in 1 or 2 extremities
   d. *No impairment*: Responds to verbal commands or has no sensory deficit.
2. *Moisture*: It is the degree to which skin is exposed to moisture (perspiration and urine).
   a. Constantly moist—skin is almost moist.
   b. Often moist—skin is often moist, and linen needs to change once a shift.
   c. Occasionally moist—linen needs to change approximately once a day.
   d. Rarely moist—skin is usually dry and linen needs to change at routine intervals.
3. *Activity*: Degree of physical activity:
   a. Bedfast-confined to the bed
   b. Severely impaired mobility, wheelchair dependent
   c. Walks occasionally
   d. Walks frequently
4. *Mobility*: Ability to change and control body position:
   a. Completely immobile—does not make changes without any assistance
   b. Very limited—slight changes occasional
   c. Slightly limited—make frequently but slight changes
   d. No limitations—major and frequent changes
5. *Nutrition*: Usual food intake:
   a. Very poor—never eats a complete meal or NPO and is on IV fluids for >5 days
   b. Probably inadequate—rarely eats a complete meal or receives less than optimum amount of liquid diet or tube feeding
   c. Adequate—eats over half of most meals or taking adequate food via tube or total parenteral nutrition (TPN)
   d. Excellent—eats most of every meal
6. *Friction and shear*:
   a. Problem—requires maximum assistance in moving the object
   b. Potential problem—requires minimum assistance
   c. No apparent problem—moves independently

Scores:
Mild risk = 15–18
Moderate risk = 13–14
High risk = 10–12
Very high risk = 9 or below

A simple screening question for PI is "Does the patient move his body? His leg?". If the answer is no or not without any help, it also predicts an increased risk of PI development.

PREVENTION

Prevention methods are used for persons at risk of PI and those with PIs for further worsening or prevention of new PI. The most common methods used for prevention include repositioning programs, skin care, nutritional support, and the use of support surfaces to reduce the pressure.

- *Repositioning and early mobilization programs*:
  - The mainstay of preventive therapy is to preserve microcirculation by reducing the pressure.

- Repositioning or turning should be done every 2–3 hours according to patient profile and support surfaces should be used for the bedridden patients; there is no clear guideline for a repositioning time interval.
- Repositioning way should redistribute the pressure and also offload the bony prominences.
- Use of 30° or lower side-lying positions is preferred for positioning and the head of the bed should be as flat as possible.
- Turning sheets, draw sheets, and pillows can be used for repositioning in the bed.
- Early mobilization should be initiated as early as the patient can tolerate to improve mobility.
- Trapeze bars can be used for repositioning by themselves.
- Heel offloading devices and water-filled gloves can be used to prevent PI at heels.
- Patients with PI should not be positioned over the PI such as the sacrum should be free from pressure if there is PI and lateral positions are preferred.

- *Support surfaces*:
  - These support surfaces redistribute the pressure more evenly and prevent PI, including specially designed beds, mattresses, mattress overlays, and cushions.
  - These bed surface areas should be sufficiently wide to allow individuals to turn.
  - Reactive support surfaces are powered and nonpowered (foam mattresses) can redistribute the pressure applied on the bony prominences, and are used at the risk of patients.
    - Powered support surfaces inflate and deflate the air cells.
  - Support surfaces should be used intraoperatively for high-risk patients [surgery duration > 3 hours, prone positioning during surgery, American Society of Anesthesiologists (ASA) scores of 3 or higher].
- *Nutrition*:
  - Nutritional screening should be done for at-risk PI individuals, a full mini-nutritional assessment version can be used as a screening tool.
  - Comprehensive nutrition assessment should be done for those who are at risk of PI and at risk of malnutrition.
  - For individuals with PI and malnourished or at risk of malnutrition, energy, and protein intake should be 30–35 kcal/kg body weight/day and 1.25–1.5 g/kg body weight/day, respectively.
  - If nutritional requirements cannot be fulfilled by normal dietary intake, high calorie, high protein nutritional supplements for PI and malnourishment or at risk of malnourishment.
  - Along with high protein, high calorie, arginine, zinc, and antioxidant or enteral formulas for stage II or more than II with malnourishment or at risk.
  - Enteral and parenteral feeding is an option if oral feeding is inadequate.
  - Adequate water and fluid intake should be provided.
- *Skin care*:
  - Skin care should be a routine for preventing PI, including attention to all bony prominences, incontinent areas, any change in skin color, excessive dryness, and cracking.
  - Excessive dry skin should be moisturized and incontinent areas should be cleaned as early as possible.
  - Excessive redden area should not be massaged, as it will impair further perfusion.

Pressure Ulcer Staging

The National Pressure Ulcer Advisory Panel's revised guidelines for PI staging are as follows:

- *Nonblanchable erythema of intact skin*:
  - It is intact skin with a localized area of nonblanchable erythema (nonblanchable erythema is the lack of a blanche response when light pressure is applied or, persistent redness in lightly pigmented skin).
  - The presence of blanchable erythema or changes in sensation, temperature, or firmness is preceding to PI.
  - Color changes of purple or maroon indicate deep tissue PI, not stage 1 PI.
  - Stage 1 PI in darkly pigmented skin: As nonblanchable erythema is difficult to appreciate in darkly pigmented skin, examine the skin changes indicating PI:
    - Discoloration compared to surrounding skin
    - Pain in the area
    - Induration
- *Partial-thickness skin loss with exposed dermis*:
  - The wound bed is viable, pink, red, moist, shiny, painful, and having serous discharge.
  - Serum-filled blister intact or ruptured is also a stage 2 PI.
  - The deeper tissues such as adipose tissue, granulation tissue, slough, and eschar are absent in stage 2 PI.
- *Full-thickness skin loss pressure injury*:
  - Adipose tissue (fat), granulation tissue, and epibole (rolled wound edges) are present

  - Slough and eschar may be visible but if slough or eschar obscures the extent of tissue loss then it will be unstageable PI
  - Heals by granulation tissue, contracture, and epithelization over the scar
- *Full-thickness loss of skin and tissue*:
  - Exposed or directly palpable fascia, muscle, tendon, ligament, cartilage, or bone in the ulcer.
  - Slough and eschar may be visible but if slough or eschar obscures the extent of tissue loss then it will be unstageable PI.
  - Epibole (rolled edges), undermining, or tunneling may occur.
- *Unstageable*:
  - Extent of the tissue damage within the ulcer cannot be determined because of the presence of slough or eschar, removal of eschar may reveal the stage of PI.
  - Stable eschar (i.e., dry, adherent, and intact eschar—without erythema or fluctuance) on an ischemic area must not be removed.
- *Deep tissue pressure injury (DTPI)*:
  - DTPI is localized area of nonblanchable deep red, maroon, or purple discoloration.
  - Skin could be intact or nonintact, epidermal separation results in a dark wound bed or blood-filled blister.
  - DTPI term should not be used in vascular, traumatic, neuropathic, or dermatologic conditions.

We should stage the PI according to the deepest layer of tissue exposed such as adipose, muscle, and bone if more than one type of tissue is exposed **(Fig. 1)**.

DIAGNOSIS

The diagnosis of PI is made by history and examination of the skin. Some noninvasive methods include high-resolution ultrasound, thermography, and surface electrical capacitance to detect early pressure changes.

- The temperature of the skin surface and tissues below the skin surfaces can be detected by thermography and both increased and decreased temperatures compared to normal are associated with PI.
- Surface electrical capacitance devices measure the water content of subepidermal skin and tissue below the skin.
- Tissue edema is found to be a risk factor for PI.

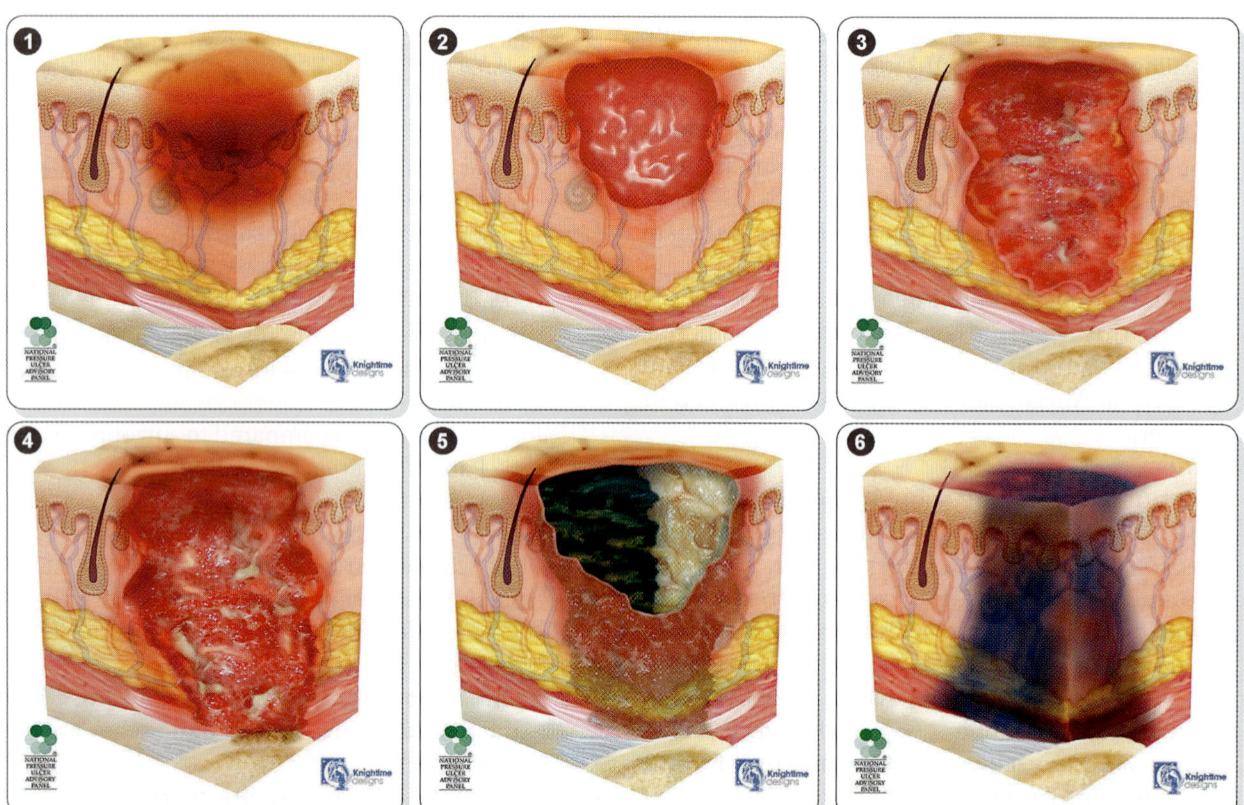

FIG. 1: National Pressure Ulcer Advisory Panel (2016) pressure ulcer staging.

PRESSURE INJURY ASSESSMENT

There are scales through which the healing of the PI is assessed, which is routinely evaluated weekly. Two evidence-based tools are used to evaluate the healing of PI, including NPIAP's Pressure Ulcer Scale for Healing tool (PUSH) and the Bates-Jensen Wound Assessment Tool (BWAT).

Pressure Ulcer Scale for Healing Tool 3.0

Directions

Observe and measure the pressure ulcer. Categorize the ulcer concerning surface area, exudate, and type of wound tissue. Record a subscore for each of these ulcer characteristics. Add the subscores to obtain the total score. A comparison of total scores measured over time indicates the improvement or deterioration in pressure ulcer healing.

Length × width: Measure the greatest length (head-to-toe) and width (side-to-side) using a centimeter ruler. Multiply these measurements (length × width) to obtain a surface area (cm^2). Always use a centimeter ruler and the same method each time the ulcer is measured.

Exudate amount: Estimate the amount of exudate (drainage) present before applying any topical agent to the ulcer. Estimate the exudate (drainage) as none, light, moderate, or heavy.

Tissue type: Types of tissue in the wound bed. Score as a "4" if there is any necrotic tissue present. Score as a "3" if any amount of slough is present and necrotic tissue is absent. Score as a "2" if the wound is clean and contains granulation tissue. A superficial wound that is re-epithelializing is scored as a "1". When the wound is closed, score as a "0".

- *4—necrotic tissue (eschar)*: Black, brown, or tan tissue that adheres firmly to the wound bed or ulcer edges and may be firmer or softer than the surrounding skin.
- *3—slough*: Yellow or white tissue that adheres to the ulcer bed in strings or thick clumps, or is mucinous.
- *2—granulation tissue*: Pink or beefy red tissue with a shiny, moist, and granular appearance.
- *1—epithelial tissue*: For superficial ulcers, new pink or shiny tissue (skin) that grows in from the edges or as islands on the ulcer surface.
- *0—closed/resurfaced*: The wound is completely covered with epithelium (new skin).
  National Pressure Injury Advisory Panel PUSH tool.

The BWAT: This tool contains 13 wound characteristics, each score ranging from 1 (best) to 5 (worst), and total scores ranging from 13 to 65.

MANAGEMENT

General Measures

Pressure injuries are the combined result of multiple factors and the main aim is to reverse the causative factor of the PI. The main component is the continuous off-loading of the pressure at the PI site by repositioning and early mobilization, for healing of the PI.

- The associated comorbidities should be treated and adequate nutrition by increasing protein and calorie intake should be ensured.
- Pressure injury pain is the most distressing symptom and must be treated adequately.
- Appropriate pain such as VAS (visual analog scale) and MPQ (McGill Pain Questionnaire) scales should be used for people with nonverbal and cognitive impairments **(Flowchart 1)**.

Dressing

Wound dressings are used to heal PIs and prevent PI. There are two types of dressings: (1) Traditional dressings, also known as inert dressing, and (2) modern dressings. Traditional dressings (gauze, cotton pads, and bandages) are not able to maintain wound bed moisture and also adhere to the granulation tissue of PI; that is why these are rarely used nowadays. Modern dressing provides a moist environment for the wound and helps to re-epithelialize the wound. Modern dressings commonly used in clinical practice include hydrogels, hydrocolloids, alginates, foams, and films **(Table 2)**.

Infected Wound

Suspicion of infection should be considered if there is delayed healing, increased size, exudate, surrounding warmth, and increased pain. Biofilm formation is considered if failure to heal despite antimicrobial therapy, increased exudate and size, and signs of infection. If patients develop confusion/delirium and anorexia, malaise, discoloration of surrounding skin spreading of the infection is suspected. The most common organisms include *Staphylococcus aureus, Proteus mirabilis, Pseudomonas aeruginosa, Enterococcus faecalis, and* Methicillin-resistant *S. aureus.* A tissue biopsy or wound bed swab should be performed to diagnose infection.

Osteomyelitis is considered if there is visible bone and soft bone on palpation. MRI is the investigation of choice for osteomyelitis diagnosis and bone biopsy should be considered. Antibiotics and the debridement of infected bone are the treatment options. Amputation is considered in large infected wounds with no perfusion supply.

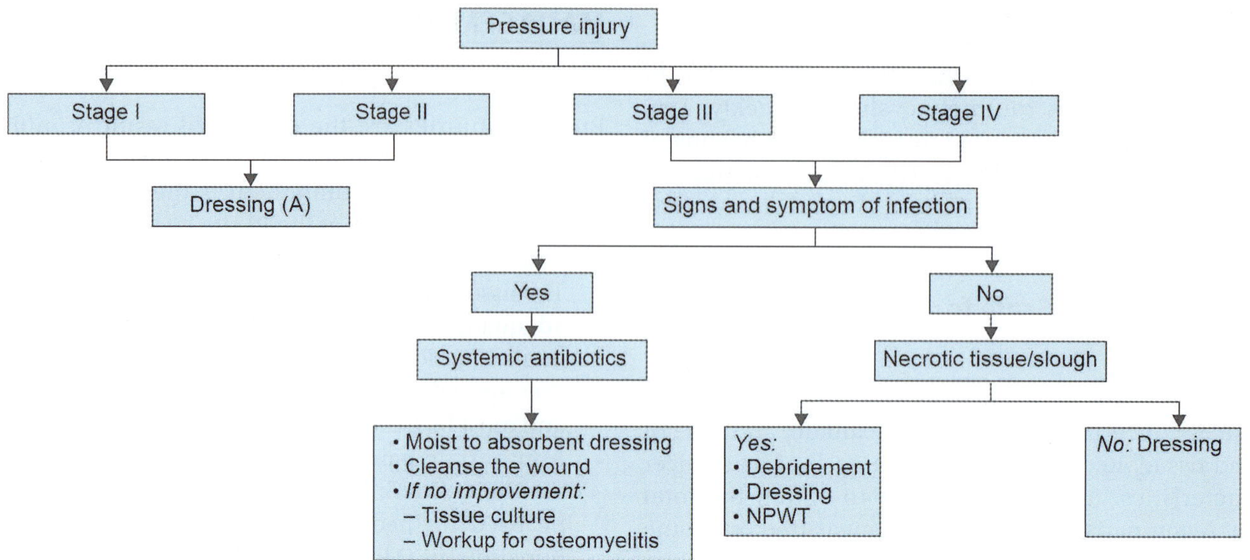

FLOWCHART 1: Wound management.
(NPWT: negative pressure wound therapy)

TABLE 2: Characteristics of modern dressings used in practice.

Dressing type	Definition	Characteristics	Uses
Hydrogel	Water—propylene glycol- or glycerin-based amorphous gels, impregnated gauze, or sheet dressings	• Reduces pain, soothing effects • Autolytic debridement • Absorbs low-moderate drainage • Not useful for infected wounds and with heavy drainage	• Management of stages II, III, IV PI, and deep wounds • It may need a secondary dressing
Hydrocolloid	Made of gelatin. Pectin, carboxymethylcellulose in the forms of wafers, paste, and powders	• Absorbs low-to-moderate wound fluid, autolysis, thermal insulation, reduces pain, bacterial barrier, and translucent to opaque • Not used for wounds with heavy exudate, sinus tracts, and infected—may injure fragile skin on removal	• As primary or secondary dressing for stages II to IV PI • Wound with slough and necrosis
Alginate	Derived from brown seaweed (calcium-sodium salts of alginic acid) in the forms of ropes, pads, and wafers	• Absorbs up to 20 times its weight, autolytic debridement, fills cavities, and pockets, and reduces pain • Not useful for dry wounds or light exudate • Need a secondary dressing	• As primary dressing for stages III and IV PI • Wounds with moderate-to-heavy exudate • Infected or noninfected wounds
Foam	Hydrophilic and nonadherent, modified polyurethane foam, in the form of wafers, pillows, and sheets	• Absorptive (moderate-to-large), autolysis • Nontraumatic removal • Thermal insulation • Antimicrobial activity • Semipermeability	• As primary (for absorption) and secondary (wounds with packing) dressings for II to IV PIs • Infected wound
Film	Polyurethane membrane allows water to vaporize and cross the barrier	• Retains moisture • Impermeable to liquid and bacteria • Autolytic debridement • May reinjure area on removal	Stage I and II PI with light or no exudates

Antibiotics are administered locally or systemically. Sepsis or cellulitis, fever, increased white blood cell counts, and osteomyelitis need systemic antibiotics. Broad-spectrum antibiotics are preferred as they increase the mortality rate due to PI-induced sepsis. Local antibiotics cadexomer iodine, silver, or PHMB are chosen to decrease the wound bed's bioburden.

Wound Cleansing and Debridement

Wound Cleansing

The main purpose of cleansing the wound is to remove the debris, microorganisms, and remnants of the previous dressings to improve healing.

- Normal saline can be used if germicidal action is not required and rinse the wound after using other cleansing solutions.
- Povidone-iodine, acetic acid (0.5%), and sodium hypochlorite (2.5%) can be used as antibacterial cleansing solutions.
- Once granulation tissue is visible, the cleansing solution should be discontinued.

Debridement

It is a process of removing all material from the wound bed that delays healing and granulation and promotes infection. This includes removing the necrotic tissue, eschar, slough, and biofilm till the granulation tissue is visible on the wound bed.

Methods of Debridement

- *Sharp debridement*: It is a surgical procedure so scalpels, curettes, scissors, and forceps are required. Vascular supply should be assessed and it should be intact.
    - Indication:
        - Need to debride extensive necrotic tissue on an urgent basis
        - The extension of the sinus tract and tunneling are not determined
        - Advance cellulitis or patient is septic due to PI
    - Contraindications: Anticoagulant therapy and bleeding disorders
- *Autolytic debridement*: Body's own phagocytic cells and proteolytic enzymes debride the necrotic tissue. Occlusive wound dressings are needed to maintain moisture, pH, and humidity.
    - Contraindicated: Untreated infection, extensive necrotic tissue, PI with sinus tract, and immunocompromised patients
- *Enzymatic debridement*: It is done by using the exogenously available proteolytic or fibrinolytic enzymes to the wound bed.
- *Biological debridement*: This debridement uses sterile fly larvae that produce the proteolytic enzymes including collagenase, allantoin, and broad-spectrum antibacterial agents to the wound bed.
    - *Contraindications*: Limb or life-threatening infection, necrotic bone and tendon tissue, exposed blood vessels, and impaired vascular supply
- *Mechanical debridement*: This debridement can remove vital and devitalized tissue. It includes wet-to-dry dressings, monofilament/microfiber debridement pads, and hydrosurgery.
    - *Wet-to-dry dressings*: Painful, remove healthy tissue too, and the need for frequent dreeing change.
    - *Monofilament/microfiber debridement*: These pads remove slough along with biofilm.
    - *Hydrosurgery*: A hydrosurgical water knife is an alternative to surgical debridement.

Negative Pressure Wound Therapy or Vacuum-assisted Closure Therapy

Vacuum-assisted closure (VAC) therapy helps to speed up wound healing in chronic wounds based on the basis that vacuum leads to wound bed cells to sense the mechanical force and this force leads to fibroblast proliferation and improves healing. This vacuum also eliminates the exudates continuously, which is useful in PI with heavy exudates. Negative pressure wound therapy (NPWT) contains a foam dressing, transparent film, and a suction device. Before applying this NPWT, the wound should be debrided, and after that, the wound is filled with a foam dressing and covered with transparent film to create a vacuum. The foam is attached to the suction device via a tubing.

Surgical Options

Surgery is needed when PI fails to heal and needs to fill the wound for further healing. For a nonhealing deep PI after all the above methods, a surgery consultation must be taken for further need of surgical reconstructions.

These methods include:

- *Direct closure*: The edges of the wound are brought together and closed after cleaning the wounds.
- *Split thickness skin grafting*: If the ulcer is superficial without exposing bone, tendon, vessels, nerve, and any heavy exudate. Skin grafting is the best method for this type of PI.
- *Local and regional flaps*: These include local transposition and rotation for local flaps. Gluteus maximus myocutaneous flap and V-Y advancement flap are the regional flap options for sacral PI.
- *Microvascular free flaps*: When local or regional flaps have failed or are not available for PI, the free flap is the best option.

Complications after surgery include infection, necrosis of the flap, bleeding, abscesses, septicemia, and osteomyelitis, but even having risks and complications surgical reconstruction is the only option to prevent the limb or life-threatening condition.

OTHER THERAPIES

- *Biophysical treatments*: Direct electric stimulation, pulsed electromagnetic field, and pulsed radio frequency energy.
- *Phototherapy treatments*: Using laser, infrared, and ultraviolet waves.
- *Hyperbaric oxygen therapy*: It increases oxygen transport to the wound area, improves angiogenesis, and lymphatic circulation, reduces inflammation and swelling, and thus helps in healing.
- *Skin substitutes*: Skin-graft substitutes include cultured dermal substitutes (CDS), cultured epidermal substitutes, and cultured skin substitutes. These improve angiogenesis and fibroplasia in wound beds.
- Cytokines and growth factors include basic fibroblast growth factor (bFGF) and granulocyte-macrophage colony-stimulating factor (GM-CSF).
- *Bone marrow/adipogenic stem cells*: Cell therapy uses live cells for therapeutic purposes. Marrow stem cells and bone marrow mononuclear cells are used for this purpose. These stem cells secret the paracrine factors that help in healing by recruiting macrophages and endothelial cells.

CONCLUSION

Pressure injury leads to increased morbidity and mortality in older adults and increased financial costs and caregiver burden. To prevent these complications, prevention is the main core element, especially in high-risk individuals. Once PI has developed, aggressive management of causative factors, associated comorbidities, and wounds are needed. Management of PI is a multidisciplinary approach including primary care physicians, nursing staff, wound care specialists, surgeons, dieticians, and physical therapists.

Self-Assessment Questionnaire

Q1. What is the pressure injury?
Q2. What are the main causes of pressure injury?
Q3. What are the methods of pressure injury prevention?
Q4. What are the stages of pressure injury?
Q5. How will we treat the different stages of pressure injury?
Q6. What different types of dressings are available for the prevention and management of pressure injury?
Q7. What are surgical reconstruction options?
Q8. What are newer therapies for the management of pressure injury?
Q9. How to treat infected pressure injury?
Q10. What are different debridement methods?

CHAPTER 19

Delirium

Yamini Ajmera

CASE VIGNETTE

Patient information: Mrs Malti Devi, a 75-year-old female, homemaker by occupation, with a history of hypertension, type 2 diabetes mellitus, lives with her husband, children, and grandchildren in a joint family setup.

Presenting complaint: Patient visits the emergency department in a confused state with reduced speech and slowness of movements. While talking to the attending doctor, the patient seemed disoriented to time and place and mistook the doctor as her distant relative.

History of present illness: Mrs Malti Devi was doing well 3 days ago, carrying out her daily routine activities at home by herself, when she developed an episode of fever in the evening, temperature around 100°F, not associated with chills. On further exploration, attendants reported an increase in urinary frequency for the past 3 days. Her condition gradually deteriorated, and she was in an acute confusional state for the past 1 day with slowness of movements and talking only when prompted.

Medical history: The patient has a history of hypertension and type 2 diabetes mellitus which are managed well on oral medications. There has not been any change in medication or dosages for the past 2 years. Her last comprehensive physical examination was conducted 1 year ago.

Social history: The patient lives with her husband, her two sons (one of whom is married), daughter-in-law, and her two grandchildren in a joint family setup.

She plays an active role in household activities and uses to perform her routine activities of daily living by herself, including helping to care for her grandchildren.

Personal history: She is a vegetarian by diet and does not have a history of alcohol or tobacco use.

Geriatric history: There is no history of forgetfulness, low mood, decreased mobility, urinary or fecal incontinence, and pressure sores.

Physical examination: During the physical examination, she is afebrile, her blood pressure is 142/88 mm Hg, and her heart rate is 78 beats per minute. She is conscious but disoriented to time, place, and person. Her neurological examination does not show any signs of focal neurological deficits.

INTRODUCTION

By virtue of socioeconomic development, the world is seeing a rapid transition in demographics, with the proportion of older people rising precipitously. In India, people aged ≥60 years are projected to rise from 8.6% in 2011 to 19% by the year 2050. Despite delirium being the most common complication affecting hospitalized older adults, with risk increasing exponentially with age, it largely remains underrecognized, poorly understood, and inadequately managed.

This chapter will focus on the nitty-gritties of delirium in the elderly and will equip future geriatricians in identifying delirium and its risk factors, devise strategies for its prevention and management, and help clinicians prognosticate about potential complications and outcomes.

DEFINITION AND CLINICAL FEATURES

The concept of delirium dates back to fifth century BC when Hippocrates first described it in acutely confused patients using terms "phrenitis" (frenzy) and "paraphrenitis" referring to acute behavioral disturbances that manifest during the state of bodily inflammation and "lethargus" to describe inertia and clouding of the senses.

The term "delirium" was coined by Aulus Cornelius Celsus in the first century AD to describe (either as a symptom or as a syndrome) mental disorders during fever or head trauma.

Delirium is currently conceptualized as a complex, reversible neuropsychiatric disorder with an acute onset and fluctuating course. It is typically characterized by disturbances in attention and cognitive domains (memory, orientation, language, visuospatial ability, or perception) with or without alteration in noncognitive domains such as sleep–wake cycle and thought process.

Core features of delirium are its limited course and external causation. However, it may persist for weeks or months if not detected or treated adequately. According to the nature of changes in psychomotor behavior, it can be divided into three subtypes:

1. Hypoactive characterized by unawareness, decreased alertness, reduced or delayed speech, lethargy, and slowed movements
2. Hyperactive where patients manifest restlessness, hypervigilance, fast or loud speech, irritability, and combativeness and are more likely to have hallucinations.
3. *Mixed*: Where symptoms fluctuate between hypoactive and hyperactive subtypes

More recently, two other "variants" have been described, i.e., the "catatonic variant" which represents an extreme form of hypoactive delirium and the "excited variant" which represents an extreme form of hyperactive delirium (mostly associated with sympathomimetic drug abuse (e.g., psychostimulants, designer drugs such as the synthetic cathinone and 3,4-methylenedioxy methamphetamine).

Subsyndromal delirium is a clinical entity representing an incomplete presentation of the syndrome characterized by the presence of one or more symptoms of delirium that fail to meet the threshold for diagnosis of delirium.

EPIDEMIOLOGY

Delirium is the most common complication affecting hospitalized patients aged 65 years and above, with risk increasing from 3% in those <65 years to 14% in those aged 65–74 years and to 36% in those ≥75 years.

In older adults, the estimated prevalence and incidence rate range from 11 to 42% and 6 to 56%, respectively, in medical wards and 32.3 to 77% and 45 to 87%, respectively, in intensive care unit (ICU) settings.

PATHOPHYSIOLOGY

Delirium may result from a wide variety of both physiological and structural insults; however, the overall mechanism is still not fully understood. Recent evidence suggests that several interacting and complementary hypotheses act together, leading to widespread disruption of neuronal networks in brain and biochemical derangement which subsequently results in complex cognitive and behavioral changes leading to delirium.

The main hypothesis involves reversible impairment of cerebral oxidative metabolism and multiple neurotransmitter abnormalities (excess of dopamine, depletion of acetylcholine). Contributing biologic factors include aging process which is associated with diminished physiological reserves causing increased vulnerability to physical stress and illnesses, neuroinflammatory processes [insults such as severe infection, trauma, and surgery lead to production of peripheral cytokines which in turn propagates into central nervous system (CNS) ultimately stimulating the release of cytokines in the brain by microglial cells], circadian rhythm dysregulation (melatonin deficiency), and aberrant stress response (pathologically sustained high levels of cortisol occur with acute stress may cause hippocampal malfunction and in turn precipitate delirium).

RISK FACTORS

In older persons, delirium has a multifactorial etiology involving a complex interrelationship between various predisposing factors and precipitating factors **(Table 1)**.

TABLE 1: Various predisposing and precipitating factors.

Predisposing factors	Precipitating factors
• Advanced age (≥75 years) • Male gender • Illiteracy • Unemployment • Neurocognitive disorders • Functional impairment • Visual impairment • Hearing impairment • Social isolation • Comorbidity burden • Polypharmacy • Depression • Malnutrition • Anemia • Frailty	• Infection • CNS insults: Stroke, meningitis • Cardiac insults: Acute coronary syndrome, heart failure • ICU admission • Prolonged hospitalization • Emergency or trauma admission • Drugs: psychoactive (sedatives or hypnotics), withdrawal states • Use of physical restraints • Use of a bladder catheter • Physiological: Electrolyte disturbances, uremia, hypoalbuminemia, hypoxia • Surgical interventions • Pain • Sleep abnormalities • Fecal or urinary retention

(CNS: central nervous system; ICU: intensive care unit)

Various biomarkers are also currently being evaluated as possible markers for delirium, including cytokines, growth factors, neurotrophic factors, and hormones. These include proinflammatory mediators such as C-reactive protein (CRP), tumor necrosis factor-alpha (TNF-α), interleukin-1β (IL-1β), interleukin-6 (IL-6), interleukin-8 (IL-8), interleukin-10 (IL-10), neopterin, S100 calcium-binding protein β (S100β), adiponectin, and neutrophil–lymphocyte ratio (NLR) which have shown a positive association with delirium in multiple studies. Delirium is also found to be negatively associated with neuroprotective factors such as insulin-like growth factor-1 (IGF-1), plasma protein C, and leptin. The presence of one copy of the apolipoprotein E (ApoE) ε4 allele has also been implicated in the development of ICU delirium in some studies.

DIAGNOSIS

The specific criteria for delirium that are currently accepted as the diagnostic standard are the Diagnostic and Statistical Manual of Mental Disorders, Fifth Edition (DSM-5) and the International Classification of Diseases, 11th Revision (ICD-11) **(Table 2)**.

To identify delirium in clinical settings, several assessment tools have been developed. The most widely used among them is the Confusion Assessment Method (CAM) which has been extensively validated and has a sensitivity of 94% and specificity of 89% with high interrater reliability. CAM variations have also been developed such as CAM-ICU and the 3-minute diagnostic interview for CAM (3DCAM) to use in ICU and general medicine settings, respectively **(Box 1)**.

TABLE 2: Criteria for delirium as per DSM-5 and ICD-11.

DSM-5	ICD-11
• Disturbance in attention and awareness • Disturbance developing over a short period of time (usually hours to few days) and often fluctuates in severity (during the course of a day) • Additional disturbance is found in cognition (e.g., memory deficit, disorientation, language, visuospatial ability, or perception) • The disturbances in A and C are not better explained by another neurocognitive disorder (preexisting, established, or evolving) and do not occur in the context of a severely reduced level of arousal, such as coma • There is evidence from the history, physical examination, or laboratory findings that the disturbance is a direct physiological consequence of another medical condition, including substance or toxin intoxication or withdrawal	• Disturbance in attention and awareness that develops over a short period of time and often fluctuates during the course of a day • It is often accompanied by impairment in cognitive domains • It may also be associated with the disturbance of the sleep–wake cycle, including reduced arousal or reversal • The symptoms are attributable to a disorder or disease not classified under mental and behavioral disorders, or to substance intoxication or withdrawal, or to a medication

(DSM-5: Diagnostic and Statistical Manual of Mental Disorders, Fifth Edition; ICD-11: International Classification of Diseases, 11th Revision)

BOX 1 Confusion Assessment Method (CAM) diagnostic algorithm.

Feature 1: Acute onset or fluctuating course: This feature is usually obtained from a family member or nurse and is shown by positive responses to the following questions: Is there evidence of an acute change in mental status from the patient's baseline? Did the (abnormal) behavior fluctuate during the day, that is, tend to come and go, or increase and decrease in severity?

Feature 2: Inattention: This feature is shown by a positive response to the following question: Did the patient have difficulty focusing attention, for example, being easily distractible, or having difficulty keeping track of what was being said?

Feature 3: Disorganized thinking: This feature is shown by a positive response to the following question: Was the patient's thinking disorganized or incoherent, such as rambling or irrelevant conversation, unclear or illogical flow of ideas, or unpredictable switching from subject to subject?

Feature 4: Altered level of consciousness: This feature is shown by any answer other than alert to the following question: Overall, how would you rate this patient's level of consciousness? [alert (normal), vigilant (hyperalert), lethargic (drowsy, easily aroused), stupor (difficult to arouse), or coma (unarousable)]

Note: The diagnosis of delirium by CAM requires the presence of features 1 and 2 and either 3 or 4.

Source:
- Copyright 2003 Sharon K Inouye.
- Inouye SK, van Dyck CH, Alessi CA, Balkin S, Siegal AP, Horwitz RI. Clarifying confusion: the confusion assessment method. A new method for detection of delirium. Ann Intern Med. 1990;113(12):941-8.

Another brief test is *4A's* test (4AT), validated in clinical settings involving dementia patients, and is easy to administer, with a sensitivity of 90% and specificity of 84%.

Behavioral checklists for symptoms of delirium, particularly for quick assessment by nursing staff:
- Delirium Observation Screening Scale
- Nursing Delirium Screening Checklist
- Neelon and Champagne (NEECHAM) Confusion Scale

Delirium severity measurement tools:
- Delirium Rating Scale-Revised-98 (DRS-R-98)
- Memorial Delirium Assessment Scale (MDAS)
- CAM-Severity (CAM-S) scale

Cognitive evaluation for delirium:
- Short Portable Mental Status Questionnaire
- Mini-Cog or Montreal Cognitive Assessment

Approach to Diagnosis

Approach to diagnosis of delirium is given in **Table 3**.

PREVENTION AND TREATMENT STRATEGIES

The treatment strategy for delirium should be tailored to the patient's medical condition, risk factors, and environmental insults. The multicomponent nonpharmacological interventions remain the mainstay in both the prevention and treatment of delirium. The most widely disseminated approach is the Hospital Elder Life Program, involving healthcare professionals, families, caregivers, and patients, and it has shown to reduce the incidence of delirium by 40% in multiple studies.

Effective approaches include the following:
- Reorientation (e.g., using orientation boards, calendars, and clocks), encouraging regular visits from family members and friends

TABLE 3: Approach to diagnosis of delirium.

Assessment	Actions
History	• Check baseline cognitive function and recent (within the past 2 weeks) changes in mental status (e.g., family, staff) or any new diagnosis • Do a complete review of systems • Review all current drugs (including over-the-counter and herbal preparations); pay special attention to new drugs and drug interactions • Review alcohol and sedative use • Assess for pain and discomfort (e.g., urinary retention, constipation, and thirst)
Vital signs	• Measure temperature, O_2 saturation, and fingerstick glucose concentration • Take postural vital signs as needed
Physical and neurological examination	• Search for signs of occult infection, dehydration, acute abdominal pain, deep vein thrombosis, and other acute illnesses • Assess for sensory impairments • Search for focal neurological changes and meningeal signs
Targeted laboratory assessment (selected tests based on clues from history and physical examination)	• Complete blood count • Toxicology screen, urinalysis • Measurement of concentrations of electrolytes and glucose • Measurement of renal, liver, and thyroid function • Cultures of urine, blood, and sputum • Measurement of drug concentrations in serum/urine • Measurement of concentrations of ammonia, vitamin B12, folate, and thiamine • Arterial blood gas • Infectious serologies: RPR, fungal, and viral markers • Electrocardiography • Chest radiography (tumor, infection) • Lumbar puncture (reserved for suspicion of meningitis/encephalitis)
Targeted neuroimaging (selected patients)—brain MRI or CT	Assess focal neurological changes (cerebrovascular accident, tumor, atrophy); suspected encephalitis or head trauma
Electroencephalography (selected patients)	Assess for occult seizures; differentiate psychiatric disorder from delirium
(RPR: rapid plasma reagin)	

- *Maintain adequate hydration and nutrition*: Ensure availability and proper fit of dentures. Seek dietician input early if needed
- *Sleep enhancement*: Avoid medical/nursing procedures and giving medication during sleep if possible
- Pain management
- Optimization of vision and hearing deficits through assistive devices
- Encourage therapeutic activities.
- Encourage early mobilization and regular ambulation. Keep walking aids (canes, walkers) readily available at all times.
- Minimize the use of physical restraints.
- Avoid unnecessary catheterization.
- Keep private rooms closer to the nurses' station for increased supervision.

Pharmacologic therapies should be reserved for severely agitated patients, psychotic individuals, or those who pose a substantial risk of harm to self or others. Treatment should begin with low doses. Currently, there are no antipsychotic medications that are approved by Food and Drug Administration for the prevention or treatment of delirium.

- Low-dose haloperidol (0.25–0.5 mg twice orally or intramuscularly) is most often used to correct behavioral changes.
- Second-generation antipsychotics (such as olanzapine, quetiapine, risperidone, ziprasidone) may also be considered based on expected side-effect profiles.
- Benzodiazepines should be refrained from use except in alcohol or benzodiazepine withdrawal-related delirium.
- *Emerging drug therapies:*
  - Dexmedetomidine, a sedative α2-agonist, which has shown some efficacy in ICU patients requiring sedation for agitated delirium
  - Melatonin and melatonin receptor agonists (ramelteon), which were regarded as the best preventive medicine for delirium in a recent meta-analysis

In a recent Cochrane review examining antipsychotics for treatment of delirium in hospitalized non-ICU patients, antipsychotics were not found to shorten the course of delirium, reduce the severity of delirium, resolve symptoms, lower the risk of dying, shorten the hospital length of stay, or improve health-related quality of life when compared to nonantipsychotic drugs or placebo.

High-risk medications that should be avoided in delirium include:

- *Anticholinergics*:
  - Antihistamines (chlorpheniramine, hydroxyzine)
  - Antiparkinsonian agents (benztropine, trihexyphenidyl)
  - Skeletal muscle relaxants (cyclobenzaprine)
  - Antipsychotics (olanzapine, clozapine)
  - Antimuscarinics (oxybutynin, solifenacin)
  - Antispasmodics (atropine, hyoscyamine)
  - Antiemetics (prochlorperazine, promethazine)
  - Antidepressants (particularly amitriptyline, desipramine, doxepin, nortriptyline, and paroxetine)
- Corticosteroids
- H2-receptor antagonists (cimetidine, famotidine, nizatidine, ranitidine)
- Meperidine
- Sedative hypnotics (benzodiazepines and barbiturates)

PROGNOSIS OF DELIRIUM

Delirium has been found to be associated with both short-term and long-term outcomes:

- *Short-term outcomes*:
  - Increased in-hospital mortality
  - Longer duration of hospital stay
- *Long-term outcomes*:
  - Postdischarge mortality
  - Reinfection
  - Admission to residential care
  - Postdischarge sleep disturbance
  - Cognitive decline
  - Functional dependency
  - Increased risk of falls

Delirium shares a complex relationship with frailty. Both are risk factors for each other and share many similarities. Both lead to deterioration in general condition, daily living skills, and cognitive function. Both entities have identical predisposing factors such as malnutrition, sarcopenia, systemic inflammation, neuroendocrine dysregulation, oxidative stress, or mobility limitations and are prototypical of multidimensional geriatric syndromes. The increased risk of experiencing delirium in older age and frailty was also demonstrated during the COVID-19 pandemic, as was the dramatic impact of delirium on mortality.

CONCLUSION

Delirium is a complex geriatric syndrome with high frequency of occurrence in geriatric patients, has a multifactorial etiology, and leads to poor health outcomes. Therefore, it warrants early identification, better management practices with focus on multidisciplinary care approach including geriatricians, nursing staff, physiotherapist, dietician and clinical psychologist, and early implementation of rehabilitation services.

Confusion Assessment Method for the intensive care unit (CAM-ICU) flowsheet.

• Acute change or fluctuating course of mental status: ○ Is there an acute change from mental status baseline? Or ○ Has the patient's mental status fluctuated during the past 24 hours?	—No→	CAM-ICU negative No delirium
↓Yes		
• Inattention: ○ Squeeze my hand when I say the letter A – Read the following sequence of letters: SAVEAHAART – Errors: No squeeze with A and squeeze on a letter other than A ○ If unable to complete letters → pictures	0–2 errors	CAM-ICU negative No delirium
↓ >2 errors		
• Altered level of consciousness Current RASS level	RASS other than zero	CAM-ICU positive Delirium present
↓RASS = Zero		
• Disorganized thinking: ○ Will a stone float on water? ○ Are there fish in the sea? ○ Does one pound weigh more than two? ○ Can you use a hammer to pound a nail? • *Command:* ○ Hold up this many fingers (hold up two fingers) ○ Now do the same thing with the other hand (do not demonstrate) Or ○ Add one more finger (if patient unable to move both arms)	>1 error 0–1 error	CAM-ICU negative No delirium

(RASS: Richmond Agitation-Sedation Scale)
Source: Copyright © 2002, E Wesley Ely, MD, MPH and Vanderbilt University, all right reserved

Self-Assessment Questionnaire

Q1. What is delirium?
Q2. How frequent is delirium?
Q3. What are the risk factors of delirium?
Q4. What is the underlying pathophysiology?
Q5. How to diagnose delirium?
Q6. How to prevent and treat delirium?
Q7. What is the prognosis of delirium?
Q8. What is the role of a geriatrician in the treatment of delirium?

FURTHER READINGS

1. Deksnytė A, Aranauskas R, Budrys V, Kasiulevičius V, Šapoka V. Delirium: its historical evolution and current interpretation. Eur J Inter Med. 2012;23(6):483-6.
2. Harrington CJ, Vardi K. Delirium: presentation, epidemiology, and diagnostic evaluation (part 1). R I Med J (2013). 2014;97(6):18-23.
3. Kukreja D, Günther U, Popp J. Delirium in the elderly: current problems with increasing geriatric age. Indian J Med Res. 2015;142(6):655.
4. Hshieh TT, Inouye SK, Oh ES. Delirium in the elderly. Clin Geriatr Med. 2020;36(2):183-99.
5. Maldonado JR. Delirium pathophysiology: an updated hypothesis of the etiology of acute brain failure. Int J Geriatr Psychiatry. 2018;33(11):1428-57.
6. Maclullich AM, Anand A, Davis DH, Jackson T, Barugh AJ, Hall RJ, et al. New horizons in the pathogenesis, assessment and management of delirium. Age Ageing. 2013;42(6):667-74.

7. Grover S, Kathiravan S, Dua D. Delirium research in India: a systematic review. J Neurosci Rural Pract. 2021;12(2): 236-66.
8. Pendlebury S, Lovett N, Smith S, Dutta N, Bendon C, Lloyd-Lavery A, et al. Observational, longitudinal study of delirium in consecutive unselected acute medical admissions: age-specific rates and associated factors, mortality and re-admission. BMJ Open. 2015;5(11):e007808.
9. Iglseder B, Frühwald T, Jagsch C. Delirium in geriatric patients. Wien Med Wochenschr. 2022;172(5-6):114-21.
10. American Psychiatric Association. Diagnostic and statistical manual of mental disorders: DSM-5. 5th edition. Washington, DC: American Psychiatric Association; 2013. p. 947.
11. World Health Organization. (2025). ICD-11: International Classification of Diseases 11th Revision. [online] Available from https://icd.who.int/en/
12. Rieck KM, Pagali S, Miller DM. Delirium in hospitalized older adults. Hosp Prac. 2020;48(sup1):3-16.
13. Burry L, Mehta S, Perreault MM, Luxenberg JS, Siddiqi N, Hutton B, et al. Antipsychotics for treatment of delirium in hospitalised non-ICU patients. Cochrane Database Syst Rev. 2018;6(6):CD005594.
14. Wu YC, Tseng PT, Tu YK, Hsu CY, Liang CS, Yeh TC, et al. Association of delirium response and safety of pharmacological interventions for the management and prevention of delirium: a network meta-analysis. JAMA Psychiatry. 2019;76(5):526-35.
15. Toft K, Tontsch J, Abdelhamid S, Steiner L, Siegemund M, Hollinger A. Serum biomarkers of delirium in the elderly: a narrative review. Ann Intensive Care. 2019;9(1):76.
16. Ajmera Y, Paul K, Khan MA, Kumari B, Kumar N, Chatterjee P, et al. The evaluation of frequency and predictors of delirium and its short-term and long-term outcomes in hospitalized older adults. Asian J Psychiatr. 2024;94:103990.

CHAPTER 20

Cardiac Fraitly and Heart Failure in Elderly

Avinash Chakrawarty, Shreya Biswal

INTRODUCTION

In India, the combination of age-related cardiovascular (CV) changes and the rising prevalence of CV disease in older adults significantly increases the risk of heart failure (HF). HF predominantly affects those over 75 years old, mirroring global trends, where this age group constitutes a significant portion of HF hospitalizations and deaths. As India's population ages, the incidence and prevalence of HF are expected to rise sharply, potentially doubling the number of older adults with HF over the next 25 years.

In addition to hospitalizations and mortality, HF causes substantial chronic disability in older adults, often necessitating long-term care. It is a common comorbidity among hospitalized older adults, especially those developing delirium, and it exacerbates major geriatric syndromes. The societal burden of HF in India's aging population is extremely high, highlighting the need for improved healthcare infrastructure, increased awareness, and better management strategies for HF among the elderly. Much of cardiac patients' management takes place in an elective care setting, and this allows greater scope for preassessment and improvement of frail patients' physiological status, prior to any treatment, procedure, or intervention.

CHANGES IN THE AGING HEART

Structural Alterations

- *Increase in cardiac mass*:
  - MRI studies show a 10% increase in cardiac mass from age 20 to 80 years in both men and women.
  - The left ventricle in healthy older adults shows an increased mass-to-volume ratio.
  - Autopsies confirm a high prevalence of left ventricular hypertrophy (LVH) in the elderly.
- *Factors contributing to LVH*:
  - Increased impedance to left ventricular (LV) ejection due to reduced elasticity and compliance of the aorta and large arteries
  - Higher systolic arterial pressures and age-related degenerative aortic valve disease with sclerosis and thickening of valve leaflets
  - Contribution of these changes to LVH is not definitively proven.
- *Cardiac changes in the very elderly*:
  - Limited and often contradictory data due to varying rates of underlying diseases
  - Coronary artery disease (CAD) is more common in males, while hypertension is more common in females.
  - Males often show reduced LV systolic function and wall motion abnormalities.
  - Females are more likely to have ventricular hypertrophy, atrial dilatation, and moderate-to-severe mitral and tricuspid valve dysfunction.
- *Impact of disease and environmental factors*:
  - Studies show less marked cardiac changes in disease-free older hearts.
  - The Framingham cohort study links LVH with higher blood pressure, overweight, smoking, and diabetes.
  - Distinguishing between changes due to intrinsic aging and those due to disease or environmental factors is challenging.
  - Lifestyle or environmental factors can influence structural changes, with exercise showing potential to partially reverse age-associated changes.

- *Microscopic and cellular changes*:
  - Decrease in myocytes with hypertrophy of remaining cells and increased interstitial fat, lipofuscin pigment, and fibroblast numbers
  - Adult myocardial cells can actively divide in response to injury.
  - Age-related valvular fibrosis and calcification, causing valvular regurgitation or stenotic gradients, are common and can lead to increased CV and total mortality.
- *Intracellular deposits and arrhythmias*:
  - Amyloid deposits are common, especially in the elderly, with high prevalence in Japanese populations.
  - Extensive amyloid infiltration can cause cardiomyopathy, HF, and arrhythmias.
  - Reduction in pacemaker and myocyte cells in conducting tissues leads to dysrhythmias such as sick sinus syndrome.
- *Biochemical changes*:
  - Alterations in sarcoplasmic reticulum and Ca^{2+} uptake, slower myosin isoenzymes, and decreased adenosine triphosphatase activity.
  - These changes result in prolonged isovolumetric relaxation, affecting diastolic function and contributing to heart failure with preserved ejection fraction (HFpEF).

Physiological Alterations

- *Systolic function and cardiac output*:
  - Minimal changes in systolic function or cardiac output at rest with healthy aging
  - Diastolic function shows deterioration with age, characterized by delayed early diastolic filling and reduced maximal flow across the mitral valve.
  - Greater proportion of ventricular filling occurs during atrial contraction in late diastole.
- *Diastolic function*:
  - Changes are largely independent of disease, but the exact cause, particularly the role of reduced LV compliance, is not fully established.
  - These changes are generally inconsequential but become significant with conditions such as atrial fibrillation (AF), leading to reduced cardiac reserve and aerobic capacity.
- *Cardiac responsiveness and heart rate*:
  - Reduced responsiveness to adrenergic stimuli, resulting in decreased intrinsic and maximal heart rates
  - Attenuated heart rate increase during exercise or stress, with reliance on dilatation and increased stroke volume for increased cardiac output.
  - Reduction in cardiac reserve and maximal cardiac output due to fewer and less-sensitive cardiac beta-receptors, similar to the effects of beta-blockade
- *Baroreceptor responses*:
  - Slowed arterial baroreceptor responses with age, leading to increased arterial pressure variability and decreased heart rate variability
  - Increased predisposition to postural hypotension and syncope in elderly individuals
- *Ischemic cardiac disease*:
  - High prevalence of clinically relevant ischemic heart disease in older adults, with many having covert or unrecognized disease
  - Atherosclerosis begins in adolescence, with ischemic heart disease incidence rising dramatically with age.
  - Up to 30% of individuals over 65 years have symptoms of ischemic heart disease, with another 30% having clinically significant but unrecognized disease.
- *Challenges in diagnosis*:
  - Communication barriers, chronic cognitive impairment, and comorbidities can mask symptoms of ischemic heart disease.
  - Older adults may have impaired perception of ischemic pain, leading to vague or atypical symptoms.
  - Myocardial infarction may present as confusion or collapse, while myocardial ischemia can cause nonspecific lethargy and reduced physical capacity.
- *Clinical consequences*:
  - Reduced cardiac homeostatic reserve makes older adults more susceptible to adverse clinical outcomes such as myocardial ischemia, HF, or arrhythmias during physiological stressors.

Age-related Changes in Organ Systems and their Impact on Heart Failure

Age-related changes in various organ systems significantly influence the likelihood of older adults developing HF and affect the clinical presentation and treatment responses.

Kidneys: Renal function declines with age, reducing glomerular filtration rate (GFR) by approximately 8 cm^3/min per decade. This impairs the ability to excrete salt and water, affects water and electrolyte balance, and reduces the effectiveness of medications that are excreted by the kidneys.

Lungs and upper respiratory tract (URT): Aging leads to a loss of elastic recoil in the lungs, decreased vital capacity, and increased ventilation–perfusion mismatching. These changes contribute to more severe hypoxemia, especially when combined with HF. Decreased mucociliary clearance.

Nervous system: The central nervous system's ability to regulate cerebral perfusion in response to decreased cardiac output diminishes with age. This impaired autoregulation increases the risk of cognitive decline and delirium in older HF patients. Additionally, the thirst mechanism becomes less effective, raising the risk of dehydration due to diuretic use. Autonomic dysfunction which encompasses loss of sympathetic or parasympathetic tone has also been implicated in a higher incidence of syncope, both neurologic and cardiologic variants.

Metabolism and drug processing: Age-related changes in the alimentary tract, liver, and kidneys alter the absorption, metabolism, and excretion of medications, affecting their efficacy and safety.

Musculoskeletal system: Frailty, sarcopenia, and HF often share risk factors that exacerbate each condition, particularly in older adults. Key factors include aging, which leads to natural declines in muscle mass, CV function, and physiological reserve, as well as chronic inflammation that accelerates muscle wasting and worsens cardiac dysfunction. Poor nutrition and a sedentary lifestyle further contribute to muscle loss and frailty while negatively impacting heart health. Additionally, comorbid conditions, hormonal changes, and cognitive decline can complicate the management of all three conditions.

These age-associated changes in organ systems collectively impact the clinical management of HF in older adults, requiring careful consideration in both diagnosis and treatment.

CLINICAL SIGNIFICANCE OF FRAILTY IN CARDIOVASCULAR DISEASE

Prognosis: Frailty is associated with poorer outcomes compared to nonfrail individuals, with its impact varying based on frailty severity. Frailty affects both CV and non-CV mortality. For example, CV mortality rates are higher in frail [hazard ratio (HR): 2.79] and prefrail (HR: 1.64) individuals aged 60 years and older compared to robust participants.

Risk association: In studies of older adults, frailty is linked to increased risk of CV disease, particularly in those with conditions such as peripheral artery disease and HF. A meta-analysis involving over 31,000 subjects found that frailty and prefrailty increase the risk of CV disease (HR: 1.70) and CV death (threefold higher risk).

Mechanisms: Several factors may link frailty to CV disease, including reduced physical activity, subclinical vascular changes, oxidative stress, DNA damage, and inflammation. Frail individuals often receive less aggressive treatment, which can exacerbate comorbidities and disability, worsening their prognosis. Non-CV mortality should also be considered when evaluating the overall risk and making clinical decisions.

QUANTIFYING FRAILTY IN OLDER ADULTS WITH HEART FAILURE

Various indices and scores, validated for predicting mortality and adverse clinical outcomes, have been developed to quantify frailty **(Table 1)**.

TABLE 1: Overview of the scales and tools for assessment of frailty relevant to heart failure patients.

Instrument	Domain of frailty/ components	Interpretation	Comments
Handgrip strength test	Physical function/ mobility	Asia Working Group for Sarcopenia (AWGS) criteria: • <26.0 kg • <18.0 kg	
Gait speed test	Physical function	*0.8 m/s* is oftentimes used to define slow gait speed	
Physical activity questionnaire	Physical function		Minnesota Leisure Time Activity, Physical Activity Scale for the Elderly (PASE), and Paffenbarger Physical Activity Questionnaire

Continued

Continued

Instrument	Domain of frailty/ components	Interpretation	Comments
Short physical performance battery (SPPB)	Physical function	• Three SPPB calculation components: 1. Ability to stand for 10 seconds with feet in three different positions (together side by side, semitandem, and tandem) 2. Two timed trials of a 3-m or 4-m walk (fastest recorded) 3. Time to rise from a chair five times • Scoring: ○ Minimum score: 0 ○ Maximum score: 12 ○ Gait and chair subtests scored from 0 to 4; cutoff scores were provided for scoring ○ Higher scores indicating better lower extremity function • Three balanced subsets: 1. Side-by-side stand scored from 0 to 1 2. Semitandem stance scored from 0 to 1 3. Tandem stance scored from 0 to 2	• A score lower than 10 indicates one or more mobility limitations • A score lower than 10 is predictive of all-cause mortality • SPPB may not be able to distinguish performance in high-functioning patients
Weight loss	Physical function/ nutritional status	Persistent, unintentional loss of >5% of weight over 6–12 months	Also, a component of Mini Nutritional Assessment
Serum albumin	Nutritional status	<2.8 g/dL	
Serum Hb	Nutritional status		
Fried Frailty Index	Multimodal	• Five self-reported criteria: (1) Weight loss, (2) exhaustion, (3) low physical activity, (4) slowness, and (5) weakness • Three stages: (1) Nonfrail (score 0), (2) prefrail (score 1–2), and (3) frail (score 3–5)	
Clinical Frailty Scale	Multimodal	• Level 1—very fit • Level 2—fit • Level 3—managing well • Level 4—living with very mild frailty • Level 5—living with mild frailty • Level 6—living with moderate frailty • Level 7—living with severe frailty • Level 8—living with very severe frailty • Level 9—terminally ill: Approaching the end of life	
Essential frailty toolset	Multiple components (four items): 1. Weakness 2. Cognitive 3. Nutritional status 4. Multisystem proxy	The tool is scored 0 (least frail) to 5 (most frail)	Now proposed for prognostication in TAVR patients
Mini Nutritional Assessment	Nutritional status	• Screening score (subtotal maximum 14 points): ○ 12–14 points: Normal nutritional status ○ 8–11 points: At risk of malnutrition ○ 0–7 points: Malnourished • Assessment score (maximum 16 points) • Malnutrition indicator score (screening + assessment score): ○ 24–30 points: Normal nutritional status ○ 17–23.5 points ○ At risk of malnutrition <17 points malnourished	

Continued

Continued

Instrument	Domain of frailty/ components	Interpretation	Comments
Geriatric Depression Scale	Cognitive function/ depression	In a 15-item questionnaire: • 0–4 indicate normal • 5–8 indicate mild depression • 9–11 indicate moderate depression • 12–15 indicate severe depression	Also available in 5-item and 30-item questionnaire
Mini–Mental State Examination	Cognitive function	Twenty-four or more (out of 30) indicates a normal cognition. Severe (≤9 points), moderate (10–18 points), or mild (19–23 points) cognitive impairment can be identified	
Addenbrooke's Cognitive Examination III (ACE-III)	Cognitive function		The optimal cutoff values to detect MCI and MNCD with ACE-III were 71 and 62 (AUC: 0.849 and 0.884), respectively, in a Hindi version of ACE-III
Electronic Medical Record	• Comorbidities • Polypharmacy • Sensory impairment • Depression		

(MCI: mild cognitive impairment; MNCD: mild neurocognitive disorder; TAVR: transcatheter aortic valve replacement)

MANAGEMENT OF HEART FAILURE IN FRAIL OLDER ADULTS

Diagnosis of HF in older adults can be more difficult than in their younger counterparts. The principal goals of HF therapy are to relieve symptoms, maintain or enhance functional capacity and quality of life, preserve independence, and reduce mortality. For frail older adults, quality of life often takes precedence over quantity of life, although individual preferences can vary widely. Given the heterogeneity in lifestyle, comorbidities, and personal goals among elderly HF patients, management must be individualized and patient centered.

DIAGNOSIS OF HEART FAILURE

Diagnosing HF in older adults is particularly challenging due to the prevalence of atypical symptoms and signs. A comprehensive clinical evaluation of symptoms and signs typically leads to an accurate diagnosis.

Chest radiography remains a crucial diagnostic tool for detecting pulmonary congestion when HF is suspected. However, its interpretation can be complicated in elderly individuals by chronic lung disease, altered chest anatomy (e.g., kyphosis), or reduced inspiratory effort.

Plasma B-type natriuretic peptide (BNP) and N-terminal proBNP (NT-proBNP) levels help differentiate dyspnea caused by HF from other conditions, such as pulmonary disorders. Elevated levels of these peptides are indicative of both systolic HF and HFpEF and correlate with treatment response and prognosis. However, BNP and NT-proBNP levels naturally increase with age, particularly in women, which can diminish their specificity and accuracy in older adults. In cases of diagnostic uncertainty, low or normal levels of these peptides can effectively rule out acute HF, while significantly elevated levels provide strong support for the diagnosis.

Effective HF management involves understanding the type of LV dysfunction (systolic vs. diastolic), identifying both primary and secondary causes, and recognizing potentially treatable precipitating or contributing factors. To distinguish between systolic and diastolic dysfunction, assessment of LV ejection fraction is crucial. This can be achieved through echocardiography, radionuclide ventriculography, magnetic resonance imaging, or contrast angiography. Echocardiography, being the most commonly used and clinically valuable noninvasive test, provides detailed information about LV chamber size, wall thickness, atrial size, right ventricular function, and the presence and severity of valvular and pericardial disorders.

It is recommended for all patients with newly diagnosed HF or those with unexplained disease progression.

Etiologies should be kept in mind while approaching a diagnosis of HF. Some common causes being: HF in older adults can arise from a variety of conditions, including:

- *CAD* includes acute myocardial infarction and chronic ischemic cardiomyopathy.
- *Hypertensive heart disease*: Features such as hypertensive heart disease and hypertensive hypertrophic cardiomyopathy
- *Valvular heart disease*: Conditions such as aortic stenosis or insufficiency, mitral stenosis or insufficiency, and prosthetic valve malfunction
- *Cardiomyopathy*: Various types including dilated (nonischemic), hypertrophic (obstructive or nonobstructive), restrictive (especially amyloid), and inflammatory myocarditis
- *Pericardial disease*: Example: Constrictive pericarditis
- *High output syndromes*: Including chronic anemia, thiamine deficiency, hyperthyroidism, and arterio-venous shunting
- *Age-related changes*: Age-related diastolic dysfunction

KEY COMPONENTS OF HEART FAILURE MANAGEMENT IN FRAIL OLDER ADULTS

- *Individualized treatment*: Personalize HF management based on each patient's unique circumstances, considering their frailty, comorbid conditions, and personal preferences
- *Comprehensive care approach*: Use a multidisciplinary team to ensure coordinated care, addressing medical, psychological, and social needs
- *Address underlying causes*: Identify and treat the underlying etiology and contributing factors of HF, such as hypertension, CAD, diabetes, and dyslipidemia
- *Symptom management*: Implement an effective therapeutic regimen to relieve symptoms and prevent exacerbations. This may include judicious use of diuretics to manage fluid overload while avoiding dehydration and renal impairment, particularly important in frail patients.
- *Enhance functional capacity*: Encourage appropriate levels of physical activity tailored to the individual's capabilities and limitations to maintain or improve functional status without overexertion
- *Medication management*: Ensure adherence to medications while monitoring for potential drug interactions and side effects. Adjust dosages as needed to minimize adverse effects, particularly considering the sensitivity of frail older adults to certain medications.
- *Lifestyle modifications*: Promote healthy lifestyle changes, including smoking cessation, limited alcohol intake, and dietary adjustments. Encourage balanced nutrition to support overall health and well-being.
- *Psychosocial support*: Provide support for mental health and social well-being, recognizing the impact of HF and frailty on psychological health. Offer resources for coping with the emotional challenges associated with chronic illness.

By focusing on a patient-centered approach and considering the unique needs of frail older adults, HF management can effectively address both medical and quality-of-life aspects, enhancing overall outcomes for this vulnerable population.

FOCUSING ON ETIOLOGY AND PRECIPITATING FACTORS IN OLDER ADULTS WITH FRAILTY

Heart failure in older adults is rarely curable, but proper treatment of the underlying causes can improve symptoms and slow disease progression. Hypertension should be aggressively managed, and CAD should be treated with medications and/or revascularization. Diabetes and dyslipidemia management should be optimized, smoking should be strongly discouraged, and regular physical activity should be prescribed. Alcohol intake should be limited to two drinks per day for men and one drink per day for women, with strict avoidance in those with suspected alcoholic cardiomyopathy.

Severe aortic stenosis is a common cause of HF in older adults, and aortic valve replacement can reduce mortality and improve quality of life, even in octogenarians, with perioperative mortality rates below 10%.

Atrial fibrillation is a frequent precipitant of HF in older adults, particularly with diastolic dysfunction. Restoring and maintaining sinus rhythm can be beneficial in recent-onset symptomatic AF. In chronic AF, controlling the ventricular rate is crucial. Bradycardia, though less common, can be treated with permanent pacemaker implantation. Identifying and treating anemia, thyroid disease, and other systemic illnesses is essential.

Medication adherence and dietary restrictions, including avoiding excessive fluid intake, are critical. Nonsteroidal anti-inflammatory drugs (NSAIDs) should be avoided as they can worsen HF by promoting sodium and water retention, interfering with angiotensin-converting enzyme (ACE) inhibitors and other antihypertensive agents, and impairing renal function. Monitoring other medications that may exacerbate HF is also important.

In frail older individuals, the presence of comorbidities and the overall decline in physiological reserve require tailored and cautious management of HF. This includes close monitoring of drug interactions, careful titration of medications, and individualized physical activity plans to enhance functional capacity without overexertion.

Pharmacotherapy

Effective therapeutic regimens for HF depend on whether the patient has predominantly systolic HF or HFpEF. Although these conditions often coexist, especially in those over 70 years, for this discussion, patients with an ejection fraction < 45% are considered to have systolic HF, while those with an ejection fraction ≥ 45% are considered to have HFpEF.

Systolic Heart Failure

Over the last three decades, significant advances have been made in treating systolic HF. While many studies have either excluded those over 75–80 years or included too few elderly subjects to draw definitive conclusions, existing data suggest that older patients respond to standard therapies similarly to younger patients. Therefore, current drug treatment recommendations for systolic HF apply equally to both age groups.

Angiotensin-converting Enzyme Inhibitors

Angiotensin-converting enzyme inhibitors are crucial for managing LV systolic dysfunction, regardless of whether HF is clinically apparent. Older patients are more likely to have potential contraindications to ACE inhibitors, such as renal dysfunction, renal artery stenosis, and orthostatic hypotension, and are at an increased risk for side effects such as worsening renal function, electrolyte disturbances, and hypotension. Despite these risks, ACE inhibitors are recommended for nearly all older patients with documented LV systolic dysfunction.

Therapy should start at a low dose and gradually increase to the effective clinical trial dosages. Blood pressure, renal function, and serum potassium levels should be closely monitored during dose titration and periodically during maintenance therapy. For those who cannot tolerate standard dosages due to side effects, reduced dosages can still provide benefits.

Angiotensin Receptor Blockers

Angiotensin receptor blockers (ARBs) have a more favorable side effect profile than ACE inhibitors and achieve similar effects on major clinical outcomes such as mortality and hospitalizations. ARBs reduce mortality and hospitalizations in patients with systolic HF who cannot tolerate ACE inhibitors. Combining an ARB with an ACE inhibitor reduces HF admissions but not mortality while increasing side effects. Thus, ACE inhibitors are the first-line therapy for systolic HF, with ARBs as a suitable alternative for intolerant patients and as adjunctive agents for those with persistent symptoms.

Hydralazine and Isosorbide Dinitrate

The combination of hydralazine 75 mg QID and isosorbide dinitrate 30–40 mg QID has been linked to decreased mortality in HF patients. Recent studies have shown that this combination reduces mortality in African-American patients with symptomatic systolic HF. It is recommended for self-declared African-Americans with advanced systolic HF, for patients intolerant to ACE inhibitors and ARBs, those with significant renal insufficiency, and as an adjunctive therapy for highly symptomatic patients despite standard treatment. However, side effects are common, and the combination is not available in a once-daily formulation.

Beta-blockers

Beta-blockers improve LV function and reduce mortality in a broad range of HF patients, including those with New York Heart Association (NYHA) class IV symptoms and up to 80 years of age. They are standard therapy for clinically stable patients without major contraindications. Older patients may be limited by a higher prevalence of bradyarrhythmias and severe chronic lung disease and may be more susceptible to fatigue and impaired exercise tolerance during long-term administration.

Carvedilol, metoprolol, and bisoprolol have shown improved outcomes in patients with systolic HF, with carvedilol being more effective than metoprolol in reducing mortality in one trial. Beta-blocker treatment should start at low dosages in stable patients on a background of ACE inhibitor and diuretic therapy, and the dose should gradually increase at 2–4-week intervals to achieve maintenance dosages. Lower dosages and slower titration may be appropriate for patients over 75 years of age.

Digoxin

Digoxin improves symptoms and reduces hospitalizations in patients with symptomatic systolic HF treated with ACE inhibitors and diuretics but does not affect total or CV mortality. The effects are similar across all ages, making it a useful drug for treating systolic HF in patients of all ages with limiting symptoms despite standard therapy.

Most older patients with preserved renal function (estimated creatinine clearance ≥ 60 cm^3/minute) benefit from a daily dose of 0.125 mg. Lower dosages are necessary for patients with renal insufficiency. Monitoring serum digoxin levels is advisable to ensure that they do not exceed 0.9 ng/mL, especially when toxicity is suspected. Side effects include arrhythmias, heart block, gastrointestinal disturbances, and altered neurological function. Contrary to common belief, older patients are not at an increased risk for digitalis toxicity, as shown in the Digitalis Investigation Group (DIG) trial.

Diuretics

Diuretics are essential for most HF patients and remain the most effective agents for relieving congestion and maintaining euvolemia. While some patients with mild HF can be managed with a thiazide diuretic, most will require a loop diuretic such as furosemide, bumetanide, or torsemide. In more severe HF or significant renal dysfunction, adding metolazone 2.5–10 mg daily may be necessary.

Diuretic dosages should be titrated to eliminate signs of pulmonary and systemic venous congestion. Common side effects include worsening renal function and electrolyte disorders. Monitoring renal function and serum electrolyte levels is essential during initiation, titration, and periodically thereafter.

Aldosterone Antagonists

Spironolactone, a potassium-sparing diuretic that antagonizes aldosterone, has been shown to reduce mortality and hospital admissions when added to standard HF therapy in patients with NYHA class III–IV systolic HF, with benefits similar across all ages. Eplerenone, a selective aldosterone antagonist, reduces mortality and sudden cardiac death in patients with LV systolic dysfunction following acute myocardial infarction and in those with NYHA class II symptoms with an LV ejection fraction ≤ 30%.

Spironolactone is contraindicated in patients with severe renal insufficiency or hyperkalemia, and up to 10% of patients may develop painful gynecomastia. Older patients on spironolactone combined with an ACE inhibitor or ARB may be at an increased risk for hyperkalemia, especially if they have preexisting renal insufficiency or diabetes, and doses above 25 mg/day should be avoided. The combined use of an ACE inhibitor, ARB, and aldosterone antagonist is not recommended.

ANGIOTENSIN RECEPTOR-NEPRILYSIN INHIBITORS IN HEART FAILURE

Overview

Angiotensin receptor-neprilysin inhibitors (ARNIs) represent a significant advancement in the treatment of HF, particularly for patients with reduced ejection fraction (HFrEF). The primary ARNI, sacubitril/valsartan, combines a neprilysin inhibitor (sacubitril) with an angiotensin II receptor blocker (valsartan). This combination provides a dual mechanism of action by enhancing natriuretic peptides through neprilysin inhibition and blocking the detrimental effects of the renin-angiotensin-aldosterone system (RAAS).

Mechanism of Action

- *Neprilysin inhibition*: Sacubitril inhibits neprilysin, an enzyme responsible for degrading natriuretic peptides, bradykinin, and other vasoactive substances. By inhibiting neprilysin, sacubitril increases the levels of these peptides, leading to beneficial effects such as vasodilation, natriuresis, and diuresis, which help reduce cardiac stress and improve overall heart function.
- *RAAS blockade*: Valsartan, an angiotensin II receptor blocker, prevents the detrimental effects of angiotensin II, including vasoconstriction, sodium retention, and aldosterone secretion. This blockade helps reduce blood pressure, decrease fluid retention, and mitigate myocardial remodeling and fibrosis.

The PARADIGM-HF trial demonstrated that sacubitril/valsartan was superior to enalapril in patients with HFrEF, significantly reducing CV death by 20% and HF hospitalizations by 21%. Additionally, patients treated with sacubitril/valsartan experienced fewer symptoms and an overall improvement in the quality of life.

Based on these findings, major guidelines, including those from the American College of Cardiology (ACC), American Heart Association (AHA), and Heart Failure Society of America (HFSA), recommend the use of sacubitril/valsartan in patients with HFrEF who remain symptomatic despite optimal medical therapy with ACE inhibitors or ARBs.

Dosing and Administration

- *Initiation*: Patients are typically started on a low dose of sacubitril/valsartan (e.g., 24/26 mg or 49/51 mg twice daily), with gradual titration to the target dose of 97/103 mg twice daily, as tolerated.
- *Monitoring*: Regular monitoring of blood pressure, renal function, and serum potassium levels is crucial, particularly during dose adjustments, to detect and manage potential side effects such as hypotension, hyperkalemia, and renal dysfunction.

Older adults may have specific considerations when initiating and managing ARNI therapy:

- *Renal function*: Given the higher prevalence of renal impairment in older adults, careful monitoring and dose adjustments may be necessary.
- *Hypotension*: Older patients are more susceptible to hypotension, necessitating cautious titration and monitoring.

- *Comorbidities and polypharmacy*: The presence of multiple comorbidities and the use of various medications may increase the risk of drug interactions and adverse effects.

HEART FAILURE WITH PRESERVED EJECTION FRACTION

Over half of elderly HF patients have preserved LV systolic function. The management of HFpEF remains largely empirical as of now. The underlying cardiac disorder and contributing conditions, such as hypertension and CAD, should be managed aggressively. Diuretics should be used cautiously to relieve congestion while avoiding overdiuresis and prerenal azotemia. Topical or oral nitrates may help reduce pulmonary congestion and orthopnea.

The findings from different relevant trials are summarized below:

- The CHARM-preserved trial found that the ARB candesartan reduced HF admissions by 16% but did not affect mortality in patients with an LV ejection fraction > 40%. The trial included patients with a mean age of 67 years, 27% of whom were ≥75 years old. However, patients with substantial comorbidities were excluded, limiting the applicability of the findings to older HF patients in clinical practice.
- The I-PRESERVE trial, which included 4,128 patients (mean age 72 years, 60% women) with HFpEF (LV ejection fraction ≥ 45%), found that irbesartan had no beneficial effect on the primary composite endpoint of all-cause mortality or CV hospitalization. Similarly, the PEP-CHF trial, involving 850 patients aged 70 years or older (mean age 76 years, 55% women), found that the ACE inhibitor perindopril had no effect on the primary outcome of mortality or HF admission, although it did reduce overall HF admissions and improve NYHA class and 6-minute walk distance at 1 year.
- The SENIORS trial included 2,128 HF patients aged ≥70 years (mean age 76 years, 35% women), who were randomized to the beta-blocker nebivolol or placebo. The primary composite endpoint was all-cause mortality or CV hospitalization. Nebivolol was associated with a 15% reduction in the primary endpoint, with no effect on mortality but reduced CV admissions. Similar results were observed in patients with LV ejection fraction >35 versus ≤35%.
- The DIG ancillary trial involved 988 patients (mean age 67 years, 41% women) with HF and LV ejection fraction > 45%, randomized to digoxin or placebo. Digoxin had no effect on the primary composite endpoint of HF death or HF hospitalization nor on all-cause mortality, CV mortality, or CV hospitalizations.
- The STEP-HFpEF trial investigated the effects of semaglutide in patients with HFpEF and obesity. The trial demonstrated that semaglutide significantly reduced body weight and improved exercise capacity compared to placebo. Patients on semaglutide also showed improvements in HF-related symptoms and quality of life. Additionally, semaglutide was associated with beneficial cardiometabolic effects, including better glycemic control and reduced blood pressure. The trial concluded that semaglutide is a promising treatment for managing HFpEF in patients with obesity, offering substantial clinical benefits.

Thus, no pharmacological intervention has been shown to reduce mortality in older patients with HFpEF, and, except for diuretics to relieve congestion, there are no class I or class IIa indications for any agents in the treatment of HFpEF. Therapy should be individualized based on comorbidities and the observed response to specific interventions.

DEVICE THERAPY IN HEART FAILURE FOR FRAIL OLDER ADULTS

For many older adults with HF, medications and lifestyle changes are effective management strategies. However, implantable devices are increasingly important for certain patient groups, including frail older adults. In this population, the advantages of these devices need to be carefully balanced with potential risks and limitations.

Cardiac pacemakers: Aging often leads to a decrease in the number of functioning sinus node pacemaker cells, resulting in conditions such as sick sinus syndrome. This syndrome can cause inappropriate sinus bradycardia and chronotropic incompetence, which may worsen HF symptoms and reduce exercise capacity. For frail older adults experiencing symptomatic sick sinus syndrome, a pacemaker can be essential. It helps manage bradycardia while allowing the continued use of beta-blockers, which are beneficial for improving ventricular function and reducing mortality in systolic HF but can exacerbate bradyarrhythmias.

Cardiac resynchronization therapy (CRT): Pacemakers have also evolved to play a significant role in managing advanced HF. Around 30% of HF patients suffer from left bundle branch block or other intraventricular conduction abnormalities, causing a prolonged QRS interval (≥120 ms) and asynchronous ventricular contractions. CRT has demonstrated benefits in improving ejection fraction, reducing LV cavity size, and boosting exercise tolerance and quality of life in trials involving patients with advanced HF (NYHA class III–IV), reduced ejection fraction, and prolonged QRS duration. Meta-analyses also indicate that CRT leads to fewer hospitalizations and better survival rates. Despite older patients being underrepresented in CRT studies, observational data suggest that CRT can significantly improve quality of life and exercise tolerance in elderly patients, including those in their 80s. Thus, CRT is a viable option for carefully selected older adults with advanced HF who have not responded adequately to conventional therapies.

Exercise

Both HF and normal aging are associated with reduced exercise capacity, partly due to sarcopenia (loss of muscle mass) and changes in skeletal muscle blood flow and metabolism. Regular physical activity improves exercise performance in both healthy older adults and those with HF. Consequently, regular exercise is now recommended for most older HF patients.

In the HF-ACTION (HF: A Controlled Trial Investigating Outcomes of Exercise Training) trial, it was found that exercise was associated with an 11% reduction in the primary endpoint and a 15% reduction in CV mortality or HF hospitalization. These benefits were consistent across age groups (≤70 vs. >70 years). Additionally, patients in the exercise group reported modest but significant improvements in quality of life that persisted for up to 4 years.

Although supervised exercise programs yield the greatest improvements in exercise performance, they are often not feasible for many older patients due to availability, travel concerns, and cost constraints. Therefore, most older HF patients should be encouraged to engage in a self-monitored home exercise program that includes stretching exercises, resistance training, and aerobic activities.

Older adults should start exercising at a comfortable pace and duration, even if it is just a few minutes of slow walking. They should gradually increase the duration (not the intensity) of exercise until they can exercise comfortably and continuously for 20–30 minutes, aiming for at least 4–5 days/week. Once this level is achieved, they can consider further increasing the duration (up to 45 minutes) or gradually increasing the intensity. However, they should avoid strenuous exercise or exercising to exhaustion.

MANAGEMENT OF COMORBIDITIES IN FRAIL OLDER ADULTS WITH HEART FAILURE

Managing HF in frail older adults requires addressing the multiple comorbid conditions that often accompany aging. These comorbidities can significantly impact the diagnosis, clinical course, treatment, and prognosis of HF.

Key considerations for managing comorbidities in frail older adults with HF are as follows:

- *Renal dysfunction*:
  - Renal function declines with age, often leading to stage III chronic kidney disease despite normal serum creatinine levels.
  - Older adults have a reduced ability to excrete excess sodium and water, contributing to volume overload.
  - Diuretics may be less effective and can cause electrolyte imbalances due to decreased renal capacity to maintain homeostasis.
  - ACE inhibitors, ARBs, and diuretics can worsen renal function, requiring careful monitoring.
- *Anemia*:
  - Common due to chronic illnesses (e.g., renal disease, malignancy), poor dietary intake, and medications causing gastrointestinal blood loss (e.g., aspirin, warfarin, and NSAIDs)
  - Contributes to reduced tissue oxygen delivery, impaired exercise tolerance, and may worsen myocardial ischemia in CAD patients
  - Anemia is an independent predictor of adverse clinical outcomes in HF patients.
- *Chronic lung disease*:
  - Reduces pulmonary function, increasing dyspnea and exercise intolerance in HF patients
  - Creates diagnostic challenges, as symptoms may overlap with HF
- *Cognitive dysfunction*:
  - Impairs self-care abilities, including adherence to dietary, medication, and activity recommendations
  - Increases risk for delirium during hospitalizations, complicating management and increasing fall risk
- *Depression and social isolation*:
  - Affects up to 20% of elderly HF patients, often leading to worse outcomes due to reduced adherence to treatments and increased adrenergic tone and arrhythmias
  - Social isolation, particularly due to spousal loss, is common and associated with higher mortality and hospitalization rates.
- *Postural hypotension and falls*:
  - Increased risk due to vascular stiffness, impaired baroreflexes, and balance issues
  - Medications such as diuretics, vasodilators, and beta-blockers can exacerbate fall risk.
- *Arthritis*:
  - Commonly treated with NSAIDs, which can worsen HF by promoting sodium and water retention and antagonizing HF medications

- NSAIDs also increase the risk of gastrointestinal bleeding and subsequent anemia.
- *Urinary incontinence*:
    - Diuretics and ACE inhibitors may worsen incontinence, leading to medication nonadherence.
    - Important to inquire about incontinence as it may be underreported
- *Sarcopenia and osteoporosis*:
    - Contribute to impaired exercise tolerance and increased fall risk
    - Medications used to treat HF may further aggravate these conditions.
    - *Sensory deprivation*: Impacts adherence to medical instructions due to hearing and vision impairments
- *Nutritional disorders*:
    - Common due to multiple factors, including dietary restrictions from various conditions and reduced appetite from chronic illness or medications
    - Advanced HF may lead to cardiac cachexia, further complicating nutritional status.
- *Polypharmacy*:
    - High prevalence in HF patients, leading to reduced adherence and increased risk of drug interactions
    - The risk of clinically significant interactions increases with the number of medications.
- *Frailty*:
    - Markedly increases with age and is characterized by weight loss, weakness, and low physical activity
    - Frailty worsens during hospitalization and rarely returns to prehospitalization levels.

Patients should stop exercising and contact their physician if they experience chest pain, undue shortness of breath, dizziness, syncope, or any other symptom indicating clinical instability. Contraindications to exercise in elderly HF patients include decompensated HF, unstable coronary disease or arrhythmias, neurological or muscular disorders that preclude participation, or any other condition rendering exercise unsafe.

MULTIDISCIPLINARY CARE IN THE CONTEXT OF FRAILTY AND HEART FAILURE IN OLDER ADULTS

Managing HF in older patients is often complicated by the presence of multiple comorbid conditions, polypharmacy, dietary concerns, and various psychosocial and financial issues. These factors frequently lead to poor outcomes, including frequent hospitalizations and reduced quality of life. To address these complexities and provide comprehensive, individualized care for older HF patients, especially those with frailty, a coordinated multidisciplinary approach is essential.

Several randomized trials and meta-analyses have shown that multidisciplinary HF disease management programs can effectively reduce hospitalizations and improve the quality of life in older patients while also lowering overall medical costs. Effective HF management programs incorporate elements such as patient and caregiver education, enhancement of self-management skills, optimization of pharmacotherapy (considering polypharmacy issues, simplifying drug regimens, and avoiding drug interactions), and close follow-up (teleconsultation and home visits). These programs typically involve a team similar to a multidisciplinary geriatric assessment team, including a nurse coordinator or case manager, dietitian, social worker, clinical pharmacist, home health representative, primary care physician, and cardiology consultant. Such a comprehensive approach is particularly important for managing frailty in older HF patients, helping to mitigate the risks and complications associated with their condition.

END-OF-LIFE CARE

The 5-year survival rate for older adults with established HF is <50%, which is worse than the prognosis for many cancers. Factors contributing to poorer outcomes include older age, severe symptoms, significant functional impairment, lower systolic blood pressure, reduced LV ejection fraction, underlying CAD, hyponatremia, anemia, impaired renal function, and cognitive dysfunction. For those with advanced HF (NYHA class III–IV symptoms), the 1-year mortality rate ranges from 25 to 50%, marking HF as a terminal illness. Additionally, HF patients face the risk of sudden arrhythmic death, even during periods of apparent stability.

In India, addressing end-of-life issues early in HF management is crucial, especially for frail older adults. Discussions about end-of-life care (EOLC) should be part of the ongoing management as the disease progresses. While these conversations can be challenging, they are essential for ensuring that patients' preferences are respected. Key measures include developing an advance directive and appointing a durable power of attorney to specify the patient's wishes regarding hospitalization, life-sustaining interventions (such as respirators and feeding tubes), and resuscitation. Continuous, open communication is necessary, as patients' views on these issues may change over time.

End-stage HF often brings significant discomfort and anxiety. Evidence from the SUPPORT study indicates that the quality of EOLC is a major concern for patients and their families. Effective EOLC should prioritize pain relief and comfort using conventional therapies along with narcotics (e.g., morphine) and sedatives (e.g., benzodiazepines). Providing emotional support through healthcare professionals, including nurses and social workers, is equally important. In India, where access to specialized care may vary, institutional or home-based hospice care should be considered for patients with terminal HF to ensure that they receive compassionate and appropriate support at the end of life.

Spiritual care, be it religious or a particular faith, is an important part of palliation so is the role of advanced directives which respect the wishes of the patients in terms of personal or family affairs.

PREVENTION OF HEART FAILURE IN FRAIL OLDER ADULTS

Given the high prevalence and poor prognosis of HF in elderly individuals, especially those who are frail, more effective prevention strategies are urgently needed. The most effective methods currently involve aggressively treating established risk factors, particularly hypertension and CAD. Numerous studies have demonstrated that even modest reductions in blood pressure can significantly decrease the incidence of HF among elderly hypertensive patients.

Several clinical trials have shown the significant impact of antihypertensive therapy on reducing the incidence of HF in older adults. Reduction rates in incident HF vary across studies, with notable results including a 22% reduction in the EWPHE trial for patients over 60 years old, a 51% reduction in the STOP-HTN trial for patients aged 70–84 years, and a 64% reduction in the HYVET trial for patients aged 80 years and older. These findings underscore the effectiveness of blood pressure management in preventing HF among the elderly, including those who are frail.

In addition to hypertension management, controlling elevated cholesterol levels with HMG-CoA reductase inhibitors (statins) has been shown to reduce the incidence of HF following an acute coronary event. Other preventative measures likely to reduce HF include smoking cessation and effective diabetes management. These strategies highlight the importance of addressing multiple CV risk factors to prevent the onset of HF in the elderly population, particularly in those who are frail. Comprehensive prevention approaches are essential for improving health outcomes and reducing the burden of HF in this vulnerable group. These strategies emphasize the importance of addressing multiple CV risk factors to prevent the onset of HF in the elderly population.

CONCLUSION

The intricate interplay between cardiac frailty and HF presents unique challenges in the diagnosis, management, and treatment of older adults. Recognizing the distinct characteristics and vulnerabilities of this population is essential for optimizing care and improving outcomes. Cardiac frailty often complicates the clinical presentation of HF, with atypical symptoms and numerous comorbidities masking or mimicking the condition. This necessitates a thorough and comprehensive approach to assessment, emphasizing the importance of individualized and patient-centered management strategies.

Therapeutic interventions, whether pharmacologic or device-based, must be tailored to accommodate the physiological changes and increased sensitivity to treatment side effects inherent in frail older adults. The judicious use of medications, careful monitoring of responses, and vigilant management of potential adverse effects are critical components of effective care. Moreover, the integration of multidisciplinary teams and the incorporation of supportive and palliative care approaches can significantly enhance the quality of life for these patients.

Future research should focus on refining diagnostic criteria, developing novel therapeutic strategies, and identifying biomarkers that can more accurately predict outcomes in this vulnerable population. By advancing our understanding of cardiac frailty and HF, we can foster a more nuanced and effective approach to treating older adults, ultimately leading to better patient outcomes and improved quality of life.

Addressing the complexities of cardiac frailty and HF requires a multifaceted and patient-centric approach, underscoring the need for continued innovation, collaboration, and dedication to advancing the care of older adults facing these intertwined health challenges.

Self-Assessment Questionnaire

Q1. What are the key structural and physiological changes in the aging heart that contribute to heart failure in older adults?

Q2. How does frailty interact with cardiovascular health and outcomes in elderly patients?

Q3. How to assess frailty in older adults with heart failure?

Q4. How do age-related changes in other organ systems (e.g., renal, nervous, musculoskeletal) affect the management of heart failure in the elderly?

Q5. What are the main pharmacological therapies for systolic heart failure, and what special considerations apply to frail older patients?

Q6. What roles do exercise and multidisciplinary care play in improving outcomes for frail older adults with heart failure?

Q7. What are the strategies to reduce the incidence of heart failure in frail elderly individuals?

CHAPTER 21

Sleep-disorders

Akshata Rao

CASE VIGNETTE

A 76-year-old female presents to the outpatient department (OPD) with her daughter, with complains of difficulty in sleeping. She reports waking up frequently during the night and having trouble falling back asleep. This has been happening for about 6 months and is affecting her daytime energy level.

Past Medical and Social History

Hypothyroidism (diagnosed 20 years ago)—currently on medication [thyroxine 100 μg OD, but has been irregular on medication, and thyroid function tests (TFTs) have not been done for more than a year].

Osteoarthritis (OA) of the knees (diagnosed 5 years ago)—treated with paracetamol and local analgesics, not compliant with advised physical therapy. Pain intensity according to Numeric Rating Scale (NRS) 5–6/10.

The patient has been living alone since she lost her husband a year ago and has lost interest in day-to-day activities and has been irregular on medications and exercises since then.

The patient's daughter has noticed that her mother is tired during the day, along with headaches and daytime sleepiness. To reduce daytime sleepiness, she consumes three to four cups of tea every day. On detailed questioning, the daughter, who has been with her mother for the past 1 week, has also noticed snoring while sleeping.

She has been having bilateral pedal edema and was recently diagnosed to have hypertension as well, for which she has been started on tablet telmisartan in combination with hydrochlorothiazide at night.

On Examination

- *Pulse*: 62 bpm
- *Blood pressure*: 160/90 mm Hg
- *Respiratory rate*: 14 cpm
- *Body mass index (BMI)*: 37 kg/m^2

Factors Contributing to Her Sleep Disorders

- *Primary sleep disorder*: Obstructive sleep apnea (OSA)
- *Secondary sleep disorders*: Mood disorder, medication side effect (diuresis), and chronic pain in the knee

Comprehensive Geriatric Care Approach to the Management of Sleep Disorder

- *Hypothyroidism needs to be addressed*: TFT testing, increase compliance, and titrate dosing of thyroxine
- Mood disorder to be treated with psychological counseling, and medications such as selective serotonin reuptake inhibitor (SSRI) if required.
- Diet and exercise for weight reduction and avoidance of caffeine
- Continuous positive airway pressure (CPAP) for OSA
- Pedal edema needs to be evaluated—it could be myxedema or due to heart failure, likely heart failure with preserved ejection fraction (HFpEF) or cor pulmonale.
- Diuretics, if required to be given during the daytime
- For chronic knee pain, physiotherapy exercises and uptitration of analgesics

INTRODUCTION

Age-related sleep disturbances are a well-documented phenomenon. The physiology of sleep demonstrably changes with advancing age, and the prevalence of primary sleep disorders, such as insomnia, sleep-disordered breathing (SDB), restless legs syndrome (RLS), rapid eye movement (REM) sleep behavior disorder (RBD), and circadian rhythm disturbances, increases significantly in older adults. Furthermore, sleep disturbances can be exacerbated by secondary conditions such as medical or psychiatric comorbidities, as well as medication side effects due to polypharmacy.

NORMAL SLEEP PATTERNS AND AGING

Normal Sleep–Wake Cycle

Sleep and wakefulness are governed by a fascinating dance between two opposing neuronal groups: (1) Sleep-promoting ventrolateral preoptic nucleus (VLPO) [using gamma-aminobutyric acid (GABA)] and (2) wake-promoting monoaminergic (MA) populations in the hypothalamus and brainstem. These groups operate in a "flip-flop" dynamic, influenced by both homeostatic sleep pressure and circadian rhythms, with orexinergic neurons acting as a key switch.

Circadian Rhythm Changes with Aging

Compared to young adults, older individuals tend to exhibit an earlier sleep schedule, for both bedtime and wake-up time (a tendency for older individuals to be "larks" rather than "owls"). This shift is influenced by the circadian rhythm, a daily internal clock regulated by the suprachiasmatic nucleus (SCN) within the hypothalamus. The natural aging process can affect various brain structures critical for regulating sleep–wake cycles, such as frontal cortical areas, the hypothalamus (specifically the SCN), and the brainstem locus coeruleus. Additionally, aging reduces retinal sensitivity to light. This decreased sensitivity disrupts circadian rhythms in older adults, making it more challenging to maintain alignment with the natural 24-hour light–dark cycle.

Normal Sleep Architecture

Sleep architecture describes the fundamental structure of normal sleep, which consists of two types: (1) Nonrapid eye movement (NREM) sleep and (2) REM sleep. Throughout a sleep period, NREM and REM sleep alternate in cycles. NREM sleep is further divided into stages N_1, N_2, slow-wave sleep (SWS), including N_3 and N_4, each characterized by distinct brain wave patterns, eye movements, and muscle tone. A typical sleep episode begins with a brief period of NREM stage 1, progresses through the stages, and then transitions to REM sleep, after which the cycle repeats. NREM sleep accounts for approximately 75–80% of total sleep time, while REM sleep makes up the remaining 20–25% . The initial NREM–REM cycle lasts around 70–100 minutes, with subsequent cycles extending to about 90–120 minutes. In normal adults, REM sleep periods lengthen as the night progresses, peaking in the final third of the sleep episode.

Changes in Sleep Architecture with Aging

As people age, the percentage of time spent in sleep stages N_1 (the lightest stage of sleep) and N_2 (a deeper stage of sleep) increases, while the percentage of time spent in SWS (the deepest stage of sleep) and REM sleep decreases. Time to fall asleep (sleep latency), time spent wake after sleep onset (WASO), and the number of arousals from sleep also increase with age **(Fig. 1)**.

Sleep Efficiency and Duration

Across the lifespan, sleep architecture undergoes a demonstrably dynamic and progressive transformation. From infancy to adulthood, there are marked alterations in sleep initiation, maintenance, and the temporal distribution of sleep stages **(Table 1)**. Notably, a consistent trend emerges. Sleep efficiency, a metric reflecting the success of sleep initiation and maintenance, exhibits a progressive decline with advancing age. This is accompanied by a rise in the number of awakenings and arousals (brief periods of wakefulness) detected by electroencephalogram (EEG). These changes lead to reduced sleep efficiency and total sleep time.

Biochemical Changes: Sleep-related Hormones and Aging (Table 2)

Light-dark cycles and sleep-wake patterns primarily regulate the 24-hour profile of melatonin. Melatonin remains low during the day, rises in the evening, stays

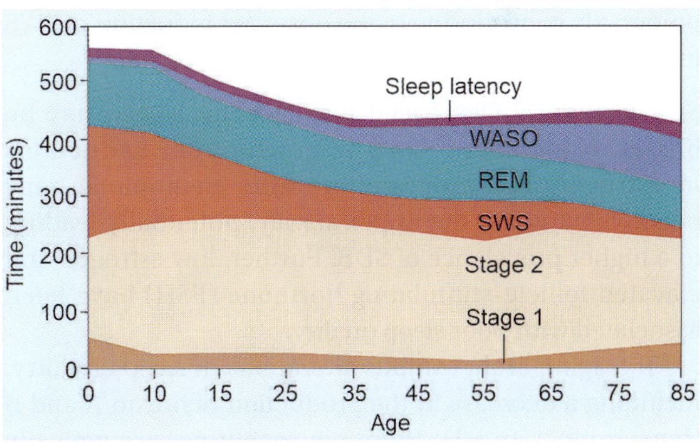

FIG. 1: Age-related changes in sleep architecture.
(REM: rapid eye movement; SWS: slow-wave sleep; WASO: wake after sleep onset)

TABLE 1: Age-related changes in sleep parameters.

Increased	Decreased
Sleep latency	Total duration of sleep
Arousal	Sleep efficiency
Wake after sleep onset (WASO)	Slow-wave sleep

TABLE 2: Changes in hormones with aging and their effect on sleep in older adults.

Hormonal changes	Sleep effects
Decreased nocturnal peak of melatonin	Increased sleep disturbances
Increased nocturnal cortisol	Reduced SWS and more awakenings
Reduced nocturnal growth hormone	Reduced SWS
Reduced testosterone	Increased sleep fragmentation/ awakening
Reduced estrogen and progesterone	Increased risk of sleep-disordered breathing

(SWS: slow-wave sleep)

elevated through sleep, and dips in the morning. However, studies show a significantly reduced nocturnal elevation of melatonin in older adults compared to younger individuals. This age-related decline in melatonin secretion may contribute to increased sleep disturbances in older populations.

Slow-wave sleep suppresses cortisol, but aging disrupts this. The circadian rhythm of cortisol flattens and remains high at night. This high nighttime cortisol may lead to less SWS and more awakenings in older adults.

The age-related decline in nocturnal growth hormone (GH) secretion might directly or indirectly influence SWS, potentially contributing to the observed reduction of SWS in older adults.

Sex hormones: Decreased testosterone levels may be linked to increased sleep fragmentation. Reductions in estrogen and progesterone after menopause may negatively impact the upper airway, potentially leading to a higher prevalence of SDB. Further, low estrogen and elevated follicle-stimulating hormone (FSH) have been associated with poor sleep quality.

The aging brain exhibits alterations in sleep circuitry, including a decrease in the production of orexin A and B (hypocretin 1 and 2). These neuropeptides are typically active during wakefulness and become inactive during sleep.

Molecular Level Changes

The complex aging process involves numerous alterations at the molecular, cellular, and genetic levels. Notably, insomnia in older adults (70–88 years) exhibits a correlation with shortened telomere length within peripheral blood mononuclear cells (PBMCs). This suggests that sleep disturbances may not only be a consequence of aging but also a potential contributor to accelerated cellular senescence in later life.

EPIDEMIOLOGY OF SLEEP DISORDERS IN THE ELDERLY—GLOBAL AND INDIAN PERSPECTIVE

Compared to the general population (15.9–22.3%), up to 50% of older adults report experiencing sleep problems in both global (30–50%) and Indian (32–52.5%) perspective. Urban populations exhibit a higher incidence of sleep disturbances compared to their rural counterparts. Additionally, research suggests a female predominance in sleep disorders in some studies, whereas some studies suggest no gender difference in sleep quality. Furthermore, a positive correlation exists between substance abuse and sleep problems. In India, early insomnia was found to be the most common pattern of insomnia.

Older adults exhibit heightened susceptibility to geriatric sleep syndrome due to several factors beyond the typical age-related alterations in sleep-wake cycles. These factors are given in **Table 3**.

Consequences of Poor Sleep

Sleep disturbances are associated with significant morbidity and mortality as well as poor consequences such as cognitive impairment, slow reaction time, balance and ambulatory difficulties, increased risk of fall, decreased quality of life, depression and anxiety, daytime sleepiness **(Flowchart 1)**.

CLINICAL PRESENTATION AND EVALUATION OF SLEEP DISORDERS IN OUTPATIENT SETTINGS

In an outpatient setting, assessing and evaluating sleep disorders in elderly individuals is paramount for determining the underlying causes, managing risk factors, and providing appropriate management. This section provides an overview of the clinical presentation and the systematic evaluation of sleep disorders in an outpatient context.

Sleep History

Asking ambulatory older individuals about their sleep regularly is the greatest way to identify sleep-wake issues. The first round of sleep assessment can be conducted using the 12 questions listed below:

1. What time do you normally go to bed at night? What time do you normally wake up in the morning?—*Circadian rhythm*

TABLE 3: Risk factors for sleep disturbances in older adults.	
Physiological cause	Age-related sleep and circadian rhythm changes
Primary sleep disorders	• Insomnia • Sleep-disordered breathing (sleep apnea) • RLS • RBD
Medical and psychological comorbidities	• *Comorbidities*: Chronic cardiopulmonary diseases, GERD, arthritis and chronic pain, BPH, and neurodegenerative diseases • *Psychiatric disorders*: Depression, anxiety disorders • *Medications*: Diuretics, beta-blockers, antidepressants
Social and environmental factors	*Diet*: Bedtime excess intake of water, caffeine intake *Social and environmental*: • Changes in daily routines: This could refer to lifestyle changes such as daytime napping or moving to a new environment post retirement. • Experiencing significant life events: Grief associated with losing a loved one or the stress of major life changes • Substance abuse • Institutionalization • Recurrent hospitalizations
Intrinsic factors • Aging brain • Altered hormone secretion • Lens and retina changes • Multimorbidity	*Extrinsic factors* • Medications • Exercise • Social activities • Life events

(BPH: benign prostatic hyperplasia; GERD: gastroesophageal reflux disease; REM: rapid eye movement; RLS: restless legs syndrome; RBD: REM sleep behavior disorder)

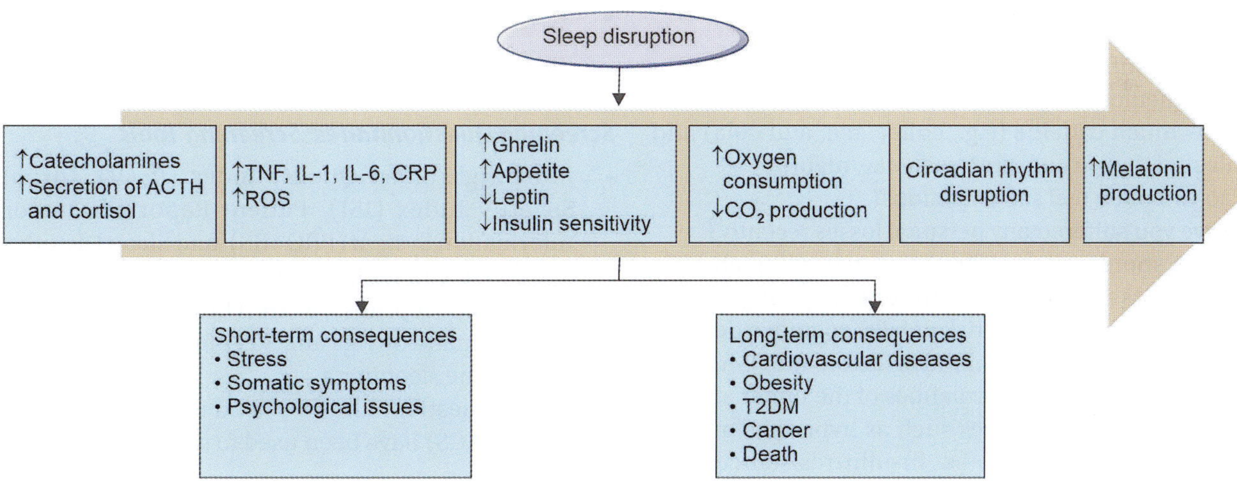

FLOWCHART 1: Consequences of sleep disruption.

(ACTH: adrenocorticotropic hormone; CRP: C-reactive protein; IL: interleukin; ROS: reactive oxygen species; TNF: tumor necrosis factor; T2DM: type 2 diabetes mellitus)

2. Do you often have trouble falling asleep at night?—*Sleep latency*
3. How many times do you wake up at night?—*Arousal*
4. If you do wake up during the night, do you usually have trouble falling back asleep?—*WASO, sleep maintenance*
5. Does your bed partner say (or are you aware) that you frequently snore, gasp for air, or stop breathing?—*OSA*
6. Does your bed partner say (or are you aware) that you kick or thrash about while asleep?—*RBD, RLS*

7. Are you aware that you ever walk, eat, punch, kick, or scream during sleep?—*NREM, parasomnia*
8. Are you sleepy or tired during much of the day?
9. Do you usually take one or more naps during the day?
10. Do you usually doze off without planning to during the day?
11. How much sleep do you need to feel alert and function well?
12. Are you currently taking any type of medication or other preparation to help you sleep?

When gathering a sleep history, it could be appropriate to follow up with questions if the initial screening indicates symptoms of a sleep complaint:

1. Do you have the urge to move your legs, or do you experience uncomfortable sensations in your legs during rest or at night?—*RLS*
2. Do you have to get up often to urinate during the night?—*OSA, benign prostatic hyperplasia (BPH), medications, congestive heart failure (CHF), atrial fibrillation (AF)*
3. If you nap during the day, how often and for how long?—*Daytime sleepiness*
4. How much physical activity or exercise do you get daily?
5. Are you exposed to natural outdoor light on most of the days?—*Circadian rhythm*
6. What medications do you take, and at what time of day and night?
7. Do you suffer any uncomfortable side effects from your medications?
8. How much caffeine (e.g., coffee, tea, and cola) and alcohol do you consume each day/night?
9. Do you often feel sad or anxious?
10. Have you suffered any personal losses recently?

History should elicit information regarding chronic pain, shortness of breath, orthopnea, quality of life (QOL), depression, anxiety, risk of falls, cognitive decline, imbalance, and Parkinsonism. Risk factors for OSA, such as obesity, anatomical abnormalities of the upper airway, and associated comorbidities such as hypertension, AF, heart failure, stroke, diabetes, insulin resistance, and hypothyroidism, need to be evaluated. Parasomnias exhibit abnormal behaviors during sleep, including bedwetting, sleepwalking, night terrors, dream anxiety attacks, and seizures. These are more common in children (except RBD), which is often seen in older adults.

Examination

Additionally crucial is a focused physical examination that is determined by the answers provided in the clinical history.

Vitals

- Hypertension—OSA, RLS, and end-stage renal disease (ESRD)
- *Pulse*: Bradycardia (hypothyroidism), hypovolemia (heart failure), and AF
- Oxygen saturation

General Examination

- Edema
- Jugular venous pressure (JVP)
- Clubbing

Head-to-toe Examination

- *Upper airway*: Nasal and pharyngeal airways
- Dental structures
- Jaw abnormalities
- Neck circumference
- Thyroid examination

Systemic Evaluation

- *Respiratory system*: Barrel-shaped chest, wheeze, crepitations
- *Cardiovascular system*: Heart failure features—basal crepitations
- *Neurological examination*: Focal neurological deficits, signs of Parkinsonism, cognitive evaluation, peripheral neuropathy, radiculopathy
- *Musculoskeletal evaluation*: Joint examination

Assessment

Screening Questionnaires: Screening Tools

- Pittsburgh Sleep Quality Index (PSQI), Insomnia Severity Index (ISI), Patient-Reported Outcomes Information System (PROMIS), and Sleep Disturbance Scale to screen for insomnia
- Epworth Sleepiness Scale (ESS) and the Essener Questionnaire on Age and Sleepiness (EQAS) to screen for daytime sleepiness
- Berlin Questionnaire (BQ) and Sleep Apnea Clinical Score (SACS) have been used to screen for OSA.

Specific Investigations in the Evaluation of Sleep Disorders

Sleep Diary with Caregiver Report

A sleep diary maintained over 1–2 weeks records bedtime, wake time, sleep latency, and nocturnal awakenings. In older adults, caregiver input adds accuracy by capturing nighttime behaviors, restlessness, or snoring that the patient may not recall.

Actigraphy

Actigraphy involves the use of a wrist-worn device that continuously records movement to estimate sleep-wake cycles over several days. It provides an objective, noninvasive assessment of sleep patterns and circadian rhythm disturbances, especially useful in outpatient and home settings.

Polysomnography

The intricate interplay of sleep cycles and stages can be elucidated through the application of electroencephalography (EEG), a technique that measures electrical patterns of brain activity. Polysomnography (PSG) is a comprehensive sleep study that evaluates various physiological parameters to diagnose SDB. It includes:

- *Respiratory monitoring*: Arterial blood oxygen saturation (SaO_2), respiratory effort (thoracic and abdominal movement), airflow (nasal and oral), and snoring
- *Sleep architecture assessment*: EEG, electrooculography (EOG), and electromyography (EMG) to characterize sleep stages and arousals
- *Cardiac and limb activity monitoring*: Electrocardiography (ECG) for heart rhythm and leg EMG to detect periodic limb movement disorder (PLMD)

Polysomnography is often followed by CPAP titration, which assesses the effectiveness of CPAP therapy in resolving SDB. While traditionally performed in a sleep laboratory setting, home sleep testing (HST) may be an option for select patients with appropriate insurance coverage.

SPECIAL INVESTIGATIONS FOR SLEEP EVALUATION

Assessment of the home environment identifies external factors that may disrupt sleep, such as noise, lighting, temperature, or uncomfortable bedding. It also includes reviewing bedroom safety, medication timing, and lifestyle habits to promote a conducive sleep setting for older adults.

Medication Review

Refer to **Table 4**.

TREATMENT OPTIONS: NONPHARMACOLOGIC AND PHARMACOLOGICAL

Sleep Hygiene Recommendations

Sleep hygiene recommendations are given in **Figure 2**.

Medications for Sleep

Hypnotic medications for older adults should be prescribed with careful consideration due to potential side

TABLE 4: Medications that contribute to sleep disturbance and their effects.

Medications contributing to sleep disturbances		Common effects on sleep
Cardiac medications	• Beta-blockers • Alpha-blockers • ACE inhibitor • Statins • Amiodarone	• Insomnia, nightmares • Palpitations, dizziness • Nocturnal cough
Psychiatry medications	SSRI, SNRI, MAO-I	Restless legs syndrome, insomnia, daytime sleepiness, decreased REM sleep
Neurological medications	• Anticonvulsant: Ethosuximide, lamotrigine • AChEI: Donepezil, galantamine, rivastigmine • Dopamine: L-DOPA, pergolide • Stimulants: Amphetamine, modafinil, caffeine	• Decreased REM and non-REM deep sleep • Increased sleep latency
Anti-infectives	Ciprofloxacin, amantadine, efavirenz, amphotericin B	Sleep latency increased
Analgesics	• NSAIDs • Opioids	• Reduction of slow-wave sleep • Respiratory depression
Corticosteroids	Prednisolone, dexamethasone	Sleep latency and maintenance, abnormal dreams
BPH	Alpha-blockers (tamsulosin, alfuzosin)	Palpitations

(AchEI: acetylcholinesterase inhibitor; ACE: angiotensin-converting enzyme; BPH: benign prostatic hyperplasia; MAO-I: monoamine oxidase inhibitor; NSAIDs: nonsteroidal anti-inflammatory drugs; REM: rapid eye movement; SNRI: serotonin–norepinephrine reuptake inhibitors; SSRI: selective serotonin reuptake inhibitor)

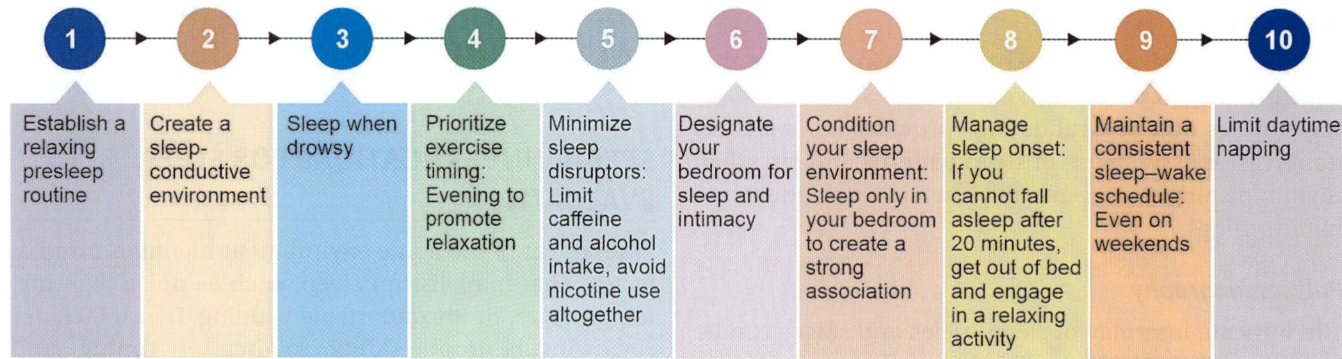

FIG. 2: Sleep hygiene recommendations.

TABLE 5: Pharmaceutical management of sleep disturbances in older adults.

Class with common adverse events	Type	Name	Dose (mg)	Half-life (hours)
Benzodiazepine • Daytime drowsiness • Increased fall risk • Mobility issues, dizziness • Cognitive impairment, delirium • Commonly used medications, such as clonazepam and alprazolam, are approved for the management of anxiety rather than sleep disturbances	Ultrashort-acting	Triazolam	0.125–0.25	2–4
	Short-acting	• Etizolam • Brotizolam	0.5–1	6
	Intermediate-acting	• Nitrazepam • Flunitrazepam • Estazolam	5–10 0.5–2 1–4	28 24 24
	Long-acting	• Flurazepam • Quazepam	10–30 15–30	65 36
Nonbenzodiazepine: • Headache, GI disturbances, dizziness, unusual night behaviors, amnesia, hallucinations with zolpidem		• Zolpidem • Zopiclone • Eszopiclone	5–10 7.5–10 1–2	2 4 7
Melatonin receptor agonist: • Headache, decreased alertness, daytime fatigue		Ramelteon	8	1–2
Dual orexin receptor antagonist: • Headache, somnolence, palpitations		Suvorexant	15	12

(GI: gastrointestinal)

effects. Short-acting medications at the lowest effective dose are preferred to minimize the risks of excessive sedation and falls. The best course of treatment might involve both behavioral therapy and medication **(Table 5)**.

Valerian, a herbal medication, quetiapine, and doxepin are also used for the management of sleep disturbances.

Management of primary sleep disorders in older adults (Table 6)

Sleep disturbance is a geriatric syndrome!

While older adults may report "not sleeping well" or experiencing early morning awakenings, these complaints often do not represent a single, defined disease. Instead, they may signify a geriatric syndrome—a cluster of interrelated factors contributing to disrupted nocturnal sleep or circadian rhythm imbalances. A geriatric syndrome, by definition, lacks a single, clear-cut cause and can arise from various factors. Impaired sleep in older adults exemplifies this concept, sharing several characteristics with other geriatric syndromes:

- *Increased prevalence with age*: The incidence of sleep problems rises significantly among older adults.
- *Distinct symptoms and outcomes*: The presentation and consequences often differ from the underlying pathologies or triggering events.
- *Multifactorial causation*: Multiple contributing factors can lead to sleep disturbances.
- *Downward trajectory*: Unattended sleep problems can contribute to a decline in overall health and physical, psychological, and social well-being.

TABLE 6: Summary of management of primary sleep disorders in older adults.

Sleep disorders	Evaluation	Nonpharmacologic management	Pharmacological management
Insomnia: Chronic insomnia is diagnosed when sleep problems (difficulty falling asleep or staying asleep) last *at least a month* and disrupt their daytime activities	*Sleep questionnaire*: • PSQI • ESS • ISI • PROMIS sleep disturbance scale • EQAS	*Cognitive-behavioral therapy*: • Sleep hygiene • Stimulus control • Sleep restriction–sleep compression, with cognitive restructuring *Other therapies*: • Massage • Exercise and physical activity • Relaxation therapy • Light therapy • Chronotherapy	• *Benzodiazepines (BZD)* • *Nonbenzodiazepines* • *Melatonin receptor agonist*
Sleep breathing disorders: Two types: 1. Obstructive sleep apnea (AHI value > 5 is diagnostic for OSA) 2. Central sleep apnea	Questionnaires • STOP-BANG • BQ • SACS • Epworth sleepiness scale (ESS) • *PSG*	• Avoidance of alcohol, sedatives, and opiates • Weight reduction • Treatment of comorbidities such as CHF	• No pharmacological treatment • Continuous positive airway pressure (CPAP) is the best approach • Oral appliances
Restless legs syndrome: Unpleasant leg sensations that disrupt sleep worse at night and improve toward morning • Primary/idiopathic • Secondary: IDA, ESRD	• Medication review: • TCA, SSRI, dopamine antagonists, lithium • Caffeine use • BMI: Obesity • Family history • Iron profile/ferritin • Renal function	• Moderate exercise • Smoking and alcohol cessation • Caffeine reduction • Stopping offending medications • Iron repletion	• *Dopaminergic agents*: Ropinirole, pramipexole • BZD • Opioids • *Anticonvulsants*: Gabapentin, carbamazepine
Circadian rhythm sleep disorders: Normal sleep, but sleep schedule is misaligned • Advanced sleep phase disorder (ASPD) • Irregular sleep–wake disorder (ISWD)	• Sleep diary • Actigraphy	• Sleep hygiene • Chronotherapy • Evening bright light therapy (7–9 PM)	Melatonin
REM sleep behavior disorder: • Dysfunction of motor neuron inhibition leading to absence of normal atonia during REM sleep • Violent motor behaviors associated with dream enactment • Most dramatic and potentially injurious	• PSG • MRI of the brain • Medications review: TCA, SSRI • Alcohol • Caffeine	Environmental safety: Remove dangerous objects from the vicinity, pad hard and sharp surfaces, to avoid falls: mattress on the floor	• Clonazepam (0.5–1 mg, 1–2 hours before bedtime) • Levodopa • Dopamine agonists • Melatonin
Summary of management of sleep disturbance with common comorbidities—usually have a bidirectional relationship with sleep			
Depression: Risk and symptom	SSRI and SNRI used for depression may increase wakefulness, reduce REM sleep time	CBT	• Mirtazapine • Trazodone • Agomelatine

Continued

Continued

Sleep disorders	Evaluation	Nonpharmacologic management	Pharmacological management
Neurodegenerative disorders: *Parkinson*: Multifactorial—nocturnal motor symptoms, RBD, nocturia, medications	PSG	Timing of medications: Selegiline and amantadine in the morning, early evening levodopa	• Melatonin • Dopamine agonist (rotigotine) • MAO-B inhibitor (rasagiline)
Dementia: Abnormal nighttime behaviors such as confusion, wandering, and agitation, leading to disrupted sleep. This leads to daytime exhaustion, resulting in daytime napping, creating a cycle	PSG: Increased latency, reduced SWS, REM sleep	• Multidomain interventions • CBT • Light therapy	• Melatonin • Trazodone
Heart failure: Orthopnea, PND	• PSG: CSA/OSA • Sleep onset latency, arousals, and early morning waking	Timing of diuretics	• ACE inhibitor • Beta-blockers ±
Chronic respiratory diseases: COPD, asthma	• Overnight pulse oximetry • PSG	• Avoid theophylline, corticosteroids • Avoid sedative hypnotics	• Optimization of respiratory disorders • Melatonin
GERD	• Nocturnal cough • PSG: Multiple arousals	• Early light dinner • Raising the head end of the bed	Proton-pump inhibitors
Nocturia: • Causes: BPH, detrusor overactivity • DM, DI, CHF, AF, venous stasis disorder, CKD, CLD	• Reduced SWS • PSA, HbA1c, LFT, KFT, electrolytes, USG with PVR	• Medication review: Diuretics, CCB, SGLT-2i • Reducing nocturnal fluid consumption	• Alpha-1 receptor antagonists • 5-alpha reductase inhibitors • Bladder relaxants
Long-term care	• Medication review • Environment review	• Bright light therapy and daytime sun exposure • Exercise activities and reduce bedtime during the day • Following the bedtime routine • Decrease nighttime noise and light	Manage: Pain, paresthesia, cough, GERD, nocturia, dyspnea

(ACE: angiotensin-converting enzyme; AF: atrial fibrillation; AHI: apnea–hypopnea index; BMI: body mass index; BPH: benign prostatic hyperplasia; BQ: Berlin Questionnaire; CCB: calcium channel blocker; CHF: congestive heart failure; CKD: chronic kidney disease; CLD: chronic liver disease; COPD: chronic obstructive pulmonary disease; CSA: central sleep apnea; DI: diabetes insipidus; DM: diabetes mellitus; EQAS: Essener Questionnaire on Age and Sleepiness; ESRD: end-stage renal disease; GERD: gastroesophageal reflux disease; HbA1c: glycated hemoglobin; IDA: iron deficiency anemia; ISI: Insomnia Severity Index; KFT: kidney function test; LFT: liver function test; MAO-B: monoamine oxidase B; MRI: magnetic resonance imaging; OSA: obstructive sleep apnea; PROMIS: Patient-reported Outcomes Information System Sleep Disturbance Scale; PSG: polysomnography; PSQI: Pittsburgh Sleep Quality Index; PVR: postvoid residual; RBD: REM sleep behavior disorder; REM: rapid eye movement; SACS: Sleep Apnea Clinical Score; SGLT-2i: sodium-glucose cotransporter-2 inhibitor; SNRI: serotonin–norepinephrine reuptake inhibitors; SSRI: selective serotonin reuptake inhibitor; SWS: slow-wave sleep; TCA: tricyclic antidepressant; USG: ultrasonography)

APPROACH TO DIAGNOSIS OF SLEEP DISORDERS BASED ON COMMON COMPLAINTS

The approach to diagnosis of sleep disorders based on common complaints is shown in **Flowchart 2**.

CONCLUSION

Sleep disturbances in older adults are highly prevalent and multifactorial, often arising from age-related physiological changes, comorbidities, medications, and psychosocial factors. Recognizing sleep disorders

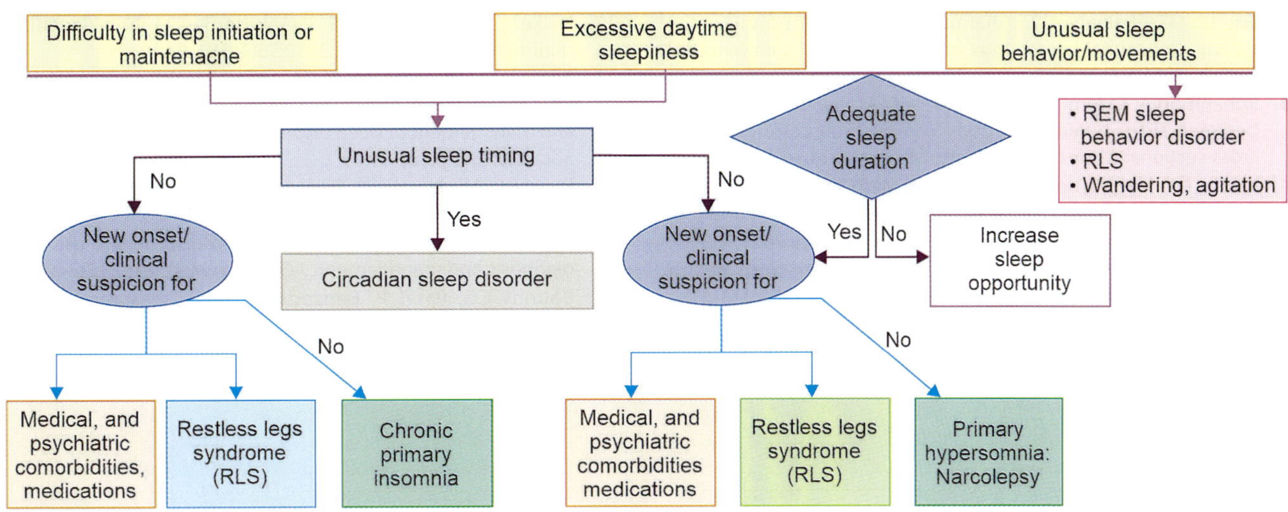

FLOWCHART 2: Approach to diagnosis of sleep disorders based on common complaints.
(REM: rapid eye movement)

as a geriatric syndrome underscores the need for a holistic, multidisciplinary approach integrating lifestyle interventions, sleep hygiene, behavioral therapy, and judicious pharmacological use. Early identification and comprehensive management not only improve sleep quality but also enhance overall physical, cognitive, and emotional well-being, thereby promoting successful aging.

Self-Assessment Questionnaire

Q1. What are the sleep disorders in the elderly and age-related changes in sleep patterns?
Q2. How common are sleep disorders in older people?
Q3. What are the risk factors for sleep disorders in older people?
Q4. What are the consequences of sleep disorders?
Q5. How do you evaluate sleep disorders in OPD?
Q6. How do you treat sleep disorders?
Q7. Is sleep impairment a geriatric syndrome?
Q8. What is the role of a geriatrician in managing sleep disorders?

FURTHER READINGS

1. Taillard J, Gronfier C, Bioulac S, Philip P, Sagaspe P. Sleep in normal aging, homeostatic and circadian regulation and vulnerability to sleep deprivation. Brain Sci. 2021;11(8):1003.
2. Institute of Medicine (US) Committee on Sleep Medicine and Research. Sleep Disorders and Sleep Deprivation: An Unmet Public Health Problem. In: Colten HR, Altevogt BM, (eds). Washington (DC): National Academies Press (US); 2006.
3. Dean GE, Weiss C, Morris JL, Chasens ER. Impaired Sleep. Nurs Clin North Am. 2017;52(3):387-404.
4. Lavoie CJ, Zeidler MR, Martin JL. Sleep and aging. Sleep Sci Pract. 2018;2(1):3.
5. Scholtens RM, van Munster BC, van Kempen MF, de Rooij SEJA. Physiological melatonin levels in healthy older people: a systematic review. J Psychosom Res. 2016;86:20-7.
6. Li J, Vitiello MV, Gooneratne N. Sleep in normal aging. Sleep Med Clin. 2018;13(1):1-11.
7. Gulia KK, Kumar VM. Sleep disorders in the elderly: a growing challenge. Psychogeriatrics. 2018;18(3):155-65.
8. Tatineny P, Shafi F, Gohar A, Bhat A. Sleep in the elderly. Mo Med. 2020;117(5):490-5.
9. Gordon NP, Yao JH, Brickner LA, Lo JC. Prevalence of sleep-related problems and risks in a community-dwelling older adult population: a cross-sectional survey-based study. BMC Public Health. 2022;22(1):2045.
10. Regati M, Vijayakumar P. Study of sleep disorders in the elderly visiting geriatrics department. J Fam Med Prim Care. 2022;11(2):614-22.
11. Sanjay TV, Thejaswini P, Vinay J, Nandini RC, Kavya U, Aparna A. Prevalence of insomnia and its associated factors among geriatric population in an urban locality of Bengaluru, Karnataka, India—a cross-sectional study. J Clin Diagn Res. 2023;17(3): LC06-10.

12. Gambhir IS, Chakrabarti SS, Sharma AR, Saran DP. Insomnia in the elderly—a hospital-based study from North India. J Clin Gerontol Geriatr. 2014;5(4):117-21.
13. Kohanmoo A, Kazemi A, Zare M, Akhlaghi M. Gender-specific link between sleep quality and body composition components: a cross-sectional study on the elderly. Sci Rep. 2024;14(1):8113.
14. Vitiello MV. Sleep in normal aging. Sleep Med Clin. 2006;1(2):171-6.
15. Mc Carthy CE. Sleep disturbance, sleep disorders and co-morbidities in the care of the older person. Med Sci. 2021;9(2):31.
16. Medic G, Wille M, Hemels ME. Short- and long-term health consequences of sleep disruption. Nat Sci Sleep. 2017;9:151-61.
17. Neikrug AB, Ancoli-Israel S. Sleep disorders in the older adult—a mini-review. Gerontology. 2010;56(2):181-9.
18. Bloom HG, Ahmed I, Alessi CA, Ancoli-Israel S, Buysse DJ, Kryger MH, et al. Evidence-based recommendations for the assessment and management of sleep disorders in older persons. J Am Geriatr Soc. 2009;57(5):761-89.
19. Reynolds AC, Adams RJ. Treatment of sleep disturbance in older adults. J Pharm Pract Res. 2019;49(3):296-304.
20. Suzuki K, Miyamoto M, Hirata K. Sleep disorders in the elderly: diagnosis and management. J Gen Fam Med. 2017;18(2):61-71.
21. Bounds CG, Patel P. Benzodiazepines. Treasure Island (FL): StatPearls Publishing; 2024.

CHAPTER 22

Elder Abuse

Mala Kapur Shankardass

CASE VIGNETTE

Patient information: Mrs Saroj Khanna, a 78-year-old, is a soft spoken, healthy, short stature, fair complexioned lady with no major ailment but a bit of hearing problem, few dental issues, weak eyesight, feels heavy- or lightheaded at times, dizzy often, and has mobility difficulty due to swelling in ankle.

Living situation: Being a widow, she lives with her son and daughter-in-law, both working, and three teenaged grandchildren, who remain busy with studies, in a joint household in an urban middle-class residential locality with limited space for her movements and daily activities, although she is the owner of the two-story house.

Primary care physician: Dr Neeraj Jain.

Presenting complaint: A few bruises on her left upper arm, remains withdrawn, lost in her thoughts, complaints of pain in the upper arm and ankle along with swelling and thus does not want to go to the kitchen for preparation of meals.

History of present illness: Bruises have been a frequent feature for the last 3 years after she became a widow. They are painful, along with recent pain in the ankle, which is troublesome and inhibits her movements. Due to swelling in the ankle, she finds it difficult to wear footwear and thus restricts her movement only to the kitchen for cooking meals and going to the toilet/bathroom. Without intake of proper medications, she is in constant pain and feels dizzy and heavy-/lightheaded due to pain.

Medical history: She has no diabetes and deficiency of vitamins is not known. She has not been tested for osteoporosis or any musculoskeletal issues nor for hypertension.

Social history: Mrs Khanna belongs to a middle-class family and has obtained education till the intermediate level. She was married for 52 years when her husband, 7 years older to her, working for a private company, passed away due to cardiac arrest. He enjoyed good health with no major ailment. A mother of four children, three sons and a daughter, Mrs Khanna stays with her eldest son and his family. Her youngest son passed away at an early age due to an accident, and the middle son who has been abroad for many years is not married. He has very little contact with her or with his siblings and has no interest in returning to the country. Her only daughter is married with two daughters; she lives in another town with her husband. The daughter used to visit her parental family every year, but after her father's death, she is not really welcome in the house by her brother and his family. She occasionally talks over phone with her mother, but conversations are limited and cordial. Mrs Khanna has no assets in her name except for the monthly rent received from the first-floor tenants, but the money is handled by her son. She is totally dependent on her son and his immediate family for her day-to-day living. She has a quaint room to herself which is dingy with no window, just enough space for her bed and to keep few of her belongings of clothes. Her jewelry is with her son, who also is in control of her savings accumulated through rent of the first floor. She cooks all the meals for everyone in the family.

Review of systems: Apart from the bruises, feeling dizzy with pain, and swelling in the ankle, Mrs Khanna does not complain of any other health concern. Her problems of weak eyesight or of not being able to eat properly or able to hear clearly are not problems for her but only signs of moving on in years. Being withdrawn, not wanting to make conversation, or not feeling stable are accepted by her as fate, connected with widowhood.

Physical examination: Examination of swelling in the ankle of Mrs Khanna indicates a fracture, confirmed by an X-ray done against the wishes of the son. Her blood pressure is high, 156/95 mm Hg, and her heart rate is 98 beats/min which is connected with her being feeling unstable and probably the cause of a fall, thus leading to the fracture of the ankle. The withdrawal symptoms—not being talkative—indicate depression.

INTRODUCTION

Worldwide, elder abuse is recognized as a social evil, a societal problem that requires combatting strategies from a public health perspective. Identified by different names in various countries, such as elder mistreatment, abuse in late life or abuse of older adults or neglect, with some experts identifying it more as a gender concern, seen to be more prominent among older widows, especially in India. Universally, as suggested by the World Health Organization (WHO), it can be defined as a single or repeated act, or lack of appropriate action, occurring within any expected trusted relationship and resulting in harm or distress to an older person. Over the years, different countries by recognizing the need for governments to protect the dignity and respect of older persons in society have adopted various legislative measures to secure the position of older persons in families in particular and also to safeguard their interests at the institutional levels against abusive situations. In the Asian context, in particular, there is a lot of emphasis on maintaining filial piety which places the responsibility of support and care of older parents and relatives on the family members. But due to various socioeconomic and demographic transformations happening in societies, many families feel caring of older members as a burden, thus leading to their neglect, abuse, and mistreatment, as seen in India. Various research studies, national surveys, and reports by nongovernmental organizations (NGOs) indicate that older adults at times are harmed by people who are supposed to care for them and with whom they are in a trusted relationship, be it family members, a friend, or neighbor, or an individual on whom an older person relies for services. Governments, through certain policy initiatives, have framed specific legislative measures which make it obligatory for families and those under whose care older persons may be due to different kinds of relationships to care and support older relatives, especially the ones who cannot manage on their own for whatever reason, be it health, economic, or sociocultural.

Most often, elder abuse is recognized as a type of domestic violence due to the fact that it happens in a domestic setting as a result of marriage or cohabitation. In much of literature, this is seen to be synonymous with intimate partner violence as it is seen to be between people who are in an intimate relationship; however in the broadest sense, in discourses on elder abuse, it involves abuse, neglect, mistreatment, exploitation, violence against older parents or any known older relative, be it a sibling or a distant family member. Some scholars term this as family violence since it is committed by family members. In this century, recognition is also given to elder abuse committed by paid or even unpaid caregivers on older persons under their care whom they help in activities of daily living. These unpaid caregivers who have no specific training in caregiving and are without any professional skill are referred to as informal caregivers whose main tasks are to assist older persons, especially when experiencing impairments related to old age, disability, or cognitive decline/mental disorder. In general, such caregivers are from the recipient's family but also can be from the social network of the older adult such as siblings or any relative. In certain cases, informal caregivers are seen to prey on older persons for the assets owned by them, which could be money, property, or any other belonging with financial/economic value. Elder abuse by paid caregivers can happen in both family and community settings, but is associated more with that occurring in institutions involved with the care of older persons such as nursing homes, senior living places, residential homes, hospitals, long-term care facilities, or medical clinics.

Abuse/neglect/mistreatment/exploitation/violence against older adults can assume multiple forms, including:

- Physical (any intentional act causing injury, discomfort, trauma to an older person by way of bodily contact)
- Verbal (oral, gestured language that is insulting, harassing, derogatory, humiliating, belittling, rebuking involving scolding, and yelling toward an older person)
- Psychological/emotional (resulting in stress, depression, anxiety, maybe due to bullying)
- Economic (the abuser controls the victim's economic resources and makes the victim depend on the abuser financially)
- Sexual (abusive sexual behavior by the perpetrator on the victim, by either using physical force or taking advantage of the victim)
- Institutional (generally perpetrated by a service provider and could be in the form of neglect, financial exploitation, misinformation, treatment, etc.)
- Combination of all of the above

Pertinently all the different forms of elder abuse are a source of mental distress for the victim, leading to reduced quality of life and setting in of various health issues which could be known to the victimized older adult or she/he may be totally unaware of the problems or may be not able to comprehend the seriousness of violation of their human rights on their well-being. Certain kinds of abuse, especially those that involve physical aspects, such as beating, bruising, disfiguring a part of the body, and those that can also cause death are seen to be more severe for the health of the victim because besides leaving a physical damage on the body of the older person, they are harmful as mental health concern having many repercussions on the psychological state of the affected older adult and hence can lead to low self-esteem, loss of confidence in self, lot of physical and mental pain, and stress. Recognition of elder abuse/neglect or mistreatment taking place is difficult to be recognized and identified unless the victim speaks up or is visible to other nonabusing people around the older victim. Clearly, multiple circumstances can be covered under elder abuse, but it does not include the general type of criminal activities meted out against older people in society, for instance, robbery, burglary, etc.

Toward the end of the 20th century and more specifically in the beginning of this century, in particular around the time of the Second World Assembly on Ageing held in Madrid in 2002, the WHO brought international attention to the growing menace of elder abuse across countries; globally, government agencies, community-based organizations (CBOs), and professional groups voiced their opinion to recognize elder abuse as a serious social problem, especially as the demographic transition toward rapidly increasing proportion of older persons in the total populations became a visible reality of various nations. In 1997, the International Network of Prevention of Elder Abuse (INPEA), with the support of many stakeholders, voiced concern about growing incidences and prevalence of elder abuse in different countries and brought attention of the United Nations to take steps to stop elder abuse. Crucial to this combating strategy was the need to recognize the hidden and silent societal issue of elder abuse by raising voices against this evil. Thus, June 15, 2006 was designated as the *World Elder Abuse Awareness Day* (WEAAD). Since then, an increasing number of events are held around this date and month in various countries, commissioned by governments, NGOs, and civil society members, to raise awareness of elder abuse and highlight ways to challenge it by bringing in partnerships between the social, medical, and legal communities.

While awareness on elder abuse is rising among the general public and experts from the field of social and medical sciences, there is consensus that as a problem, elder abuse and its associated forms have significant adverse consequences on the well-being of the affected older person. The impacts of elder abuse on the overall health of the victim are becoming a growing concern, especially as they are seen to increase the risk of premature mortality and many different types of morbidities, some coexisting, thus making the issue crucial for tackling it through responses from the sociolegal and health systems. Families, social community workers, and medical and legal professionals need to strategize combating mechanisms, probably in partnership for addressing abuse of older adults but many experts are of the opinion that the medical and related specialist workers need to rise above others in identifying cases of elder abuse through health assessments including diagnosis based on medical and psychological parameters.

EPIDEMIOLOGY, WITH A FOCUS ON INDIAN DATA/LITERATURE

Global epidemiological data suggests elder abuse being a widespread problem across countries, being better recognized and documented than others in some nations. In general, experts assessing the problem of elder abuse ascertain an estimated prevalence of 5–10% among older populations, with commonality of the abuser being more often than someone not known to the victim, for instance a family member, in most cases adult children who are supposedly responsible for taking care of the older parent(s)/relatives or a friend, neighbor, caregiver, or staff of an institution where the victim may be residing.

In India, a national survey that was conducted as part of the Longitudinal Aging Study Wave 1 during 2017–2018 by using cross-sectional data for assessing the prevalence of elder abuse in the country indicates results on elder abuse/mistreatment and associated covariates with variations across states as overall 5.2% of older adults, defined as 60 years and above having experienced abuse in the year prior to the survey with 3% among this proportion stating it being perpetrated by family members within their own households. Among the types of elder abuse experienced, verbal abuse, i.e., showing disrespect toward the older adult, was most frequent. The survey indicates that the prevalence of verbal abuse can be as high as 66.6% within the household. Survey findings also reveal a high prevalence of neglect experienced by older persons within households where an abusive environment exists, being 47.5%. Consequently, emotional/psychological abuse is also seen to be a significant matter of concern as data shows it to be 36.8% in households that are identified as being abusive toward older adults. Crucially higher education level of the older adult provides protection against elder abuse, seen particularly among women. Older adults without a spouse, with functional limitations, and having multiple morbidities, were more likely to experience abuse and neglect from family members and were also at a greater risk of facing abusive situations by care providers. Significantly, survey findings reveal that older adults who experienced abuse, including neglect and mistreatment, were two times more likely to have depressive symptoms. This could be a reason for victims of elder abuse not raising a voice against their plight or seeking any help.

These findings clearly point toward urgent attention required to combat elder abuse in the Indian society, as much it should be a priority globally too by treating the concern as a public health problem. We should not ignore the fact that various other studies conducted by researchers and a few NGOs, including a national-level large NGO HelpAge India, show similar trends, pointing toward the increasing incidences and prevalence of elder abuse in the Indian society, quite similar to trends seen in other countries too. Most of the increases relate to a rise in the population of older persons and growing ageism seen in societies that are making older adults more vulnerable to abusive environments while living in community settings or in institutional settings. In addition, lack of protection and safeguarding of interests of aging populations in different countries increases the risk of elder abuse. It is important that policies for older persons take into account mechanisms to identify the occurrence of abuse and consequential impacts on the well-being of older persons and then find strategies to manage it by looking at solutions which can place older adults in a better, less abusive situation. At the community level, it is difficult to recognize that in a family, an older person is getting abused, but if and when the victim for some reason comes for examination at a medical clinic or at the hospital, the medical personnel attending can make attempts to identify if the patient is an abusive environment. The process of recognizing the occurrence of elder abuse needs to be handled carefully and further managed in seeking solutions to address the concern and remove the victim away from abusive circumstances.

It is a very significant development that the Indian government has adopted legislative measures to address the concern of abuse and neglect of older persons in society. India has a distinctive legislation supporting traditional family values of care for older persons. The Maintenance and Welfare of Parents and Senior Citizens Act, enacted in 2007 and now being amended, has a broad scope covering all Indians except those residing in Jammu and Kashmir and Himachal Pradesh (HP) since the HP government has its own legislation for maintenance of seniors in the family. Under this legislation, the sons and daughters-in-law, and daughters and sons-in-law have a legal obligation to support parents and grandparents, and if this does not happen, then a cap of a monthly allowance of ₹10,000 has to be paid to the parent(s) for their well-being. The Act also includes societal provisions to care for older persons in terms of developing and supporting "Old Age Homes" in each district. Significantly, while the Act has put the responsibility to care for older people on the family members, it also has been expanded in scope to include the maintenance of physical and mental health of older persons and thus attempts to prevent elder abuse. The legislation has provisions for older adults to report abuse and pertinently includes consideration for including emotional forms of abuse. The Act also calls for enhanced measures for institutions to be involved with care of older adults and also has recommendations for home care services for older persons. A critical review of the legislation in place indicates that social, medical, and legal responses to address elder abuse have to go hand in hand. The role of medical practitioners in identifying elder abuse and working with stakeholders in reducing abuse or eliminating the abusive environment is extremely critical and needs urgent attention. Generally, it is observed by experts working on elder abuse issues that medical practitioners are often not properly equipped to diagnose elder abuse as they often do not have adequate training on this subject. Thus, the following discussion becomes extremely relevant in this context.

CLINICAL PRESENTATION

It is important that when an older adult comes or is brought to the medical clinic for a checkup, the medical practitioner should become cautious of elder abuse if any bruises are seen on the body of the older adult for which any immediate health cause cannot be physiologically verified; also if the older person is reluctant to speak up about health concerns or cannot provide explanation about the health condition, then probing on the health issues should be undertaken. In many cases, the accompanying person would do all the talking which also can be a warning sign for the practitioner to not take all that is being told about the patient at face value. In the case of Mrs Khanna, she is brought to the medical clinic for a checkup by her son as she is in a lot of pain and her ankle is swollen. The reason for these symptoms to be troubling the patient, as indicated by her son, is related to a fall that Mrs Khanna had a couple of days ago. However, how the fall took place could not be explained logically by the son. When the cause of the health concern needing treatment is under doubt, it also becomes a reason for the medical practitioner to go deeper into the matter. To understand the extent of the injury and have a proper diagnosis done, the medical practitioner must do proper medical investigations.

The first step toward beginning the process of investigations is that the medical practitioner must try to talk directly with the patient by building her confidence to reveal all issues related to the problem. The medical practitioner should insist on talking to the patient alone so that there is no intimidation from the accompanying person/relative. In the case of Mrs Khanna, the facts placed about her fall and bruises before the doctor do not tally with her son's version, and also the extent of injury seems inappropriate to the kind of causes for the problem. The medical practitioner, suspecting fracture based on the extent of pain and swelling, gets an X-ray done, and it reveals not a minor fall as claimed by the son nor does it correlate with the kind of fall that Mrs Khanna states to have happened. It is crucial that the doctor does further investigations to understand that if the fall was minor, then having a fracture instead of a sprain means that either Mrs Khanna has deeper problems which could be related to osteoporosis or bone health as a result of certain deficiencies and aging process. This requires proper treatment and more detailed investigations on the health status of Mrs Khanna.

While detailed investigations are needed to assess the chronicity of deterioration of bone health, what is relevant and crucial for investigation if the patient is a victim of elder abuse is to probe deeper to know if the fall was a result of a push meant to harm Mrs Khanna purposely to abuse her for certain specific reasons or there could be a clinical cause related to issues of gait. In case that is the cause, then additional examinations of various health parameters of Mrs Khanna need to be done. Absence of proper care and neglect of the health of Mrs Khanna in itself indicate that she is a case of elder abuse as her family members are ignoring her health and not providing proper health care for her. Further, it is necessary for the medical practitioner to also assess the cause of bruises, whether they are also signs of abusive behavior toward Mrs Khanna. It must be investigated if the patient is physically tortured and her skin is getting bruised due to physical violent behavior meted out against her.

The criticality of the issue is that while taking history and conducting physical examination of the patient, the physician should attempt to detect signs of abuse and recognize whether these are subtle characteristics of underlying abuse that the victim and the perpetrator may be trying to cover up in a normal setting.

What is required for a doctor to be trained to identify an abusive environment and consequently make attempts to prevent it is an important aspect dealt with in the next section of this chapter.

EXAMINATION

Detection of elder abuse is not easy, but it is pivotal for the medical community to adopt measures that can help in the detection and diagnosis of abuse occurring so that prompt interventional action can take place and the patient's risk of any further mistreatment, neglect, abuse, and violence taking place can be stopped. The medical practitioner, when consulted by a patient or for the older person, should conduct an examination confidently that works toward ascertaining the incidence of abuse. This is pertinent as symptoms of elder abuse can be mimic of those found in other medical conditions. For instance, burn marks can resemble dermatitis, and bruises which might appear to be caused by the impact of certain medications, such as anticoagulants, nonsteroidal anti-inflammatory drugs (NSAIDs), or cortisones, could in fact be due to physical injury inflicted on the person. In addition, a fracture that may be due to osteoporosis might have happened because of a strong push given to the person. Further, a doctor must be able to understand the depressive nature of the patient and correlate it with a case of depressive disorder, a common ailment for older persons, or is it fear and threat from the perpetrator of abuse that leads to withdrawal symptoms and an uncommunicative nature. It is crucial that the healthcare provider differentiates between abusive symptoms and medical parameters to appropriately chalk out a treatment plan.

The steps recommended as a diagnostic method and a resource for identifying elder abuse are as follows:

1. Take patient history and uncover potential risk factors.
2. Identify signs of current abuse and try to understand its pattern.
3. Make a note of follow-up consultations if they happen, and whether they are as per practitioners' suggestions or being skipped.
4. Record frequency of injuries.
5. Judge the promptness of seeking medical care and hesitation in leaving the victim alone with the practitioner.
6. Understand the reluctance of the patient tin seeking help due to a fear of increased abuse and further intense repercussions.
7. Gain trust of the patient, be nonjudgemental and sympathetic to the patient, and build confidentiality.

Screening Tools for Identifying Abuse

Across countries, a number of screening tools are used for history taking of the patient when suspected of abuse based on standardized questions related to occurrence, frequency, and intensity of symptoms related to injury. One of the common screening tools is Elder Abuse

Suspicion Index that is administered to cognitively stable patients, where with the help of a questionnaire six dichotomous answers in "yes/no" mode are asked from the patient. This tool is seen to show specificity of abuse of 75% when answers are yes relating to neglect, harm/injury, and violence against the victim. The advantages of using this tool are that it can be used in clinics and primary care setups, which are generally the first contact point between the suspected victim and the medical care provider, and a quick assessment an done within a short time. However, this tool provides a one-sided assessment of the elder abuse situation by looking at the caregiver of the victim as a suspected perpetrator but without a chance of evaluating the extent of the role of the supposed abuser.

Another popular screening tool being recommended in literature is the Elder Assessment Instrument, which involves many evaluation items, generally 44 appropriate questions covering social habits, medical history, emotional neglect aspects, psychological parameters, and many more related to other aspects of day-to-day interactions. The questionnaire takes about 15 minutes to administer, is easy to do, and each question is scored on a Likert scale ranging from 1 (no evidence) to 4 (evidence). This tool has a number of disadvantages such as not showing overall scoring system to indicate the intensity of abuse and difficult to validate subcategories to assess abuse; however, overall it has a sensitivity of 71% and specificity of 93% which points toward its useful utility.

Besides the elder abuse assessment tools mentioned in the preceding text, the use of older adult psychological abuse measures is fruitful in dealing with abuse cases. This takes into account the level of risk factors leading to abuse by including isolation, insensitivity, show of disrespect, intimidation, and threats toward the victim and has 92% reliability in assessment. It is important that the medical practitioners make use of these tools which are being more widely used in certain countries abroad, where the issue of elder abuse is dealt with in a more serious manner. In India, the awareness on the need to detect, diagnose, and manage elder abuse is of recent origin but it is an important field that requires the medical professionals to play an active role in dealing with elder abuse as through investigations, physical examination, and correlating symptoms with other medical conditions, suspicion of elder abuse can be confirmed.

As physical abuse and emotional/psychological abuse are more common forms and are related to when financial and sexual abuse may happen, physical examination of older adults calls for action and the medical practitioner is most equipped for that. Thus, following suspicion of abuse, relatives of an older person who may want to help should take the suspected victim for a checkup at a medical clinic where a comprehensive physical examination encompassing the patient's entire body should be done by the healthcare worker in order to detect signs of abuse. Following this, there could be a need for more detailed investigations, especially to see abuse due to neglect of taking care of health parameters.

MANAGEMENT

Once elder abuse is confirmed, taking the next steps of getting the victim out of the abusive environment is important, and for these various legal and social remedial steps should be taken by the healthcare worker. Of course, to begin with, the caretaker should be approached and counseled to stop abuse. A community or social worker or an NGO should also be approached to keep a watch on the victim so that further abuse is stopped from happening. A legal practitioner and law enforcement agency should also be consulted and brought into loop so that relief measures can be adopted to safeguard the victim. Significantly, the older adult who is being abused needs to be encouraged to speak out against abuse and helped in moving out of the abusive environment. Dealing with elder abuse requires input from the older person, family members who are not abusing, community and social workers, and medical and legal professionals. However, the role of the medical professional is most crucial as detection and identification of abuse is possible more by their contribution; thus, it is important that medical practitioners adopt a proactive role in combating elder abuse.

CONCLUSION

With rapid growth of oldest cohort in India, along with disintegration of joint family, elder abuse is getting recognied as a pressing societal and public health concern.

This chapter calls for urgent and collaborative action from families, communities, medical professionals, and legal systems to identify, prevent, and address elder abuse in both domestic and institutional settings. The manifestation of abuse can be physical, emotional, financial, and psychological forms with detrimental consequences for the overall health and well-being of the elderly.

The Maintenance and Welfare of Parents and Senior Citizens Act is a legal safeguard to older adults, but effective implementation and awareness at the community and institutional levels are critical.

Geriatrician may plays a pivotal role in detecting and managing cases of elder abuse, and there is a need to enhance their training and proactive response to such situations.

Self-Assessment Questionnaire

Q1. Define elder abuse as per the World Health Organization (WHO).

Q2. What are the primary forms of elder abuse?

Q3. How demographic and socioeconomic changes contributed to the increasing incidence of elder abuse in India?

Q4. What legal provisions are included in the Maintenance and Welfare of Parents and Senior Citizens Act, 2007, to prevent elder abuse in India?

Q5. What are the warning signs a geriatrician must notice to diagnose possible elder abuse during examination or history taking?

Q6. Describe the multidisciplinary strategies to manage elder abuse.

Q7. Why is elder abuse often underreported, and what measures can improve early detection and prevention within families and communities?

FURTHER READINGS

1. Bagga A, Sakurkar A. Abuse and violence in the lives of older women: its impact on their mental health. HelpAge India Res Dev J. 2011;17(3):7-19.
2. Bansod DW, Phad S, Kundu J. Elder abuse and its implications on health status of the elderly in India. In: Shankardass MK (Ed). Ageing issues in India: practices, perspectives and policies. Singapore: Springer; 2021. pp. 361-80.
3. HelpAge India. (2018). Elder abuse in India—2018: changing cultural ethos and impact of technology. [online] Available from https://www.helpageindia.org/documents/research/research-reports
4. Jahangir S, Nikhil PNN, Bailey A, Datta A. Contextualizing elder abuse and neglect in institutional and home settings: case studies from India. In: Shankardass MK, Rajan SI (Eds). Abuse and neglect of the elderly in India. Singapore: Springer; 2018. pp. 175-88.
5. Government of India. (2007). The Maintenance and Welfare of Parents and Senior Citizens Act, Bill no. 56 (2007). [online] Available from https://www.indiacode.nic.in/handle/123456789/2033?sam_handle=123456789/1362. [Last accessed May, 2025].
6. Government of India. (2019). The Maintenance and Welfare of Parents and Senior Citizens Amendment, Bill no. 374 (2019). [online] Available from https://prsindia.org/files/bills_acts/bills_parliament/2019/Maintenance%20and%20Welfare%20of%20Parents%20and%20Senior%20Citizens%20(Amendment)%20Bill,%202019.pdf. [Last accessed May, 2025].
7. Patel K, Bunachita S, Chiu H, Suresh P, Patel UK. Elder abuse: a comprehensive overview and physician-associated challenges. Cureus. 2021;13(4):e14375.
8. Shankardass MK. Maintenance and Welfare Bill, 2007 as adult protection legislation: a critical assessment. HelpAge India-Res Dev J. 2007;13(3).
9. Shankardass MK. Elder abuse and adult protection. In: Johnson CS, Rajan SI (Eds). Aging and health in India. Jaipur: Rawat Publications; 2010: pp. 187-209.
10. Shankardass MK. Elder abuse prevention in Asia: some challenges and age-friendly initiatives in selected countries. J AARP Int. 2010 pp. 1-6.
11. Shankardass MK. Addressing elder abuse: review of societal responses in India and selected Asian countries. Int Psychogeriatr. 2013;25(8):1229-34.
12. Shankardass MK. (2016). Elder abuse: Stop it, prevent and manage it. The Asian Age. [online] Available from https://www.asianage.com/life-and-style/elder-abuse-stop-it-prevent-and-manage-it-793. [Last accessed May, 2025].
13. Shankardass MK. Perspectives on abuse and neglect of the elderly in India. In: Shankardass MK, Rajan SI (Eds). Abuse and neglect of the elderly in India. Singapore: Springer; 2018. pp. 13-30.
14. Shankardass MK. Where the elderly are vulnerable to abuse. Hindustan Times, 2018 May 9.
15. Shankardass MK. Perspectives on elder abuse and mistreatment from selected countries and regions: a preamble. In: Shankardass MK (Ed). International Handbook of Elder Abuse and Mistreatment. Singapore: Springer; 2020. pp. 1-12.
16. Shankardass MK. Reflections on elder abuse and mistreatment in India. In: Shankardass MK (Ed.). International handbook of elder abuse and mistreatment. Singapore: Springer; 2020. pp. 371-84.
17. Shankardass MK. What do we know of elder abuse in the Indian context? In: Shankardass MK, (Ed). Handbook of Aging, Health and Public Policy: Perspectives from Asia. Singapore: Springer Nature; 2022. p. 1-13.
18. Sathya T, Selvamani Y, Nagarajan R. Elder abuse/mistreatment and associated covariates in India: results from the Longitudinal Aging Study in India wave 1, 2017–2018. Epidemiol Health. 2022;44:e2022017.

CHAPTER 23

Diseases of Aging Eye

Ananya Parampalli Ravindra, Yogita Gupta, Radhika Tandon

CASE VIGNETTE

Patient information: Mrs GS is a 76-year-old homemaker with a history of type 2 diabetes and hypertension.

Living situation: She lives with her husband, Mr RS, a 78-year-old retired schoolteacher.

Presenting complaint: Mrs GS, a 76-year-old female, presents with a complaint of gradual, painless, and progressive diminution of vision in both her eyes over the past 5 years.

History of presenting illness: The patient was apparently well until about 5 years ago when she developed complaints of gradually painless progressive diminution of vision in both her eyes; the right eye was comparatively worse, with no associated complaints of glare, colored haloes around lights, photophobia, or any obvious blind spots or scotomas. She gives a history of usage of over-the-counter eye drops which claimed to improve vision but found no benefit with the same.

Medical history: She was diagnosed with type 2 diabetes at the age of 55 years, after which she has been on oral hypoglycemic agents, with which she is reasonably compliant but admits that she forgets to take them once in a while. She got her blood sugars tested last week, and her fasting blood glucose was 200 mg/dL and glycated hemoglobin level was 8.8%. Her blood pressure, on the other hand, is well controlled on medications.

Review of systems: She denies any other systemic issues than occasional episodes of weakness.

Physical examination: Her blood pressure is 124/78 mm Hg, heart rate was 80 beats/min, examination of respiratory, cardiovascular and neurological systems reveal no obvious abnormalities.

Ocular examination: Visual acuity in the right eye was 6/60 and that in the left eye was 6/24, with normal intraocular pressures (IOPs) of 12 and 14 mm Hg in the right and left eyes, respectively. The orbits, eyelids, adnexa, and extraocular movements were within normal limits, and direct and consensual pupillary reactions were normal. Slit-lamp biomicroscopy revealed clear corneas, deep anterior chambers, and immature senile cataracts (right > left). Fundus evaluation showed mild nonproliferative diabetic retinopathy (NPDR) changes with no macular edema.

Management: An endocrinology referral was sought to optimize the blood sugar levels, after which she was taken up for right eye phacoemulsification under topical anesthesia, and an enhanced monofocal intraocular lens was implanted. A week later, the same surgery was performed in the fellow eye. She was advised strict blood sugar control and an annual fundus review in view of mild NPDR without macular edema.

Treatment outcomes: Her postoperative visual acuity was 6/6 in both eyes, and with well-controlled blood pressure and sugar levels, no worsening of retinopathy was noted on follow-up.

The patient had a successful outcome of cataract surgery on both eyes with an improvement in quality of life.

INTRODUCTION

Senescence manifests in every organ of the human body, including the eye, due to several theorized mechanisms operating at cellular and organ levels, which may be programmed or unprogrammed, along with neuroendocrine degeneration and accumulation of cellular waste products and genetic damage to cells. In healthy conditions, the eye functions like a sophisticated and precise camera system; light enters through transparent tear film and cornea (the frontmost part of the eye) and then passes through aqueous humor, pupil ("aperture" of the eye), crystalline lens, and vitreous humor and finally focuses an image on the light-sensitive retina (screen) of the eye. The image signals ("afferent pathway") are sent from both eyeballs through neurons to the brain's visual cortex via the optic nerve for further visual processes to produce a three-dimensional (3D) binocular image of the object being viewed. The normal visual function gets disturbed in case of age-related deviations or dysfunction in the eye.

With aging, several changes are noted in the eye which result in worsening of vision **(Box 1)**. A change in vision is often the first sign noted by individuals while aging. In the fifth decade of life, most individuals notice that the reading distance, where they can see the nearby objects comfortably, has changed for them. The lens fibers and zonules develop stiffening with age. As a result, the eye loses the power of accommodation and is unable to focus on near objects ("presbyopia"). Lens, which is clear in healthy conditions, loses its transparency due to opacification of lens fibers and capsule and develops "senile cataracts" as one ages. Other ocular pathological processes related to aging may result in visual impairment. For example, age-related macular degeneration (ARMD), which affects the central part of the retina (the "macula") causes deterioration of the most precise central field of vision, leading to inability to recognize faces or perform reading activities.

BOX 1 Physiological changes in the eye related to aging.

- The corneal transparency is reduced due to weakening of corneal endothelial cell pump
- The lens becomes denser and lens transparency reduces
- The lens fibers and zonules stiffen with age, leading to difficulty in accommodation
- The pupil's reactions to light become slower
- The binocular functions of eye, such as depth perception, are weaker
- The ocular surface is drier due to reduced tear secretion
- The eyelid skin and tissues are more lax, leading to dropping of eyelid (senile ptosis)
- The orbital fat decreases in amount, which leads to a sunken appearance of eyeballs (deep-set eyes)
- The fine details such as color hues and different tones are difficult to discern as there is a decrease in the number of nerve cells that transmit visual signals from the eyes to the brain
- The vitreous condensations are seen [posterior vitreous detachments (PVDs)], which may present as floaters

A thin line exists between pathological and physiological processes of aging, and most commonly geriatric physicians see features of both of these. The eye may be involved in any disease process occurring in the other bodily systems, and conversely, ocular disease can be heralded by systemic manifestations of tissue dysfunction. In addition, drugs used to treat systemic disease may have ocular adverse effects, and likewise, systemic absorption of topically applied eye drops can manifest as systemic adverse effects.

The study of geriatric ocular changes has become important in the last century due to an increase in life expectancy and a concurrent increase in the number of older persons worldwide. Globally, more than 250 million people have visual impairment, with over 80% of them being 50 years of age or older. The Longitudinal Aging Study in India (LASI, 2017–2019) estimated that blindness was six times more prevalent (3.8%) in those aged over 60 years than among older adults aged 45–59 years (0.6%). The survey conducted in India for Rapid Assessment of Avoidable Blindness (RAAB, 2015–2019) made an estimate that visual impairment of moderate to severe degree (MSVI) in the total study population was seen in 2.19%, while that calculated only in people aged ≥ 50 years was a whopping 11.77%; blindness was seen in 0.36% in all age groups, whereas that in people aged 50 years or older was 1.99%.

Disease processes in the elderly are complex and often compounded by problems such as cognitive impairment, hearing impairment (presbycusis), locomotor disabilities, mobility challenges due to osteoporosis, arthritis, etc., depression, and other comorbidities. These necessitate more specific attention from the caregiver's part as compared to younger patients with similar ophthalmic problems.

EYE DISEASES IN THE GERIATRIC POPULATION

Disease burden: The India Study of Age-related Eye Disease (IndEye) was a large population-based study of people aged ≥ 60 years in rural and urban areas of North and South India (population size > 2,000) which estimated the age- and gender-specific prevalence of age-related pathologies (ARMD, lens opacities) and their associations. The overall prevalence of cataracts was found to be 70.3–73.3% in the population aged ≥ 60 years (unoperated cataract being ~52.9%) and higher in those aged ≥ 70 years (62.7% in the North and 63.3% in the South) as compared to those aged 60–69 years (92.3% in North and 87% in South).

The Cataract and Sun Exposure (CASE) and Sun Exposure, Environment, and Dry Eye Disease (SEED) studies were population studies performed in India

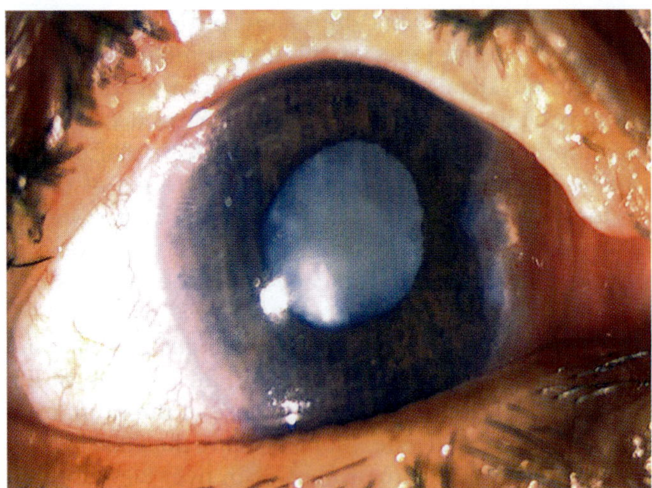

FIG. 1: A representative image of an elderly patient's eye with nasal pterygium and senile cataract.

among geographically diverse populations aged ≥40 years. They studied the effect of age as an intrinsic factor on the prevalence of eye diseases such as cataract, dry eye disease (DED), and pterygium among 9,735 individuals (mean age 54.5 ± 0.1 years; range 40–99, males 45.5%) across randomly sampled villages in coastal, plains, and hilly areas of India. They reported that the prevalence of cataract and DED increased with age, irrespective of other factors (such as topography, sun exposure, gender, and comorbidities). **Figure 1** shows the eye of an elderly individual, with a nasal pterygium encroaching onto the cornea, and senile mature cataract. **Table 1** summarizes the prevalence of common eye diseases in various age brackets.

TABLE 1: Prevalence of eye diseases with increasing age as reported by large population studies from India.

Age group	Cataract	Dry eye disease	Pterygium
Overall in 40+ years	33.3	26.2%	13.2%
Effect of increasing age	Increases	Increases	Increases
40–49 years	6.5	20.7 (19.5–22.0)	11.1 (10.1–12.1)
50–59 years	24.9	26.8 (25.1–28.6)	13.7 (12.3–15.1)
60–69 years	60 • 62.7 (north) • 63.3 (south) OR 1–2.57)	29.1 (27.1–31.1)	15.8 (14.2–17.4)
70+ years	90.1 • 92.3 (north) • 87 (south) OR 8.04 (6.48–9.97)	37.2 (34.5–39.8) *1.8* times higher than that in 40–49 years	14.7 (12.8–16.6)

(OR: odds ratio)

DISEASES OF THE EYE IN THE ELDERLY

Refractive Errors

Epidemiology: All over the world, uncorrected refractive errors are the leading causes of moderate and severe visual impairment. Refractive errors can be myopia, hyperopia, or presbyopia. A landmark Australian study (Blue Mountains Eye Study) placed the prevalence of Myopia (spherical equivalent of <–0.5 D) at 15% and that of hyperopia [standard error (SE) of >+0.5 D] at 57% in the age group of 49–97 years, and a landmark American study (Beaver Dam) estimated that the prevalence of myopia and hyperopia was 26.2% and 49%, respectively, in the age bracket of 43–84 years.

As the world's population is aging, by the year 2050, when 21% of the world's population will be 60 years or older, presbyopia may become the most common cause of visual impairment and blindness, with its predicted global prevalence being 1.8 billion. Currently, the prevalence of presbyopia in India is estimated to be about 42.9% in the age group of over 35 years and that in the West is estimated to be nearly 80% by the age 45–55 years.

Pathophysiology: Alterations in the refractive index of the lens and the accommodative apparatus are said to be responsible for the same **(Figs. 2 to 4)**. Residual refractive errors in postcataract surgery patients, if not rehabilitated, also lead to visual impairment. Population-based studies report that residual refractive errors are seen in about 11–42% of patients.

These then call for nonsurgical and in intolerable cases, surgical corrections. Spectacle correction forms the backbone of nonsurgical management of residual refractive errors.

Presbyopia is an entirely separate class, referring to the loss of the ability of the visual system to focus on objects at different distances due to age-induced worsening accommodation, usually starting at the age of 40 years (and becomes nearly universal by the age of 65 years), occurring due to age-related changes in the lens and its capsule along with the ciliary and zonular apparatus.

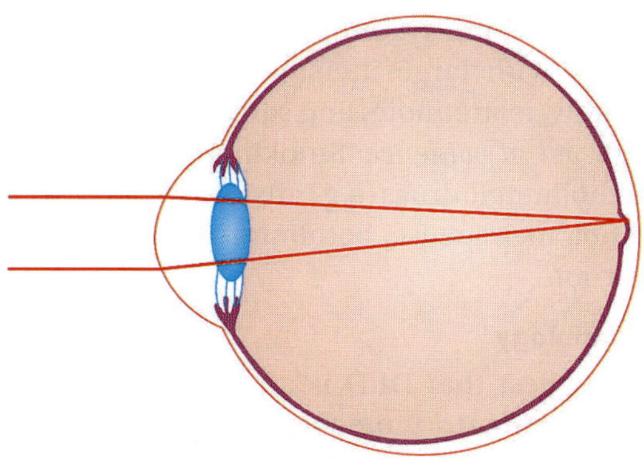

FIG. 2: A line drawing showing rays of light coming from infinity being focused on the fovea by the refractive apparatus of the eye, representing emmetropia.

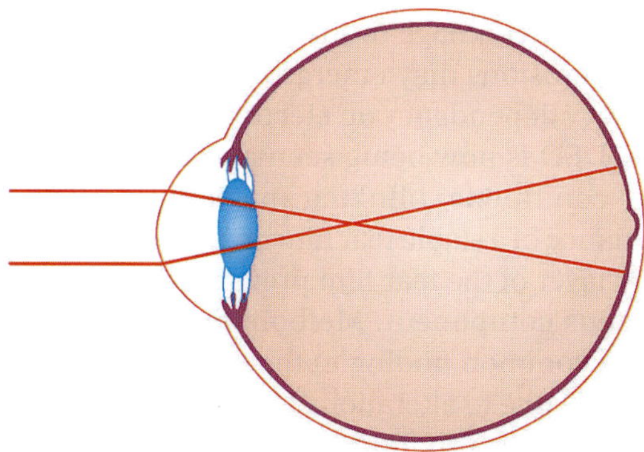

FIG. 3: A line drawing showing rays of light coming from infinity being focused before the fovea by the refractive apparatus of the eye, representing the condition of myopia or shortsightedness.

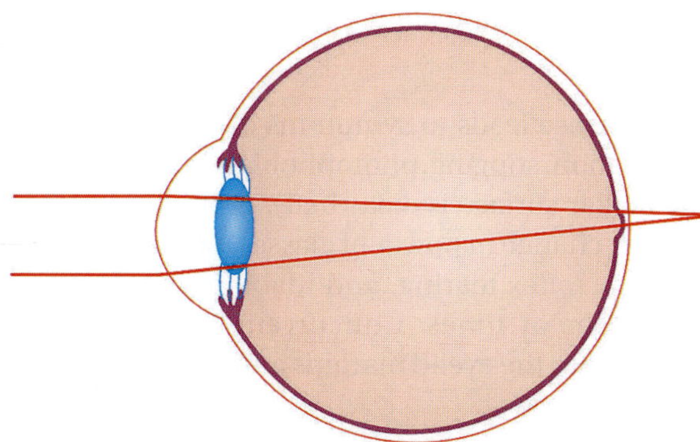

FIG. 4: A line drawing showing rays of light coming from infinity being focused beyond the fovea by the refractive apparatus of the eye, representing the condition of hypermetropia.

Risk factors: Older age, a history of glaucoma surgery and cataract surgery, male sex, and a higher level of education have been seen to be associated with myopia whereas female sex and lower level of education have a higher risk of hyperopia. Racial factors are also implicated, e.g., myopia is more common in Asians than in the West, and longer mean axial length corresponds to a higher prevalence of myopia in Chinese as compared to Indians. Risk factors for presbyopia also include female sex and a higher level of education.

Treatment options: Treatment options for myopia, hyperopia, and astigmatism include spectacles, contact lenses (CLs), cornea-based LASER vision correction such as flap-based corneal ablations [LASER in situ keratomileusis (LASIK)], lenticule extraction surgery such as small incision lenticule extraction (SMILE), surface ablation (photorefractive keratectomy), and phakic intraocular lenses (IOLs).

Presbyopic treatment options are as follows:

- *Optical aids*:
  - *Spectacles*: Near-vision glasses, having a single focal point and correct eyesight at one particular distance only, making them ideal to give additional converging power for near after cataract surgery has adequately dealt with distance correction, but necessitate removal to view distant objects.

    Now we have bifocal lenses having a top zone for distance correction and a bottom zone with additional converging (plus) power for near correction. Trifocal lenses incorporate an in-between zone for intermediate vision. Progressive addition spectacle lenses (PALs) have a continuous and smooth increase in plus power, providing a smooth transition from distance to near vision or vice versa without causing any image jump and without noticeable lines separating the zones.
  - *CLs*: CLs, also available in monofocal and multifocal designs, provide spectacle independence, though they require additional safety and hygiene measures. Enhanced monovision and monovision employ correcting one eye for distance viewing and the other with a bifocal or multifocal CLs (enhanced monovision) or a near vision monofocal lens (monovision).
- *Pharmacological management*: Topical pilocarpine eye drops, which constrict the pupil, improve near visual acuity and depth of focus by pinhole optics.
- *Surgical options*: Monovision LASIK, wherein the dominant eye is corrected for distance vision and the fellow eye for near, LASER blended vision (e.g., Presbyond), presbyopic phakic IOLs, and refractive lens exchange are the various surgical options available for presbyopia. These modalities are neither very popular nor always practical in the geriatric age group. In patients nearing or crossing 60 years of age, the opportunity to consider surgical options for spectacle independence arises at the time of cataract surgery when the choice of IOL and selection of

appropriate design and dioptric power is planned to provide good vision for distance and near to the extent of managing activities of daily living without glasses as far as possible.

Cornea and Ocular Surface Disorders

Dry Eye Disease

Dry eye disease is a "multifactorial disease of the tears and ocular surface that results in symptoms of discomfort, visual disturbance, tear film instability with potential damage to the ocular surface. It is accompanied by increased osmolarity of the tear film and subacute inflammation of the ocular surface."

As one ages, glandular changes in the meibomian glands and lacrimal glands lead to altered tear film composition and DED.

Epidemiology

Dry eye disease is a global public health problem. The prevalence of DED in ≥40 years age group is estimated as 25–35% and is also reported to increase with increasing age. There is a reported risk for severe DED in elderly persons aged ≥40 years [odds ratio (OR) 1.73] compared to those aged 21–40 (OR 1.46) and <20 (OR 1) years. In a large epidemiological study, Tandon et al. reported that the prevalence of DED was highest in ≥70 years (37.2%) and lowest in 40–49 years (20.7%) age groups.

Risk factors

Common risk factors for DED are older age, female gender, autoimmune diseases, screen (mobile, computers) use, thyroid abnormalities, hypertension, and diabetes. Additionally, systemic medications including analgesics (aspirin, ibuprofen), antiarrhythmics/bronchodilators (atropine, ipratropium), antihistamines (diphenhydramine, azelastine), anti-Parkinson (levodopa, benzopyrene), antihypertensives (atenolol, hydrochlorothiazide), and hormone replacement therapies cause dry eye, and likewise, topical eye drops, especially antiglaucoma and antiallergics tend to cause or worsen DED.

As per the level of evidence, the risk factors can be classified as follows:

- *High level of evidence*: Increased age, female gender, corneal refractive surgeries, collagen vascular disease, irradiation, hematopoietic stem cell transplantation, vitamin A deficiency, hepatitis C, androgen insufficiency, postmenopausal estrogen therapy, and antihistamines
- *Moderate level of evidence*: Medications (antidepressants, selective serotonin reuptake inhibitors, diuretics, and beta-blockers), diabetes mellitus (DM), HIV infection, systemic chemotherapy, cataract surgery with large incision, keratoplasty, low air humidity, isotretinoin, and sarcoidosis
- *Low level of evidence*: Smoking, Hispanic ethnicity, anticholinergic drugs (e.g., anxiolytics, antipsychotics), alcohol, menopause, botulinum toxin injection, acne, and gout

Pathophysiology

Studies suggest that DED is an inflammatory disease, and an inflammatory mechanism is theorized for the pathogenesis of DED. In DED, the ocular surface and tear film show increased levels of proinflammatory cytokines, chemokines, matrix metalloproteinases, etc., and increased infiltration by helper T cells. These propagate an inflammatory cascade in the tear film, which leads to damage to the ocular surface. Superficial epithelial erosions may emerge consequently. In today's era of heavy dependency on electronic gadgets and digital devices, DED is now being seen as a lifestyle disease. In healthy conditions, blinking mechanisms help in the maintenance of a stable tear film on the ocular surface and the lipid layer of the tear film prevents the evaporation of its aqueous component. Meibomian gland dysfunction (MGD), a common finding in the elderly population, can lead to DED due to alterations in the lipid layer of the tear film. Tear film is also found to be hyperosmolar in DED. In the natural course, there may be chronic sequelae, e.g., conjunctival scarring, ocular surface fibrosis, and corneal opacification, if DED is left untreated. DED related to increased screen time occurs because of factors such as reduced blink rate and altered blinking dynamics.

Symptoms

Dry eye disease leads to symptoms of burning or foreign body sensation, stinging, photophobia, visual disturbances (as the ocular surface is disturbed), problems in focusing on objects, change in power of glasses, occasional redness of the eyes, reflex tearing, and inability to tolerate wind or room fans at times. Concurrent MGD presents as discharge from the eyelid margins and redness of the eyes.

Types

Dry eye disease can be classified as "aqueous-deficient/AD" (dry eye with reduced tear production) or "hyperevaporative" (dry eye with increased evaporation of tear film). Most (80%) DED cases have mixed forms, while only 10% have solely AD-DED.

Staging: DED can be mild or moderate or severe, based on the visual symptoms, level of discomfort, severity of DED, frequency of symptoms, condition of lids, meibomian glands, clinical examination findings, and values of clinical tests such as tear break-up time and Schirmer score.

Management

Management approach of DED involves primarily the identification of triggering factors (e.g., heavy screen use) or underlying systemic/ocular disease leading to DED. It is mostly managed conservatively using tear substitutes/artificial tears, anti-inflammatory agents (topical corticosteroids, topical cyclosporine), oral antibiotics (tetracycline, e.g., doxycycline, azithromycin), and omega fatty acids. Besides, counseling for the maintenance of eyelid hygiene is given to the DED patients. Rarely, surgeries may be required for very severe DED having damaged ocular surface.

Prevention

Dry eye disease can be prevented, to an extent, by certain lifestyle changes, including reducing the use of electronic devices and overall duration of screen exposure, adjusting distance from screens, glare-reducing matte screen filters, adjusting brightness and contrast settings, and taking regular breaks with screen use, i.e., every 20 minutes, shifting eyes to look at a distant object (placed at least 20 feet away), for at least 20 seconds ("20-20-20 rule").

Pterygium

Pterygium is an ocular surface disorder common in tropical countries of the world. It is defined as a triangular fibrovascular overgrowth of subconjunctival tissue encroaching on to the cornea within the palpebral fissure **(Fig. 1)**, on the medial and/or lateral aspects, leading to corneal astigmatism (due to induced flattening of the cornea in the horizontal axis) and can lead to low vision in elderly individuals.

Risk Factors

Pterygium has an association with risk factors such as exposure to sunlight, particularly ultraviolet (UV) radiation, increased outdoor activity, and geographic areas situated nearer to the equator.

Pathophysiology

Ultraviolet radiations may damage the limbal stem cells (LSCs) of the cornea by affecting their proliferation. Damage to LSCs leads to invasion of the limbus and peripheral cornea by fibroblasts resulting in opacification or haziness of the peripheral cornea. The opacity or fibrovascular growth can slowly reach the center of the cornea. UV rays may also cause *p53* gene mutations (tumor suppressor gene), and this can result in abnormal pterygium epithelium. Genetic mechanisms and inflammatory agents such as cytokines, growth factors, antiapoptotic mechanisms, extracellular tissue remodeling, and viral infections are involved in the pathogenesis of pterygium. It is a recurrent disease, with recurrence commonly seen after surgery.

Symptoms

Pterygium is associated with gradual painless progressive diminution of vision and once it encroaches the corneal center, it causes loss of vision. Pterygium presents as blurring of vision (due to underlying refractive error), redness, lacrimation, irritation of the eye, and foreign body sensation and causes a cosmetic blemish. Large pterygia can restrict extraocular movements, though seen rarely.

Staging

Pterygium can be grades I–II (limited to the limbus and peripheral cornea) or grade III (pterygium encroaching the center of the cornea crossing the pupillary margin). Several grading systems are well established for pterygium.

Types

Pterygium can be progressive (thick, fleshy, vascular, and increasing progressively in size) or atrophic (thin, avascular, and static in size).

Management

Pterygium is preferably managed by surgical means: Pterygium excision plus conjunctival autograft or primary closure. The decision for surgery is taken for reasons such as the pterygium encroaching corneal center, cosmesis, severe corneal astigmatism, chronic pain, or discomfort. Artificial tear drops and decongestants are given for temporary relief in the preoperative period. Other management modalities are bare sclera technique, simple excision, conjunctival rotational autograft, limbal conjunctival autotransplant, LSC transplantation, amnion membrane grafting, lamellar or full-thickness keratoplasty, mitomycin C application, etc. Surgical management has a recurrence rate of 15–20%.

Preventive Measures

Avoidance of risk factors such as sunlight exposure can possibly lead to the prevention of pterygium, to some extent. This can be achieved by eye protection using sunglasses, covering the face with shields, and wearing a cap/hat to limit overall eye exposure to sunlight.

Corneal Dystrophies

Dystrophies are inherited disorders affecting any layer of the cornea, usually progressive, bilateral conditions without systemic effects. Some may be asymptomatic throughout a patient's lifetime and be diagnosed incidentally, while others may progress and cause substantial visual disturbances requiring intervention. Fuchs' endothelial corneal dystrophy (FECD) is an endothelial dystrophy causing a slow loss of endothelial cells and development of guttae (excrescences of Descemet's membrane), leading to corneal decompensation and loss of deturgescence, further leading to edema, scarring, and visual loss. **Figures 5A and B** show a case of corneal decompensation due to Fuchs' dystrophy, with stromal edema and epithelial cysts and bullae.

Epidemiology

Guttata without corneal edema may occur in up to 4% of patients older than 40 years old in the Western world, and FECD has been seen to be the most common bilateral corneal dystrophy, accounting for up to a third of all corneal transplants performed in the United States. A study from the Indian subcontinent placed the incidence of FECD at 0.08%, with a female predominance (65.53%), and the most common age group being the seventh decade of life.

Risk Factors

Age is the most important risk factor, with patients older than 40 years developing the disease most often. Female sex also has a relation, with female-to-male ratio being 2.5:1–3:1. An early onset form occurring in patients <40 years old and with 1:1 incidence of males:females with mutations in the gene *COL8A* in the chromosomal position 1p34.3–p32.3 (FCD1) has also been described.

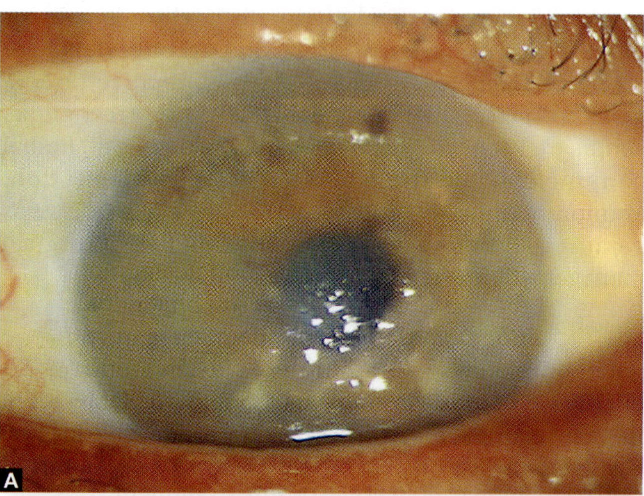

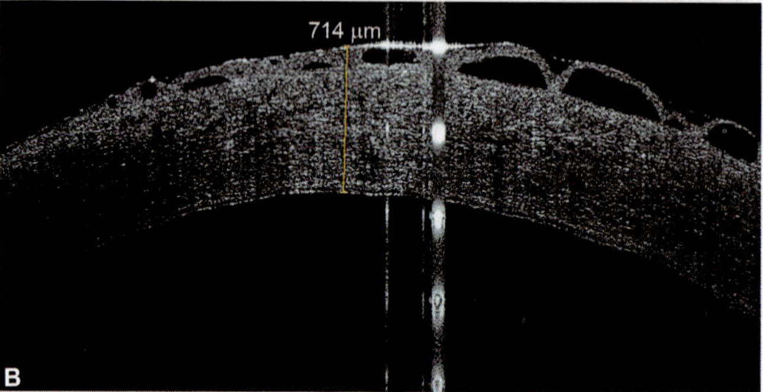

FIGS. 5A AND B: (A) A case of corneal decompensation due to Fuchs' dystrophy; (B) Anterior segment optical coherence tomography image of the cornea.

Figure 5A shows a case of corneal decompensation due to Fuchs' dystrophy, leading to stromal edema and epithelial cysts and bullae. **Figure 5B** shows the anterior segment optical coherence tomographic image of this cornea, with increased corneal thickness due to stromal edema, and multiple epithelial bullae.

Pathophysiology

The pathophysiology of Fuchs' endothelial dystrophy (FED) involves several proposed mechanisms involving channelopathies in the corneal endothelium like mutations in *SLC4A11*, oxidative stress due to exposure of the cornea to UV rays, apoptosis of endothelial cells, and epithelial–mesenchymal transition.

Symptoms and Staging

- *Stage 1*: Manifests around the fourth decade of life and is asymptomatic; is clinically indistinguishable from central corneal guttata (and thus only identified after the patient progresses to later stages)
- *Stage 2*: Corneal edema due to endothelial decompensation, with patients complaining of painless blurring of vision and glare; characteristically worse upon waking up in the morning (due to reduced evaporation and increased hydration of cornea underneath closed eyelids)
- *Stage 3*: Epithelial bullae develop, causing further deterioration of vision **(Figs. 5A and B)**. Episodes of pain may occur due to rupture of bullae, causing exposure of naked nerve endings.
- *Stage 4*: Subepithelial scarring occurs, and patients experience significant vision loss. This stage may be less painful than the previous but requires full-thickness transplants, in contrast to the previous stages in which posterior lamellar transplants suffice.

Implications

At present, nearly 300 million people aged 30 years and above are estimated to be suffering from FECD, and a substantial increase of 41.7% in this number, placing it at 415 million by the year 2050. It is currently the most common indication for corneal transplantation in the United States, with almost 36% of those performed in the United States in 2016 in a study.

Management

Medical treatment such as hyperosmotic saline (drops or ointment) can promote corneal dehydration (a handheld hairdryer can also be used by patients themselves for the same purpose) and improve vision in early stages, while phototherapeutic keratectomy, anterior stromal puncture, and amniotic membrane transplants can be used to relieve pain in the bullous keratopathy stage. Definitive management involves corneal transplants, endothelial transplants [posterior lamellar keratoplasties such as Descemet stripping automated endothelial keratoplasty (DSAEK), Descemet membrane endothelial keratoplasty (DMEK), or deep lamellar endothelial keratoplasty (DLEK)] or penetrating keratoplasty in cases with significant scarring of the stroma in which an endothelial keratoplasty will not suffice.

Prevention

Fuchs' endothelial corneal dystrophy is not preventable, but currently studies are underway to promote endothelial function and prevent the progression of FECD using Rho kinase (ROCK) inhibitor Y-27632, which improves adhesion and proliferation of endothelial cells and gene therapies (adenovirus vector therapy, *CRISPR* gene editing).

Age-related Cataracts

Cataract refers to the opacification of the lens or its capsule **(Fig. 6)**. Senile cataracts are the most common cause of avoidable blindness globally, with most cases aged over 60 years. These are related to aging and are affected by environmental factors such as exposure to sunlight or UV radiation. It is almost universally seen in individuals aged >70 years.

Epidemiology

The overall prevalence of cataract in ≥40 years age group in India is reported as 33.3%. The prevalence increases with age and is as high as 90.1% in those aged ≥70 years. The age-wise prevalence of cataract is reported in the literature as follows: 6.5% in 40–49 years, 24.9% in 50–59 years, 60% in 60–69 years, and 90.1% in 70+ years **(Table 1)**.

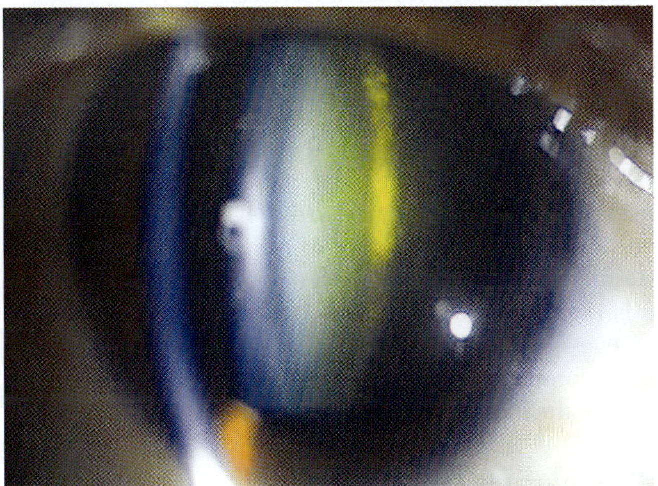

FIG. 6: Slit-lamp biomicroscopic image of a senile cataract showing nuclear sclerosis with posterior subcapsular cataract.

The India Study of Age-related Eye Disease (IndEye) reported increased odds of having lens opacification with increasing age. The OR was 8.04 (6.48–9.97) for ≥70 years and 2.57 (2.23–2.96) for 65–69 years, as compared to those aged 60–64 years. The likelihood of cataracts was reported as higher in women (OR 1.8) than men.

Risk Factors

Cataract is known to have a significant association with smoking and indoor kitchen smoke exposure. Higher sun exposure is an identified risk factor for cataract development, especially in rural areas of India.

Types

Senile cataracts can be classified based on morphology as cortical cataract, nuclear cataract, or posterior subcapsular cataract (PSC). Cortical cataract affects the peripheral cortex of the lens. Nuclear or sclerotic cataracts affect the lens nucleus, causing a gradual myopic shift due to an increase in the refractive index of the lens. This leads to a temporary improvement in the near vision in the presbyopes, a condition referred to as the "second sight of the elderly." The PSCs are a collection of modified epithelial cells called "Wedl cells" or "bladder cells" situated just anterior to the posterior capsule of the lens. PSCs cause the maximum visual dysfunction on account of being the closest to the nodal point of the eye, a point located just anterior to the center of the posterior lens capsule.

Pathophysiology

Senile cataracts occur due to loss of transparency of the lens due to oxidative damage in lens proteins. There is a proven role of free oxygen radical damage and reduced glutathione in the pathogenesis of cataract in the lens. In diabetics, chronic hyperglycemia leads to the development of cataract, secondary to the deposition of sorbitol and advanced glycation end products and reduced superoxide dismutase.

Symptoms

Blurred vision (painless gradual progressive loss of vision), change in power of glasses, polyopia (seeing two or more images), and photophobia are its symptoms. In advanced stages, intumescent cataract can lead to phacomorphic glaucoma, which presents as an acute painful red eye due to raised IOP.

Staging

In the cortical type of senile cataract, the first stage is "lamellar separation," where the separation of cortical lens fibers by fluid is seen. This leads to a grayish appearance of the pupil in elderly persons and causes reflections and scattering of light. The next stage is "incipient stage," where wedge-shaped spoke-like opacities (*cuneiform* opacities) are seen in the cortex of the lens approaching its center, with clear areas in between. These lead to changes in refraction, visual deterioration, and polyopia (multiple images seen). As the peripheral cuneiform opacities reach the central visual axis, visual disturbances increase, and visual acuity falls. In later stages, the lens opacities increase in density and number and become more diffuse in distribution. Lens fibers become hydrated and the lens appears swollen (*intumescent* cataract). In the initial stages when a clear lens area is visible between the pupillary margin and lens opacity, it is referred to as *immature* cataract. In advanced stages, the cataract is said to be *mature*, in which the entire cortex and nuclear parts are opacified, and there is no clear lens area between the pupillary margin and the cataract with no iris shadow. If cataracts are not operated in time, i.e., before reaching maturity, the natural course of the disease leads to *hypermature cataracts*, where the cortex becomes inspissated and shrunken, sometimes yellow in appearance, and the capsule thickens into dense, white calcific mass. Hypermature cataracts are mostly associated with degenerated and weak lens zonules and, hence, they have a higher predisposition for complications such as zonular dehiscence, posterior capsular rupture, and vitreous loss during cataract surgery.

In senile nuclear cataracts, there is nuclear sclerosis while the cortex is clear. It blurs the distance vision more than the near vision. The nuclear cloudiness increases in intensity as nuclear cataract advances. Its appearance changes from transparent (in healthy conditions) to amber color or dark brown (cataracta brunescens) or even black at times (cataracta nigra or black cataract). When mature, the lens cortex and capsule also opacify. At this stage, there is severe impairment of vision.

The Lens Opacities Classification System III (LOCSIII) is internationally used for grading cataracts using slit-lamp and retroillumination images. In LOCSIII, the grades of nuclear color and opalescence (NO and NC) range from NO1 to NO6 and NC1 to NC6; cortical cataracts are graded from C1 to C5 and PSCs from P1 to P5.

Implications

Cataract leads to vision impairment and blindness. There is strong evidence for an increased risk of falls (almost three-fold higher), and hip fractures are noted in elderly persons with cataract due to visual disability caused by cataracts. In older adults awaiting cataract surgeries, a substantial risk of falls and fall injury is reported. Low vision, secondary to cataract, has been found to have an association with depression or cognitive impairment in approximately 25–33% of patients. Individuals with cataracts specifically have an increased depression risk (65–78% increase in risk) as per several cohort studies.

Management

Cataract is surgically removed, with cataract surgery being the most common ophthalmic surgery worldwide. There is no proven medical treatment for senile cataracts. The decision to operate depends upon the patient's handicap in daily activities and their visual needs. A cataract is operated mostly at immature stages for successful outcomes.

The current standard of care for the management of cataracts is *microincision cataract surgery with an IOL implantation using the phacoemulsification technique*. Modern cataract surgery has evolved over decades. Previously, surgeries done for cataract removal were extracapsular cataract extraction (ECCE) or intracapsular cataract extraction (ICCE). In today's era, ECCE has different methods for cataract removal: Conventional ECCE, small incision cataract surgery (SICS), and phacoemulsification or femtosecond laser-assisted cataract surgery (FLACS). IOL implantation is performed during cataract surgery for visual rehabilitation of the patient. The type of IOL implanted depends upon the visual needs, vision potential, and other comorbidities of the patient and may be monofocal (successful for rehabilitation of distance vision) or multifocal (focal point for near and distance and/or intermediate vision). Enhanced monofocal lenses and extended depth of focus (EDoF) lenses are a new addition to our armamentarium to provide excellent distance visual acuity along with improved intermediate vision.

The *Motiya Bind Mukti Abhiyan* and National Programme for Control of Blindness and Visual Impairment (NPCBVI) are free cataract surgery campaigns launched by the Government of India to tackle the avoidable blindness caused by cataracts, as part of national visual rehabilitative services.

Preventive Measures

Lens opacification with aging is almost universal and is an inevitable phenomenon. However, lens clouding is known to develop earlier (even in presenile age) in patients with risk factors such as uncontrolled diabetes, dyslipidemias, deranged calcium and parathyroid levels, hypothyroidism, and in cases with exposure to radiation or oral/topical steroid use. Hence, for primary and secondary prevention, it is important to get a routine evaluation of the eye by an eye specialist. This would help in the early detection and prompt treatment of senile cataracts and would also reduce the incidence of surgical complications.

Glaucoma

With increasing age, the eye undergoes multiple changes in the lens, its zonular apparatus, the trabecular meshwork, and the optic nerve, causing a reduction in the outflow of aqueous humor and a reduction in the area of trabecular meshwork available for filtration, leading to increase in IOP along with associated changes in the optic nerve and causing visual field defects. More than 60 million people have glaucoma, which is now the second most common cause of blindness and the most common cause of irreversible blindness worldwide, and the age-standardized prevalence of glaucoma is approximately 3.5% in the population aged > 40 years.

Primary Open-angle Glaucoma

The most common subtype of glaucoma is primary open-angle glaucoma (POAG), defined as the chronic, progressive, and irreversible optic neuropathy of multifactorial etiology characterized by an open angle of the anterior chamber, typical optic nerve head changes, retinal nerve fiber layer (RNFL) thinning, and progressive loss of peripheral vision, for which increased IOP is a risk factor.

Epidemiology

About 68.56 million people worldwide are estimated to be suffering from POAG currently. The prevalence of the same in older adults aged ≥ 80 years is 9.2%.

Pathophysiology

Primary open-angle glaucoma is a result of age-related changes in the trabecular meshwork (including obstruction by glycosaminoglycans, endothelial cell loss, and reduction in phagocytic activity of the same), reduced ocular perfusion pressure (with relation to systemic vascular diseases), and loss of neurotrophic factors, causing ganglion cell loss, optic nerve damage, and resultant loss of visual field.

Risk Factors

Older age, African race (four-fold higher risk), family history (9.2 times higher risk of developing OAG in first-degree relatives of glaucoma patients), myopia, and low ocular perfusion pressure have been implicated in the development of POAG. Genetic factors such as *MYOC* (myocilin) and *OPTN* (optineurin) genes, usage of corticosteroids, and of course high IOP play important roles.

Symptoms

Though asymptomatic in the early stages, visual field defects may be noticed by observant patients. But as the disease progresses, there is severe constriction of the visual field leaving only a tunnel of vision.

Management

Diagnosis is made based on ophthalmoscopic findings of increased cupping of the optic nerve head, thinning and loss of RNFL, and optic disk hemorrhages. Tonometry or measurement of IOP and perimetry (visual field examination) play the most important roles in assessing these patients. Slowing disease progression and preserving quality of life are the most important goals for glaucoma treatment. Reduction of IOP is by far the only proven method to treat glaucoma, for which we have the option of medical management, lasers, and surgeries including implants.

Lens-induced Glaucomas

Lens-induced glaucomas can be open-angle glaucomas or angle-closure glaucomas.

Phacomorphic Glaucoma

A cataractous lens increases in anteroposterior thickness leading to contact between its anterior surface and the posterior aspect of the iris, causing pupillary block, which blocks the flow of aqueous from the posterior chamber (where it is released into after production in the ciliary body) to the anterior chamber (from where it is drained). This aqueous trapped in the posterior chamber pushes the iris forward, leading to a shallow anterior chamber and high IOP, referred to as an acute angle closure attack. When this condition is brought about by an intumescent cataract, it is known as phacomorphic glaucoma **(Fig. 7)**.

Symptoms: An elderly patient, usually with a history of poor vision in that eye (due to a long-standing cataract), with normal anterior chamber depth in the fellow eye (distinguishing this condition from primary angle closure, in which the fellow eye also has a shallow anterior chamber), presents with complaints of acute-onset severe pain and redness in that eye and very high IOPs.

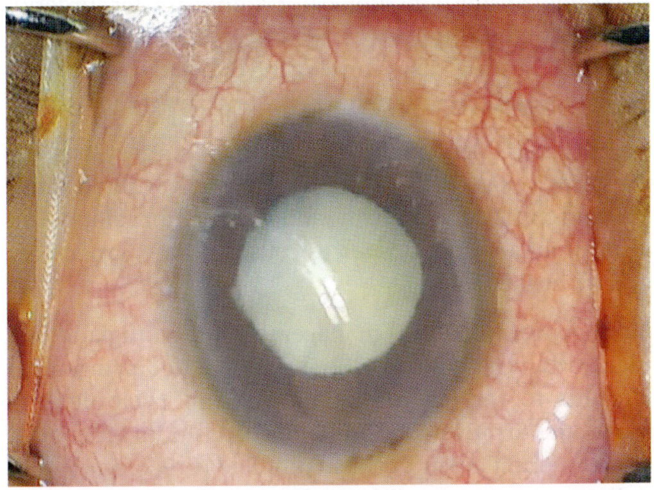

FIG. 7: An intumescent cataract causing pupillary block with high intraocular pressures and shallow anterior chamber, with mild corneal edema.

Management: The initial management is to reduce the IOP and provide symptomatic relief, for which intravenous and oral hyperosmotic agents such as mannitol (IV) and glycerol (oral) can be given. Topical antiglaucoma medications such as beta-blockers and carbonic anhydrase inhibitors are also started, and the patient is taken up for cataract extraction, which is the definitive treatment.

Phacolytic Glaucoma

A senile hypermature Morgagnian cataract can develop microleaks via its anterior capsule, with extrusion of high molecular weight proteins as well as macrophages and other inflammatory cells into the anterior chamber, clogging the outflow system and causing phacolytic glaucoma.

Symptoms: Though the presenting symptoms are similar to those mentioned in phacomorphic glaucoma, the diagnosis is made by the presence of significant cell-flare reaction in the anterior chamber, along with white lens particles, but without keratic precipitates (KPs) (which distinguish this from another condition, phacoanaphylactic glaucoma, discussed below), pseudohypopyon or a collection of protein deposits at the inferior angle as a result of gravity, high IOP with corneal edema, mature cataract but open angles on gonioscopy (distinguishing it from phacomorphic glaucoma).

Management: Initial management consists of cycloplegics to control pain, steroids to reduce inflammation, and aqueous suppressants to reduce IOP, but the definitive treatment is cataract extraction. Failure to manage on time may lead to a painful blind eye.

Lens Particle Glaucoma

If the lens capsule is disrupted by trauma (or after surgery), lens particles themselves or macrophages that have engulfed these particles can clog the trabecular meshwork impeding outflow and giving rise to lens particle glaucoma.

Symptoms: A patient with a history of surgery/trauma presents weeks or months after the event with elevated IOP and cortical matter in the anterior chamber along with signs of inflammation, such as cells and flare, synechiae, and corneal edema.

Management: Medical management with antiglaucoma medications to control IOP and associated symptoms; steroids to reduce inflammation; and cycloplegics/mydriatics to prevent the formation of posterior synechiae, seclusio pupillae, or occlusio pupillae is recommended. Failure to improve with medical management or the presence of a large amount of obviously unresorbable lens matter warrants surgical removal of the same.

Phacoantigenic/Phacoanaphylactic Glaucoma

Phacoanaphylactic is a misnomer since the underlying mechanism is not an allergic or anaphylactic reaction but an arthus-type immune complex reaction, against lens proteins which are immune-privileged antigens sequestered within the lens capsule but brought in contact with the immune system following a complicated cataract surgery or trauma, which has caused retention of these proteins in the vitreous cavity which then gets released slowly (usually 1–14 days after the antecedent event).

Symptoms: Intense anterior chamber reaction with cells, flare, KPs, usually of the mutton-fat kind, posterior synechiae, with or without anterior vitritis are its symptoms.

Treatment: Treatment is similar to that mentioned in lens particle glaucoma.

Prevention: The only preventive method for lens-induced glaucomas is early cataract surgeries before the development of complications.

Pseudoexfoliation Syndrome

Another condition known to have a direct relationship with age is pseudoexfoliation (PEX) syndrome, a systemic condition associated with a mutation in the *LOXL1* gene, with deposition of fibrillary (pseudoexfoliative) basement membrane material at various sites including the anterior segment of the eye and the trabecular meshwork, impeding aqueous outflow, causing PEX glaucoma.

Epidemiology

Pseudoexfoliative glaucoma accounts for 25% of cases of open-angle glaucoma worldwide. PEX has been seen to have a cumulative probability of developing in PEG in 15% of cases within 10 years. Though found in all geographic populations, the prevalence of PEX varies markedly based on race, with as low as 0% in Inuits and as high as 38% in Navajo Indians. An Indian population-based study found that of those identified as POAG, exfoliation was present in 26.7%, and that the prevalence of PXF was 6.0%.

Pathophysiology

Pseudoexfoliation material arises from the abnormal accumulation of elastic microfibrils made of fibrillin-1, fibulin-2, lysyl oxidase, vitronectin, clusterin, and other proteins. It deposits on anterior segment structures such as iris pigment epithelium, anterior lens capsule, zonular fibers, and corneal endothelium.

Risk Factors

Increasing age (which is the strongest risk factor), some races (discussed above), people living in high altitudes, smoking, and low antioxidant consumption are the known risk factors.

Symptoms

Patients are often asymptomatic but may present with loss of peripheral visual field from secondary glaucoma or PEG. Diagnosis is made clinically, on observing white, flaky, dandruff-like PEX material along the pupillary margin and anterior lens capsule (central disk and peripheral ring of fibrillary with a clear intermediate zone maintained by abrasion due to pupillary constriction and dilation, called target sign). Gonioscopy shows PEX deposits in the angles, with hyperpigmentation of Schwalbe's line (Sampaolesi line). PEG shows elevated IOP and associated changes in the optic nerve head.

Management

Cataract surgery is especially challenging in these cases due to poor pupillary dilation, zonular weakness, and subluxation of the lens predisposing to increased risk of nucleus drop, vitreous loss, and postoperative dislocation of bag–IOL complex, preexisting endothelial damage, and usage of high energy during phacoemulsification leading to postoperative corneal edema. IOP can be controlled by topical medications and selective laser trabeculoplasty or in uncontrolled pressures, trabeculectomy may be needed.

Prevention

Regular visits to the ophthalmologist for IOP monitoring, perimetry and optimization of antiglaucoma medications, and early cataract surgery before the development of severe zonulopathy with risks explained play an important role in the management. The possibility of late decentration of the IOL due to progressive zonular weakness needs to be explained.

Retinal Disorders

Population aged 40 years and above have been reported to be suffering from retinal disorders at a rate of around 5.35–21.02% in various studies. These include macular diseases, such as ARMD, macular hole, cystoid macular edema (CME), and epiretinal membrane (ERM), and vascular disorders, such as diabetic retinopathy (DR), vascular occlusions [central retinal vein occlusion (CRVO), central retinal artery occlusion (CRAO), branch retinal vein occlusion (BRVO), and branch retinal artery occlusion (BRAO)], and hypertensive retinopathy.

Age-related Macular Degeneration

Age-related macular degeneration (AMD) is an acquired degeneration of the retina causing significant central visual impairment through both non-neovascular [drusen and retinal pigment epithelium (RPE) abnormalities] and neovascular (choroidal neovascular membrane formation) derangement.

Epidemiology

Age-related macular degeneration is estimated to affect 1.4–3.1% of the Indian population, and much higher in the Western population, to the extent of 12.33% in Europeans, 7.53% in Africans, and 7.38% in Asians, and an estimate has been made that by the year 2040, the number of cases may reach 113 million.

Risk Factors

Along with the obvious risk factor of increasing age, as suggested by the name, cigarette smoking, hyperopia, hypercholesterolemia, and genetic factors (complement factor H) have also been observed to increase the risk of developing the disease.

Pathophysiology

Failure of RPE to function, causing abnormal misfolded proteins and lipids to accumulate and form drusen, which then triggers chronic inflammation in the subretinal space, leading to neovascularization and ultimately scarring.

Symptoms

These patients present with gradual painless, progressive diminution of vision, unless complicated by a submacular hemorrhage, which can cause acute worsening of visual loss. Metamorphopsia (distortion of vision) and scotomas (blind spots) may also be experienced by observant patients. The hallmark features of AMD are drusen (lipid and protein-rich extracellular deposits) and pigmentary changes, both of which are features of nonexudative or dry AMD and additional subretinal neovascularization in exudative or wet AMD.

Routine dilated fundus examinations are required to pick up worsening or development of neovascularization, which can also be recognized in investigative modalities such as fundus fluorescein angiography (FFA), optical coherence tomography (OCT) **(Fig. 8A)**, or optical coherence tomography angiography (OCTA) **(Fig. 8B)**.

Figure 8A shows loss of foveolar contour with pigment epithelial detachments and drusen (seen as undulations of the hyperreflective RPE) on OCT, and **Figure 8B** shows neovascularization on OCTA.

Treatment

Treatment of dry AMD is mainly by antioxidant and mineral supplementation, as advised by age-related eye disease studies (AREDS/AREDS2), which is a combination of:

- 500 mg of vitamin C
- 400 international units (IUs) of vitamin E
- 80 mg of zinc as zinc oxide
- 2 mg of copper as cupric oxide
- 10 mg lutein
- 2 mg zeaxanthin

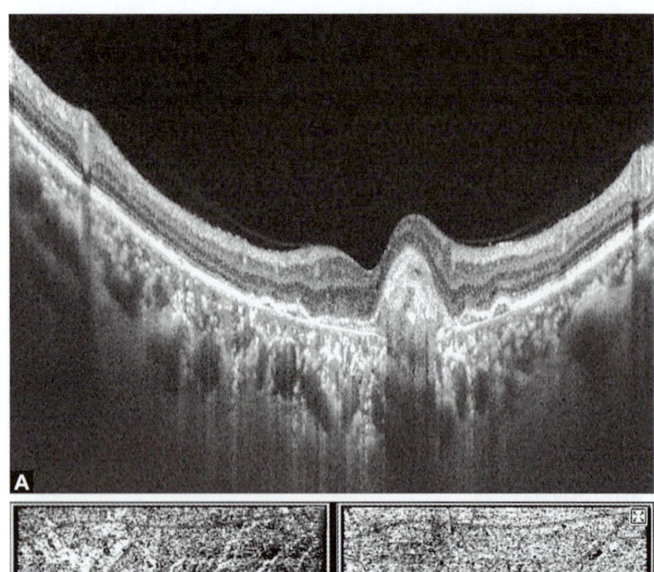

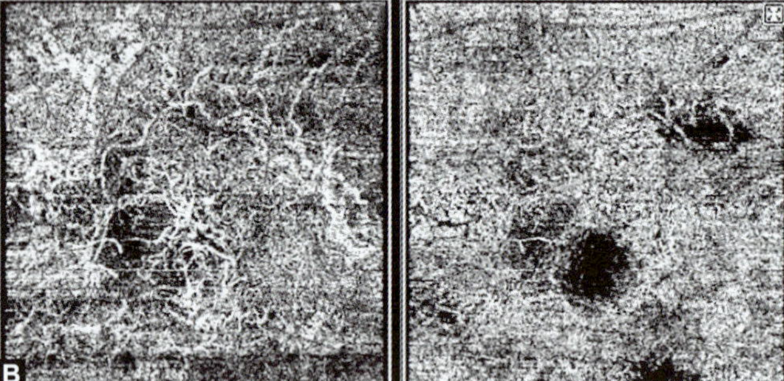

FIGS. 8A AND B: (A) Loss of foveolar contour with pigment epithelial detachments and drusen; (B) Neovascularization on OCTA.
(OCTA: optical coherence tomography angiography)

Treatment of exudative AMD involves intravitreal injections of anti-vascular endothelial growth factor (anti-VEGF) agents such as bevacizumab, ranibizumab, aflibercept, and brolucizumab. A port delivery system (PDS) supplying constant doses of ranibizumab (Susvimo) has recently been approved by the FDA. Faricimab, which is a bispecific antibody against both VEGF and angiopoietin-2, has also been recently approved.

Implications

Patients with AMD are at a greater risk for cognitive impairment and Alzheimer's disease than normal controls. Additionally, AMD is associated with a 20% increased risk of overall mortality and 46% higher risk for cardiovascular disease.

Prevention

Avoidance of smoking and inculcating a healthy lifestyle with dietary modification and inclusion of antioxidants (vitamins A, C, and E, lutein, zeaxanthin, omega-3 fatty acids, and regular physical exercise to avoid obesity) have been shown to help.

Macular Hole

A partial- or full-thickness defect in the neurosensory retina at the center of the macula (fovea), called a macular hole, occurs idiopathically (IMH) mostly in the age group of sixth or seventh decade of life, more commonly in females.

Epidemiology

The prevalence of the same in India is 1.7–2.7 per 1,000 population and that found in a landmark study, the Baltimore Eye Survey, was 3.3 per 1,000 population.

Risk Factors

Increasing age, female sex, myopia, trauma, or ocular inflammation increase the likelihood of the development of MH.

Pathophysiology

The most extensively accepted hypothesis is the exertion of direct anterior–posterior traction as well as tangential traction by the posterior vitreous cortex on the fovea by abnormal vitreomacular adhesions (VMAs).

Symptoms and Signs

Typically, the patient experiences a reduction in visual acuity and metamorphopsia, which progresses to a central scotoma as the disease progresses. An OCT can show a defect in the neurosensory retina at the fovea and is also used to stage the disease and can also show vitreoretinal adhesion and traction, which are said to be the prelude to a full-thickness hole.

Stages

The International Vitreomacular Traction Study (IVTS) Group classified the stages based on OCT as follows:

- *VMA*: No distortion of the foveal pit; subdivided based on the area of attachment between the retina and hyaloid as focal (≤1,500 μm) or broad (>1,500 μm)
- *Vitreomacular traction (VMT):* Distortion of the foveal pit or intraretinal structural changes noted in the absence of a full-thickness macular hole (FTMH); subdivided based on the area of attachment between the retina and hyaloid as focal (≤1,500 μm) or broad (>1,500 μm)
- *FTMH*: Full-thickness defect from the internal limiting membrane (ILM) to the RPE. These can be described based on three factors:
    i. *Size (horizontal diameter at narrowest point)*: Small (≤250 μm), medium (250–400 μm), and large (>400 μm)
    ii. *Cause*: Primary or secondary (associated with any other ocular pathology)
    iii. Presence or absence of VMT

Management

Vitreomacular adhesion and asymptomatic VMT may be observed, due to the possibility of spontaneous closure. The surgical technique employs peeling the ILM around the hole to reduce traction and limit the proliferation of cells to form an ERM (discussed later), and the peeled flap of ILM may even be laid on top of or plugged in the macular hole to form a scaffold for proliferation of glial cells to promote closure. Of late, other materials to promote the closure of macular holes are being studied, including the human amniotic membrane, autologous lens capsule (obtained during cataract surgery), autologous serum, autologous whole blood, autologous platelet-rich plasma, and thrombin. Postsurgical positioning of the patient also plays an important role; prone or face-down positioning is suggested for the gas tamponade to act.

Complications if management is delayed: In general, better postoperative visual outcomes are associated with good preoperative visual outcomes. A higher likelihood of anatomical closure is also associated with smaller-sized holes as compared to larger ones. These imply that delay in management would mean poorer postoperative results.

Implications

Since patients with MH have an inherently abnormal vitreoretinal interface, they might have a higher risk of retinal tears or detachment intraoperatively.

Prevention

There is no proven measure for the prevention of IMH.

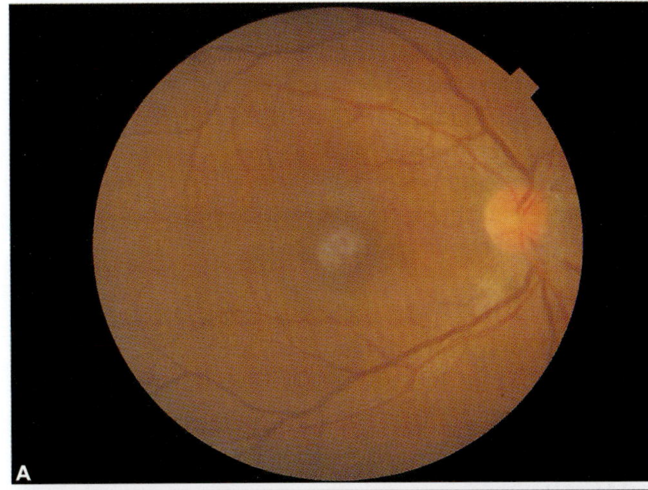

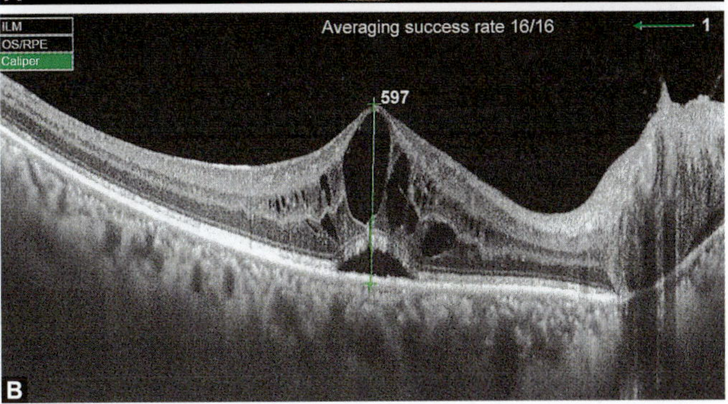

FIGS. 9A AND B: (A) A pseudocolor fundus photograph of an eye with cystoid macular edema; (B) Optical coherence tomography image of the same eye.

Cystoid Macular Edema

Cystoid macular edema is cyst-like spaces in the macula oriented radially (also known as petaloid fashion), occurring as a sequel to intraocular inflammation, retinal venous occlusions (RVOs) (discussed below), DR, in which it is one of the most common causes of vision loss and is referred to as diabetic macular edema (DME), or following cataract surgeries (also called Irvine–Gass syndrome).

Pathophysiology

Disruption of the balance between the osmotic force, hydrostatic force, capillary permeability, and vascular compliance leads to accumulation of fluid in cystoid spaces (petaloid pattern) within the inner layers of the retina, most commonly the watershed area between the retinal and choroidal circulation, the outer plexiform layer (OPL), which at the central retina is called the Henle's fiber layer **(Figs. 9A and B)**.

Figure 9A shows a pseudocolor fundus photograph of an eye with CME, with dull foveal reflex and loss of foveal contour, and **Figure 9B** shows the optical coherence tomographic image of the same, with intraretinal clear spaces containing fluid distributed in a petaloid fashion, with loss of foveal depression and increased central macular thickness.

Risk Factors

Diabetes, intraocular inflammation (uveitis), cataract surgeries, especially complicated ones with insult to the posterior capsule, other ocular surgeries, and laser procedures are risk factors.

Epidemiology

It has been seen that about 20% of patients who undergo uncomplicated cataract surgeries develop CME over 3–12 weeks postoperatively, but only 1% of these are clinically significant.

Symptoms

Patients present with a reduction in visual acuity as well as altered visual functions such as color vision and contrast sensitivity. Metamorphopsia, micropsia (perceiving objects as being smaller in size than they actually are), and central scotoma (blind spot) may also be noticed by observant patients.

Management

Most cases are self-limiting, with spontaneous improvement with treatment of the underlying disorder. Nonsteroidal anti-inflammatory drugs, carbonic anhydrase inhibitors, and corticosteroids, along with laser photocoagulation, are recommended; in cases with persistent DME, vitrectomy is of help. Intravitreal steroid injections and anti-VEGF injections are also seen to be effective.

Epiretinal Membrane

Epiretinal membrane refers to an avascular membrane over the ILM at the macular area. It is synonymously known as surface wrinkling retinopathy or epiretinal gliosis or epimacular proliferations.

Epidemiology

It most commonly occurs idiopathically in the elderly (over 50 years of age) at an incidence of 7% in the Blue Mountains Eye Study, with only 1.9% in persons < 60 years of age but as much as 9.3% in people aged > 80 years. The prevalence of the same in the Indian population is comparable—7.6%.

Pathophysiology

Though the most common cause of ERM is idiopathic, secondary ERMs are often seen post trauma, ocular surgery, laser, or in patients with underlying retinal pathology such as DR, RVOs, chronic macular edema with or without intraocular inflammation, or retinal detachment, wherein PVD causes insult to or dehiscence in the ILM, and microglial cells, hyalocytes, and laminocytes interact and transdifferentiate into fibroblast-like cells to form a cellophane-like sheet.

Symptoms

It causes a reduction in visual acuity along with distortion of images (metamorphopsias, micropsias, or macropsias). It would be advisable for patients to monitor themselves periodically with Amsler grid charts, and an OCT would show a hyperreflective layer over the ILM.

Management

Asymptomatic ERMs may be observed but those causing symptoms would require a vitrectomy along with peeling of the ERM as well as the ILM since it is the ILM that forms the scaffold for the proliferation of fibroblasts and glial cells that form the ERM. On the other hand, some workers also believe that ILM peeling might cause damage to muller cells.

Diabetic Retinopathy

Diabetic retinopathy is the most frequent microvascular complication of DM (the others being nephropathy and neuropathy) and the most widespread cause of blindness in working adults in the West.

Symptoms

Though asymptomatic in the initial stages, progression may be accompanied by diminution of vision, floaters, and partial or total vision loss.

Stages

The Early Treatment Diabetic Retinopathy Study group classified the disease into NPDR associated with microaneurysms (focal dilatations of capillary walls), hemorrhages (superficial flame-shaped or deep dot and blot hemorrhages), hard exudates (lipoproteins and lipid-filled macrophages) and soft exudates or cotton-wool spots (focal arteriolar infarcts in the nerve fiber layer), intraretinal microvascular abnormalities (IRMAs), venous beading or looping and arterial narrowing and obliteration and proliferative DR (PDR) associated with the development of new vessels over the optic disk (NVD) or elsewhere (NVE), which may develop vitreous hemorrhage (VH) or neovascular glaucoma (NVG) and painful blind eye from neovascularization of iris (NVI) and angles (NVA).

Management

Diabetic macular edema is currently managed with intravitreal anti-VEGF agents such as bevacizumab (off-label), ranibizumab, aflibercept, pegaptanib and brolucizumab, and long-acting corticosteroid implants (dexamethasone, fluocinolone acetonide). PDR is managed with laser photocoagulation and in high-risk cases or advanced diabetic eye disease with nonresolving vitreous hemorrhage or tractional retinal detachment, vitrectomy is advisable.

Implication

Since good systemic control remains the cornerstone of treatment, the importance of regular visits to the endocrinologist with a strict diabetic diet and monitoring of blood sugars cannot be stressed enough.

Retinal Vascular Occlusions

Retinal Arterial Occlusions

Retinal arterial occlusions, including vascular transient monocular visual loss (TMVL) or transient ischemic attacks or amaurosis fugax, BRAOs, CRAOs, and ophthalmic artery occlusions (OAOs), are more than just causes of visual loss; they are harbingers of cerebral ischemic strokes and cardiac events, due to shared vascular risk factors. Interestingly, CRAO also conforms to the definition of ischemic stroke, "an episode of neurological dysfunction caused by focal cerebral, spinal or retinal infarction."

Epidemiology: The incidence of CRAO is about 0.85–10 cases per 100,000, but that of asymptomatic BRAO is much higher, amounting to about a cumulative 10-year incidence of 2.9% in those ≥ 49 years old.

Pathophysiology: These occur due to acute disruption of blood flow causing ischemia to the areas supplied by the vessel, which are visualized as whitish retinal discoloration, sometimes with visible emboli within the vasculature. Giant cell arteritis is a common association and needs to be ruled out.

Symptoms: Acute CRAO presents with sudden severe painless monocular visual loss. However, the presence of a cilioretinal artery may preserve central vision. OAO is particularly devastating, with loss of even perception of light, with relative afferent pupillary defect (RAPD) in that eye. BRAOs in the periphery may be asymptomatic, and those involving central retinal vasculature may present with a diminution of vision.

Management: Ocular massages to dislodge the emboli, anterior chamber paracentesis, and thrombolysis when platelet-fibrin thrombi are suspected are recommended; vasodilators and inhalation of carbogen (95% oxygen, 5% carbon dioxide) have been tried, but prognosis usually remains poor.

Implications: Immediate internist and cardiology evaluation to look for and initiate treatment for systemic conditions such as hypertension, arteriosclerotic cardiovascular disease, and giant cell arteritis plays the most important role in the prevention of undue systemic complications such as stroke in the near future.

Retinal Venous Occlusions

Retinal vein occlusions refer to thrombosis within the CRVO posterior to the lamina cribrosa, or one of its tributaries, called BRVO. CRVO may be nonischemic (perfused, with <10 disk areas of retinal capillary nonperfusion) or ischemic (nonperfused, having >10 disk areas of retinal capillary nonperfusion).

Epidemiology: The prevalence of RVO in the developed nations is 5.20 per 1,000 and that specifically of CRVO is 0.8 per 1,000.

Pathophysiology: Virchow's triad postulates that the following factors predispose a person to developing vascular thrombosis: Increased coagulability of blood, change in blood flow in the vessels, and injury to the vessel wall/endothelial damage. Any cause of these can predispose to clot formation. Anatomically, retinal veins and arteries share a common adventitial sheath, and the thickening of arterial walls due to atherosclerosis can also lead to compression of the vein. Back pressure due to venous occlusion leads to the finding of dilation and tortuosity of veins downstream along with extensive hemorrhages and RNFL infarcts.

Symptoms: Nonischemic CRVO, which is more common than the ischemic variety, to about 70% of cases of CRVO, present with good visual acuity (often better than 6/60 or 20/200), and ischemic CRVO, though forming only about 30% of cases, present with poor visual acuity.

These eyes show varying degrees of venous dilation or tortuosity, retinal hemorrhages, cotton-wool patches, macular edema, and retinal nonperfusion on fluorescein angiography. Ischemic CRVO patients have a high risk of NVG due to the development of new vessels (as a result of the release of proangiogenic factors such as VEGF by the ischemic retina) in 50% of eyes, usually by 3 months, giving it the name 100-day glaucoma.

Management: It mainly includes intravitreal anti-VEGF or steroid injections or implants to control macular edema and prevent the development of new vessels.

CONCLUSION

Age-related senescence in vision and its complex system pose a significant challenge to the older adults due to their high prevalence, complexity and inaccessibility to optimum healthcare. Age-related ophthalmological problems like presbyopia, cataract, glaucoma, macular degeneration, and dry eye disease commonly result in progressive vision loss, affecting independence and quality of life. Early detection through regular screening, timely intervention, and control of systemic comorbidities like diabetes and hypertension are crucial for preventing visual impairment. Surgical advancements have improved outcomes for common conditions like cataract and retinal disorders, but awareness, caregiver vigilance, and promoting access to ophthalmic care, especially for rural older adults, are vital to preserving vision and enhancing well-being in the elderly.

Self-Assessment Questionnaire

Q1. What are the causes of gradual, painless reduction of vision in the elderly?

Q2. What are the causes of acute loss of vision in the elderly?

Q3. What are the adverse effects that systemic medications prescribed to the elderly have on the eye?

Q4. List names of some ophthalmic medications with systemic side effects.

Q5. What are the implications of poor vision in the elderly?

Q6. How does one ensure good eye care for the elderly?

FURTHER READINGS

1. Balcombe NR, Sinclair A. Ageing: definitions, mechanisms and the magnitude of the problem. Best Pract Res Clin Gastroenterol. 2001;15(6):835-49.
2. Lin JB, Tsubota K, Apte RS. A glimpse at the aging eye. NPJ Aging Mech Dis. 2016;2(1):16003.
3. Vashist P, Talwar B, Gogoi M, Maraini G, Camparini M, Ravindran RD, et al. Prevalence of cataract in an older population in India. Ophthalmology. 2011;118(2-19):272-78.e2.
4. Tandon R, Vashist P, Gupta N, Gupta V, Sahay P, Deka D, et al. Association of dry eye disease and sun exposure in geographically diverse adult (≥40 years) populations of India: The SEED (sun exposure, environment and dry eye disease) study—second report of the ICMR-EYE SEE study group. Ocul Surf. 2020;18(4):718-30.
5. Vashist P, Tandon R, Murthy GVS, Barua CK, Deka D, Singh S, et al. Association of cataract and sun exposure in geographically diverse populations of India: the CASE study. First Report of the ICMR-EYE SEE Study Group. PLoS One. 2020;15(1):e0227868.
6. Tandon R, Vashist P, Gupta N, Gupta V, Yadav S, Deka D, et al. The association of sun exposure, ultraviolet radiation effects and other risk factors for pterygium (the SURE RISK for pterygium study) in geographically diverse adult (≥40 years) rural populations of India—3rd report of the ICMR-EYE SEE study group. PLoS One. 2022;17(7):e0270065.
7. Attebo K, Ivers RQ, Mitchell P. Refractive errors in an older population: the Blue Mountains Eye Study. Ophthalmology. 1999;106(6):1066-72.
8. Wang Q, Klein BE, Klein R, Moss SE. Refractive status in the Beaver Dam Eye Study. Invest Ophthalmol Vis Sci. 1994;35(13):4344-7.
9. Holden BA. Global vision impairment due to uncorrected presbyopia. Arch Ophthalmol. 2008;126(12):1731.
10. Malhotra S, Vashist P, Kalaivani M, Rath RS, Gupta N, Gupta SK, et al. Prevalence of presbyopia, spectacles coverage and barriers for unmet need among adult population of rural Jhajjar, Haryana. J Family Med Prim Care. 2022;11(1):287-93.
11. Zebardast N, Friedman DS, Vitale S. The prevalence and demographic associations of presenting near-vision impairment among adults living in the United States. Am J Ophthalmol. 2017;174:134-44.
12. Kanthan GL, Mitchell P, Burlutsky G, Wang JJ. Intermediate- and longer-term visual outcomes after cataract surgery: the Blue Mountains Eye Study. Clin Exp Ophthalmol. 2011;39(3):201-6.
13. Lavanya R, Wong TY, Aung T, Tan DTH, Saw SM, Tay WT, et al. Prevalence of cataract surgery and post-surgical visual outcomes in an urban Asian population: the Singapore Malay Eye Study. Br J Ophthalmol. 2009;93(3):299-304.
14. Hofstetter HW. A comparison of Duane's and Donders' tables of the amplitude of accommodation*. Optom Vis Sci. 1944;21(9):345.
15. Hashemi A, Khabazkhoob M, Hashemi H. High prevalence of refractive errors in an elderly population; a public health issue. BMC Ophthalmol. 2023;23:38.
16. Tan CSH, Chan YH, Wong TY, Gazzard G, Niti M, Ng TP, et al. Prevalence and risk factors for refractive errors and ocular biometry parameters in an elderly Asian population: the Singapore Longitudinal Aging Study (SLAS). Eye (Lond). 2011;25(10):1294-301.
17. Patel I, West SK. Presbyopia: prevalence, impact, and interventions. Community Eye Health. 2007;20(63):40-1.
18. The definition and classification of dry eye disease: report of the definition and classification subcommittee of the International Dry Eye WorkShop (2007). Ocul Surf. 2007;5(2):75-92.
19. Titiyal JS, Falera RC, Kaur M, Sharma V, Sharma N. Prevalence and risk factors of dry eye disease in North India: ocular surface disease index-based cross-sectional hospital study. Indian J Ophthalmol. 2018;66(2):207-11.
20. Hasan ZAIY. Dry eye syndrome risk factors: a systemic review. Saudi J Ophthalmol. 2022;35(2):131-9.
21. Messmer EM. The pathophysiology, diagnosis, and treatment of dry eye disease. Dtsch Arztebl Int. 2015;112(5):71-82.
22. Stern ME, Schaumburg CS, Pflugfelder SC. Dry eye as a mucosal autoimmune disease. Int Rev Immunol. 2013;32(1):19-41.
23. Stevenson W, Chauhan SK, Dana R. Dry eye disease: an immune-mediated ocular surface disorder. Arch Ophthalmol. 2012;130(1):90-100.
24. Al-Mohtaseb Z, Schachter S, Lee BS, Garlich J, Trattler W. The relationship between dry eye disease and digital screen use. Clin Ophthalmol. 2021;15:3811-20.
25. Pterygium throughout the world. Med J Aust. 1966;1(1):25.
26. Sarkar P, Tripathy K. Pterygium. Treasure Island, FL: StatPearls Publishing; 2024.
27. Di Girolamo N, Chui J, Coroneo MT, Wakefield D. Pathogenesis of pterygia: role of cytokines, growth factors, and matrix metalloproteinases. Prog Retin Eye Res. 2004;23(2):195-228.
28. Maheshwari S. Pterygium-induced corneal refractive changes. Indian J Ophthalmol. 2007;55(5):383-6.
29. Sarnicola C, Farooq AV, Colby K. Fuchs endothelial corneal dystrophy: update on pathogenesis and future directions. Eye Contact Lens. 2019;45(1):1-10.
30. Altamirano F, Ortiz-Morales G, O'Connor-Cordova MA, Sancén-Herrera JP, Zavala J, Valdez-Garcia JE. Fuchs endothelial corneal dystrophy: an updated review. Int Ophthalmol. 2024;44(1):61.
31. Das AV, Chaurasia S. Clinical profile and demographic distribution of Fuchs' endothelial dystrophy: an electronic medical record–driven big data analytics from an eye care network in India. Indian J Ophthalmol. 2022;70(7):2415-20.
32. Nanda GG, Alone DP. REVIEW: current understanding of the pathogenesis of Fuchs' endothelial corneal dystrophy. Mol Vis. 2019;25:295-310.
33. Aiello F, Afflitto GG, Ceccarelli F, Cesareo M, Nucci C. Global prevalence of Fuchs endothelial corneal dystrophy (FECD) in adult population: a systematic review and meta-analysis. J Ophthalmol. 2022;2022:3091695.
34. Koizumi N, Okumura N, Ueno M, Kinoshita S. New therapeutic modality for corneal endothelial disease using Rho-associated kinase inhibitor eye drops. Cornea. 2014;33 Suppl 11:S25-31.
35. Hashemi H, Pakzad R, Yekta A, Aghamirsalim M, Pakbin M, Ramin S, et al. Global and regional prevalence of age-related cataract: a comprehensive systematic review and meta-analysis. Eye (Lond). 2020;34(8):1357-70.
36. Sihota, Tandon R. Parson's Diseases of the Eye—E-Book. Centro Rio de Janeiro: Elsevier Health Sciences; 2014. p. 641.
37. Atalay E, Oğurel T, Derici MK. The role of oxidative damage in cataract etiopathogenesis. Ophthalmol Eye Dis. 2023;15:25158414231168813.
38. Pollreisz A, Schmidt-Erfurth U. Diabetic cataract—pathogenesis, epidemiology and treatment. J Ophthalmol. 2010;2010:608751.
39. Ivers RQ, Cumming RG, Mitchell P, Attebo K. Visual impairment and falls in older adults: the Blue Mountains Eye Study. J Am Geriatr Soc. 1998;46(1):58-64.
40. Palagyi A, McCluskey P, White A, Rogers K, Meuleners L, Ng JQ, et al. While we waited: incidence and predictors of falls in older adults with cataract. Invest Ophthalmol Vis Sci. 2016;57(14):6003-10.
41. McCarty CA, Fu CL, Taylor HR. Predictors of falls in the Melbourne visual impairment project. Aust N Z J Public Health. 2002;26(2):116-9.

42. Cox A, Blaikie A, MacEwen CJ, Jones D, Thompson K, Holding D, et al. Visual impairment in elderly patients with hip fracture: causes and associations. Eye (Lond). 2005;19(6):652-6.
43. Mencucci R, Stefanini S, Favuzza E, Cennamo M, Vitto CD, Mossello E. Beyond vision: cataract and health status in old age, a narrative review. Front Med (Lausanne). 2023;10:1110383.
44. Redruello-Guerrero P, Rivera-Izquierdo M, Jiménez-Gutiérrez C, Láinez-Ramos-Bossini AJ, Yela R, López-Marín I. Improvement of intermediate vision with new monofocal intraocular lenses: a systematic review and meta-analysis. Eur J Ophthalmol. 2023;33(3):1308-19.
45. Jonas JB, Aung T, Bourne RR, Bron AM, Ritch R, Panda-Jonas S. Glaucoma. Lancet. 2017;390(10108):2183-93.
46. Zhang N, Wang J, Li Y, Jiang B. Prevalence of primary open angle glaucoma in the last 20 years: a meta-analysis and systematic review. Sci Rep. 2021;11:13762.
47. Distelhorst JS, Hughes GM. Open-angle glaucoma. Am Fam Physician. 2003;67(9):1937-44.
48. Wolfs RC, Klaver CC, Ramrattan RS, van Duijn CM, Hofman A, de Jong PT. Genetic risk of primary open-angle glaucoma. Population-based familial aggregation study. Arch Ophthalmol. 1998;116(12):1640-5.
49. Weinreb RN, Aung T, Medeiros FA. The pathophysiology and treatment of glaucoma. JAMA. 2014;311(18):1901-11.
50. Boland MV, Ervin AM, Friedman DS, Jampel HD, Hawkins BS, Vollenweider D, et al. Comparative effectiveness of treatments for open-angle glaucoma: a systematic review for the U.S. Preventive Services Task Force. Ann Intern Med. 2013;158(4):271-9.
51. Ritch R, Schlötzer-Schrehardt U. Exfoliation syndrome. Surv Ophthalmol. 2001;45(4):265-315.
52. Forsius H. Prevalence of pseudoexfoliation of the lens in Finns, Lapps, Icelanders, Eskimos, and Russians. Trans Ophthalmol Soc UK (1962). 1979;99(2):296-8.
53. Faulkner HW. Pseudo-exfoliation of the lens among the Navajo Indians. Am J Ophthalmol. 1971;72(1):206-7.
54. Krishnadas R, Nirmalan PK, Ramakrishnan R, Thulasiraj RD, Katz J, Tielsch JM, et al. Pseudoexfoliation in a rural population of southern India: the Aravind Comprehensive Eye Survey. Am J Ophthalmol. 2003;135(6):830-7.
55. Nirmalan PK, Katz J, Robin AL, Tielsch JM, Namperumalsamy P, Kim R, et al. Prevalence of vitreoretinal disorders in a rural population of southern India: the Aravind Comprehensive Eye Study. Arch Ophthalmol. 2004;122(4):581-6.
56. Thapa SS, Thapa R, Paudyal I, Khanal S, Aujla J, Paudyal G, et al. Prevalence and pattern of vitreo-retinal diseases in Nepal: the Bhaktapur glaucoma study. BMC Ophthalmol. 2013;13:9.
57. Hamati J, Prashanthi S, Narayanan R, Sahoo N, Das AV, Rani PK, et al. Prevalence of age-related macular degeneration and associated factors in Indian cohort in a tertiary care setting. Indian J Ophthalmol. 2023;71(10):3361-6.
58. Likhar N, Mothe RK, Kanukula R, Shah C, Dang A. The prevalence of age-related Macular degeneration in Indian Population: a systematic review. Value in Health. 2015;18(3):A180.
59. Kulkarni SR, Aghashe SR, Khandekar RB, Deshpande MD. Prevalence and determinants of age-related macular degeneration in the 50 years and older population: a hospital based study in Maharashtra, India. Indian J Ophthalmol. 2013;61(5):196-201.
60. Wong WL, Su X, Li X, Cheung CMG, Klein R, Cheng CY, et al. Global prevalence of age-related macular degeneration and disease burden projection for 2020 and 2040: a systematic review and meta-analysis. Lancet Global Health. 2014;2(2):e106-16.
61. Shirley M. Faricimab: first approval. Drugs. 2022;82(7):825-30.
62. Woo SJ, Park KH, Ahn J, Choe JY, Jeong H, Han JW, et al. Cognitive impairment in age-related macular degeneration and geographic atrophy. Ophthalmology. 2012;119(10):2094-101.
63. McGuinness MB, Karahalios A, Finger RP, Guymer RH, Simpson JA. Age-related macular degeneration and mortality: a systematic review and meta-analysis. Ophthalmic Epidemiol. 2017;24(3): 141-52.
64. Di Carlo E, Augustin AJ. Prevention of the onset of age-related macular degeneration. J Clin Med. 2021;10(15):3297.
65. Sen P, Bhargava A, Vijaya L, George R. Prevalence of idiopathic macular hole in adult rural and urban south Indian population. Clinical Exper Ophthalmol. 2008;36(3):257-60.
66. Nangia V, Jonas JB, Khare A, Lambat S. Prevalence of macular holes in rural central India. The Central India Eye and Medical Study. Graefes Arch Clin Exp Ophthalmol. 2012;250(7):1105-7.
67. Rahmani B, Tielsch JM, Katz J, Gottsch J, Quigley H, Javitt J, et al. The cause-specific prevalence of visual impairment in an urban population. The Baltimore Eye Survey. Ophthalmology. 1996;103(11):1721-6.
68. Duker JS, Kaiser PK, Binder S, de Smet MD, Gaudric A, Reichel E, et al. The International Vitreomacular Traction Study Group classification of vitreomacular adhesion, traction, and macular hole. Ophthalmology. 2013;120(12):2611-9.
69. Ray S, D'Amico DJ. Pseudophakic cystoid macular edema. Semin Ophthalmol. 2002;17(3-4):167-80.
70. Mitchell P, Smith W, Chey T, Wang JJ, Chang A. Prevalence and associations of epiretinal membranes. The Blue Mountains Eye Study, Australia. Ophthalmology. 1997;104(6):1033-40.
71. Koh V, Cheung CY, Wong WL, Cheung CM, Wang JJ, Mitchell P, et al. Prevalence and risk factors of epiretinal membrane in Asian Indians. Invest Ophthalmol Vis Sci. 2012;53(2):1018.
72. Eisma JH, Dulle JE, Fort PE. Current knowledge on diabetic retinopathy from human donor tissues. World J Diabetes. 2015;6(2):312-20.
73. Early Treatment Diabetic Retinopathy Study Research Group. Early photocoagulation for diabetic retinopathy. ETDRS report number 9. Ophthalmology. 1991;98(5 Suppl):766-85.
74. Sacco RL, Kasner SE, Broderick JP, Caplan LR, Connors JJB, Culebras A, et al. An updated definition of stroke for the 21st century: a statement for healthcare professionals from the American Heart Association/American Stroke Association. Stroke. 2013;44(7): 2064-89.
75. Rumelt S, Dorenboim Y, Rehany U. Aggressive systematic treatment for central retinal artery occlusion. Am J Ophthalmol. 1999;128(6):733-8.
76. Cugati S, Wang JJ, Rochtchina E, Mitchell P. Ten-year incidence of retinal emboli in an older population. Stroke. 2006;37(3):908-10.
77. Klein R, Moss SE, Meuer SM, Klein BEK. The 15-year cumulative incidence of retinal vein occlusion: the Beaver Dam Eye Study. Arch Ophthalmol. 2008;126(4):513-8.
78. Kumar DR, Hanlin E, Glurich I, Mazza JJ, Yale SH. Virchow's contribution to the understanding of thrombosis and cellular biology. Clin Med Res. 2010;8(3-4):168-72.
79. Havens SJ, Gulati V. Neovascular glaucoma. Dev Ophthalmol. 2016;55:196-204.
80. Raharja A, Whitefield L. Clinical approach to vision loss: a review for general physicians. Clin Med (Lond). 2022;22(2):95.
81. Syed MF, Rehmani A, Yang M. Ocular side effects of common systemic medications and systemic side effects of ocular medications. Med Clin North Ame. 2021;105(3):425-44.

CHAPTER 24

Mild Cognitive Impairment

Arunansu Talukdar, Akshata Rao

CASE VIGNETTE

Patient: Mr Sengupta, a 68-year-old, retired, hypertensive, lives with wife.

Presenting complaints: Since the past year, he frequently forgts important events, lost things, struggles with words, and neglected bills. Since recently, he has been forgetting medications, becomes easily irritated, and sometimes feels low. He functions cognitively well, and his daily activities are intact. Initially minor, his forgetfulness has worsened, raising concerns about dependency.

Medical: Hypertension that is managed with medication.

Social: He lives with his wife and son stays abroad. He assists with chores. There is no history of alcohol or tobacco use.

Review of systems: No significant symptoms such as chest pain, visual disturbances, dizziness, or urinary incontinence are noted.

Physical examination: Blood pressure (BP) 135/82 mm Hg, heart rate (HR) 76 bpm. No focal deficits are found in the neurological examination. Musculoskeletal examination shows no rigidity, bradykinesia, tremor, or gait disturbance. No hallucinations, speech issues, or unexplained falls are seen.

INTRODUCTION

Aging causes deterioration in various aspects of cognitive function. Our brain, such as the rest of our body, changes as we grow older. Many people notice a progressive increase in forgetfulness as they age. It may take longer to find a proper word or to recall a person's name.

Mild cognitive impairment (MCI) is a condition in which memory problems and/or other cognitive difficulties (e.g., ability to think, learn, remember, use judgment, and make decisions) are noticeable. MCI is more severe than aging-related alterations. People who have MCI could be conscious that their mental or memory skills have "slipped." It is evident to close friends, family, work colleagues, and others. Yet, these impairments are not severe enough to interfere with day-to-day tasks of everyday living, as they have intact activities of daily living (ADLs) and usually take care of themselves.

Mild cognitive impairment is the preclinical and transitional stage between healthy aging and dementia that may be a potential "target" for interventions designed to delay progression to dementia, which takes place between the normal decreases in memory and reasoning that occur with age and the more serious decline of dementia. MCI causes cognitive changes that are serious enough to be noticed by the person affected and by family members and friends. MCI can cause memory, language, thinking, and judgment issues.

Several MCI subtypes have been identified. They differ in terms of the cognitive abilities that are affected. Individuals with amnestic MCI have severe memory abnormalities that can occur alone (*amnestic MCI single domain*) or in combination with deficits in other cognitive domains *(amnestic MCI multiple domain)*. Individuals with nonamnestic forms of MCI perform normally on memory tasks but have significant deficits in one other cognitive domain, such as language, executive functioning, or visuospatial abilities (*nonamnestic MCI single domain*) or impairments in two or more of these cognitive domains (*nonamnestic MCI multiple domain*). It has been proposed that these four clinical subgroups may have distinct underlying causes, one of which could be approaching dementia or Alzheimer's disease (AD).

Mild cognitive impairment may be associated with an increased risk of dementia caused by AD or other brain

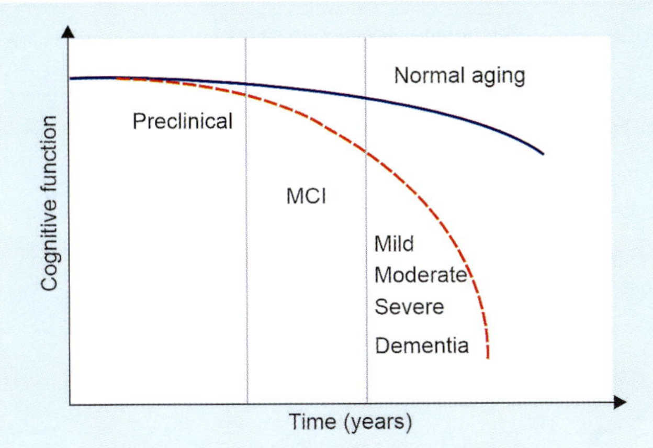

FIG. 1: Progression from normal aging to Alzheimer's disease or another dementia.
(MCI: mild cognitive impairment)

illnesses **(Fig. 1)**. For the treatment of AD, early diagnosis or increased-risk identification may be very helpful. However, some patients with MCI may never deteriorate. In addition, some can eventually get better with time.

EPIDEMIOLOGY

Prevalence and Global Perspective

The prevalence of MCI varies widely ranging from 3 to 42% across the population. In the Longitudinal Aging Study in India-Diagnostic Assessment of Dementia (LASI-DAD) study, the prevalence of mild neurocognitive disorder, weighted to the population, is 17.6%, while that of a major neurocognitive disorder stands at 7.2%. Evidences from researchers show that individuals with MCI are more likely to develop AD or a related dementia than individuals without it. The annual progression rate from MCI to AD is reported to range between 10 and 15%. According to research, hereditary variables may play a role in who will develop MCI, just as they do in Alzheimer's and similar dementias. Studies are being conducted to explore why some persons with MCI develop Alzheimer's while others do not. Cognitive decline is a natural part of getting older. Cognitive changes in MCI are more significant than those seen in normal aging, but not severe enough to require considerable lifestyle adjustments. Although there may be progression from normal aging to MCI to dementia, this does not always occur. Not everyone with MCI develops dementia. According to some research, up to 40% of people who match the criteria for MCI recover within a year. Mood swings and drug side effects can mimic MCI. *About 10–15% of people with MCI will develop dementia during the first year, and approximately 50% (25–80%) will have dementia within 5 years.* This is a greater incidence rate than that of people without MCI. However, it is important to note that MCI does not invariably lead to dementia.

Risk Factors for Cognitive Impairment

The 2024 update to the Lancet Commission on dementia prevention, intervention, and care identifies 14 modifiable risk factors that, if addressed, could prevent or delay nearly half of all dementia cases worldwide **(Fig. 2)**.

Mild Cognitive Disorder in Indian Elderly

Over 138 million Indian adults are aged 60 years and older. It is expected that they will constitute 20% of the population of India by 2050. Along with expanding population come different concerns related to aging, including medical diseases and health conditions. MCI is one of them. From different studies focused on MCI in India, it has been seen that the prevalence is between 15 and 33%.

Gender Discrepancies

Studies have shown that MCI is more prevalent among females than in males. In India, a higher risk of development of cognitive impairment in females is often linked with lower levels of early-life human capital investments in their education and nutrition compared to males.

- *Urban versus rural variances*: There is evidence that show that there is a difference in the prevalence of MCI in rural and urban areas. Different factors, such as socioeconomic status, malnutrition, and environment of the surroundings, make the rural population more susceptible to MCI.
- *Chronic health conditions*: Older people are often burdened with chronic health conditions, diabetes and hypertension being common ones. It has been found that diabetes, hypertension, and stroke are significant risk factors for MCI.
- *Malnutrition*: Prevalence of malnutrition has been found to be high among the elderly, and there is a positive relation between malnutrition and cognitive impairment. It plays an important role in the progression of cognitive decline in an individual. Hence, early recognition and treatment are important preventive measures.
- *Psychosocial factors*: They also have the potential to contribute to cognitive impairment. It has been seen that older age, low educational level, smoking, depressive symptoms, lower social support, and living alone all these factors are associated with an increased risk of cognitive impairment.

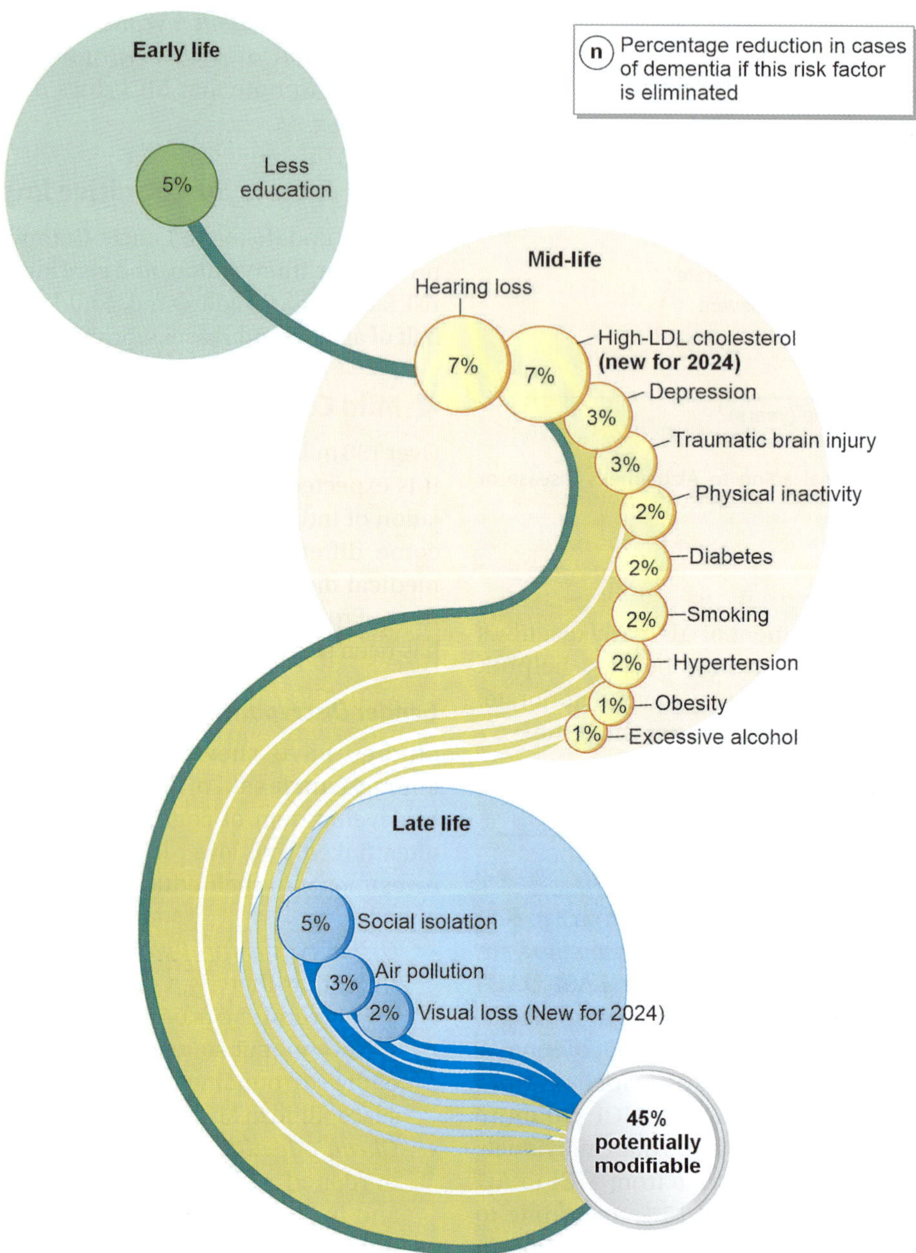

FIG. 2: Fourteen modifiable risk factors for cognitive impairment.
(LDL: low-density lipoprotein)

CLINICAL PRESENTATION

The main sign of MCI is a slight decline in cognitive abilities, such as:

- *Memory problems*: The individual may forget recent occurrences or keep asking the same questions and telling the same stories. He may forget the names of acquaintances and family members, as well as appointments or planned events. He also misplaces things more frequently than usual. He loses his train of thought, or he may not be able to follow the plot of a book or movie.
- *Language issues*: The individual is having word-finding difficulties. He may also have difficulty understanding written or spoken information. He has difficulty with following instructions.
- *Attention*: He may become more easily distracted or lose focus than usual. He has trouble following up with a conversation. The individual finds it hard to make decisions, finish a task, or follow instructions.

- *Reasoning and judgment*: The person may have difficulties solving problems, making judgments, and an inability to take appropriate decisions.
- *Visual depth perception*: The individual strains to perceive a thing in three dimensions, judge distances, or negotiate stairs.

A person with MCI may also experience *depressive symptoms, anxiety, short temper, aggression*, and a *lack of interest* while doing tasks. Patients with MCI generally maintain daily function but may experience cognitive decline, taking longer to complete tasks without needing help. Reliable informants are helpful for assessment. If patients continue normal activities such as driving or managing finances, they likely do not meet dementia criteria. The clinician must assess cognitive changes, confirm objective evidence, ensure that daily function is intact, and rule out dementia. To gain a better understanding about the difference between major cognitive impairment and MCI, the diagnostic criteria of major neurocognitive disorder and mild neurocognitive disorder according to Diagnostic and Statistical Manual of Mental Disorders, Fifth Edition (DSM-5) are mentioned in **Boxes 1 and 2**.

If MCI is confirmed, the clinician should determine if memory is a key factor. If memory is impaired, amnestic MCI applies; if memory is intact, nonamnestic MCI is more appropriate. According to Petersen et al., clinicians can use progression criteria from a **Flowchart 1** to better understand the diagnosis of MCI. When a patient reports cognitive concerns, it is important to confirm their history with someone familiar with the patient. Cognitive concern signals a change in performance, not lifelong low cognitive function. Without formal longitudinal data, clinical history becomes essential. Clinicians should focus on specific cognitive changes, especially recent memory loss (within 6 months to a year), such as forgetfulness about events, appointments, or conversations. Repeating oneself may indicate worsening deficits, highlighting changes in memory or cognition.

BOX 1 **DSM-5 diagnostic criteria of major neurocognitive disorder.**

- *A*: Evidence of significant cognitive decline from a previous level of performance in one or more cognitive domains (complex attention, executive function, learning and memory, language, perceptual–motor, or social cognition) based on:
  - Concern of the individual, a knowledgeable informant, or the clinician that there has been a significant decline in cognitive function.
  - A substantial impairment in cognitive performance, preferably documented by standardized neuropsychological testing or, in its absence, another quantified clinical assessment.
- *B*: The cognitive deficits interfere with independence in everyday activities (i.e., at a minimum, requiring assistance with complex instrumental activities of daily living such as paying bills or managing medications).
- *C*: The cognitive deficits do not occur exclusively in the context of a delirium.
- *D*: The cognitive deficits are not better explained by another mental disorder (e.g., major depressive disorder, schizophrenia).

Specify whether due to: Alzheimer's disease, frontotemporal lobar degeneration, Lewy body disease, vascular disease, traumatic brain injury, substance/medication use, HIV infection, prion disease, Parkinson's disease, Huntington's disease, another medical condition, multiple etiologies, or unspecified.

(DSM-5: Diagnostic and Statistical Manual of Mental Disorders, Fifth Edition)

BOX 2 **DSM-5 diagnostic criteria of mild neurocognitive disorder.**

- *A*: Evidence of modest cognitive decline from a previous level of performance in one or more cognitive domains (complex attention, executive function, learning and memory, language, perceptual–motor, or social cognition) based on:
  - Concern of the individual, a knowledgeable informant, or the clinician that there has been a mild decline in cognitive function.
  - A modest impairment in cognitive performance, preferably documented by standardized neuropsychological testing or, in its absence, another quantified clinical assessment.
- *B*: The cognitive deficits do not interfere with capacity for independence in everyday activities (i.e., complex instrumental activities of daily living such as paying bills or managing medications are preserved, but greater effort, compensatory strategies, or accommodation may be required).
- *C*: The cognitive deficits do not occur exclusively in the context of a delirium.
- *D*: The cognitive deficits are not better explained by another mental disorder (e.g., major depressive disorder, schizophrenia).

Specify whether due to: Alzheimer's disease, frontotemporal lobar degeneration, Lewy body disease, vascular disease, traumatic brain injury, substance/medication use, HIV infection, prion disease, Parkinson's disease, Huntington's disease, another medical condition, multiple etiologies, or unspecified.

(DSM-5: Diagnostic and Statistical Manual of Mental Disorders, Fifth Edition)

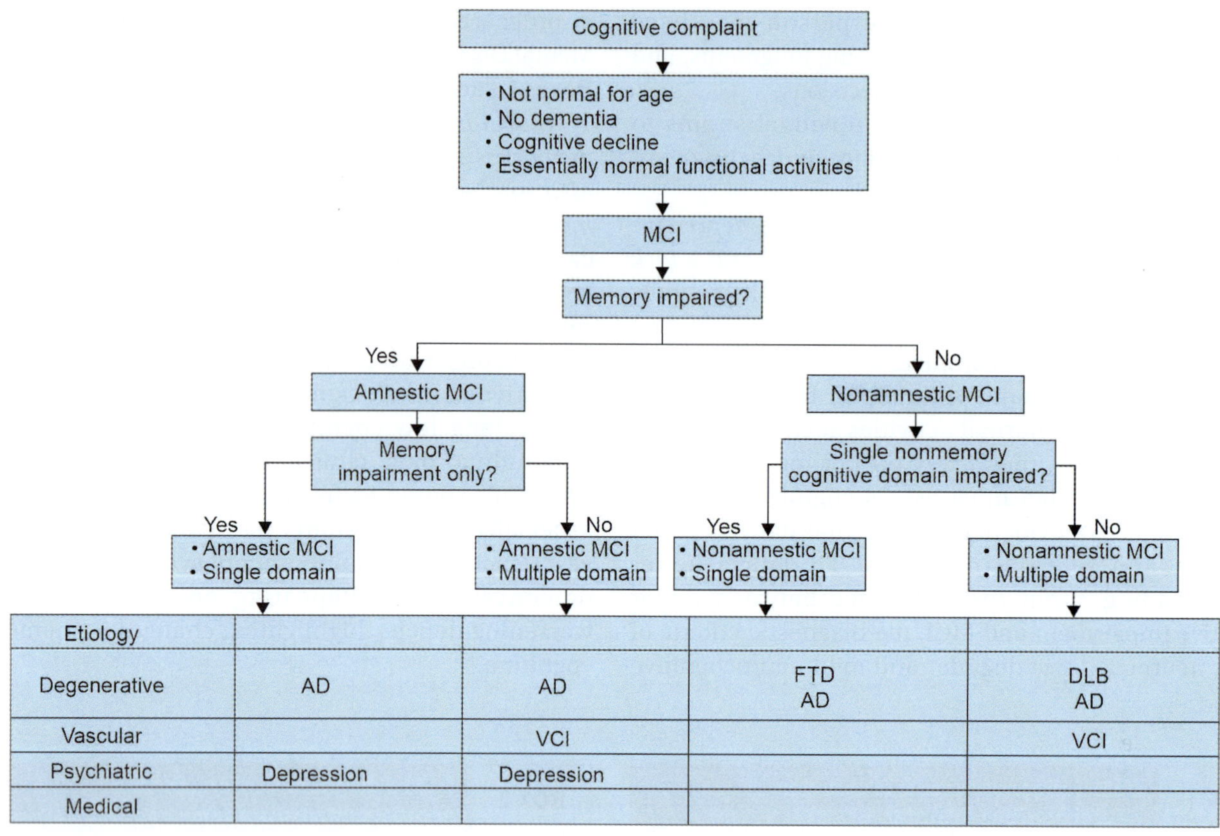

FLOWCHART 1: Clinical evaluation and diagnosis of cases with MCI.

(AD: Alzheimer's disease; DLB: dementia with Lewy bodies; FTD: frontotemporal disorders; MCI: mild cognitive impairment; VCI: vascular cognitive impairment)

EVALUATION AND INVESTIGATION

The primary objectives are to differentiate MCI from dementia or normal aging, as well as to identify types of MCI that are reversible and may be caused by other disorders. The focus should be placed on functional status, cognitive functions, medications, psychiatric or neurological abnormalities, and laboratory testing.

- Comprehensive history and physical examination
- *Cognitive assessment*: Screening followed by detailed assessment
- Functional status assessment
- Neuropsychological assessment
- *Biomarker evaluation*: Imaging, cerebrospinal fluid (CSF), and blood

Comprehensive History

Cognitive Functioning

A history of cognitive changes over time, confirmed by reliable informants, is critical for detecting the first diagnostic criterion, deterioration in cognitive function. Differences in symptom severity reported by patients and informants may stem from a lack of insight or emotional factors. Clinicians should evaluate the overall severity of cognitive impairment and determine whether it is restricted to memory or also affects other areas such as attention and concentration. Often, patients may mention memory issues when they are experiencing difficulties with attention or language. Therefore, it is essential to identify the full range of cognitive changes through domain-specific history and assessments.

After a detailed cognitive history, the clinician must focus on the possible etiology. Degenerative, vascular, psychological, or medical factors may explain the symptoms and guide further diagnostic steps. A slow, progressive onset suggests a degenerative cause, while vascular risk factors and cerebral ischemia point to vascular etiology. The onset, duration, progression, and nature of cognitive symptoms are crucial in determining the cause. Rapid decline over weeks or months is unusual for Alzheimer's-related MCI and may indicate other causes, such as neoplasms, metabolic issues, or prion diseases.

A review of symptoms should probe vision and hearing impairments, sleep apnea, behavioral or personality changes (which may suggest depression, thyroid disease, or frontotemporal dementia), visual hallucinations (Lewy-body dementia, severe depression with psychotic features), numbness or tingling in the extremities (neuropathy), dizziness when standing (orthostatic hypotension), changes in speech [stroke, Parkinson's disease (PD)], and changes in gait [stroke, normal pressure hydrocephalus (NPH), PD]. Other medical diseases, such as uncompensated heart failure, poorly managed diabetes, or chronic obstructive pulmonary disease, must always be examined by the clinician as determinants of cognitive impairment. Some of these medical comorbidities are treatable or manageable, and their medications can cause clinical symptoms.

Comprehensive Neurological Examination

Orthostatic hypotension, extraocular movements, vision, hearing, speech, focal weakness, the ability to stand from a chair, and gait can help identify potential contributors to cognitive decline, such as stroke, PD, NPH, or neuropathy caused by toxins or vitamin deficiency.

Cognitive Assessment Tools

Some of the commonly used screening tools for the detection of cognitive impairment are given in **Figure 3**.

The Mini-Mental State Examination (MMSE) and Montreal Cognitive Assessment (MoCA) are commonly used for screening, with the MoCA designed for MCI detection in about 10 minutes. Delayed recall is impaired in MCI. Studies show MoCA's attention tasks (digit span, sustained attention, serial 7s) distinguish Alzheimer's from MCI. Clinicians may consider the Mini-cog test, as it has acceptable test performance characteristics and can be completed in ≤3 minutes. Clinicians can use Addenbrooke's cognitive examination-III (ACE-III), informant questionnaire on cognitive decline in the elderly (IQCODE), the dementia severity rating scale (DSRS), and the Ascertain Dementia 8-item Questionnaire (AD8) to obtain standardized information on cognitive function from informants.

Mini-Cog: Mini-Cog was developed by Borson et al. in 2000. It is a short cognitive impairment-screening exam that combines a short memory test and an executive clock-drawing test. This enables fast screening for short-term memory problems and other cognitive functions that are reduced in patients with MCI. The ranges are mentioned below:

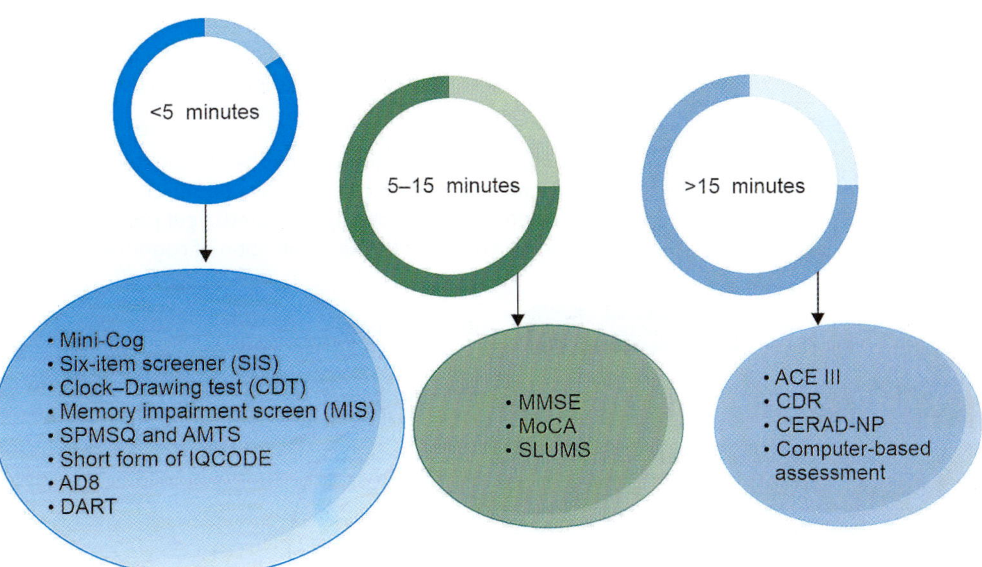

FIG. 3: Commonly used screening tools for the detection of cognitive impairment.

(ACE III: Addenbrooke's cognitive examination III; AD8: ascertain dementia-8 questionnaire; AMTS: abbreviated mental test score; CDR: clinical dementia rating; CERAD-NP: Consortium to Establish a Registry for Alzheimer disease neuropsychological battery; IQCODE: informant questionnaire on cognitive decline in the elderly; MMSE: mini-mental state examination; MoCA: Montreal cognitive assessment; SLUMS: St. Louis University mental status exam; SPMSQ: short portable mental status questionnaire)

<table>
<tr><td colspan="2">Mini-Cog©</td><td colspan="4">Instructions for administration and scoring:
ID: Date:</td></tr>
<tr><td colspan="6">Step 1: Three-word registration</td></tr>
<tr><td colspan="6">Look directly at the person and say "Please listen carefully. I am going to say three words that I want you to repeat back to me now and try to remember. The words are (select a list of words from the versions below). Please say them for me now." If the person is unable to repeat the words after three attempts, move on to step 2 (clock drawing).</td></tr>
<tr><td colspan="6">The following and other word lists have been used in one or more clinical studies. For repeated administrations, use of an alternative word list is recommended.</td></tr>
<tr><td>Version 1
Banana
Sunrise
Chair</td><td>Version 2
Leader
Season
Table</td><td>Version 3
Village
Kitchen
Baby</td><td>Version 4
River
Nation
Finger</td><td>Version 5
Captain
Garden
Picture</td><td>Version 6
Daughter
Heaven
Mountain</td></tr>
<tr><td colspan="6">Step 2: Clock drawing</td></tr>
<tr><td colspan="6">Say "Next, I want you to draw a clock for me. First, put in all of the numbers where they go," When that is completed, say "Now, set the hands to 10 past 11."</td></tr>
<tr><td colspan="6">Use a preprinted circle (see next page) for this exercise. Repeat instructions as needed as this is not a memory test. Move to step 3 if the clock is not complete within 3 minutes.</td></tr>
<tr><td colspan="6">Step 3: Three-word recall</td></tr>
<tr><td colspan="6">Ask the person to recall the three words you stated in step 1. Say "What were the three words I asked you to remember?" Record the word list version number and the person's answers below.
Word list version: Person's answers:</td></tr>
<tr><td colspan="6">Scoring</td></tr>
<tr><td>Word recall</td><td>(0–3 points)</td><td colspan="4">1 point for each word spontaneously recalled without cueing.</td></tr>
<tr><td>Clock draw</td><td>(0 or 2 points)</td><td colspan="4">Normal clock–2 points. A normal clock has all numbers placed in the correct sequence and approximately correct position (e.g., 12, 3, 6, and 9 are in anchor positions) with no missing or duplicate numbers. Hands are pointing to the 11 and 2 (11:10). Hand length is not scored.
Inability or refusal to draw a clock (abnormal) = 0 points</td></tr>
<tr><td>Total score</td><td>(0–5 points)</td><td colspan="4">Total score = Word Recall score + Clock Draw score
A cut point of <3 on the Mini-Cog has been validated for dementia screening, but many individuals with clinically meaningful cognitive impairment will score higher. When greater sensitivity is desired, a cut point of <4 is recommended as it may indicate a need for further evaluation of cognitive status.</td></tr>
</table>

Clock drawing ID:_______ Date:___________

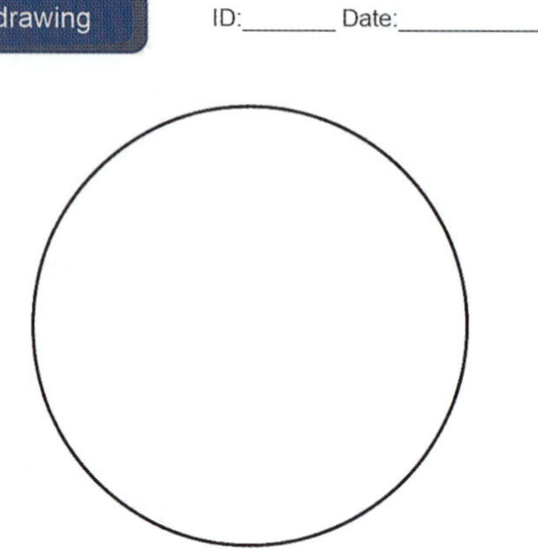

Source: Mini-Cog. (2025). Mini-Cog©—Quick Screening for Early Dementia Detection. [online] Available from https://mini-cog.com/. [Last accessed May, 2025].

- 0–2 indicates a higher likelihood of clinically important cognitive impairment.
- 3–5 indicates a lower likelihood of dementia but does not rule out some degree of cognitive impairment.

Montreal cognitive assessment: MoCA was developed by Ziad Nasreddine. It is a highly sensitive tool that can be used for the early detection of MCI as well as to detect early signs of dementia. It assesses a broad array of cognitive domains, such as visuospatial, attention/executive functioning, and language. The maximum possible score is 30 and a score of 26 or above is considered normal. The severity range is mentioned below:

Montreal Cognitive Assessment (MoCA) version 7.1 original version		**Name:** **Education:** **Sex:**		**Date of birth:** **Date:**			
Visuospatial/executive E End, A, 5, B, 2, 1 Begin, D, 4, 3, C		Copy cube		Draw clock (Ten past eleven) (3 points) [] Contour [] Numbers [] Hands			√5
Naming				√3			
Memory: Read list of words, subject must repeat them. Do 2 trials, even if 1st trial is successful. Do a recall after 5 minutes.		Face	Velvet	Church	Daisy	Red	*No points*
	1st trial						
	2nd trial						
Attention: Read a list of digits (1 digit/sec).	Subject has to repeat them in the forward order [] 2 1 8 5 4 Subject has to repeat them in the backward order [] 7 4 2						√2
Read list of letters. The subject must tap with his hand at each letter A. No points if ≥2 errors [] FBACMNAA JKLBAFAKDEA A A JAMOFA AB							√1
Serial 7 subtraction starting at 100 [] 93 [] 86 [] 79 [] 72 [] 65 4 or 5 correct subtractions: *3 pts*, 2 or 3 correct: *2 pts*, 1 correct: *1 pt*, 0 correct: *0 pt*							√3
Language	*Repeat*: I only know that John is the one to help today [] The cat always hid under the couch when dogs were in the room []						√2
Fluency/name maximum number of words in 1 minute that begin with the letter F (N ≥11 words) []							√1
Abstraction	Similarity between, e.g., banana-orange = fruit [] train-bicycle [] watch-ruler						√2
Delayed recall	Has to recall words *With no cue*	Face []	Velvet []	Church []	Daisy []	Red []	Points for *uncued* recall only √5
Optional	Category cue						
	Multiple choice cue						
Orientation	[] Date [] Month [] Year [] Day [] Place [] City						√6
Normal ≥26/30 Administered by:				Total √30 Add 1 point if ≤12 years education			
Source: ©Nasreddine Z. (2025). MoCA Test—Montreal Cognitive Assessment. [online] Available from https://www.mocacognition.com/the-moca-test/. [Last accessed May, 2025].							

Severity ranges:

- 18–25 = Mild cognitive impairment
- 10–17 = Moderate cognitive impairment
- <10 = Severe cognitive impairment

Addenbrooke's cognitive examination: The ACE was developed by Hodges et al. ACE-III is the test's current version. This comprises 19 tasks that assess five different cognitive domains: Language, attention, memory, fluency, and visuospatial processing. This is a detailed test, which takes around half an hour to complete and is scored out of 100. The score needs to be interpreted in the context of the patient's overall history and examination, but a score of 88 and above is considered normal; below 83 is abnormal; and between 83 and 87 is inconclusive. A score of <82 indicates likely dementia. The test gives helpful details on domains of function:

- Attention–marked out of 18
- Memory–marked out of 26
- Fluency–marked out of 14
- Language–marked out of 26
- Visuospatial–marked out of 16

Addenbrooke's cognitive examination–ACE-III Indian English						
Name: Date of birth: Hospital no. or address: Languages known: Native language:		Date of testing: ____/____/____ Tester's name:________ Age at leaving full-time education:________ Occupation:________ Handedness:________				
Attention						
• *Ask*: What is the	Day	Date	Month	Year	Season	Attention (score 0–5)
• *Ask*: Which	No./Floor	Street/Hospital	City	State	Country	Attention (score 0–5)
Attention						
• *Tell*: "I'm going to give you three words and I'd like you to repeat them after me: lemon, key and ball." After subject repeats, say "Try to remember them because I'm going to ask you later." • Score only the first trial (repeat 3 times if necessary). • Register number of trials:________					Attention (score 0–3)	
Attention						
• *Ask the subject*: "Could you take 7 away from 100? I'd like you to keep taking 7 away from each new number until I tell you to stop." • If subject makes a mistake, do not stop them. Let the subject carry on and check subsequent answers (e.g., 93, 84, 77, 70, 63— score 4). • Stop after five subtractions (93, 86, 79, 72, 65).					Attention (score 0–5)	
Memory						
• *Ask*: "Which 3 words did I ask you to repeat and remember?"________					Memory (score 0–3)	
Fluency						
• *Letters* *Say*: "I'm gong to give you a letter of the alphabet and I'd like you to generate as many words as you can beginning with that letter, but not names of people or places. For example, if I give you the letter 'C', you could give me words like 'cat, cry, clock' and so on. But you can't give me words like Catherine or Canada." Do you understand? Are you ready? You have 1 minute. The letter I want you to use is the letter "P"					Fluency (score 0–7)	
					>14	7
					11–14	6
					8–10	5
					6–7	4
					3–5	3
					2	2
					1	1
					0	0
					Total	Correct

Continued

Continued

• *Animals* *Say*: "Now can you name as many animals as possible. It can begin with any letter."				Fluency (score 0–7)

Total	Correct
>16	7
14–16	6
11–13	5
8–10	4
6–7	3
3–5	2
1–2	1
0	0

Memory

- *Tell*: "I'm going to give you a name and address and I'd like you to repeat the name and address after me. So you have a chance to learn, well be doing that 3 times. I'll ask you the name and address later."

Score only the third trial.

Memory (score 0–7)

	1st trial	2nd trial	3rd trial
Sunil Kumar Singh 52 Station Road Gandhinagar, Prayagraj, Uttar Pradesh, India	________ ________ ________ ________	________ ________ ________ ________	________ ________ ________ ________

Memory

- Name the current Chief Minister __________________
- Name the Prime Minister of India__________________
- Name the actor who was a hero in the film "Mera Naam Joker"__________________
- Name the Father of our Nation__________________

Memory (score 0–4)

Language

- Place a pencil and a piece of paper in front of the subject. As a practice trial, ask the subject to "Pick up the pencil and then the paper." If incorrect, score 0 and do not continue further.
- If the subject is correct on the practice trial, continue with the following three commands below:
  i. Ask the subject to "Place the paper on top of the pencil"
  ii. Ask the subject to "Pick up the pencil but not the paper"
  iii. Ask the subject to "Pass me the pencil after touching the paper"

Note: Place the pencil and paper in front of the subject before each command.

Language (score 0–4)

Language

- Ask the subject to write two (or more) complete sentences about his/her last holiday/weekend/festival. Write in complete sentences and do not use abbreviations.
- Give 1 point if there are two (or more) complete sentences about the one topic and give another 1 point if grammar and spelling are correct.

Language (score 0–3)

Language

- Ask the subject to repeat "caterpillar": "eccentricity": "unintelligible": "statistician"

Score 2 if all are correct, score 1 if 3 are correct, and score 0 if 2 or less are correct

Language (score 0–2)

Language	
• Ask the subject to repeat: **'All that glitters is not gold'**	**Language** [Score 0–1] ☐
• Ask the subject to repeat: **'A stitch in time saves nine'**	**Language** [Score 0–1] ☐

Language	
• Ask the subject to name the following pictures:	**Language** [Score 0–12] ☐

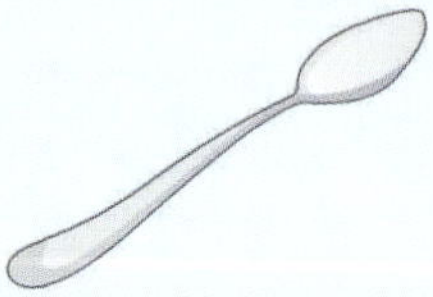

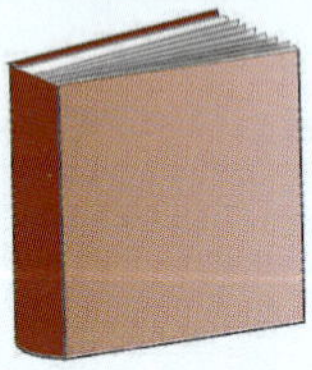

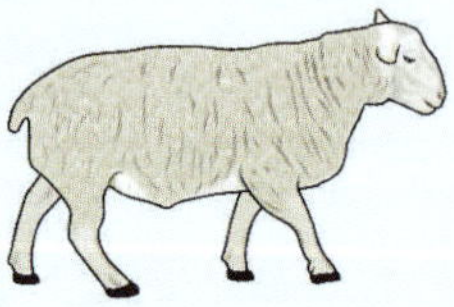

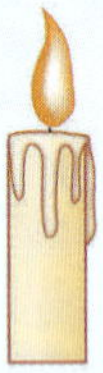

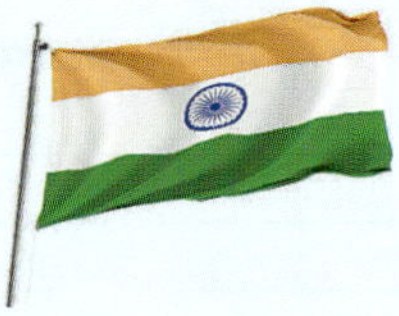

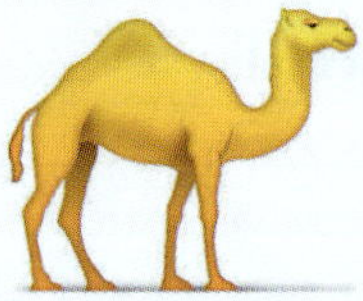

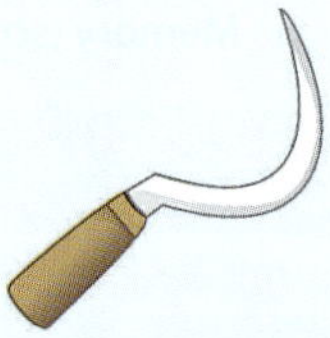

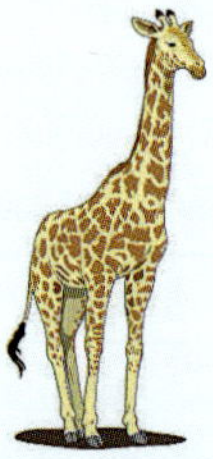

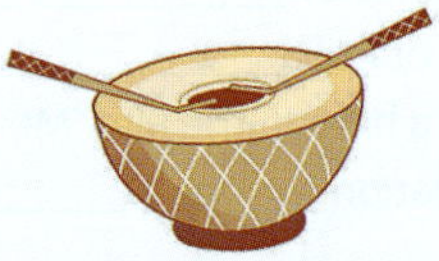

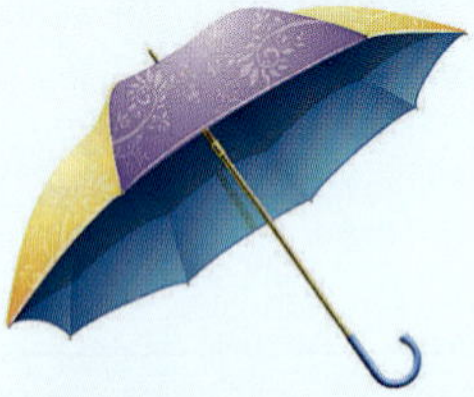

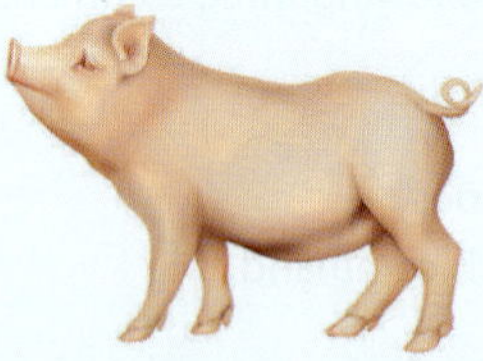

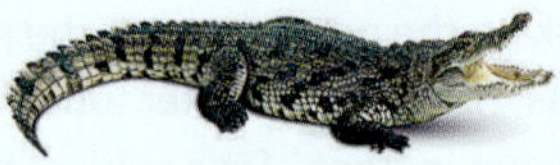

Language	
• *Using the pictures above, ask the subject to:* – Point to the one which is used in rain – Point to the one which emits light – Point to the one which is associated with farming – Point of the one which is found in desserts	**Language** [Score 0–4] ☐

Continued

Continued

Language	
• Ask the subject to read the following words (score 1 only if all correct) **sew** **pint** **soot** **dough** **height**	**Language** [Score 0–1]

Visuospatial abilities	
• *Infinity diagram:* Ask the subject to copy this diagram	**Visuospatial** [Score 0–1]
• *Wire cube:* Ask the subject to copy this drawing (for scoring, see instructions guide)	**Visuospatial** [Score 0–2]
• *Clock:* Ask the subject to draw a clock face with numbers and the hands at ten past five (for scoring see instruction guide: circle = 1, numbers = 2, hands = 2 if all correct)	**Visuospatial** [Score 0–5]

Continued

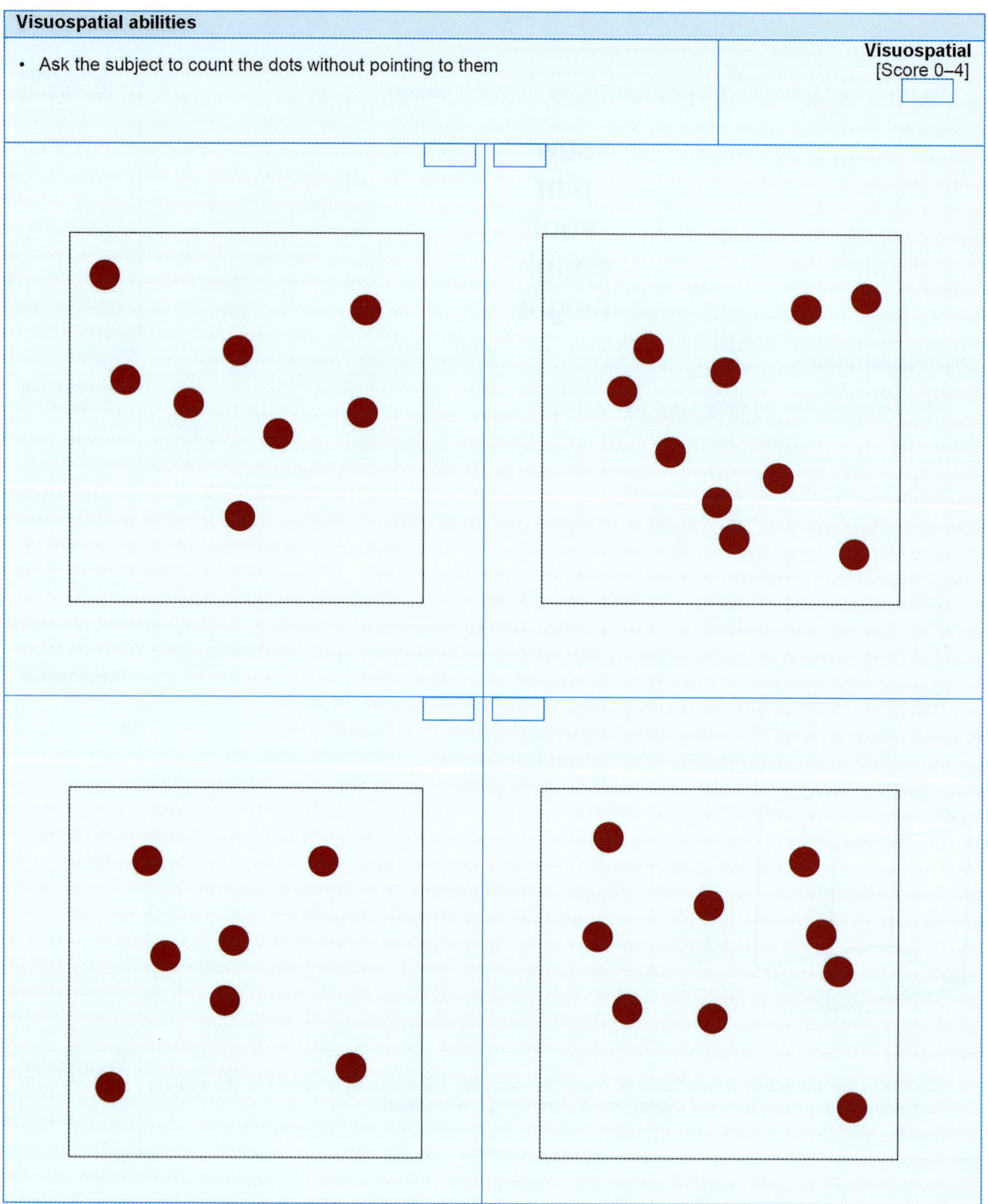
Visuospatial abilities
• Ask the subject to count the dots without pointing to them
Visuospatial
[Score 0–4]

Continued

Continued

Visuospatial abilities			
• Ask the subject to identify the letters			Visuospatial (score 0–4)
Memory			
• Ask "Now tell me what you remember about that name and address we were repeating at the beginning."			
Sunil Kumar Singh 52 Station Road Gandhinagar Prayagraj, Uttar Pradesh, India	....		Memory (score 0–7)
Memory			
This test should be done if the subject failed to recall one or more items above. If all items were recalled, skip the test and score 5. If only part was recalled, start by ticking items recalled in the shadowed column on the right-hand side; and then test not recalled items by telling the subject "ok, I'll give you some hints: was the name X, Y or Z?" and so on. Each recognised item scores one point, which is added to the point gained by recalling.			Memory (score 0–5)
Sum Kumar Sharma	Sunk kumar Singh	Rakesh Yadav	Recalled
25	52	37	Recalled
Market Road	Sastri Marg	Station Road	Recalled
Prakash Nagar	Gandh Nagar	Patel Nagar	Recalled
Prayagraj	Gwalior	Indore	Recalled
Scores			
Total ACE-III score			/100
Attention			/18
Memory			/26
Fluency			/14
Language			/26
Visuospatial			/16
Source: sydney.edu.au			

Functional Status Assessment

The assessment of functional status determines whether a patient is independent (MCI) or whether cognitive decline is severe enough to require consistent assistance with daily activities (dementia). The functional activities questionnaire (FAQ) is a brief, standardized instrument used by therapists to acquire instrumental activities of daily living (IADLs) information from informants. Using the FAQ, patients with MCI have more IADLs that "require assistance" compared to those with normal cognition (2.7 vs. 0.1, $p < 0.01$). A cut point of ≥6 points on the FAQ was found to have an accuracy of 85% for discriminating patients with MCI from those with dementia.

Neuropsychological Assessment

Neuropsychological testing is valuable in distinguishing a patient's cognitive symptoms from normal aging by assessing whether cognitive function is appropriate for their age, gender, and education level. When applied effectively, it provides a more sensitive measure of early cognitive changes indicative of neurodegenerative processes. Cognitive impairment can also occur in mental illnesses such as major depressive disorder (MDD) or generalized anxiety disorder (GAD), with depression often linked to cognitive decline in older adults—a relationship that is likely bidirectional. In cases of suspected MCI, clinicians should conduct a comprehensive neuropsychological evaluation and assess for depression. The Geriatric Depression Scale (score ≥ 6) can screen for depression, while the neuropsychiatric inventory helps informants report depressive and behavioral symptoms.

Biomarker Evaluation

Imaging in Mild Cognitive Impairment

The clinical progression mirrors the topographic spread of neuronal degeneration on imaging, starting from the hippocampus and medial temporal lobe, moving to the posterior cingulate cortex, lateral temporal cortex, and finally affecting the frontal, temporal, parietal neocortex, sensorimotor areas, and the occipital cortex in typical AD. Since MCI is a precursor transitional phase in the cognitive continuum, various imaging findings are noted. In MCI, brain imaging techniques such as MRI, diffusion tensor imaging (DTI), functional MRI (fMRI) (resting-state and task-related), positron emission tomography (PET), and magnetic resonance spectroscopy (MRS) can provide important insights:

- *MRI*: Atrophy, especially in the medial temporal lobe (hippocampus, amygdala, and parahippocampal regions such as entorhinal region)
- *fMRI*: Altered connectivity in key networks. Reduced resting-state activity in the PCC, right angular gyrus, and right PHG. Decreased activation was mainly detected in frontoparietal and default mode networks in task-based fMRI
- *PET*: Amyloid plaque accumulation and reduced glucose metabolism in specific brain regions such as inferior parietal lobules, posterior cingulate cortex, and precuneus
- *DTI*: White matter tract changes, particularly in the hippocampus, indicating early microstructural damage
- *MRS*: Raised myoinositol (mI) concentration and altered choline/creatine ratio (Cho/Cr) along with reduced N-acetylaspartate (NAA) level in precuneus and hippocampus

These findings help in early diagnosis and monitoring of MCI progression toward AD **(Fig. 4)**

Cerebrospinal fluid biomarkers: Three key CSF biomarkers—(1) total tau, (2) phospho-tau, and (3)

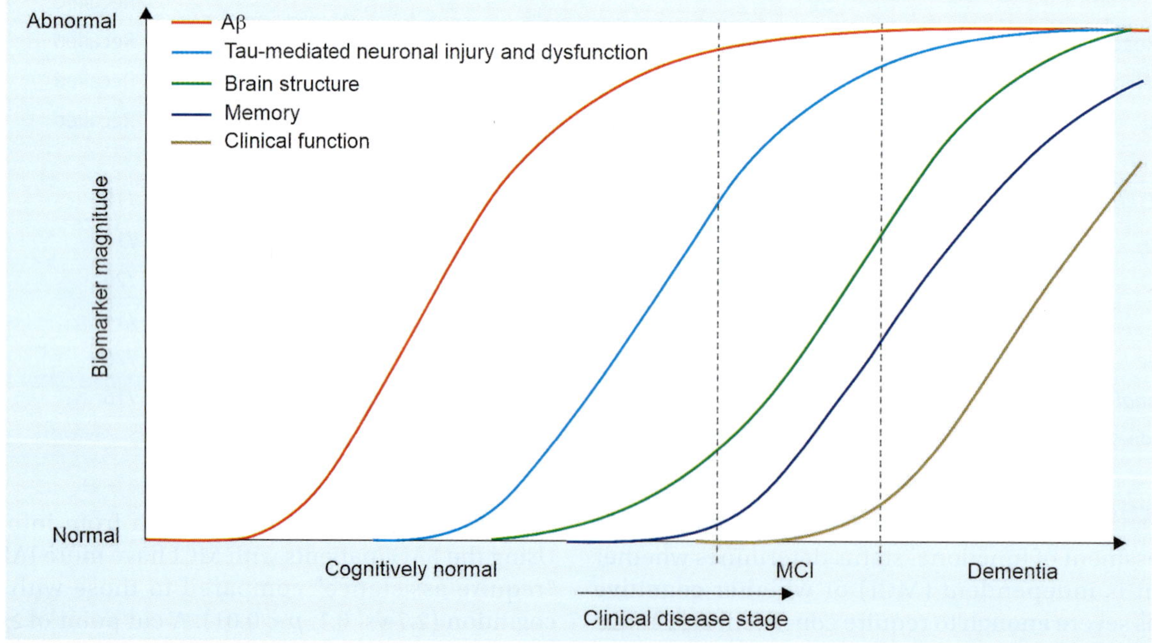

FIG. 4: Graph showing sequential changes in biomarkers and functional changes across the cognitive continuum from normal cognition to MCI and dementia.
(MCI: mild cognitive impairment)

amyloid beta 42 (Aβ42)—are considered the most accurate for early diagnosis of AD and predicting its progression in patients with MCI. Additionally, emerging biomarkers such as soluble amyloid precursor protein (APP), apoptotic proteins, secretases, and inflammatory and oxidative markers show promising potential for future advancements.

Blood biomarkers: Various blood markers, such as neurofilament light (NfL), glial fibrillary acidic protein (GFAP) , p-Tau181, plasma Aβ42/40 ratio, and t-Tau, are currently under investigation as potential biomarkers to predict the conversion from MCI to AD. These markers could help in improving early detection and monitoring disease progression.

MANAGEMENT

Diagnosis and management of MCI is given in **Flowchart 2** and **Box 3**.

TREATMENT OPTIONS

Reviewing various guidelines, Chen et al. found that there are varying recommendations for diagnostic criteria, the use of biomarkers, and cognitive tests. Treatment approaches primarily focus on nonpharmacological interventions, such as cognitive training and lifestyle modifications, with limited pharmacological options.

Nonpharmacological Options

Dietary Interventions

Diets such as the Mediterranean diet, which emphasizes fruits, vegetables, whole grains, and healthy fats, have been linked to better cognitive health. In a recent systematic review, Devranis et al. found that adhering to the Mediterranean diet for 10 weeks showed improvements in global cognition, while the ketogenic diet benefited diabetic patients by enhancing verbal recognition. The Mediterranean-DASH Intervention for Neurodegenerative Delay (MIND) diet, specifically effective for obese individuals, improved working memory, verbal recognition, memory, and attention.

Psychotherapy and Psychoeducation

Psychotherapeutic interventions including cognitive rehabilitation, reminiscence therapy, cognitive behavioral therapy, problem-solving therapy (PST), and interpersonal therapy (IPT) are recommended as well as psychoeducational interventions including cognitive rehabilitation, cognitive training (episodic memory strategies as well as exercises to increase attentional control, computer-based cognitive training), mindfulness-based stress reduction (MBSR), behavioral activation, and problem-focused coping strategies. These activities promote mental stimulation, such as learning new skills or engaging in intellectually challenging tasks, and help in cognitive restructuring. There is empirical support for

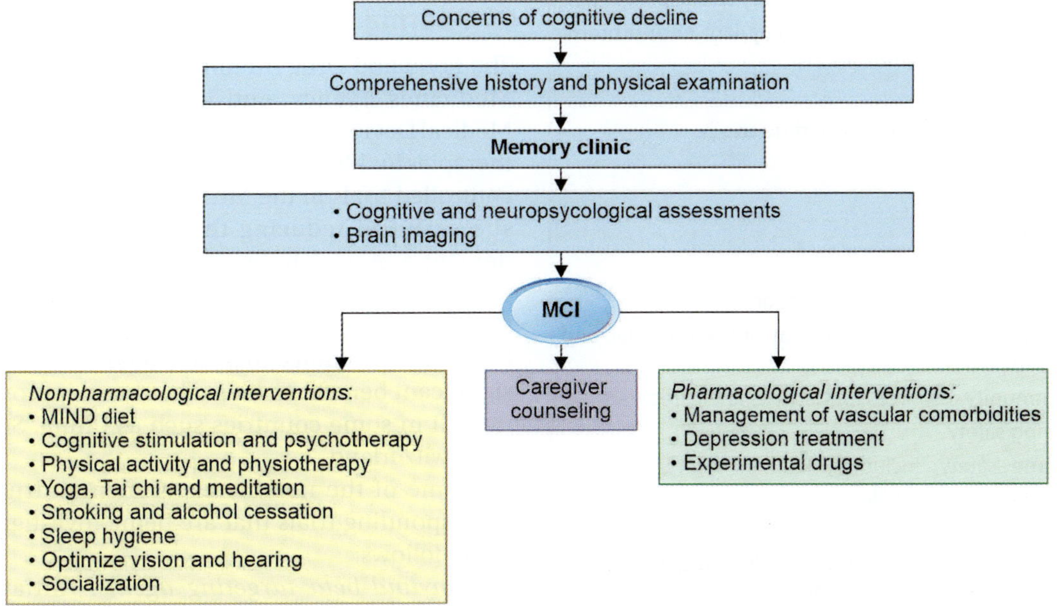

FLOWCHART 2: Suggested approach to the diagnosis and management of mild cognitive impairment.

(MIND: Mediterranean–DASH Intervention for Neurodegenerative Delay; MCI: mild cognitive impairment)

Source: Adapted from Langa KM, Levine DA. The diagnosis and management of mild cognitive impairment: a clinical review. JAMA. 2014;312(23):2551-61.

the beneficial effects of psychotherapy on depressive symptoms and quality of life.

Physical Exercise

Regular physical activity has been shown to have positive effects on cognitive function and overall brain health by reducing vascular risk factors and specific cognitive effects. At the molecular level, aerobic exercise is thought to regulate the activation of microglia and astrocytes, which are key in brain inflammation and neurogenesis. It also promotes the release of exercise-related factors such as irisin, cathepsin B, CLU, and GPLD1, which may enhance synaptic plasticity and provide neuroprotective effects. Exercise training has shown to improve cognitive symptoms related to attention and executive function.

Physiotherapy and Occupational Therapy

Physiotherapy and occupational therapy involve exercises improving motor coordination, gait training. Physical exercise therapy has shown to improve strength, step length, balance, mobility, walking endurance, flexibility, and ADLs. It has also shown to reduce decline in global cognition and working memory.

Occupational therapy focuses on enhancing daily functioning and independence through targeted interventions. It aims to improve cognitive abilities, such as memory and attention, while supporting participation in meaningful activities such as self-care, work, and leisure. Therapists may introduce strategies for organizing tasks, maintaining routines (rehabilitation strategies), and using compensatory techniques to cope with cognitive challenges, adaptations in physical and social environment, and caregiver skill training.

Mind-body practices such as yoga and tai chi have been shown to be safe and beneficial for the physical and mental well-being and improving sleep quality of people with MCI.

Social Engagement

Encouraging social interactions and maintaining social relationships can help improve cognitive function and delay progression.

Sleep

There is a bidirectional relationship between MCI and sleep disorders. Sleep is essential for memory consolidation and helps in clearing metabolites such as Aβ, reducing fatigue, and supporting brain function. Improved sleep reduces oxidative stress, which helps lower Aβ accumulation and promotes better cognitive health.

BOX 3 Treating and counseling patients with MCI.

Control of vascular risk factors and prevention of stroke and subclinical brain injury:
- *Hypertension present*: Control blood pressure and avoid hypotension
- *Diabetes present*: Control severe hyperglycemia and avoid severe hypoglycemia
- Statin if indicated for primary or secondary stroke prevention
- *Atrial fibrillation present*: Initiate anticoagulant or antithrombotic therapy. If no contraindications

Beneficial behaviors:
- Abstain from heavy alcohol or illicit drug use
- Engage in mental activity
- Engage in physical activity
- Stop smoking

Social needs:
- Encourage and facilitate social interactions
- Discuss living will, durable power of attorney, financial, and long-term care plans
- Provide community resources for patients and caregivers
- Discuss driving safety
- Discuss home safety, including kitchen safety, firearms, poisons, and potential fall risks

Prognosis and follow-up:
- Discuss current evidence and uncertainty regarding MCI prognosis with the patient and family
- Arrange follow-up approximately every 6 months to assess changes in cognitive function and potential evolving needs for social support

(MCI: mild cognitive impairment)

Pharmacological Interventions

The Food and Drug Administration (FDA), the European Medicines Agency, and Japan's Pharmaceuticals and Medical Devices Agency have all rejected pharmacological therapies for MCI. There have been numerous randomized controlled trials in the MCI spectrum, but none has been successful in reducing the progression of MCI to AD dementia. Acetylcholinesterase inhibitors, memantine, *Ginkgo biloba* (EGb 761), anti-inflammatory drugs (NSAIDs), statins, platelet aggregation inhibitors, etc., have all been studied in MCI, but none of them has shown significant benefit. *G. biloba* has been approved for usage in MCI in some countries such as China, Spain, Russia, and Switzerland.

Some of the notable experimental drugs and their corresponding trials that are being investigated for MCI are as follows:

- *Amyloid-beta targeting agents*: Antiamyloid-beta monoclonal antibody:
    - *Aducanumab (ADUHELM)*: EMERGE and ENGAGE trials, though its approval and efficacy have been controversial

    - *Lecanemab (Leqembi)*: Has shown promise in trials such as the Clarity AD study
    - *Donanemab*: TRAILBLAZER-ALZ trial
- *Tau-targeting agents*:
    - *Gantenerumab*: A monoclonal antibody targeting amyloid and tau. The phase 3 GRADUATE I and II trials are ongoing.
    - *Tilavonemab*: An anti-tau monoclonal antibody. Clinical trials did not show a significant benefit.
- *Neuroinflammation modulators*:
    - *Lecanemab*
    - Anti-inflammatory agents: Research is ongoing with various compounds.
- *Neuroprotection and cognitive enhancement*:
    - *Lynx1 inhibitors*: Investigational drugs targeting Lynx1, a protein involved in cognitive decline. These are still in early preclinical or phase 1 trials.
    - *Nootropics*: Nootropics, known as the "smart drugs," are a diverse class of substances that enhance brain function without directly acting on neurotransmitters or receptors. Instead, they improve the brain's supply of glucose and oxygen, have antihypoxic properties, and protect brain tissue from neurotoxicity. These effects contribute to better cognitive performance and neuroprotection, making nootropics popular for enhancing mental clarity, memory, and focus.
- *Hormonal and metabolic modulators*:
    - *Estradiol*: Hormone replacement therapy is being explored in MCI patients, particularly in trials assessing its impact on cognitive function.
    - *Ketone esters*: Compounds such as ketone ester supplements are under investigation in clinical trials for their effects on cognitive performance.
- *Gene therapy and stem cell approaches*:
    - *Gene therapy (BDNF)*: Various gene-editing strategies are in preclinical stages, targeting genetic factors associated with MCI and early-onset AD.
    - *Stem cell therapy*: Clinical trials are investigating the use of stem cells for neurodegenerative conditions, including MCI. For example, trials are exploring the potential of mesenchymal stem cells in neurodegeneration.

ROLE OF CAREGIVER

A caregiver is any family member or friend who provides instrumental or emotional support to someone without receiving financial compensation. Caregivers play a crucial role in managing MCI in the form of monitoring patients' symptoms, medication adherence, routine maintenance and cognitive stimulation, safety management, emotional support, and coordination of care plan. Around 36% of caregivers for people with MCI experience a significant burden, impacting them emotionally, physically, socially, and financially. Objectively, caregivers take on new roles such as managing finances and daily tasks, while subjectively, they struggle with emotional distress from witnessing the memory decline. This leads to increased anxiety, depression, and a lower quality of life. This experience can lead to heightened anxiety, depression, and a reduced quality of life. To address the needs of this population, interventions focusing on cognitive, psychological, and multidimensional aspects have proven effective in mitigating caregiver burden.

PREVENTION

As the population ages, prevention and treatment of cognitive impairment in the elderly have become more crucial. MCI cannot be prevented. However, research has found that some lifestyle factors may lower the risk of getting MCI.

Several studies have adopted a multifactorial intervention approach, incorporating regular exercise, a healthy diet, and the management of vascular risk factors, psychosocial stress, and depression. Notable examples include the "Finnish Geriatric Intervention Study to Prevent Cognitive Impairment and Disability (FINGER)," "Multidomain Alzheimer Preventive Trial (MAPT)," and others such as Prevention of Dementia by Intensive Vascular Care (preDIVA), "SCD-Well", "Medit-Ageing" project, and Body, Brain, Life for Cognitive Decline (BBL-CD). These approaches offer a promising strategy for preventing cognitive decline and developing tailored therapeutic interventions across different stages of cognitive impairment.

CONCLUSION

Mild cognitive impairment can be considered as a transitional and noticeable stage between normal aging and dementia, gives the geriatrician an opportunity to assess and treat the older adults. It has few subtypes as per the domains of memory involvement and various risk factors. MCI can be reversible with early intervention and does not necessarily progress to dementia. Geriatrician needs to proactively screen for early memory loss or MCI in their clinic for their every clients. Diagnosis and management of MCI focus on multidisciplinary comprehensive assessment, nonpharmacological interventions, lifestyle modifications, and supporting caregivers. While effective pharmacological treatments remain limited, preventive approaches, including exercise, healthy diet, and managing risk factors, offer promise in delaying cognitive decline among the elderly.

ACKNOWLEDGMENTS

The author thanks Dr Himadri Das, Dr Suman Maity, Dr Partha Mondal, Dr Bhaskar Roy Chowdhury, Dr Subhadip Mukhopadhyay, Dr Soubhik Mondal, Ms Subhasree Roy, Ms Hiya Basu, Ms Upasana Ghosh and Ms Raksha Banka, Department of Geriatric Medicine, Medical College, Kolkata, West Bengal, India for their time and contribution to prepare this chapter.

Self-Assessment Questionnaire

Q1. How can mild cognitive impairment (MCI) be differentiated from normal aging and dementia in terms of functional status?

Q2. What are the major clinical subtypes of MCI, and how do they differ in presentation?

Q3. How do vascular and metabolic disorders contribute to the development of cognitive decline in older adults?

Q4. What are the typical reversible causes of cognitive impairment that must be ruled out before diagnosing MCI?

Q5. Discuss how imaging and biomarker studies aid in the diagnosis and prognosis of MCI.

Q6. What lifestyle interventions have been proven to delay or prevent the progression from MCI to dementia?

Q7. What are the limitations of current pharmacological treatments for MCI?

FURTHER READINGS

1. Aisen PS, Cummings J, Jack CR, Morris JC, Sperling R, Frölich L, et al. On the path to 2025: understanding the Alzheimer's disease continuum. Alzheimer's Res Ther. 2017;9:60.
2. Anderson ND. State of the science on mild cognitive impairment (MCI). CNS Spectr. 2019;24(1).
3. Gross AL, Nichols E, Angrisani M, Ganguli M, Jin H, Khobragade P, et al. Prevalence of DSM-5 mild and major neurocognitive disorder in India: results from the LASI-DAD. PLOS ONE. 2024;19(2):e0297220.
4. Albert MS, DeKosky ST, Dickson D, Dubois B, Feldman HH, Fox NC, et al. The diagnosis of mild cognitive impairment due to Alzheimer's disease: recommendations from the National Institute on Aging-Alzheimer's Association workgroups on diagnostic guidelines for Alzheimer's disease. Alzheimers Dement J Alzheimers Assoc. 2011;7(3):270-9.
5. Tábuas-Pereira M, Baldeiras I, Duro D, Santiago B, Ribeiro MH, Leitão MJ, et al. Prognosis of early-onset vs. late-onset mild cognitive impairment: comparison of conversion rates and its predictors. Geriatrics. 2016;1(2):11.
6. Irwin C, Tjandra D, Hu C, Aggarwal V, Lienau A, Giordani B, et al. Predicting 5-year dementia conversion in veterans with mild cognitive impairment. Alzheimer's Dement Diagn Assess Dis Monit. 2024;16(1):e12572.
7. Livingston G, Huntley J, Liu KY, Costafreda SG, Selbæk G, Alladi S, et al. Dementia prevention, intervention, and care: 2024 report of the Lancet standing commission. Lancet. 2024;404(10452):572-628.
8. Government of India. (2020). Longitudinal Ageing Study in India (LASI). [online] Available from https://www.iipsindia.ac.in/sites/default/files/LASI_India_Report_2020_compressed.pdf. [Last accessed May, 2025].
9. Das SK, Bose P, Biswas A, Dutt A, Banerjee TK, Hazra AM, et al. An epidemiologic study of mild cognitive impairment in Kolkata, India. Neurology. 2007;68(23):2019-26.
10. Sosa AL, Albanese E, Stephan BC, Dewey M, Acosta D, Ferri CP, et al. Prevalence, distribution, and impact of mild cognitive impairment in Latin America, China, and India: A 10/66 population-based study. PLOS Med. 2012;9(2):e1001170.
11. Angrisani M, Jain U, Lee J. Sex differences in cognitive health among older adults in India. J Am Geriatr Soc. 2020;68(S3):S20-8.
12. Sachdev PS, Blacker D, Blazer DG, Ganguli M, Jeste DV, Paulsen JS, et al. Classifying neurocognitive disorders: the DSM-5 approach. Nat Rev Neurol. 2014;10(11):634-42.
13. Petersen RC, Caracciolo B, Brayne C, Gauthier S, Jelic V, Fratiglioni L. Mild cognitive impairment: a concept in evolution. J Intern Med. 2014;275(3):214-28.
14. Petersen RC. Mild cognitive impairment. Contin Lifelong Learn Neurol. 2016;22(2 Dementia):404-18.
15. Bhattarai B, Nagaraj H. Mild cognitive impairment: an overview. Neurorehabilitation and Physical Therapy. IntechOpen; 2023.
16. McCarten JR. Clinical evaluation of early cognitive symptoms. Clin Geriatr Med. 2013;29(4):791-807.
17. Holsinger T, Deveau J, Boustani M, Williams JW. Does this patient have dementia? JAMA. 2007;297(21):2391-404.
18. Folstein MF, Folstein SE, McHugh PR. Mini-mental state. J Psychiatr Res. 1975;12(3):189-98.
19. Nasreddine ZS, Phillips NA, Bédirian V, Charbonneau S, Whitehead V, Collin I, et al. The Montreal Cognitive Assessment, MoCA: a brief screening tool for mild cognitive impairment. J Am Geriatr Soc. 2005;53(4):695-9.
20. Lin JS, O'Connor E, Rossom RC, Perdue LA, Eckstrom E. Screening for cognitive impairment in older adults: a systematic review for the US. Preventive Services Task Force. Ann Intern Med. 2013;159(9):601-12.
21. Jorm AF. A short form of the Informant Questionnaire on Cognitive Decline in the Elderly (IQCODE): development and cross-validation. Psychol Med. 1994;24(1):145-53.
22. Cm C. Performance of the dementia severity rating scale: a caregiver questionnaire for rating severity in Alzheimer's disease. Alzheimer Assoc Disord. 1996;10:31-9.
23. Galvin JE, Roe CM, Powlishta KK, Coats MA, Muich SJ, Grant E, et al. The AD8. Neurology. 2005;65(4):559-64.
24. Borson S, Scanlan J, Brush M, Vitaliano P, Dokmak A. The Mini-Cog: a cognitive "vital signs" measure for dementia screening in multi-lingual elderly. Int J Geriatr Psychiatry. 2000;15(11):1021-7.

25. Senda M, Terada S, Takenoshita S, Hayashi S, Yabe M, Imai N, et al. Diagnostic utility of the Addenbrooke's Cognitive Examination – III (ACE-III), Mini-ACE, Mini-Mental State Examination, Montreal Cognitive Assessment, and Hasegawa Dementia Scale-Revised for detecting mild cognitive impairment and dementia. Psychogeriatrics. 2020;20(2):156-62.
26. Noone P. Addenbrooke's Cognitive Examination-III. Occup Med. 2015;65(5):418-20.
27. Pfeffer RI, Kurosaki TT, Harrah CH Jr, Chance JM, Filos S. Measurement of functional activities in older adults in the community 1. J Gerontol. 1982;37(3):323-9.
28. Petersen RC. Clinical practice. Mild cognitive impairment. N Engl J Med. 2011;364(23):2227-34.
29. Brown PJ, Devanand DP, Liu X, Caccappolo E. Alzheimer's disease neuroimaging initiative. Functional impairment in elderly patients with mild cognitive impairment and mild Alzheimer disease. Arch Gen Psychiatry. 2011;68(6):617-26.
30. Yesavage JA, Brink TL, Rose TL, Lum O, Huang V, Adey M, et al. Development and validation of a geriatric depression screening scale: a preliminary report. J Psychiatr Res. 1982;17(1):37-49.
31. Cummings JL, Mega M, Gray K, Rosenberg-Thompson S, Carusi DA, Gornbein J. The neuropsychiatric inventory. Neurology. 1994;44(12):2308-14.
32. Talwar P, Kushwaha S, Chaturvedi M, Mahajan V. Systematic review of different neuroimaging correlates in mild cognitive impairment and Alzheimer's Disease. Clin Neuroradiol. 2021;31(4):953-67.
33. Weiner MW, Veitch DP, Aisen PS, Beckett LA, Cairns NJ, Cedarbaum J, et al. Impact of the Alzheimer's Disease Neuroimaging Initiative, 2004 to 2014. Alzheimers Dement J Alzheimers Assoc. 2015;11(7):865-84.
34. Papaliagkas V, Kalinderi K, Vareltzis P, Moraitou D, Papamitsou T, Chatzidimitriou M. CSF Biomarkers in the early diagnosis of mild cognitive impairment and Alzheimer's Disease. Int J Mol Sci. 2023;24(10):8976.
35. Silva-Spínola A, Lima M, Leitão MJ, Bernardes C, Durães J, Duro D, et al. Blood biomarkers in mild cognitive impairment patients: relationship between analytes and progression to Alzheimer's disease dementia. Eur J Neurol. 2023;30(6):1565-73.
36. Langa KM, Levine DA. The diagnosis and management of mild cognitive impairment: a clinical review. JAMA. 2014;312(23): 2551-61.
37. Chen YX, Liang N, Li XL, Yang SH, Wang YP, Shi NN. Diagnosis and treatment for mild cognitive impairment: a systematic review of clinical practice guidelines and consensus statements. Front Neurol. 2021;12.
38. Devranis P, Vassilopoulou E, Tsironis V, Sotiriadis PM, Chourdakis M, Aivaliotis M, et al. Mediterranean diet, ketogenic diet, or MIND diet for aging populations with cognitive decline: a systematic review. Life. 2023;13(1):173.
39. Rostamzadeh A, Kahlert A, Kalthegener F, Jessen F. Psychotherapeutic interventions in individuals at risk for Alzheimer's dementia: a systematic review. Alzheimer's Res Ther. 2022;14(1):18.
40. Huang B, Chen K, Li Y. Aerobic exercise, an effective prevention and treatment for mild cognitive impairment. Front Aging Neurosci. 2023;15.
41. Li H, Su W, Dang H, Han K, Lu H, Yue S, et al. Exercise training for mild cognitive impairment adults older than 60: a systematic review and meta-analysis. J Alzheimers Dis. 88(4):1263-78.
42. Lam FM, Huang MZ, Liao LR, Chung RC, Kwok TC, Pang MY. Physical exercise improves strength, balance, mobility, and endurance in people with cognitive impairment and dementia: A systematic review. J Physiother. 2018;64(1):4-15.
43. Law CK, Lam FM, Chung RC, Pang MY. Physical exercise attenuates cognitive decline and reduces behavioural problems in people with mild cognitive impairment and dementia: a systematic review. J Physiother. 2020;66(1):9-18.
44. Graff MJL, Vernooij-Dassen MJFJ, Hoefnagels WHL, Dekker J, De Witte LP. Occupational therapy at home for older individuals with mild to moderate cognitive impairments and their primary caregivers: a pilot study. OTJR Occup Ther J Res. 2003;23(4):155-64.
45. Smallfield S, Metzger L, Green M, Henley L, Rhodus EK. Occupational therapy practice guidelines for adults living with Alzheimer's disease and related neurocognitive disorders. Am J Occup Ther. 2024;78(1):7801397010.
46. Karamacoska D, Tan T, Mathersul DC, Sabag A, de Manincor M, Chang D, et al. A systematic review of the health effects of yoga for people with mild cognitive impairment and dementia. BMC Geriatr. 2023;23(1):37.
47. Wang X, Si K, Gu W, Wang X. Mitigating effects and mechanisms of Tai Chi on mild cognitive impairment in the elderly. Front Aging Neurosci. 2023;14:1028822.
48. Randhi B, Gutlapalli SD, Pu J, Zaidi MF, Patel M, Atluri LM, et al. Sleep disorders in mild cognitive impairment. Cureus. 15(3):e36202.
49. Karakaya T, Fußer F, Schröder J, Pantel J. Pharmacological Treatment of Mild Cognitive Impairment as a Prodromal Syndrome of Alzheimer´s Disease. Curr Neuropharmacol. 2013;11(1):102-8.
50. Kasper S, Bancher C, Eckert A, Förstl H, Frölich L, Hort J, et al. Management of mild cognitive impairment (MCI): The need for national and international guidelines. World J Biol Psychiatry. 2020;21(8):579-94.
51. Florian H, Wang D, Arnold SE, Boada M, Guo Q, Jin Z, et al. Tilavonemab in early Alzheimer's disease: results from a phase 2, randomized, double-blind study. Brain J Neurol. 2023;146(6):2275-84.
52. Fink HA, Jutkowitz E, McCarten JR, Hemmy LS, Butler M, Davila H, et al. Pharmacologic interventions to prevent cognitive decline, mild cognitive impairment, and clinical Alzheimer-type dementia. Ann Intern Med. 2018;168(1):39-51.
53. Shenkarev ZO, Shulepko MA, Bychkov ML, Kulbatskii DS, Shlepova OV, Vasilyeva NA, et al. Water-soluble variant of human Lynx1 positively modulates synaptic plasticity and ameliorates cognitive impairment associated with α7-nAChR dysfunction. J Neurochem. 2020;155(1):45-61.
54. Kang M, Lee DB, Kwon S, Lee E, Kim WJ. Effectiveness of nootropics in combination with cholinesterase inhibitors on cognitive function in mild-to-moderate dementia: a study using real-world data. J Clin Med. 2022;11(16):4661.
55. Yoon BK, Chin J, Kim JW, Shin MH, Ahn S, Lee DY, et al. Menopausal hormone therapy and mild cognitive impairment: a randomized, placebo-controlled trial. Menopause. 2018;25(8):870-6.
56. Bohnen JLB, Albin RL, Bohnen NI. Ketogenic interventions in mild cognitive impairment, Alzheimer's disease, and Parkinson's disease: a systematic review and critical appraisal. Front Neurol. 2023;14:1123290.
57. ClinicalTrials.gov. (2024). A clinical trial of AAV2-BDNF gene therapy in early Alzheimer's disease and mild cognitive impairment. [online] Available from https://clinicaltrials.gov/study/NCT05040217. [Last accessed May, 2025].
58. Domingues NS, Verreault P, Hudon C. Reducing burden for caregivers of older adults with mild cognitive impairment: a systematic review. Am J Alzheimer's Dis Demen. 2018;33(7): 401-14.

CHAPTER 25

Major Neurocognitive Disorder

Ananta Aryal, Gaurav Sharma

CASE VIGNETTE

Mr P, a 72-year-old male with a known case of diabetes mellitus and hypertension, was brought to the geriatric outpatient department (OPD) by his son and daughter-in-law with a history of change in behavior for the past 6 months. Mr P worked as a shopkeeper for 30 years and has now retired for the last 2 years when he had difficulty in calculating. His son tells history that there was some financial loss as his father could not recall lending money. Initially, the family thought his miscalculation and forgetfulness were due to his old age. 6 months back, he forgot his way on returning home from the nearby temple, and his neighbor helped him. Now, Mr P does not recognize his son and calls him brother. He says he wants to go to his home even when he is at home. His daughter-in-law gets embarrassed when Mr P tells the relatives visiting him that he has not been served food, although he just had food. Three days back, he urinated in the corner of his kitchen, which made the son and daughter-in-law bring him to the OPD.

He is conscious and oriented on assessment, and his vitals are stable. The systematic examination was normal. His Mini-Mental State Examination (MMSE) score was 16/30. No other neurological deficit. His random blood sugar (RBS) was 160 mg/dL and HbA1c—7.2%, with electrolytes within normal limits. His vitamin B12 was 256 pg/mL. His MRI of the brain shows diffuse cerebral atrophy with reduced volume of the hippocampus.

INTRODUCTION

Dementia is typically defined as a clinical syndrome of cognitive decline that is sufficiently efficient to interfere with social or occupational functioning. The nomenclature of the word major cognitive disorder started in 2011, the National Institute on Aging and the Alzheimer's Association (NIA-AA) released and cosponsored revised clinical diagnostic guidelines for dementia, dementia due to Alzheimer's disease (AD), mild cognitive impairment (MCI), and a theoretical framework for defining the preclinical stages of AD. In 2013, the American Psychiatric Association published the Diagnostic and Statistical Manual of Mental Disorders, Fifth Edition (DSM-5). Within this edition, the term "dementia" was replaced with "major neurocognitive disorder (MNCD)" and the term "MCI" with "mild neurocognitive disorder."

DIAGNOSTIC AND STATISTICAL MANUAL OF MENTAL DISORDERS, FIFTH EDITION MAJOR NEUROCOGNITIVE DISORDER DIAGNOSTIC CRITERIA

A. Evidence of significant cognitive decline from a previous level of performance in one or more cognitive domains (complex attention, executive function, learning and memory, language, perceptual-motor, or special cognition) based on:
   - Concern of the individual, a knowledgeable informant, or the clinician that there has been a significant decline in cognitive function.
   - A substantial impairment in cognitive performance, preferably documented by standardized neuropsychological testing or, in its absence, another quantified clinical assessment.

B. The cognitive deficits interfere with independence in everyday activities (i.e., at a minimum, requiring assistance with complex instrumental activities of daily living such as paying bills or managing medications).

C. The cognitive deficits do not occur exclusively in the context of delirium.

D. The cognitive deficits are not better explained by another mental disorder (e.g., major depressive disorder and schizophrenia).

Specify whether due to: AD, frontotemporal degeneration, Lewy body disease, vascular disease, traumatic brain injury (TBI), substance/medication use, HIV infection, prion disease, Parkinson's disease, Huntington's disease, multiple etiologies, and unspecified.

Specify:
- *Without behavioral disturbance*: If the cognitive disturbance is not accompanied by any clinically significant behavioral disturbance.
- *With behavioral disturbance (specify disturbance)*: If the cognitive disturbance is accompanied by a clinically significant behavioral disturbance (e.g., psychotic symptoms, mood disturbance, agitation, apathy, or other behavioral symptoms).

Specify current severity:
- *Mild*: Difficulties with instrumental activities of daily living (e.g., housework and managing money)
- *Moderate*: Difficulties with basic activities of daily living (e.g., feeding and dressing)
- *Severe*: Fully dependent

EPIDEMIOLOGY AND RISK FACTORS

There has been an increased incidence and prevalence of MNCD with the increase in the number of older population worldwide. MNCD stands out as one of the most debilitating diseases in old age, accounting for approximately one sixth of all disability-adjusted life years in individuals aged 60 years and above. Someone in the world develops MNCD every 3 seconds. There are over 55 million people worldwide living with MNCD in 2020. This number will almost double every 20 years, reaching 78 million in 2030 and 139 million in 2050. This rise is particularly notable in low- and middle-income countries, with studies indicating a concerning trend in India, regarding dementia prevalence among older adults. Available prevalence studies in India demonstrate variability, ranging from 1.4 to 9.1%. Presently, an estimated 3.01 million individuals in India are affected by dementia.

In India, the prevalence of MNCD mirrors the global trend of rising dementia cases, particularly among the elderly population. Studies reveal a significant burden of MNCD among older adults in India, with prevalence rates ranging from 1.4 to 9.1%. Hospital-based investigations further highlight the substantial prevalence of MNCD, underscoring the urgent need for enhanced awareness, early detection, and effective management strategies.

Alzheimer's disease constitutes the most common cause of MNCD, accounting for 70–80% of all cases, occurring either sporadically or in familial forms. Vascular dementia (VaD) represents approximately 15% of all MNCD cases and exhibits an incidence rate that escalates with age, doubling every 5.3 years.

Lewy body dementia (LBD) contributes to around 5% of MNCD cases, although epidemiological data may not fully reflect its prevalence due to underdiagnosis. Parkinson's disease dementia (PDD) constitutes approximately 10% of MNCD cases.

Frontotemporal dementia (FTD), attributed to 25% of MNCD cases in individuals older than 65 years, emerges as the second most common cause of MNCD in individuals younger than 65 years. However, epidemiological studies on FTD encounter limitations, partly due to challenges in its identification.

Creutzfeldt–Jakob disease, rare and occurring in about one to two cases per million per year globally, rounds up the spectrum of MNCD disorders.

ALZHEIMER'S DISEASE

Alzheimer's disease is the fifth most common leading cause of death in the United States from 2019 to 2023. Risk factors are related to genetic and nongenetic markers. AD is characterized by widespread cortical atrophy and the deposition of amyloid plaques and neurofibrillary tangles of hyperphosphorylated tau protein.

FRONTOTEMPORAL DEMENTIA

It is more prevalent in the fifth to seventh decades of life. Hallmark of the disease is the focal atrophy of frontal, insular, and/or temporal cortex.

Pathophysiology

Microscopic findings include gliosis, microvacuolation, and neuronal loss. Glial inclusion contains either tau or TDP-43 in 90% of cases. The pathophysiology of FTD lies in loss of TDP-43 function resulting in mis-splicing events which lead to mRNA degradation which further rise to dysfunctional peptides. Sometimes exhibited as prion-like properties due to selective involvement of the anterior frontal and temporal neocortex by pathologically intraneural cytoplasmic inclusions (pick bodies).

VASCULAR DEMENTIA

Risk factors include cardiovascular risk factors such as hypertension, dyslipidemia, atrial fibrillation, and coronary artery disease. Patient with a history of cardiovascular disease (CVD) and stroke raises the suspicion of the disease.

Pathophysiology of the disease lies in the ischemic changes ranging from small vessel disease to large strokes caused by either blockage of blood flow, or bleeding results in deprivation of oxygen, and thus, function is disrupted. Relevance of site, size, and number of lesions:

- In pure VaD infarct size—100 cm^3
- In AD + CVD, size of infarct is 50 cm^3

The majority of patients with intermediate volume lesion (50–100 cm^3) present with cognitive impairment.

Subtypes of cerebral vascular disease associated with vascular components to cognitive impairment and dementia are given as follows:

- *Large cerebral stroke*: There is an irreversible injury to the cerebral cortex, subcortical white matter, or other subcortical and infratentorial structures which results in cognitive impairment.
- *Cerebral small vessel disease*: Two common age-related cerebral small vessel diseases are as follows:
    i. Arteriosclerosis—plasma protein deposition in the vessel wall
    ii. Cerebral amyloid angiopathy—beta-amyloid deposition in small cerebral arteries and capillaries

LEWY BODY DEMENTIA

Lewy body dementia, which appears as PDD or dementia with Lewy bodies (DLBs), is the second leading cause of neurodegenerative dementia after AD. DLB is characterized by dementia, psychosis, and features of Parkinsonism, and there is fluctuation of symptoms with time and vary among different individuals.

Pathophysiology

Lewy bodies, the hallmark of DLB, are intracellular cytoplasmic inclusions found within neurons that can be stained using periodic acid–Schiff (PAS) and ubiquitin. However, they are now primarily detected using antibodies against the presynaptic protein α-synuclein. These depositions of pathologic propagation from the periphery to the brain from the enteric nervous system through the vagus nerve to the heart, lower brainstem, substantia nigra, limbic system, and lastly to cerebral cortex relate to the symptom evolution.

There are decreased levels of acetylcholine in the temporal and parietal cortex resulting in visual hallucinations (a prominent feature of LBD), while upregulation of muscarinic M1 receptors in the temporal lobe results in delusions.

Lewy body dementia is poorly understood, and its clinical features overlap with other more common disorders, such as Parkinson's disease and AD; hence, it is underdiagnosed. Studies have shown that DLB accounts for up to 20–30% of all dementia cases. It is prevalent in Asian, African, and European races. Its incidence increases with increasing age and is more common in men. A family history of LBD and Parkinson's disease increases a patient's risk of having DLB.

Types of Dementia with Lewy Body

- *DLBs*: Dementia occurring first or within 1 year of movement disorder.
- *PDD*: Dementia occurs in a patient who receives a diagnosed of Parkinson's disease and then develops dementia symptoms after 1 year or more of the diagnosis.

Huntington's disease: It is caused by an autosomal dominant inherited gene mutation.

Prion-related dementias: It is caused by misfolded prions, infectious proteinaceous particles, leading to syndromes such as Creutzfeldt-Jakob disease and Kuru.

Human immunodeficiency virus infection: Associated with the development of neurocognitive disorders due to macrophage activation and toxic inflammation leading to neurodegeneration.

Alcohol consumption: Particularly high doses and prolonged use are associated with multiple cytotoxic processes in the brain.

CLINICAL FEATURES OF MAJOR NEUROCOGNITIVE DISORDER

The clinical course of MNCD is progressive, with symptoms worsening over time and eventual loss of independence in activities of daily living. The initial presentation of patient depends upon the cause of MNCD. However, the advanced stage is similar in all types of dementia, patients requiring assistance in both basic and instrumental activities of daily living. AD begins with recent memory impairment with intact remote memory; FTD may start with behavioral issues or difficulty in language but memory may be preserved in the early stage; DLB may begin with fluctuation in cognitive decline, hallucinations, and features of Parkinsonism; VaD may present with difficulty in executive functions; and PDD is characterized by Parkinsonism followed by cognitive impairment.

Alzheimer's Disease

The cognitive decline begins 7.5 years prior to diagnosis of AD. Typical AD dementia initially presents with an episodic memory impairment reflecting the selective vulnerability of the medial temporal lobe to AD pathology. Episodic memory relates to our ability to remember information specific to a time and place when that memory was formed (e.g., What did you eat for dinner? What did you do on a trip?). Semantic memory dysfunction can be an early feature of AD but occurs after episodic memory involvement. Executive function (planning, organization, problem solving, and set switching) decline occurs in mild AD. Language disturbance often occurs in the mild-moderate stage of AD dementia. Initial complaints often include word-finding difficulty. In time, other features of aphasia may develop, and in the late stages, language output can be limited. Decline in visuospatial skills is common, often manifesting early with the complaint of becoming lost or being disorientated in unfamiliar places.

- *Semantic* memory dysfunction: *Category fluency test*—impaired early
- *Executive functions* such as planning, organization, and problem solving are mild till late in disease course (compared to bvFTD).
- *Language* disturbance: Seen at mild-moderate stage, word-finding difficulty, aphasia, and limited language output
- *Visuospatial skills*: May manifest early, complaint of becoming lost or being disoriented in unfamiliar places. Several abilities were preserved till the very late stage.
- *Motor learning* (procedural) motor and sensory skills

Occasionally, AD can present with focal cortical syndromes without memory loss initially.

The three most commonly described atypical presentations are as follows:

1. Posterior cortical atrophy (PCA)
2. Logopenic aphasia (LPA)
3. Frontal variant of AD

Frontotemporal Dementia

There are chiefly three variants of FTD syndrome as described:

1. *Behavioral variant (bvFTD)*: Most common variant that presents with apathy, disinhibition, compulsivity, loss of empathy, and overeating.
2. *Primary progressive aphasia (PPA)*: It consists of semantic and nonfluent/agrammatic variants.
   a. Semantic variant: Patients slowly lose the ability to decode word, object, person specific, and emotions.
   b. Nonfluent/agrammatic: Inability to produce words, with prominent speech impairment
3. FTD is also closely related to motor neuron disease (MND), most closely associated with behavioral variant type.

Vascular Dementia

Clinical features of vascular dementia include:

- *Behavioral symptoms*: Memory, slowed thinking, depression, and anxiety
- *Locomotor problems*: Gait disturbance, dysarthria, and autonomic dysfunction
- *Loss of executive function*: Problem solving, working memory, judgment, and reasoning
- Visual orientation problem, hallucination

Diagnostic triad of VaD is given as follows:

- Dementia syndrome—with memory and/or executive function impairment
- Vascular cause—postictus or subcortical ischemia
- *Adequate relationship*:
  - Temporal (immediate, subacute, and insidious)
  - Functional (lesion to the structure of cognitive integration)

Lewy Body Dementia

Parkinson's disease dementia and DLB typically present with significant impairments in executive function, attention, and visuospatial abilities, while episodic memory is usually preserved. Cognitive declines are severe enough to affect daily activities compared to parkinsonian symptoms.

Clinical symptoms can range from psychosis in the form of visual hallucinations, fluctuating cognition, rapid eye movement sleep behavior disorder (RBD), and Parkinsonism. Fluctuating attention is another characteristic feature. Rapid eye movement (REM) sleep behavior can be in the form of skeletal muscle paralysis; patients may enact dreams, sometimes injuring themselves or their bed partners. Highly sensitive to infectious or metabolic disturbances.

The difference between DLB and PDD can be done by the symptom onset and duration. Patient presenting with long-standing PD manifesting dementia are mostly PDD, whereas when the dementia and the neuropsychiatric symptoms precede or coemerge with the Parkinsonism, the patient is diagnosed with DLB.

Autonomic dysfunction such as orthostatic hypotension, syncopal events, erectile dysfunction, and constipation can be early features of DLB too sometimes challenging to differentiate with multiple system atrophy (MSA).

Complications

- Increased susceptibility to infections, including respiratory and urinary tract infections
- Malnutrition and dehydration due to forgetfulness or inability to perform activities of daily living
- Falls and related injuries, resulting from impaired balance and gait instability
- Worsening of preexisting medical conditions due to neglect or failure to adhere to treatment regimens
- Development of pressure ulcers and skin breakdown, particularly in immobile or bedridden individuals
- Increased risk of medication errors and adverse drug reactions due to cognitive deficits

Examination

History is an important part of MNCD diagnosis; however, all patients with cognitive impairment should have a systemic examination with a focus on the neurological system. A complete neurologic examination is performed to look for signs of other diseases that could cause dementia, such as Parkinson's disease or multiple strokes.

Evaluation and Investigations

The detailed history and examination are followed by a cognitive/mental state examination, which should include the following domains of cognition:

- Executive function
- Attention and concentration
- Recent and remote memory
- Language
- Praxis (i.e., ability to perform skilled motor tasks without nonverbal prompting)
- Visuospatial function

There are many mental state examination tools but standardized tools such as Mini–Mental State Examination (MMSE), Montreal Cognitive Assessment (MoCA), and Addenbrooke's Cognitive Examination-III (ACE-III). These tools can have education, language, and social constraints which can be minimized by using locally adaptable standard tools.

NEUROIMAGING AND BIOMARKERS ADVANCEMENTS

Neuroimaging studies, including magnetic resonance imaging (MRI) or computed tomography scans, may show cortical atrophy, ventricular enlargement, or white matter changes consistent with vascular pathology.

Laboratory investigations may be conducted to rule out metabolic or infectious causes of cognitive decline, including complete blood count, electrolyte panel, thyroid function tests, and serological markers for infectious diseases.

Magnetic Resonance Imaging of the Brain

In the early stages of AD, an MRI scan of the brain may be normal. In later stages, MRI may show a decrease in the size of different areas of the brain (mainly affecting the temporal and parietal lobes).

Frontotemporal Dementia

Magnetic resonance imaging finding of the disease in anatomic localization of the disorder is mostly atrophy of medial and orbital frontal and anterior insula in behavioral FTD. The anterior temporal region in the semantic variant and lateral frontal and precentral gyrus of the dominant hemisphere in nonfluent/agrammatic PPA **(Table 1)**.

Lewy Body Dementia

Magnetic resonance imaging finding: Polysomnography shows RBD with atonia. Cerebrospinal fluid (CSF) shows either alpha-synuclein oligomers (RT-uIC) or CSF or blood levels of phospho-tau 217, iodine-123-meta-iodibenylguanidine (MIBG) cardiac scintigraphy showing cardiac postganglionic sympathetic denervation.

The field of biomarkers has moved on and has made some significant changes **(Table 2)**.

TABLE 1: Key differences between dementia and pseudodementia.

Feature	Dementia	Pseudodementia
Definition	A chronic, progressive neurodegenerative disorder characterized by cognitive decline, often irreversible	A condition mimicking dementia, usually related to depression, with reversible cognitive impairment
Onset	Gradual, with progressive worsening over months or years	Abrupt, often following a depressive episode
Cause	Neurodegenerative disorders (e.g., Alzheimer's disease, vascular dementia)	Primarily due to underlying depression or other psychiatric conditions
Mood changes	Mood may fluctuate but is usually secondary to cognitive decline	Mood symptoms (e.g., depression, sadness) are prominent and primary

Continued

Continued

Feature	Dementia	Pseudodementia
Memory complaint	Patients may not be aware or may minimize cognitive deficits; family often reports memory issues	Patients are acutely aware and often complain about memory loss, sometimes exaggerating it
Attention and concentration	Often impaired in later stages	Typically preserved; issues usually stem from lack of motivation rather than true cognitive dysfunction
Response to testing	Shows effort but may struggle due to true cognitive deficits	Often gives "I don't know" answers or poor effort, with inconsistencies in performance
Progression	Gradual worsening over time; irreversible	Typically reversible with treatment for the underlying psychiatric condition
Insight	Poor insight into their cognitive deficits as the disease progresses	Good insight into memory issues and often anxious about cognitive decline
Response to treatment	Limited; symptomatic treatments may slow progression but not reverse the condition	Cognitive symptoms improve significantly with antidepressant therapy and psychotherapy
Example conditions	Alzheimer's disease, vascular dementia, and Lewy body dementia	Depression-related cognitive impairment, sometimes called "depressive pseudodementia"

TABLE 2: Differences between cortical and subcortical dementia.

Feature	Cortical dementia	Subcortical dementia
Primary brain region affected	Cortex (outer layer of the brain)	Subcortical structures (e.g., basal ganglia, thalamus, and white matter)
Examples of disorders	Alzheimer's disease, frontotemporal dementia	Parkinson's disease dementia, Huntington's disease, and progressive supranuclear palsy
Onset	Gradual, often starting with memory loss	Gradual but usually slower than cortical dementia; motor symptoms often precede cognitive decline
Cognitive features	Prominent deficits in memory, language, and executive function	Impaired processing speed, attention, and executive function with less memory impairment early on
Memory impairment	Early, severe memory impairment, especially episodic memory	Mild memory impairment early on, with difficulties more related to retrieval than storage
Language and speech	Often affected, with issues like aphasia and word-finding difficulties	Less affected; language generally intact until later stages
Motor symptoms	Minimal until late stages; apraxia may occur	Early motor symptoms (e.g., bradykinesia, tremor, and rigidity) are common
Mood and behavior changes	Less frequent early on; apathy or irritability in later stages	Depression, apathy, and mood changes are common early signs
Processing speed	Typically preserved until advanced stages	Slowed processing speed is a key feature
Insight	Often impaired, especially in later stages	Insight may remain intact longer, especially early in the disease course
Response to testing	Marked deficits in memory and language tests	Slower responses, with deficits in motor and psychomotor tests

PREVENTION AND MANAGEMENT

A 2024 report of the *Lancet* Standing Commission was released recently and had some of the changes to prevent dementia **(Fig. 1)**. The evidence is suggestive of and has become more stronger than before that tackling the many risk factors for dementia [i.e., less education, hearing loss, hypertension, smoking, obesity, depression, physical inactivity, diabetes, excessive alcohol consumption (i.e., >21 UK units, equivalent to >12 US units), TBI, air pollution, and social isolation] reduces the risk of developing dementia.

A new compelling evidence suggests that untreated vision loss and high low-density lipoprotein (LDL) cholesterol are risk factors for dementia. New evidence

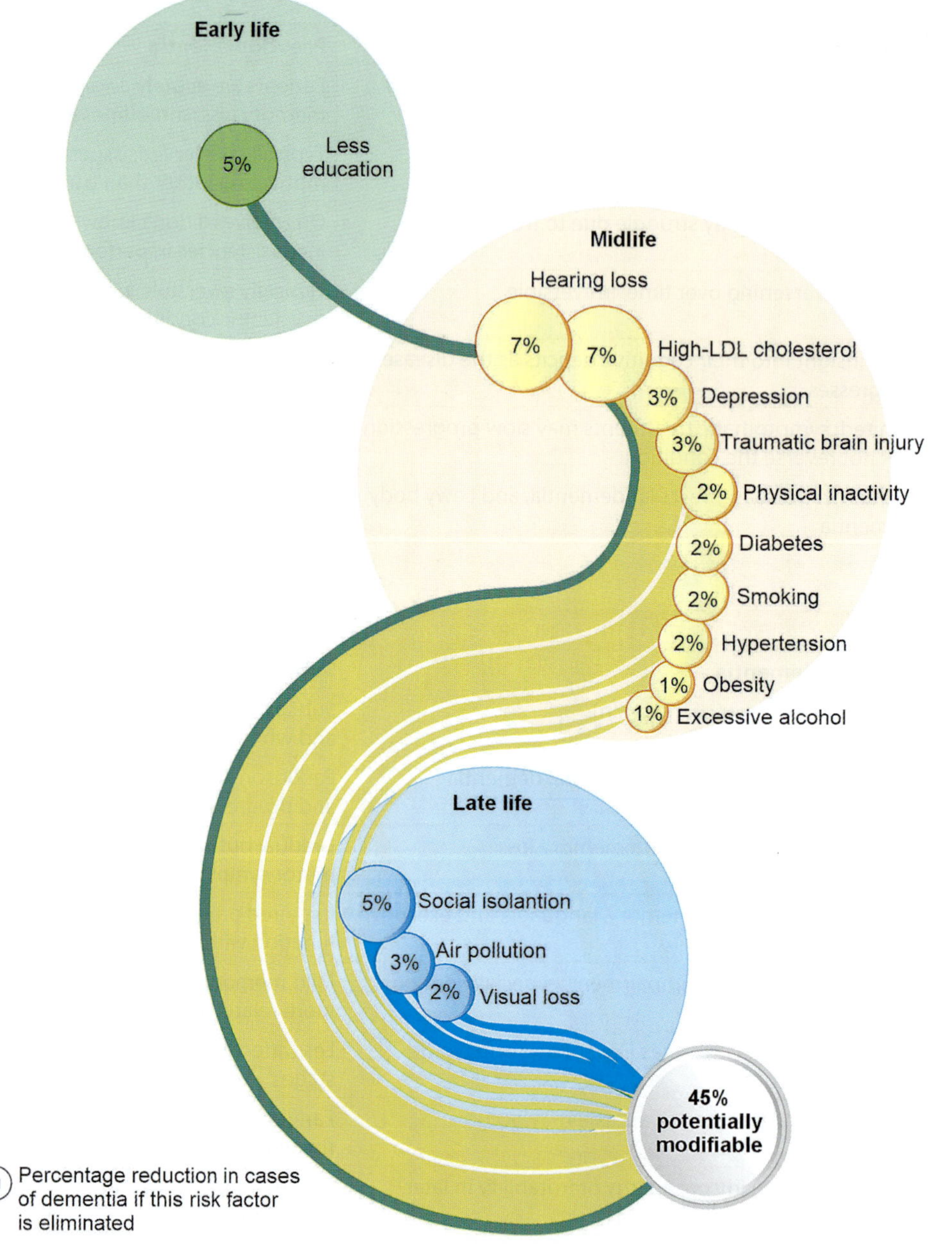

FIG. 1: Population attributable fraction of potentially modifiable risk factors for dementia, Lancet Commission 2024. (LDL: low-density lipoprotein)

suggests that reducing the risk of dementia increases the number of healthy years of life and compresses the duration of ill health for people who develop dementia.

There have been many studies about the risk factors and the evidence surrounding it. A follow-up study found that a diet for brain health (Mediterranean-DASH Diet Intervention for Neurodegenerative Delay—MIND diet score in upper 40% of cohort distribution), late-life cognitive activities (composite score in upper 40%), moderate or vigorous physical activity (≥150 min/week), no smoking, and light to moderate alcohol consumption (women 1–15 g/day; men 1–30 g/day) were associated with a longer life expectancy among men and women, and they lived a larger proportion of their remaining years without Alzheimer's dementia.

A lot depends on neuropathology of the brain as well, which is often taken as nonmodifiable risk factor, but studies suggest people who are physically healthier are better able to withstand the effects of neuropathology than people who are physically unhealthy or frail.

Modifiable risk factors to prevent dementia include:

- *High blood pressure*: There are evidence that supports the benefits of antihypertensive treatment in late-mid and later life to lower the risk of dementia.
- *Education*: A systematic review and meta-analyses comprehending Latin American and Caribbean populations revealed dementia was almost twice as prevalence in the population with no formal education than those receiving at least >1 year of formal education. A Chinese study found rising incidence and prevalence of dementia in aging population, which were found most to be in participants having attained <6 years of education. Similar reductions in dementia prevalence were noted in increased education in a diverse US population. However, there are some studies, meta-analysis comprising 92 articles concluded that there is no substantial association between educational attainment and changes in cognitive performance.
- *Cognitive stimulation (CS)*: A multicohort study found that cognitive stimulating jobs were associated with lowering risk of dementia than those with nonstimulating jobs. The ability to increase cognitive reserve by these stimulations is postulated to be due to higher concentration of circulating proteins to allow brain repair through axonogenesis and synaptogenesis.
- *Hearing loss and hearing aids*: Lancet Commission included hearing loss as one of 14 major risk factors in the incidence of dementia. Further, five meta-analyses determined the association between hearing loss and subsequent dementia. Study published in 2024 comprised 50 studies, suggesting risk of dementia increases by 16% for each 10 dB worsening of hearing. Psychosocial factors such as loneliness, depression, and social isolation are believed to be influenced by hearing loss and are thought to play a role in the relationship with dementia.
- *Diabetes*: Onset of diabetes is said to be more significant where midlife diabetes is a risk factor for dementia but might not be a risk in those whose diabetes onset is in late life. Mechanism postulated to play a role in such includes microvascular and macrovascular complications, decreased insulin signaling in the central nervous system (CNS) leading to increased amyloid B toxicity, tau hyperphosphorylation, oxidative stress, and neuroinflammation.
- *Depression*: There are already enough evidences linking depression with dementia. New meta-analysis further strengthens this association. The link between depression and dementia is taken as bidirectional and often depression too can only be symptom of evolving dementia. Though depression can occur in all age groups and be a risk factor of dementia, association of late-life depression is thought to be of preclinical dementia.
- *Traumatic brain injury*: It is found that TBI is one of the significant risk factors of dementia with association of nearly 70% with increased risk. Such risk factor is more increased in the case of contact sport such as rugby, ice hockey, and wrestling. The plausible mechanisms involved in the causation are axonal injury promoting early generation of proteinopathies (e.g., hyperphosphorylated tau and amyloid B), microglial activation, and cortical atrophy.
- *Smoking*: As identified previously, late-life smoking is associated with an increased risk of dementia; new evidence appears that a larger duration of smoking such as midlife and early-life smoking appears to be stronger risk factor. It is also suggested as in a Korean study that former smokers have a lower risk than those continuing smoking.
- *Cardiovascular risk factors*: In China, a 10-year study of 29,072 people (mean age 72 years) found that slow memory decline was linked to being in a healthy group, defined by having at least four of six factors: (1) A healthy diet, (2) regular physical exercise, (3) active social contact, (4) cognitive activity, (5) not smoking, and (6) minimal alcohol consumption.
- *Low-density lipoprotein*: The risk of increase in LDL cholesterol is found to be associated with all-cause dementia with stronger risk factor in people younger than 65 years at baseline. Excess brain cholesterol is associated with increased stroke risk and deposition of brain amyloid B and tau, suggesting a potential mechanism for link of dementia. This gives a potential window of statin for the treatment of dementia due to their link in anti-inflammatory and antioxidant properties, as well as reducing cholesterol levels. However, more studies are needed to increase the quality of evidence and incorporate in clinical practice.
- *Physical inactivity, exercise, and fitness*: A systematic review and meta-analysis consisting of 58 studies explored the link and found a decreased risk of all-cause dementia in short and long follow-ups of at least 20 years. The type of activity responsible for the risk reduction includes moderate-intensity continuous training or high-intensity interval training twice a week. Exercise appears to help cognition by changes in blood flow and function, reduction of hypertension and increased nitric oxide, and reduced neuroinflammation.

TREATMENT

Alzheimer's Disease

Pharmacological Interventions

- *Cholinesterase inhibitors*:
  - Mechanism: Enhance cholinergic transmission by inhibiting the enzyme acetylcholinesterase, which breaks down acetylcholine
  - For example:
    - Donepezil: Approved for all stages of AD, typically well tolerated, with side effects such as nausea, diarrhea, and insomnia
    - Rivastigmine: Available in oral and transdermal patch forms, commonly used in mild-to-moderate AD
    - Galantamine: Dual mechanism involving acetylcholinesterase inhibition and nicotinic receptor modulation, used in mild-to-moderate AD
  - Considerations: Titrate doses slowly to minimize gastrointestinal side effects
- *N-methyl-D-aspartate (NMDA) receptor antagonists:*
  - Memantine:
    - Mechanism: Regulates glutamatergic signaling to prevent excitotoxicity
    - Indications: Moderate-to-severe AD, either as monotherapy or in combination with cholinesterase inhibitors
    - Side effects: Dizziness, headache, and confusion
- *Emerging therapies:*
  - Antiamyloid agents: Recent advancements include monoclonal antibodies targeting amyloid-beta, such as lecanemab and aducanumab.
    - Indications: Early or mild AD with confirmed amyloid pathology
    - Challenges: High costs, potential side effects such as amyloid-related imaging abnormalities (ARIA)
  - Tau-based therapies: Targeting tau protein aggregation; ongoing clinical trials
- *Management of neuropsychiatric symptoms:*
  - Depression: Selective serotonin reuptake inhibitors (SSRIs) (e.g., sertraline) are commonly used.
  - Agitation and psychosis:
    - Atypical antipsychotics (e.g., quetiapine and olanzapine) may be used with caution due to risks such as increased mortality.
    - Nonpharmacological approaches are preferred first-line interventions.

Nonpharmacological Interventions

- *CS and rehabilitation*:
  - Typically classified as CS, cognitive training (CT), and cognitive rehabilitation (CR)
  - Regular activities to enhance memory, problem-solving, and language skills
  - Cognitive stimulation therapy (CST) involves different sessions of themed activities usually related to tasks, including money use, word games, word association, object categorization, current affairs, and famous faces which is typically taken twice weekly; such CST has provided a robust evidence-based body of data, especially in mild and moderate dementia.
  - Programs such as reminiscence therapy and reality orientation therapy
- *Behavioral interventions*:
  - Tailored strategies to manage challenging behaviors, such as agitation or wandering
  - Environmental modifications to reduce triggers (e.g., minimizing noise and clutter)
  - Occupational therapy: This uses a combined approach, including activity simplification, environmental modification, adaptive aids, problem-solving strategies, skill training, and caregiver education.
- *Caregiver education and support*:
  - Training in communication strategies and managing challenging behaviors
  - Access to support groups and respite care to reduce caregiver burden

Lifestyle Modifications

- *Dietary interventions*:
  - Mediterranean diet: Rich in fruits, vegetables, whole grains, and healthy fats
  - Nutritional supplements (e.g., omega-3 fatty acids, vitamin E) lack robust evidence for cognitive benefits but may be considered on a case-by-case basis.
- *Physical activity*:
  - Regular aerobic exercise (e.g., walking, swimming) to improve vascular health (by reducing blood pressure, arterial stiffness, oxidative stress, systemic inflammation, enhancing endothelial dysfunction) and cognition. Documented to improve physical health, well-being, as well as enhance performance in the activities of daily living. Exercise also preserves neurons and promotes neurogenesis, synaptogenesis, and neuronal plasticity.

- *Cognitive engagement*:
  - Activities such as puzzles, reading, and social interaction to maintain mental stimulation
- *Sleep hygiene*:
  - Management of sleep disturbances through structured routines, limiting daytime naps, and melatonin when necessary
- *Psychological therapy*: Depression and anxiety are very common in people with dementia; use of cognitive-behavioral therapy, psychodynamic therapy, interpersonal therapy, and supportive counseling are the main psychotherapeutic approaches which have shown evidence.

Palliative Care Considerations

- *Advanced care planning*:
  - Early discussions about goals of care and advanced directives with patients and families
- *Symptom management*:
  - Comprehensive care for late-stage AD, focusing on pain management, nutritional support, and prevention of infections
- *End-of-life care*:
  - Hospice care to ensure comfort and dignity in terminal stages

Multidisciplinary and Individualized Care

- Integration of neurologists, geriatricians, psychiatrists, and allied health professionals
- Personalized treatment plans based on disease stage, comorbidities, and patient/family preferences

Multidimensional stimulation therapy (MST) with combined CS, recreational activities, and physical exercises demonstrated more effective intervention in improving both behavioral and functional outcomes in AD patients.

Complementary and Alternative Medicine

- *Aromatherapy*: A part of phytotherapy is based on the use of essential oils from fragrant plants to relieve health problems and improve quality of life (QoL). It has the potential effects of relaxation and improvement of pain and sleep as well as reduction of depressive symptoms. However, the data are equivocal, and more high-quality randomized controlled trials (RCTs) need to be explored.
- *Music therapy*: It includes the use of music; sound as a nonverbal communication tool to induce educational, rehabilitative, or therapeutic effect. These may include singing, listening, improvising, or playing along on musical instruments. The theoretical basis shows activation of the large number of cortical and subcortical areas involved in emotional processing. Also, it improves communicative and relational processes, which becomes an efficient tool for rehabilitation. However, recent RCTs and meta-analysis do not yield any addition to pharmacotherapy effect.
- *Massage and touch*: Evidence suggests that it may result to reduce behavioral and psychological symptoms of dementia (BPSD), improve appetite, sleep and communication problems, and to some extent counteract cognitive decline.

Frontotemporal Dementia

Pharmacological Interventions

- *Behavioral variant FTD (bvFTD)*:
  - SSRIs:
    - For example: Sertraline, fluoxetine, and citalopram
    - Indications: Reduce disinhibition, compulsive behaviors, and irritability
    - Evidence: Some studies suggest modest improvement in behavioral symptoms.
  - Atypical antipsychotics (used with caution):
    - For example: Quetiapine and olanzapine
    - Indications: Severe agitation or psychosis
    - Risks: Extrapyramidal symptoms and increased mortality in older adults necessitate judicious use.
- *Language variants (PPA):*
  - No specific pharmacological therapies target language deficits directly.
  - Symptom management may include SSRIs for associated behavioral symptoms.
- *Cholinesterase inhibitors and memantine:*
  - Evidence: Generally not effective in FTD and may worsen symptoms in some patients
  - Current role: Not recommended as standard treatment
- *Experimental therapies:*
  - Antitau agents and progranulin-enhancing therapies are under investigation.
  - Potential future role for genetic therapies in familial cases is linked to mutations (e.g., progranulin or C9orf72).

Nonpharmacological Interventions

- *Behavioral and environmental modifications*:
  - Create structured routines to minimize confusion and agitation
  - Simplify the living environment to reduce triggers for problematic behaviors
  - Positive reinforcement for desired behaviors

- *Speech and language therapy*:
  - Focus: Augmentative and alternative communication strategies for patients with progressive aphasia
  - Techniques: Use of picture boards, electronic devices, and structured language exercises
  - Goal: Maximize functional communication for as long as possible
- *Occupational therapy*:
  - Strategies to maintain functional independence in daily activities
  - Assistive devices to address limitations in motor function or apathy

Supportive Measures

- *Caregiver education and training*:
  - Training caregivers to manage challenging behaviors, including apathy, disinhibition, and compulsive actions
  - Providing resources for support groups and respite care
- *Counseling*:
  - Address emotional and psychological stress in both patients and caregivers
- *Legal and financial planning*:
  - Early referral for guardianship, power of attorney, and financial planning due to early-onset and rapid progression

Lifestyle Modifications

- *Dietary management*:
  - Address compulsive overeating or food-related behaviors often seen in FTD
- *Physical activity*:
  - Regular physical exercise to manage apathy and maintain overall health
- *Sleep hygiene*:
  - Interventions to improve disrupted sleep patterns, including structured routines and relaxation techniques

Future Directions and Research

- *Genetic counseling and testing*:
  - Indicated for familial cases with mutations in genes such as progranulin (GRN), microtubule-associated protein tau (MAPT), or C9orf72
  - Role in identifying at-risk family members and guiding potential future therapies
- *Targeted therapies*:
  - Development of tau and TDP-43 protein-targeted therapies
  - Trials involving progranulin replacement in GRN mutation carriers

Palliative Care Considerations

- *Symptom management*:
  - Focus on QoL, particularly in the advanced stages
  - Address feeding difficulties, mobility issues, and recurrent infections
- *End-of-life care:*
  - Ensure comfort and dignity, with discussions on advanced directives and hospice care

Vascular Dementia

Pharmacological Interventions

- *Management of cognitive symptoms*:
  - Cholinesterase inhibitors:
    - For example: Donepezil and rivastigmine
    - Evidence: May provide modest cognitive benefits, particularly in mixed dementia (VaD with concurrent Alzheimer's pathology)
  - Memantine:
    - Indication: Moderate-to-severe VaD; benefits observed in some studies, though the evidence is less robust compared to AD.
- *Control of vascular risk factors*:
  - Antihypertensives:
    - Goal: Maintain optimal blood pressure to prevent further cerebrovascular events
    - Evidence: Intensive blood pressure control reduces the risk of recurrent stroke and cognitive decline.
  - Antiplatelet or anticoagulant therapy:
    - For example: Aspirin, clopidogrel, or warfarin (if indicated)
    - Indication: Prevent secondary ischemic events, particularly in patients with large-vessel disease or cardioembolic sources
    - Caution: Avoid in hemorrhagic strokes unless indicated for other reasons
  - Lipid-lowering agents:
    - For example: Statins (e.g., atorvastatin and rosuvastatin)
    - Indication: Reduce LDL cholesterol and atherosclerotic burden
  - Diabetes management:
    - Use of oral hypoglycemic agents or insulin to achieve glycemic control
    - Avoid hypoglycemia, which can worsen cognitive impairment.
- *Symptom management*:
  - Mood disorders: SSRIs (e.g., sertraline) for depressive symptoms
  - Sleep disturbances: Melatonin or short-term use of sedative-hypnotics

Nonpharmacological Interventions

- *Cognitive rehabilitation:*
  - Goal: Improve memory, attention, and problem-solving skills
  - Techniques: Structured tasks, memory aids, and computerized cognitive training programs
- *Physical therapy*:
  - Focus: Improve mobility, balance, and prevent falls
  - Programs: Aerobic exercises, strength training, and tailored physiotherapy
- *Lifestyle modifications*:
  - Dietary interventions:
    - Emphasize a heart-healthy diet: Mediterranean or dietary approaches to stop hypertension (DASH)
  - Smoking cessation:
    - Immediate and long-term benefits in vascular health and cognitive decline prevention
  - Regular physical activity:
    - Activities: Walking, swimming, and yoga
    - Benefits: Enhances vascular health and neuroplasticity
  - Alcohol moderation:
    - Avoid excessive alcohol intake; low-to-moderate consumption may have cardiovascular benefits
- *Social engagement*:
  - Encourage participation in group activities and social events to reduce isolation and depression

Preventive Strategies

- *Stroke prevention*:
  - Antiplatelet or anticoagulation therapy in high-risk patients
  - Management of atrial fibrillation and carotid artery disease
- *Control of modifiable risk factors*:
  - Aggressive management of hypertension, hyperlipidemia, and diabetes
  - Regular monitoring of vascular health with periodic checkups

Supportive Measures

- *Caregiver education*:
  - Training on managing cognitive and behavioral symptoms
  - Techniques for communication and ensuring patient safety
- *Environmental modifications*:
  - Fall-proofing the home, using assistive devices, and labeling items to aid memory
- *Community resources*:
  - Access to support groups and adult daycare centers

Dementia with Lewy Bodies

Pharmacological Interventions

- *Cognitive symptoms*:
  - Cholinesterase inhibitors:
    - For example: Rivastigmine (most evidence-based) and donepezil
    - Mechanism: Enhance cholinergic transmission to improve cognitive function and neuropsychiatric symptoms
    - Benefits: Improved attention, hallucinations, and cognitive stability
    - Side effects: Nausea, vomiting, and potential exacerbation of bradycardia
  - Memantine:
    - Role: Limited evidence but may provide cognitive and behavioral benefits in some patients
- *Parkinsonism*:
  - Levodopa (L-Dopa):
    - Indication: Alleviation of Parkinsonian motor symptoms such as rigidity and bradykinesia
    - Challenges: May exacerbate hallucinations and delusions
    - Dosage: Start with the lowest effective dose and titrate cautiously
  - Dopamine agonists:
    - Generally avoided due to a higher risk of psychosis in DLB patients
- *Psychosis and hallucinations*:
  - Atypical antipsychotics (used with caution):
    - Preferred agents: Quetiapine or clozapine
    - Avoid: Typical antipsychotics (e.g., haloperidol) and risperidone due to high sensitivity in DLB, leading to severe extrapyramidal symptoms or neuroleptic malignant syndrome
    - Dosing: Use the lowest effective dose for the shortest possible duration
  - Cholinesterase inhibitors may also reduce hallucinations and delusions.
- *RBD*:
  - Clonazepam:
    - Indication: Alleviates violent or disruptive behaviors during REM sleep
    - Caution: Risk of sedation, falls, and respiratory depression
  - Melatonin:
    - An alternative to clonazepam with a lower side effect profile

- *Autonomic dysfunction*:
  - Orthostatic hypotension:
    - Management: Fludrocortisone, midodrine, or nonpharmacological measures such as compression stockings and increased salt intake
  - Constipation:
    - Use of laxatives or stool softeners as needed
  - Urinary symptoms:
    - Anticholinergic agents are generally avoided due to potential worsening of cognitive symptoms.
- *Sleep disturbances*:
  - Nonpharmacological measures (e.g., maintaining a consistent sleep schedule) are first line.
  - Melatonin or sedative-hypnotics for short-term management

Nonpharmacological Interventions

- *Cognitive stimulation*:
  - Activities tailored to improve cognitive function, reduce apathy, and enhance engagement
  - For example: Puzzles, memory games, and music therapy
- *Occupational therapy*:
  - Strategies to maintain independence in daily living activities
  - Training in the use of assistive devices for motor symptoms
- *Physical therapy*:
  - Focus: Improve mobility, gait, and reduce the risk of falls
  - Techniques: Balance training, strength exercises, and adaptive movement techniques
- *Environmental modifications*:
  - Creating a safe and low-stimulation environment to reduce hallucination triggers and agitation
  - Use of nightlights and labeled items to help with orientation

Supportive Measures

- *Caregiver education and support*:
  - Training in managing behavioral symptoms and understanding the fluctuating course of DLB
  - Access to support groups and respite care services
- *Multidisciplinary care*:
  - Involvement of neurologists, geriatricians, psychiatrists, and palliative care specialists
- *Legal and financial planning*:
  - Early guidance on advanced care planning, including durable power of attorney and guardianship

Lifestyle Modifications

- *Dietary adjustments*:
  - Encourage a balanced diet, emphasizing hydration and fiber to manage autonomic symptoms such as constipation
- *Regular physical activity*:
  - Light exercises such as walking or yoga to maintain cardiovascular health and mobility
- *Cognitive engagement*:
  - Encourage social interactions and participation in mentally stimulating activities

NEW TECHNOLOGIES

- *Global positional system (GPS)*: The development of this technology can allow people with dementia to stay outdoors in a safe and secure way. Tracking technology can promote perceived safety and security among caregivers and relatives of people with dementia.
- *Surveillance and management of high-risk behaviors*: It can play a role to replace more severe physical restraints. Acoustic sensors in bedroom/living room can record noise or patient movement.
- Body-worn gyroscopes measuring angular velocity to measure the acceleration of the trunk and inertial sensors may detect fall when it occurs.
- Shoe insole that delivers vibration may also prevent falls and improve gait and balance.
- Virtual reality (VR) and gaming have potential applications of VR systems to assess and train AD patients.
- Telemedicine can provide follow-up care to help people with dementia to maintain their independence and ameliorate clinical outcomes in reduced access to health services **(Table 3)**.

TABLE 3: Summary of the level of evidence, main positive outcomes, and limitations of the nonpharmacological treatment for Alzheimer's disease and dementia.

Treatment	Subtype	Evidence	Main positive outcomes	Limitations
Exercise and motor rehabilitation		Moderate	• Reduction of BPSD • Improvement of ADL	• Limited evidence for cognition, QoL, depression, mortality, and caregiver burden • Few comparative studies exploring the most effective exercise intervention • Unclear duration and intensity of activity

Continued

Continued

Treatment	Subtype	Evidence	Main positive outcomes	Limitations
Cognitive intervention	CS	Moderate	• Improvement of general cognitive function • Small effect on mood and QoL of patients and caregivers	• Unclear long-term effect on cognition • Heterogeneity of the outcomes
	CT	Small	Enhancement of performance in trained and similar tasks	• No generalization effect to daily function • Low-quality studies
	CS + CT	Small	Improvement of general cognitive function	• Heterogeneity of treatment • Heterogeneity of dementia severity • Few high-quality RCTs
	CST	Moderate	• Improvements of general cognitive function and specific cognitive domains • Small effect on QoL • Improvement of caregiving relationship • Small effect on depressive symptoms and QoL of caregivers	• Not all services offer this treatment • Unclear effect on BPSD and ADL
Occupational therapy		Small	• Improvement of ADL, social participation, and QoL • Reduction of BPSD and depression • Reduction of caregiver burden	• Unclear optimal duration • Unclear long-term effect • Mixed approaches • Few high-quality RCTs
Psychological therapy		Small	• Reduction of depression, anxiety, and apathy • Enhancement of patient's well-being	• No comparative studies between different psychological treatments • No long-term studies • Few high-quality RCTs
Multicomponent/ multidimensional strategies		Small	• Reduction of BPSD • Improvement of some cognitive domains • Delayed institutionalization • Reduction of caregiver burden	• Persistence of effect • Generalization to everyday life • Limited implementation and dissemination • Few high-quality RCTs
Aromatherapy		Very small	• Reduction of BPSD and sleep disturbances • Improvements in motivational behavior	• Severe methodological issues • Few high-quality RCTs
Music therapy		Small	• Reduction of depression • Improvement in communication, social participation, relations, and cognition	• Unclear long-term effect • Small sample size • Low-quality studies
Art therapy		Very small	• Reduction of BPSD • Improvement of attention • Improvement of social behavior and self-esteem	• Unclear long-term effect • No RCTs
Massage and touch		Very small	• Reduction of BPSD • Improvement of mood, sleep, and appetite	• Small sample size • Low-quality studies

(ADL: activities of daily living; BPSD: behavioral and psychological symptoms of dementia; CS: cognitive stimulation; CST: cognitive stimulation therapy; CT: cognitive training; QoL: quality of life; RCT: randomized controlled trial)

CONCLUSION

MNCD, including dementia, is becoming increasingly prevalent with the aging global population, posing significant challenges to healthcare systems due to its impact on functional independence and quality of life. Alzheimer's disease remains the leading cause of MNCD along with vascular dementia, Lewy body dementia, and frontotemporal dementia also representing major subtypes. Early detection, patient-centred care, and multidisciplinary management—including both pharmacological and nonpharmacological interventions—are essential for improving outcomes.

The role of caregiver education, environmental modification, and the use of therapies like cognitive stimulation, exercise, and occupational therapy is emphasized, alongside advances in pharmacologic options and emerging technologies. Geriatrician along with multidisciplinary team needs to focus on supporting patients and caregivers through individualized, care critical in reducing the burden of MNCD and improving the quality of life.

Self-Assessment Questionnaire

Q1. What are the DSM-5 diagnostic criteria for major neurocognitive disorder, and how do they differ from mild neurocognitive disorder?

Q2. What are the major modifiable risk factors for dementia identified in the 2024 Lancet Standing Commission report?

Q3. Which neuroimaging findings help differentiate Alzheimer's disease, frontotemporal dementia, and Lewy body dementia?

Q4. How can cognitive stimulation therapy (CST) improve outcomes in mild to moderate dementia?

Q5. What are the pharmacological and nonpharmacological management strategies for Alzheimer's disease?

Q6. How can emerging technologies such as GPS tracking, telemedicine, and virtual reality enhance dementia care and patient safety?

FURTHER READINGS

1. Halter JB, Ouslander JG, Studenski S (Eds). Hazzard's Geriatric Medicine and Gerontology, 8th edition. New York; Chicago; San Francisco; Athens; London: McGraw Hill; 2022. p. 1790.
2. Sachdev PS, Blacker D, Blazer DG, Ganguli M, Jeste DV, Paulsen JS, et al. Classifying neurocognitive disorders: the DSM-5 approach. Nat Rev Neurol. 2014;10(11):634-42.
3. Ahmad FB, Cisewski JA, Anderson RN. Leading Causes of Death in the US, 2019-2023. JAMA. 2024;332(12):957-8.
4. Livingston G, Huntley J, Liu KY, Costafreda SG, Selbæk G, Alladi S, et al. Dementia prevention, intervention, and care: 2024 report of the Lancet standing Commission. Lancet. 2024;404(10452):572-628.
5. Wallace LMK, Theou O, Darvesh S, Bennett DA, Buchman AS, Andrew MK, et al. Neuropathologic burden and the degree of frailty in relation to global cognition and dementia. Neurology. 2020;95(24):e3269-79.
6. Peters R, Xu Y, Fitzgerald O, Aung HL, Beckett N, Bulpitt C, et al. Blood pressure lowering and prevention of dementia: an individual patient data meta-analysis. European Heart J. 2022;43(48):4980-90.
7. Ribeiro F, Teixeira-Santos AC, Caramelli P, Leist AK. Prevalence of dementia in Latin America and Caribbean countries: systematic review and meta-analyses exploring age, sex, rurality, and education as possible determinants. Ageing Res Rev. 2022;81:101703.
8. Ding D, Zhao Q, Wu W, Xiao Z, Liang X, Luo J, et al. Prevalence and incidence of dementia in an older Chinese population over two decades: the role of education. Alzheimer's Dement. 2020;16(12):1650-62.
9. Hayward MD, Farina MP, Zhang YS, Kim JK, Crimmins EM. The importance of improving educational attainment for dementia prevalence trends from 2000 to 2014, among older non-Hispanic Black and White Americans. J Gerontol B Psychol Sci Soc Sci. 2021;76(9):1870-9.
10. Seblova D, Berggren R, Lövdén M. Education and age-related decline in cognitive performance: systematic review and meta-analysis of longitudinal cohort studies. Ageing Res Rev. 2020;58:101005.
11. Kivimäki M, Walker KA, Pentti J, Nyberg ST, Mars N, Vahtera J, et al. Cognitive stimulation in the workplace, plasma proteins, and risk of dementia: three analyses of population cohort studies. BMJ. 2021;374:n1804.
12. Yu RC, Proctor D, Soni J, Pikett L, Livingston G, Lewis G, et al. Adult-onset hearing loss and incident cognitive impairment and dementia—a systematic review and meta-analysis of cohort studies. Ageing Res Rev. 2024;98:102346.
13. Amidei CB, Fayosse A, Dumurgier J, Machado-Fragua MD, Tabak AG, van Sloten T, et al. Association between age at diabetes onset and subsequent risk of dementia. JAMA. 2021;325(16):1640.

14. Stafford J, Chung WT, Sommerlad A, Kirkbride JB, Howard R. Psychiatric disorders and risk of subsequent dementia: systematic review and meta-analysis of longitudinal studies. Int J Geriat Psychiatry. 2022;37(5):gps.5711.
15. Gardner RC, Bahorik A, Kornblith ES, Allen IE, Plassman BL, Yaffe K. Systematic review, meta-analysis, and population attributable risk of dementia associated with traumatic brain injury in Civilians and Veterans. J Neurotrauma. 2023;40(7-8):620-34.
16. Zhong G, Wang Y, Zhang Y, Guo JJ, Zhao Y. Smoking is associated with an increased risk of dementia: a meta-analysis of prospective cohort studies with investigation of potential effect modifiers. PLoS One. 2015;10(3):e0118333.
17. Jeong SM, Park J, Han K, Yoo J, Yoo JE, Lee CM, et al. Association of changes in smoking intensity with risk of dementia in Korea. JAMA Netw Open. 2023;6(1):e2251506.
18. Jia J, Zhao T, Liu Z, Liang Y, Li F, Li Y, et al. Association between healthy lifestyle and memory decline in older adults: 10 year, population based, prospective cohort study. BMJ. 2023;380:e072691.
19. Wee J, Sukudom S, Bhat S, Marklund M, Peiris NJ, Hoyos CM, et al. The relationship between midlife dyslipidemia and lifetime incidence of dementia: a systematic review and meta-analysis of cohort studies. Alzheimers Dement (Amst). 2023;15(1): e12395.
20. Olmastroni E, Molari G, De Beni N, Colpani O, Galimberti F, Gazzotti M, et al. Statin use and risk of dementia or Alzheimer's disease: a systematic review and meta-analysis of observational studies. Eur J Prev. Cardiol. 2022;29(5):804-14.
21. Iso-Markku P, Kujala UM, Knittle K, Polet J, Vuoksimaa E, Waller K. Physical activity as a protective factor for dementia and Alzheimer's disease: systematic review, meta-analysis and quality assessment of cohort and case–control studies. Br J Sports Med. 2022;56(12):701-9.
22. Huuha AM, Norevik CS, Moreira JBN, Kobro-Flatmoen A, Scrimgeour N, Kivipelto M, et al. Can exercise training teach us how to treat Alzheimer's disease? Ageing Res Rev. 2022;75: 101559.

CHAPTER 26

Obesity in Elderly

Swarup Das

CASE VIGNETTES

Case Vignette 1

A 65-year-old female patient with a 10-year history of hypertension, diabetic with body mass index (BMI) of 50 kg/m^2 presents to the outpatient department (OPD). She has uncontrolled hypertension, diabetes, fatigue, and difficulty in doing daily activities. How to approach this patient?

Case Vignette 2

A 75-year-old female patient with a 10-year history of hypertension, diabetic with BMI of 35 kg/m^2 presents to OPD. She has uncontrolled hypertension, fatigue, and difficulty in doing daily activities. She also had a fear of fall. How to approach this patient?

INTRODUCTION

Obesity is defined as an unhealthy excess of body fat, which enhances the risk of morbidity and mortality. Obesity is a global epidemic and has also become a major problem in an aging population. Obesity is associated with an increased risk of multiple health problems, including hypertension, type 2 diabetes, dyslipidemia, obstructive sleep apnea, nonalcoholic fatty liver disease (NAFLD), degenerative joint disease, sarcopenia, and increased risk of malignancies in older adults. So, it is important to identify, evaluate, and treat patients for obesity and associated comorbid conditions.

WHAT IS THE PREVALENCE OF OBESITY?

Global prevalence: According to global data, the overall age-adjusted prevalence of obesity in the United States is estimated to be 35% among men and 40.4% among women. In geriatric population, there are 37.1% of men and 33.6% of women are classified obese. A systematic analysis for the Global Burden of Disease Study revealed a worldwide increase in the prevalence of overweight and obesity by 27.5% between 1980 and 2013.

Prevalence in India: According to a report of the Longitudinal Aging Study in India (LASI), a higher proportion of older adults aged 45–59 years are overweight and obese (24% and 9%) than elderly aged 60 years and above (17% and 6%). More elderly people were overweight and obese in urban areas (27% and 12%) than in rural areas (12% and 3%).

WHAT IS THE RELATION OF AGING AND OBESITY?

Aging is associated with significant changes in body composition. After the age of 30 years, individuals tend to show a progressive decrease in fat-free mass (FFM), such as muscle and bone, and an increase in fat mass. Moreover, data from some studies suggest an accelerated loss of FFM in women after they reach age 60 years. FFM attains its peak during the third decade of life, whereas fat mass reaches its peak during the seventh decade and is followed by a subsequent decline. Aging is also associated with the redistribution of body fat. The intra-abdominal fat increases, whereas the subcutaneous fat and total body fat decrease with aging. Some hormonal changes with aging include a reduced production of the anabolic hormones, growth hormone, insulin-like growth factor 1, testosterone, and dehydroepiandrosterone (DHEA), without a concomitant decline in the catabolic hormone cortisol.

WHAT IS THE PATHOPHYSIOLOGY OF OBESITY?

Here is a detailed look at the various aspects contributing to the pathophysiology of obesity **(Fig. 1)**.

Genetic Factors

- *Leptin and leptin receptor genes*: Leptin produced by adipose tissue regulates appetite and energy balance. Mutations in the leptin gene or its receptor can lead to severe obesity.
- *Melanocortin 4 receptor gene*: It plays a critical role in energy homeostasis and appetite regulation and causes obesity.

Environmental Factors

- *Diet*: High-calorie diets rich in fats and sugars promote weight gain.
- *Sedentary lifestyle*: It reduces energy expenditure, contributing to weight gain.
- *Socioeconomic status*: Lower socioeconomic status is associated with higher obesity rates due to limited access to healthy foods and recreational activities.

Physiological Factors

- *Hormonal regulation*: Hormones such as insulin, ghrelin, and adiponectin play roles in appetite regulation and fat storage.
- *Insulin resistance*: It leads to higher insulin levels, promoting fat storage.
- *Ghrelin*: This is known as the hunger hormone, which stimulates appetite. Elevated levels can lead to increased food intake.
- *Adiponectin*: Usually decreased in obesity, adiponectin helps regulate glucose levels and fatty acid breakdown.
- *Adipose tissue*: Beyond storing fat, adipose tissue acts as an endocrine organ, secreting various cytokines and adipokines (e.g., TNF-α and IL-6) that influence metabolism and inflammation. Chronic low-grade inflammation is common in obesity and contributes to insulin resistance and metabolic syndrome.

Neural and Behavioral Factors

Hypothalamus: It regulates hunger and satiety. Dysfunctions in hypothalamic signaling can lead to overeating. The brain's reward systems, involving neurotransmitters such as dopamine, can promote overeating. Stress, emotional factors, and certain behavioral patterns (e.g., binge eating) are also implicated in obesity.

Gut Microbiota

Dysbiosis: Imbalance in gut microbiota known as dysbiosis, which can contribute to weight gain and obesity by affecting nutrient absorption and energy regulation.

Metabolic Factors

Nonexercise activity thermogenesis (NEAT): Low NEAT levels contribute to a positive energy balance and weight gain.

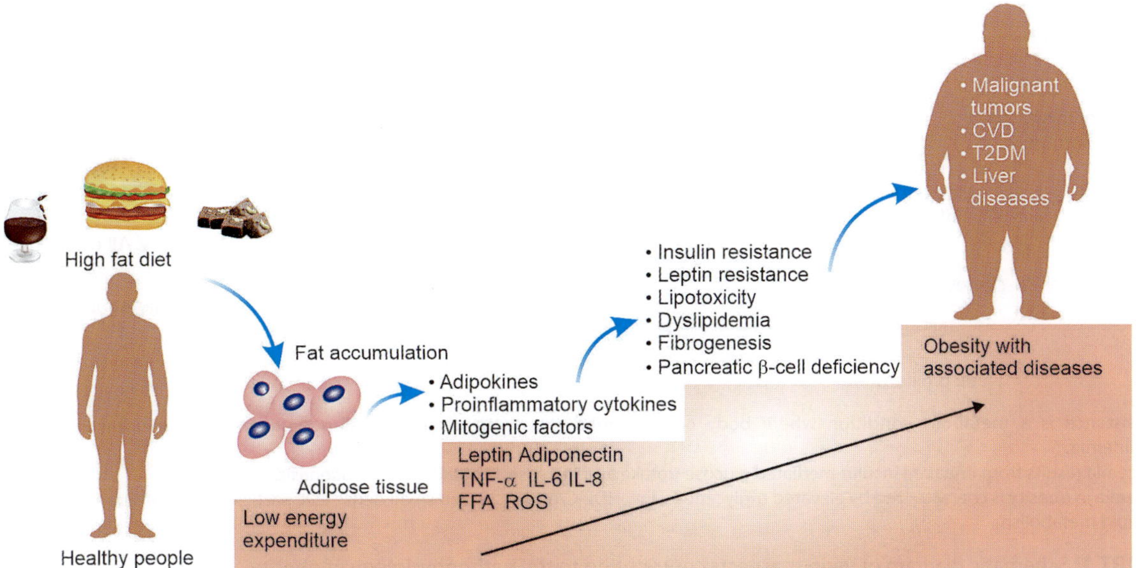

FIG. 1: Pathophysiology of obesity and associated diseases.

(CVD: cardiovascular disease; FFA: free fatty acid; IL: interleukin; ROS: reactive oxygen species; T2DM: type 2 diabetes mellitus; TNF: tumor necrosis factor)

Source: Jin X, Qiu T, Li L, Yu R, Chen X, Li C, et al. Pathophysiology of obesity and its associated diseases. Acta Pharm Sin B. 2023;13(6):2403-24.

Endocrine Disruptors

Exposure to certain chemicals, known as obesogens (e.g., bisphenol A and phthalates), can interfere with lipid metabolism and energy balance, promoting weight gain and obesity.

NEUROHORMONAL REGULATION OF OBESITY

Long-term energy stores are regulated by adipose tissue leptin, adiponectin, and the pancreas (insulin), and glucagon-like peptide (GLP), glucose-dependent insulinotropic polypeptide (GIP), and oxyntomodulin (OXM) are sensitize to insulin. Short-term eating is controlled by hypothalamus, hindbrain, where the nucleus tractus solitarius (NTS) receives input from vagal afferent, stimulated by secretin (SCT) and cholecystokinin (CCK).

WHAT IS THE RELATION BETWEEN OBESITY AND METABOLIC SYNDROME?

Obesity is closely linked to metabolic syndrome, a group of metabolic disorders that increase the risk of cardiovascular disease, type 2 diabetes, and other conditions. Obesity is an exaggeration of normal adiposity and is a central player in the pathophysiology of diabetes mellitus, insulin resistance, dyslipidemia, hypertension, and atherosclerosis, largely because of its secretion of excessive adipokines. Obesity is a major contributor to the metabolic dysfunction involving lipid and glucose, but on a broader scale, it influences organ dysfunction involving cardiac, liver, pulmonary, endocrine, and reproductive functions. Finally, obesity contributes to immune dysfunction from the effects of its secretion of inflammatory adipokines and is a major risk factor for many cancers. Because of the accelerating effects it has on the worsening of metabolic syndrome and cancer, obesity has the potential to be profoundly detrimental to our species if major methods of prevention and/or effective treatment are not realized.

WHAT IS THE ROLE OF LIPOTOXICITY AND INFLAMMATION ON OBESITY?

White adipose tissue (WAT) releases prefatty acids and adipokines, which are lipotoxic and inflammatory and result in diverse effects, outlined in the left-hand columns.

Their correlation to the metabolic syndrome is shown on the right-hand column, whereas all the effects culminate in atherosclerosis on the bottom, as shown in **Flowchart 1**.

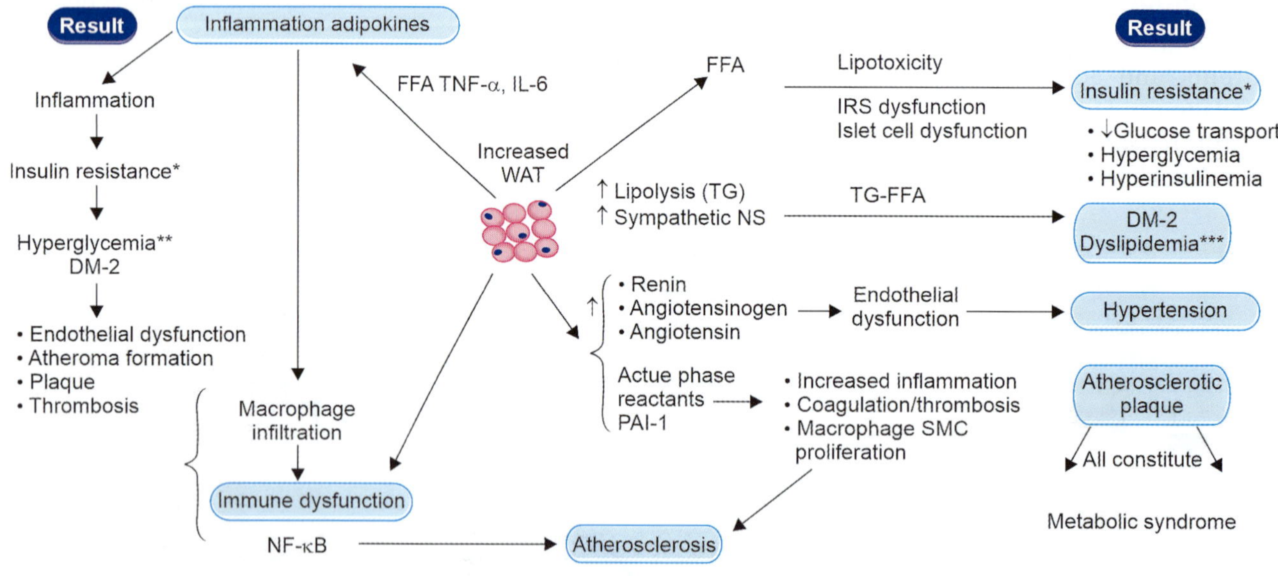

*Insulin resistance is a metabolic condition where body cells respond poorly to insulin, causing reduced glucose uptake and compensatory hyperinsulinemia.

**Hyperglycemia results from impaired insulin-mediated glucose uptake and increased hepatic gluconeogenesis.

***Dyslipidemia in obesity is characterized by elevated triglycerides, low HDL-C, and increased small dense LDL particles due to altered free fatty acid flux and hepatic lipid metabolism.

FLOWCHART 1: Schematic diagram of various aspects contributing to the pathophysiology of obesity.

(CVD: cardiovascular disease; DM: diabetes mellitus; FFA: free fatty acid; IL-6: interleukin-6; IRS: insulin receptor substrate; NF-κB: nuclear factor kappa-light-chain-enhancer of activated B cells; NS: nervous system; PAI-1: plasminogen activator inhibitor-1; SMC: smooth muscle cells; T2DM: type 2 diabetes mellitus; TG: triglyceride; TNF: tumor necrosis factor; WAT: white adipose tissue)

Source: Redinger RN. The pathophysiology of obesity and its clinical manifestations. Gastroenterol Hepatol (N Y). 2007;3(11):856-63.

HOW TO MEASURE AND STAGE OBESITY?

Obesity is measured using several methods that assess body fat and body composition **(Table 1)**.

- Body mass index (BMI) is calculated as weight in kilograms divided by height in meters squared (kg/m^2).
    - *Advantages*: Simple, cost-effective, and widely used
    - *Limitations*: Does not distinguish between muscle and fat mass; may not accurately reflect body fat distribution.
- Waist circumference is measured around the narrowest part of the waist, usually just above the belly button. Increased risk is measured by waist circumference >102 cm (40 inches) for men and >88 cm (35 inches) for women.
- *Waist-to-hip ratio (WHR)*: The waist circumference is divided by the hip circumference. Increased risk is measured by WHR > 0.90 for men and >0.85 for women.
- Body fat percentage can be measured using various techniques, such as:
    - *Skinfold measurements*: Uses callipers to measure the thickness of skinfolds at specific body sites.
    - *Bioelectrical impedance analysis (BIA)*: Estimates body fat by measuring the resistance of body tissues to a small electrical current.
    - *Dual-energy X-ray absorptiometry (DEXA)*: Uses X-rays to differentiate between bone, muscle, and fat tissues.
    - Other methods are *MRI and CT*.

TABLE 1: Nutritional status based on the WHO and "Asian criteria" values.

Nutritional status	WHO criteria BMI (kg/m^2) cutoff	Asian criteria BMI (kg/m^2) cutoff
Underweight	<18.5	<18.5
Normal	18.5–24.9	18.5–22.9
Overweight	25–29.9	23–24.9
Preobese	-	25–29.9
Obese	≥30	≥30
Obese type 1 (obese)	30–40	30–40
Obese type 2 (morbid obese)	40.1–50	40.1–50
Obese type 3 (super obese)	>50	>50

(BMI: body mass index; WHO: World Health Organization)

Source: Haam JH, Kim BT, Kim EM, Kwon H, Kang JH, Park JH, et al. Diagnosis of obesity: 2022 update of clinical practice guidelines for obesity by the Korean Society for the Study of Obesity. J Obes Metab Syndr. 2023;32(2):121-9.

WHAT ARE THE COMPLICATIONS OF OBESITY IN ELDERLY?

A detailed look at the major complications of obesity is given as follows:

- *Metabolic complications*:
    - *Type 2 diabetes mellitus (T2DM)*: Obesity is a major risk factor for insulin resistance, which can lead to type 2 diabetes.
    - *Dyslipidemia*: Obesity often leads to an abnormal lipid profile, including elevated levels of triglycerides and low-density lipoprotein (LDL) cholesterol and reduced high-density lipoprotein (HDL) cholesterol.
    - *Hypertension*: Excess body weight increases blood volume and resistance in blood vessels, contributing to high blood pressure.
- *Cardiovascular complications*: Coronary artery disease and heart failure risks are increased with obesity.
- *Respiratory complications*: Risk of obstructive sleep apnea and type 2 respiratory failure increases with obesity.
- *Gastrointestinal complications*: Common complications are NAFLD and gastroesophageal reflux disease (GERD).
- *Musculoskeletal complications*: Obesity significantly impacts the musculoskeletal system, leading to various complications that affect mobility, function, and quality of life. Addressing obesity through weight management, physical activity, and dietary changes is crucial for preventing and managing these complications. The common complications include:
    - Osteoarthritis (OA) and degenerative spine disease, osteoporosis, sarcopenia and sarcopenic obesity (SO), and tendinopathy
    - Late-onset rheumatoid arthritis, gout, plantar fasciitis, etc.

Flowchart 2 shows the relation between obesity and its metabolic complications.

WHAT ARE THE MALIGNANCIES THAT ARE COMMON IN AN ELDERLY PATIENT WITH OBESITY?

Obesity is also associated with an increased risk of several types of malignancy. Commonly associated malignancies with obesity are mentioned in **Figure 2**.

Reproductive and Urological Complications

Increased risk of erectile dysfunction due to vascular issues and hormonal changes. Excess weight can weaken pelvic floor muscles and increased risk of urinary incontinence.

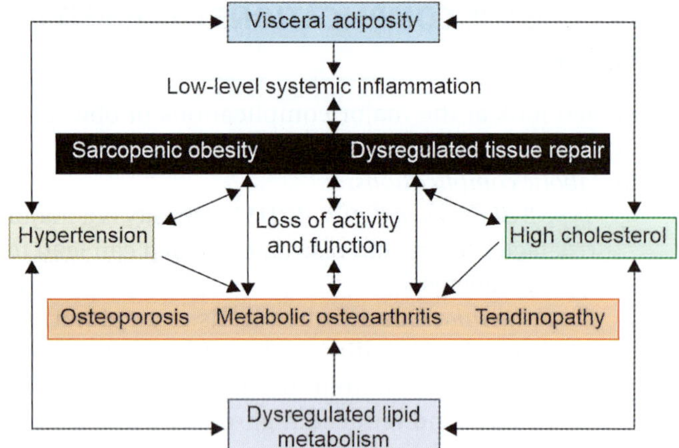

FLOWCHART 2: Obesity and metabolic complications.

Source: Collins KH, Herzog W, MacDonald GZ, Reimer RA, Rios JL, Smith IC, et al. Obesity, metabolic syndrome, and musculoskeletal disease: common inflammatory pathways suggest a central role for loss of muscle integrity. Front Physiol. 2018;9:112.

Psychological Complications

Obesity is linked to higher rates of mental health issues of depression and anxiety.

Geriatric Syndromes

- *Mobility impairment*: Obesity exacerbates mobility issues, leading to decreased independence and increased risk of falls.
- *Cognitive impairment*: Obesity is associated with an increased risk of cognitive decline and dementia.
  Figure 3 summarizes obesity and its complication.

WHAT ARE THE MECHANISM OF MORTALITY IN OBESITY?

Adipose tissue is recognized as a source of inflammatory mediators producing cytokines such as *tumor necrosis*

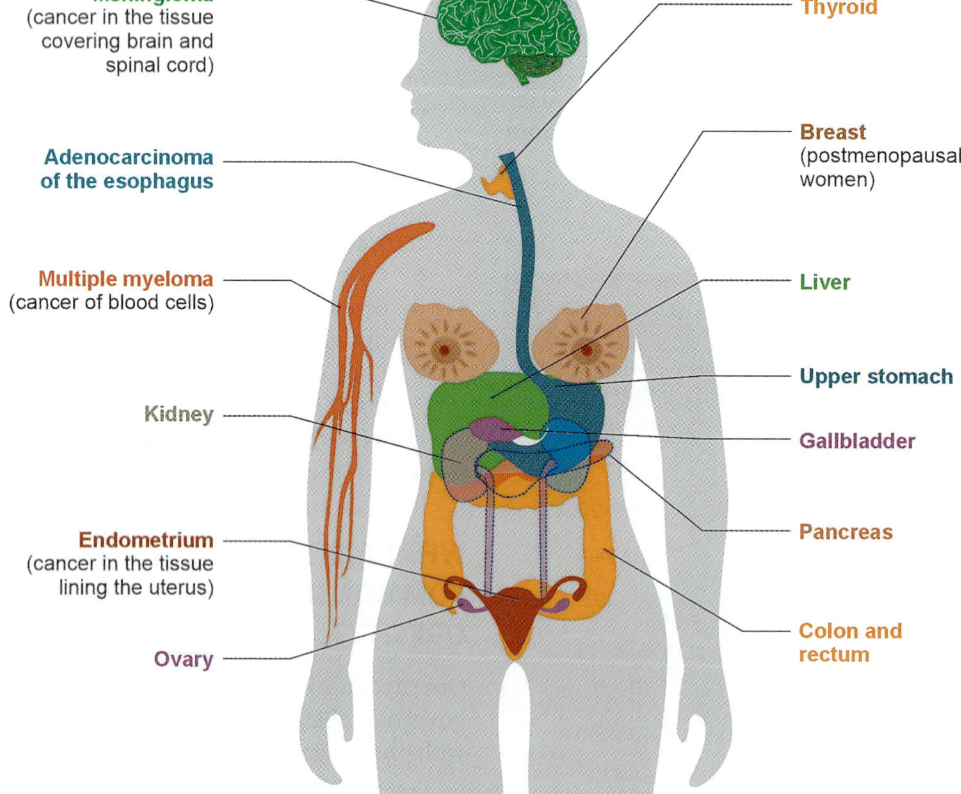

FIG. 2: Common malignancies associated with obesity.

Source: Centers for Disease Control and Prevention. (2025). Obesity and Cancer. [online] Available from https://www.cdc.gov/cancer/risk-factors/obesity.html. [Last accessed May, 2025].

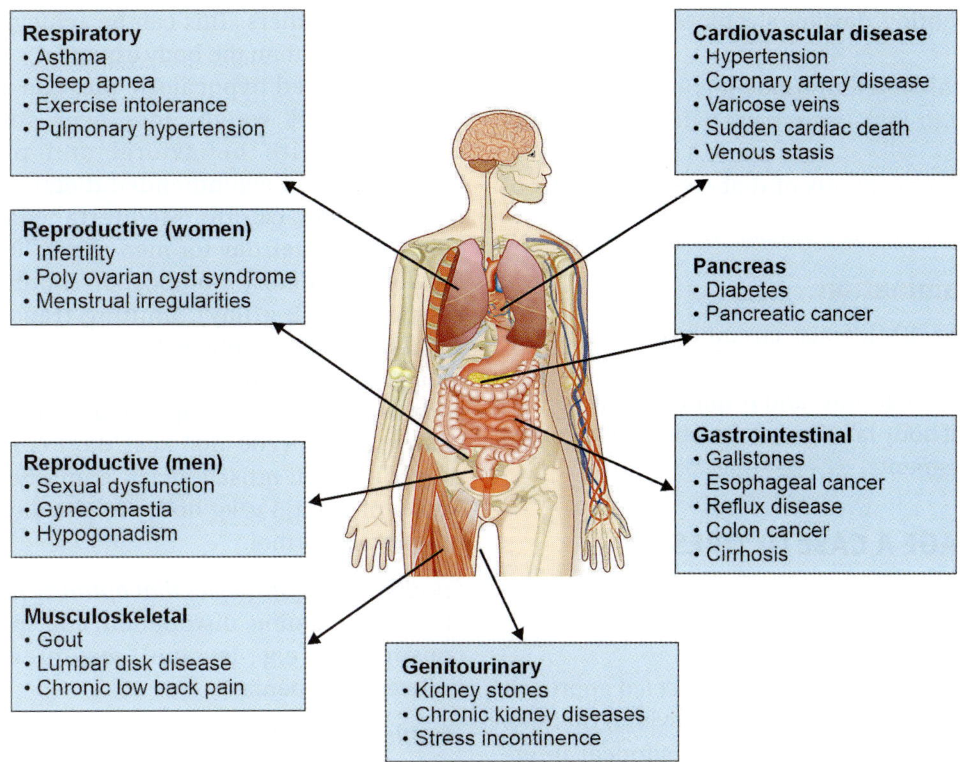

FIG. 3: Schematic diagram of obesity and its complications.

Source: Kumar M, Kaushik D, Kaur J, Proestos C, Oz F, Oz E, et al. A critical review on obesity: herbal approach, bioactive compounds, and their mechanism. Appl Sci. 2022;12(16):8342.

factor-α and interleukin-6. It appears that the relationship between obesity, insulin resistance, and atherosclerosis may depend partially on the increased production and release of these inflammatory mediators from adipose tissue. It is postulated that the visceral fat is most responsible for producing these deleterious cytokines, which in turn lead to diabetes, coronary artery disease, and malignant disease, more commonly seen in older adults. More research is needed to better characterize this new area of study.

Evaluation of a Case of Obesity in Elderly

Taking a comprehensive history is a critical step in evaluating and managing a patient with elderly obesity.

History Taking

- *Demographics*: Age, sex, ethnicity, and occupation
- Age of onset and duration of obesity
- *Treatment history*: History of previous weight loss attempts, including diets, medications, and surgeries. Any ongoing medications that may contribute to weight gain (e.g., corticosteroids, antipsychotics, and antidepressants).
- *Known comorbidities*: T2D, hypertension, dyslipidemia, coronary artery disease, sleep apnea, GERD, and OA
- *Dietary pattern*: Daily intake, meal frequency, snacking habits, and consumption of sugary beverages, or presence of binge eating episodes
- *Physical activity*: Current and past levels of physical activity, including type, frequency, duration, and intensity of exercise
- Barriers to exercise such as physical limitations, lack of time, or lack of access to facilities. Sedentary behavior history in the past
- *Psychosocial history*: History of depression, anxiety, or lack of support from family, friends, and social networks
- *Family history*: Family history of obesity, metabolic disorders, and related conditions such as diabetes, hypertension, and cardiovascular disease
- Overall quality of life

Systemic Complaints

- *Cardiovascular*: Chest pain, palpitations, and shortness of breath

- *Respiratory*: Snoring, daytime sleepiness, and difficulty breathing
- *Gastrointestinal*: Heartburn, bloating, and constipation
- *Musculoskeletal*: Joint pain, back pain, and mobility issues
- *Endocrine*: Complications of diabetes, symptoms of hypothyroidism

Physical Examination

- Weight, height, BMI, waist circumference, and hip circumference
- Blood pressure, heart rate, and respiratory rate
- Distribution of body fat, signs of metabolic syndrome
- Mobility assessment

HOW TO MANAGE A CASE OF OBESITY IN ELDERLY?

Multidimensional Approach

Management of obesity involves a multifaceted approach that includes lifestyle modifications, behavioral therapy, pharmacotherapy, and, in some cases, surgical interventions. A detailed overview of the key components of obesity management is described here.

Lifestyle Modifications

Dietary Changes

Caloric restriction: Reducing caloric intake is an essential process for weight loss in elderly rather than physical activity and others. This can be achieved by consuming fewer calories than the body expends.

A structured hypocaloric diet can achieve approximately 8–10% weight loss over six months when combined with behavioral and physical activity interventions. Recommended dietary patterns include a low-fat, low-calorie, Mediterranean diet, providing 1,500–1,800 kcal/day for men and 1,200–1,500 kcal/day for women. Dietary modification should include sodium restriction (<2 g/day), limiting trans fats and added sugars to <10% of total calories, and portion-controlled meals. In older adults with obesity, particularly those with or at risk for sarcopenic obesity, a less restrictive caloric deficit (200–500 kcal/day) is recommended to prevent loss of muscle mass, combined with a protein intake of 1.0–1.5 g/kg body weight/day, provided renal function is normal.

Specific feeding strategies that optimize protein anabolism: The source, timing, distribution, and specific amino acid constituents (e.g., leucine), may prevent weight-loss-induced sarcopenia.

Healthy eating: Adopting balanced eating patterns, such as the Mediterranean diet, DASH diet, or plant-based diets, which emphasize fruits, vegetables, whole grains, lean proteins, and healthy fats. Learning to manage portion sizes to avoid overeating. Limiting foods high in sugars and unhealthy fats that contribute to excess calorie intake **(Fig. 4)**.

Negative effects of calorie restriction: With calorie restriction, negative effects are also common in elderly such as

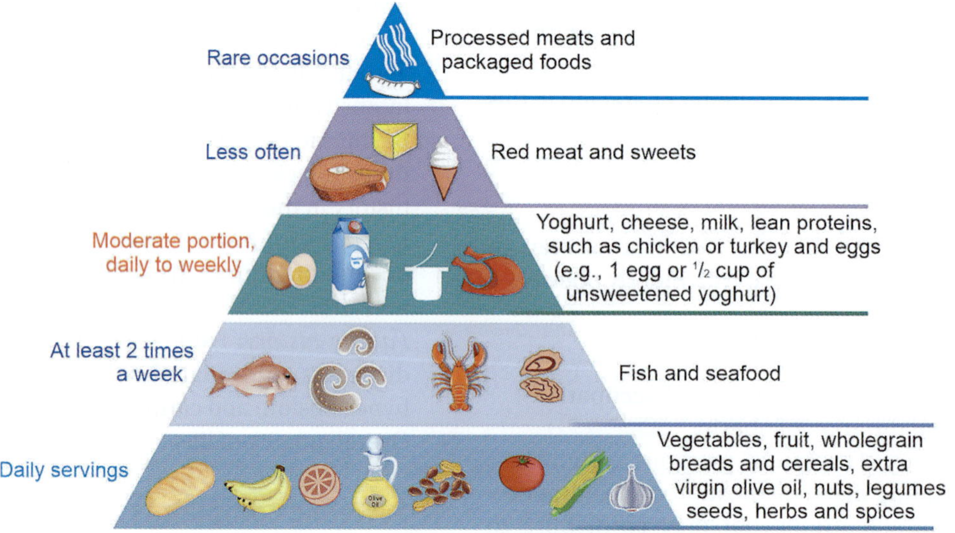

FIG. 4: Mediterranean diet.

Source: Adapted from the Healthy Eating Pyramid by Nutrition Australia (2015).

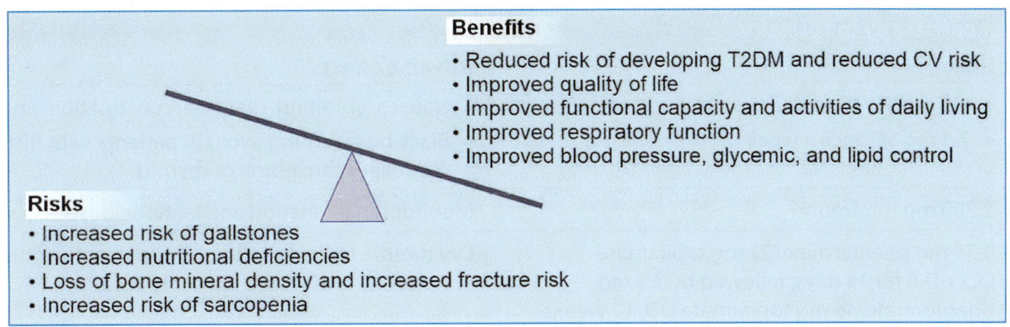

FIG. 5: Risk and benefits of weight loss in elderly.

Source: McKee AM, Morley JE. Obesity in elderly. In: Feingold KR, Ahmed SF, Anawalt B (Eds). Endocrinology. South Dartmouth (MA): MDText.com, Inc.; 2000.

malnutrition and vitamin deficiency, sarcopenia, frailty, depression, fatigue, reduced hormonal levels, reduced immunity, and osteoporosis **(Fig. 5)**.

Physical Activity

- *Regular exercise:* Engaging in at least *150 minutes of moderate-intensity or 75 minutes of high-intensity exercise* per week, including activities such as walking, cycling, swimming, or strength training.
- *Increased daily activity*: Incorporating more physical activity into daily routines, such as taking stairs instead of elevators, walking or biking for short trips, and engaging in active hobbies.

Though an elderly person has more chances of geriatric syndromes such as sarcopenia, frailty, depression, chronic fatigue, reduced hormonal levels, and reduced bone density which causes difficulty in doing physical activity.

Behavioral Therapy

Cognitive behavioral therapy helps individuals identify and change negative thought patterns and behaviors related to food and activity.

WHAT ARE THE PHARMACOTHERAPY AVAILABLE?

- Orlistat reduces fat absorption in the intestines.
- Lorcaserin acts on serotonin receptors to promote satiety.
- *Phentermine-topiramate*: A combination that suppresses appetite and increases feelings of fullness.
- *Naltrexone-bupropion*: A combination that influences appetite and reward pathways in the brain.
- *Liraglutide*: A GLP-1 receptor agonist that helps control blood sugar and appetite **(Table 2)**.

SURGICAL INTERVENTIONS

Bariatric Surgery

For individuals with severe obesity (BMI ≥ 40 kg/m^2 or BMI ≥ 35 kg/m^2 with obesity-related comorbidities) who have not achieved significant weight loss through other methods, bariatric surgery can be an effective option.

Common procedures include:

- *Gastric bypass*: It reduces the size of the stomach and bypasses part of the small intestine, limiting food intake and nutrient absorption.
- *Sleeve gastrectomy*: It removes a portion of the stomach, reducing its size and capacity.
- *Adjustable gastric banding*: It places a band around the upper part of the stomach to create a small pouch that limits food intake.
- *Biliopancreatic diversion with duodenal switch*: It combines stomach reduction with bypassing a significant portion of the small intestine.

Comprehensive Weight Management

Multidisciplinary approach involves a team of healthcare providers, including physicians, dietitians, psychologists, and exercise specialists, to provide comprehensive and coordinated care. Continuous monitoring of progress and regular follow-up visits to adjust the treatment plan as needed and to provide ongoing support and motivation. Personalized treatment plan to address individual health needs and risks associated with obesity.

Public Health and Policy Interventions

Community programs initiatives to promote physical activity and healthy eating in schools, workplaces, and communities.

Flowchart 3 summarizes obesity management algorithm.

TABLE 2: Pharmacotherapy for obesity.

Drugs	Dose	Adverse effects
• Liraglutide • Semaglutide	• 0.6 mg SC OD increase up to 3 mg, once a week • 2.4 mg SC once a week	• Nausea, vomiting, diarrhea, constipation, and hypoglycemia • Black box warning avoid in patients with history of medullary carcinoma of thyroid
Metformin	2,500 mg maximum	Monitor renal function and lactic acidosis
Phentermine–topiramate	3.75 mg phentermine/23 mg topiramate OD 1-0-0 for 14 days, followed by 7.5 mg phentermine/46 mg topiramate OD, 12 weeks	Dry mouth, taste disturbance, and constipation
Bupropion-naltrexone	90 mg/8 mg once daily, titrated up to two tablets twice daily over 4 weeks	• Nausea, constipation, headache, and vomiting • Black box warning for patients with suicidal tendency and uncontrolled HTN
Orlistat	120 mg three times daily with fat-containing meals	Cramps, flatulence, fecal incontinence, and fat-soluble vitamin deficiency
Dapagliflozin	10 mg daily	Increased risk of genitourinary infections, bone fractures, hypersensitivity, and use limited in CKD
Tirzepatide	Start 2.5 mg S/C once weekly; titrate to 5–15 mg weekly as tolerated	Nausea, vomiting, constipation, decreased appetite; rare pancreatitis; Caution in history of medullary thyroid carcinoma or MEN2

(CKD: chronic kidney disease; HTN: hypertension; SC: subcutaneous)

Source: Tchang BG, Aras M, Kumar RB, Aronne LJ. Pharmacological treatment of overweight and obesity. In: Feingold KR, Ahmed SF, Anawalt B (Eds.). South Dartmouth (MA): MDText.com, Inc.; 2000.

WHAT IS SARCOPENIC OBESITY?

Sarcopenic obesity is a condition characterized by the coexistence of sarcopenia (loss of muscle mass and strength) and obesity.

Pathophysiology

Aging is associated with changes in body composition. Percentage of body fat increases until 80 years and then reaches a plateau. The distribution of body fat also changes with age, with reduction in appendicular fat and an increase in trunk fat. Fat also begins to infiltrate nonfatty tissues. Loss of muscle mass is accompanied and often preceded with loss of muscle strength. SO results from the combination of mechanisms that drive both sarcopenia and obesity.

Clinical Features

Increases fat mass and reduce muscle mass, reduce grip strength and functional impairment. The diagnosis of sarcopenic obesity involves assessing both components: obesity assessment by BMI, waist circumference and techniques like DEXA and BIA.

Sarcopenia is assessed using a combination of muscle mass, muscle strength, and physical performance parameters. Muscle mass can be accurately measured by dual-energy X-ray absorptiometry (DEXA), which is the most widely used and validated method in clinical and research settings. Bioelectrical impedance analysis (BIA) provides a simple, portable, and cost-effective alternative for estimating skeletal muscle mass in large populations, while magnetic resonance imaging (MRI) and computed tomography (CT) offer gold-standard assessments of muscle quantity and quality, including fat infiltration and cross-sectional area. Muscle strength is commonly assessed using grip strength dynamometry. Physical performance assessed through tests like gait speed, short physical performance battery (SPPB), timed up and go (TUG) test.

Complications

It includes same as obesity complications such as metabolic disorders, increased risk of cardiovascular disease, with functional decline and increased mortality. A meta-analysis found that sarcopenic obese persons were more than 2.5 times more likely to develop IADL disability compared to persons without SO.

Management

Sarcopenic obesity requires a multifaceted approach that addresses both muscle loss and excess fat: Lifestyle modifications by resistance training and aerobic exercise help reduce fat mass and improve cardiovascular health. Balance and flexibility exercises are important for reducing fall risk and improving functional abilities.

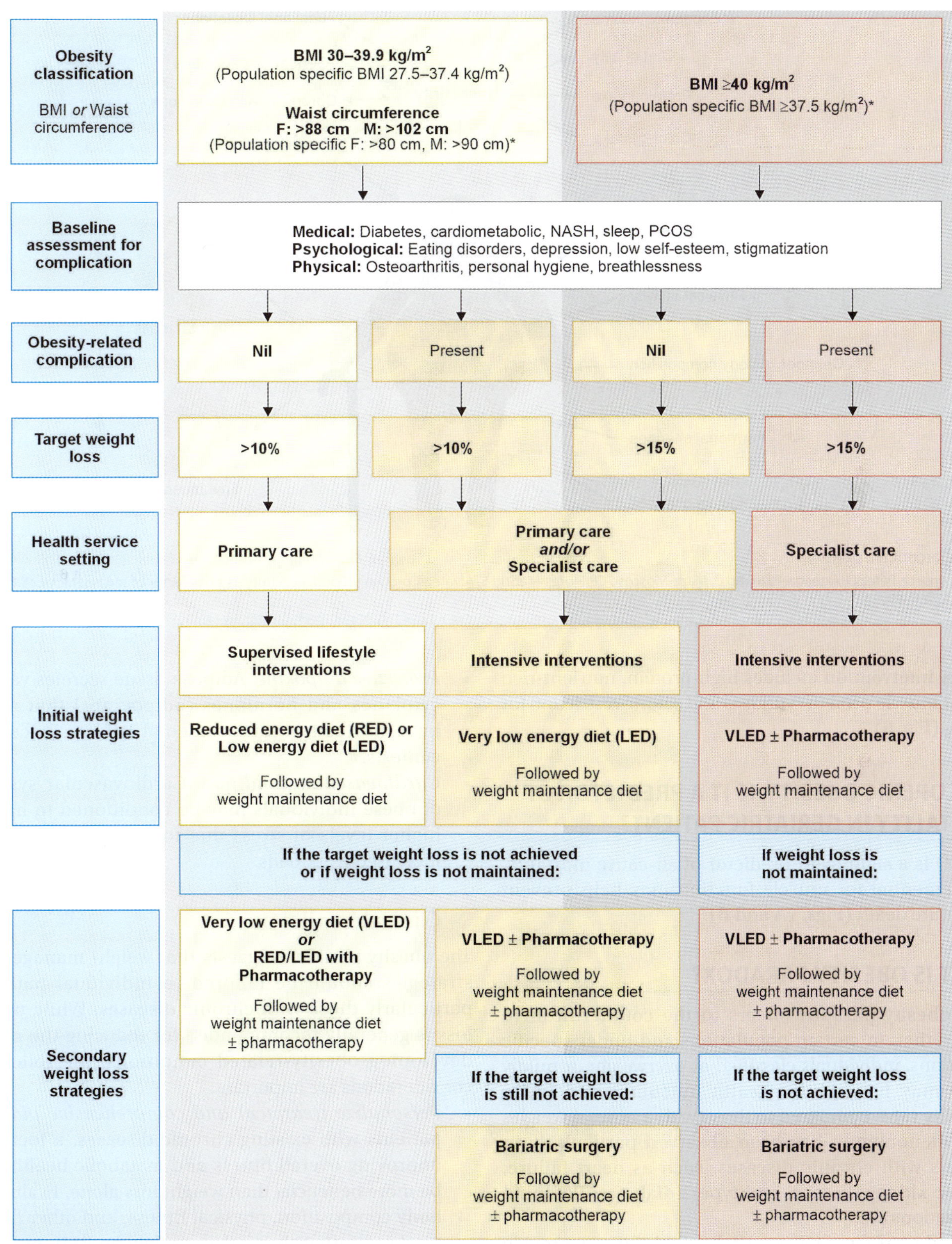

*Cut-offs apply to Asian population and recommended for Australian indigenous population.

FLOWCHART 3: Summary of obesity management.

(PCOS: polycystic ovary syndrome)

Source: Markovic TP, Proietto J, Dixon JB, Rigas G, Deed G, Hamdorf JM, et al. The Australian obesity management algorithm: a simple tool to guide the management of obesity in primary care. Obes Res Clin Pract. 2022;16(5):353-63.

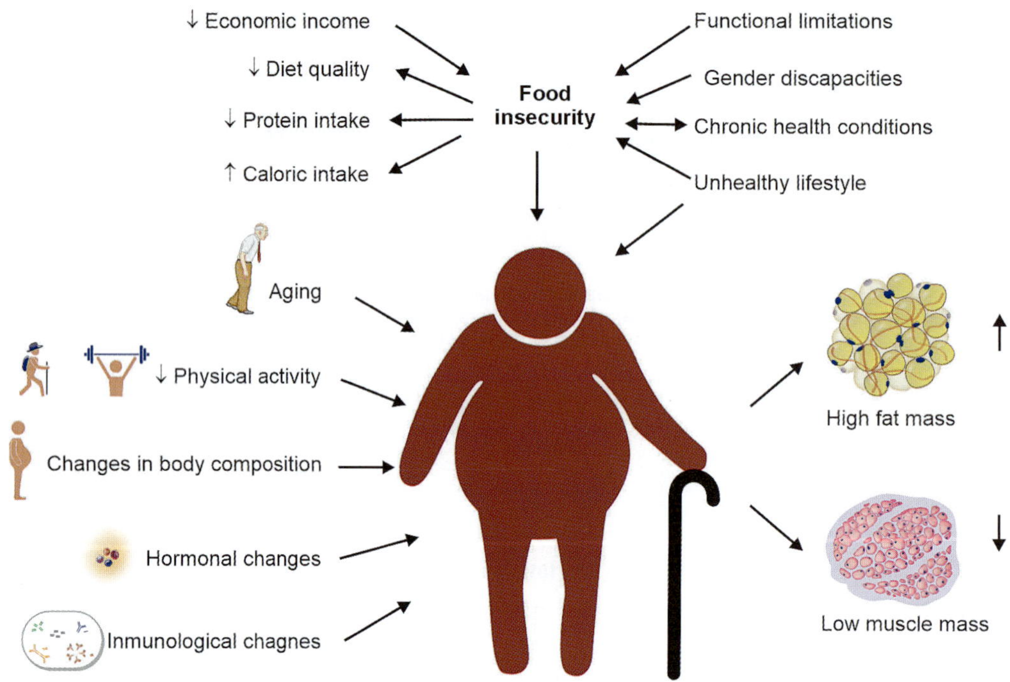

FIG. 6: Sarcopenic obesity.

Source: Fonseca-Pérez D, Arteaga-Pazmiño C, Maza-Moscoso CP, Flores-Madrid S, Álvarez-Córdova L. Food insecurity as a risk factor of sarcopenic obesity. Front Nutr. 2022;9:1040089.

Dietary intervention includes high-protein, nutrient-rich diet for muscle protein synthesis and caloric restriction for fat loss **(Fig. 6)**.

SARCOPENIC OBESITY, IS IT A PREDICTOR OF MORTALITY IN GERIATRIC PATIENT?

Yes, SO is a significant predictor of all-cause mortality, and screening for muscle function may help prevent premature death **(Figs. 7A and B)**.

WHAT IS OBESITY PARADOX?

The "obesity paradox" refers to the counterintuitive finding that, in certain populations and under specific conditions, individuals classified as overweight or mildly obese may have better health outcomes and lower mortality rates compared to those with a normal weight. This phenomenon has been observed particularly in patients with chronic diseases, such as heart failure, chronic kidney disease, and type 2 diabetes. Potential explanations are:

- *Good nutritional reserve*: Higher body fat may provide energy reserves during severe illness, offering a survival advantage.
- *Protective adipokine*: Adipose tissue secretes various cytokines and hormones (adipokines) that might have protective cardiovascular effects in certain contexts.
- *Cardiovascular condition*: Cardiovascular systems of obese individuals may be conditioned to handle higher levels of stress due to chronic exposure to increased workloads.

Clinical Implications

The obesity paradox suggests that weight management strategies should be tailored to individual patients, particularly those with chronic diseases. While weight loss is generally recommended for reducing the risk of developing obesity-related conditions, the following considerations are important:

- *Personalize treatment and comprehensive plan*: In patients with existing chronic diseases, a focus on improving overall fitness and metabolic health may be more beneficial than weight loss alone. Evaluating body composition, physical fitness, and other health markers, rather than relying solely on BMI, provides a more accurate assessment of health risks and benefits.

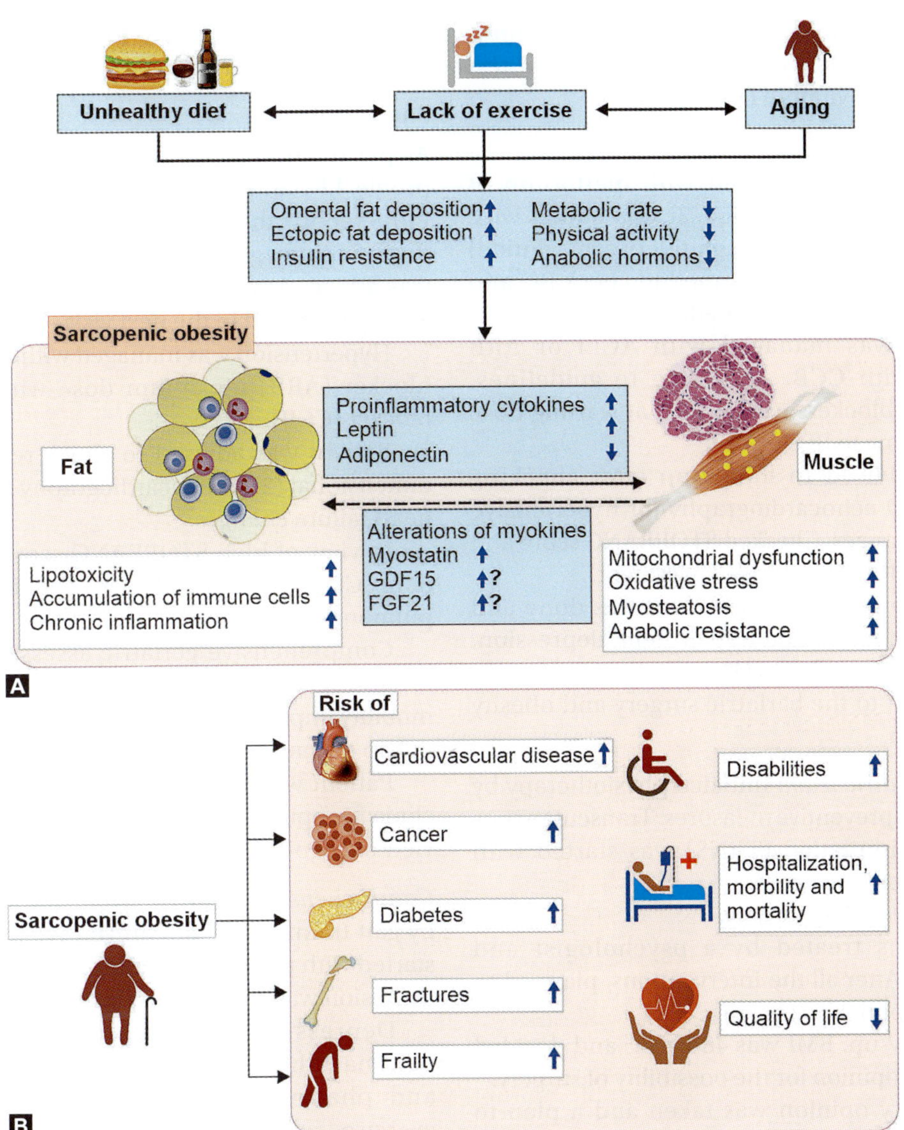

FIGS. 7A AND B: Sarcopenic obesity: A predictor of mortality.

(FGF: fibroblast growth factor; GDF: growth differentiation factor)

Source: Wei S, Nguyen TT, Zhang Y. Ryu D, Gariani K. Sarcopenic obesity: epidemiology, pathophysiology, cardiovascular disease, mortality, and management. Front Endocrinol (Lausanne). 2023;14:1185221.

- *Adequate nutrition*: Ensuring adequate nutrition and preventing unintentional weight loss are critical in managing chronic diseases, as malnutrition can exacerbate health problems.

HOW TO APPROACH A GERIATRIC OBESE PATIENT?

Case Vignette 1

A 65-year-old female patient with a 10-year history of hypertension, diabetic with BMI of 50 kg/m^2 presents to OPD. She has uncontrolled hypertension, diabetes, fatigue, and difficulty in doing daily activities. How to approach this patient?

Intervention

Nonpharmacological

Patient was advised to follow a low salt diabetic diet by a dietitian. Physiotherapy opinion was given with 20 minutes of free hand exercise in the morning and a 20-minute walk in the evening.

Investigations: Complete blood count (CBC), fasting blood sugar (FBS), postprandial blood sugar (PPBS) and glycosylated hemoglobin (HbA1c), urine albumin–

creatinine ratio (ACR), liver function test (LFT), kidney function test (KFT), lipid profile, thyroid function test (TFT), iron profile, and vitamin D.

Pharmacological

According to reports, maximized with metformin at a tolerated dose of 2 g/day. SGLT-2i was added with metformin. Also, GLP-1 analog (liraglutide or semaglutide) was added at the initial dose. Planned to check BG and start insulin in a further visit if needed.

Hypertension was managed with ACEI or ARB maximum dose with CCB. According to guidelines, diuretics and beta-blockers were added at starting dose and titrated according to BP.

Patient was advised to follow-up after checking retinopathy and 2D echocardiography for hypertensive and heart failure changes. Checked STOPBANG score and sleep study done. CPAP was advised overnight.

Comprehensive geriatric assessment was done and found a high risk of fall, vision impairment, depression, and mobility impairment due to OA.

Patient was sent to the bariatric surgery and obesity clinic for an opinion.

Comprehensive geriatric team: Initiated physiotherapy by gait training and fall preventive measures. Transcutaneous electrical nerve stimulation (TENS) was started with pharmacotherapy for OA knee.

Vision was corrected by surgery.

Depression was treated by a psychologist and pharmacotherapy. After all the interventions, planned to follow-up after 3 months.

Again, on follow-up, BMI was 48 kg/m^2 and decided to bariatric surgery opinion for the possibility of surgery.

Bariatric surgery opinion was taken and a plan to sleeve gastrectomy after preanesthetic clearance, and all medications were adjusted.

After 3 monthly follow-up, patient had weight reduction of 20% and improvement of diabetic status and controlled hypertension and other complications.

Case Vignette 2

A 75-year-old female patient with a 10-year history of hypertension, diabetic with BMI of 35 kg/m^2 presents to OPD. She complains of fatigue, weakness, and history of fall four times in last 2 months. She also had a fear of fall, causing an inability to do daily basic activities. How to approach this patient?

Intervention

Nonpharmacological

Patient was advised to follow a low-salt diabetic diet by the dietitian.

Investigations: CBC, FBS, PPBS, and HbA1c, Urine ACR, LFT, KFT, lipid profile, TFT, iron profile, and vitamin D.

Pharmacological

As per reports, the patient had normal Hb, normal iron profile, LFT and KFT were also normal. According to FBS, PPBS reports that metformin was maximized at tolerated dose. Sodium–glucose cotransporter-2 inhibitor (SGLT2i) was added. Advised to follow-up and plan to add GLP-1 analog if needed in the next visit.

Hypertension was managed with angiotensin receptor blocker (ARB) maximum dose with calcium channel blocker (CCB).

Patient was advised to check retinopathy and two-dimensional (2D) echocardiography for hypertensive and heart failure changes.

In view of high STOPBANG score, a sleep study was done. CPAP was advised overnight after discussion with a pulmonologist.

Comprehensive geriatric assessment was done and found high risk of fall, vision impairment, depression, mobility impairment due to neuropathy, and forgetfulness due to degenerative and vascular causes.

Patient was sent to the bariatric surgery and obesity clinic for opinion, advised to do medical management in view of cognitive impairment and less life expectancy.

Comprehensive geriatric team: Initiated physiotherapy by gait training and fall preventive measures. TENS was started with pharmacotherapy for OA knee.

Vision was corrected by surgery.

Depression was treated by a psychologist and pharmacotherapy. Forgetfulness details were assessed and pharmacotherapy was added with cognitive exercise.

Nerve conduction velocity (NCV) was done, and suggestive of diabetic sensory neuropathy and pharmacotherapy was prescribed.

She was advised to follow-up after 4 weeks.

She persistently had fear of fall and weakness, so sarcopenia SARC-F screening tool was found to be positive.

Physiotherapy team was again approached to do resistant exercise. DEXA scan was done suggestive of severe osteoporosis. It was managed with calcium, monthly vitamin D, and bisphosphonate therapy. A high-protein diet was given after consulting with a dietitian. Advised to follow-up after 8 weeks.

On follow-up, 5% weight loss, power improved, and able to walk without fear.

After 3 monthly follow-up, patient had weight reduction of 10% and improvement of diabetic status and controlled hypertension and other complications.

RESEARCH IN ELDERLY OBESITY

Research in the elderly is scant. There is no clear BMI target in this age group. With aging, there is a reduction in muscle mass, height loss, and an increase in abdominal obesity, none of which are accounted for in the BMI. The main goal in older adults with obesity is to improve physical function and minimize the impact of obesity-related complications.

In individuals with BMI 30–40 kg/m^2 and BMI ≥40 kg/m^2 without complications, the aims of treatment are to maintain health and physical function, prevent weight gain, and generate a more moderate intentional weight loss. In individuals with a BMI ≥ 40 kg/m^2 with obesity-related complications, more intensive therapies are indicated, but maintaining physical function, favorable body composition, and quality nutrition may require specific lifestyle programs. When engaging older adults in intensive therapies, cardiovascular fitness should be considered.

CONCLUSION

The landscape of the population is certainly changing and is marked by two significant trends: (1) An increasingly elderly population and (2) an ongoing obesity epidemic. This will undoubtedly impact families, social structures, and healthcare costs. Physicians will need to balance the complications of obesity to decide on the best patient-centered approach. Effective management requires a comprehensive, individualized approach that incorporates lifestyle changes, behavioral therapy, medical treatment, and possibly surgical intervention. A supportive environment and multidisciplinary care are essential to achieving and maintaining weight loss and improving overall health outcomes.

Self-Assessment Questionnaire

Q1. What are the significant age-related changes in body composition that contribute to obesity in older adults?

Q2. How does adipose tissue function as an endocrine organ, and what are the metabolic consequences of its dysregulation?

Q3. What is the relationship between obesity and metabolic syndrome in elderly individuals?

Q4. Define sarcopenic obesity, and its impact on mortality in older adults?

Q5. How to manage obesity in the elderly?

Q6. Describe how calorie restriction should be modified in older adults to prevent adverse effects such as sarcopenia or frailty.

Q7. What are the standard pharmacological options for obesity management, and which precautions are necessary in elderly patients?

FURTHER READINGS

1. Halter JB, Ouslander JG, Studenski S, High KP, Asthana S, Supiano MA, et al, editors. Hazzard's Geriatric Medicine and Gerontology. 7th ed. New York: McGraw-Hill Education; 2017. Available from https://accessmedicine.mhmedical.com/content.aspx?bookid=1923§ionid=143987228
2. Jameson JL, Fauci AS, Kasper DL, Hauser SL, Longo DL, Loscalzo J, editors. Harrison's Principles of Internal Medicine. 21st ed. New York: McGraw Hill; 2022.
3. Michel JP, Beattie BL, Martin FC, Walston J, editors. Oxford Textbook of Geriatric Medicine. 3rd ed. Oxford: Oxford University Press; 2017.
4. McKee AM, Morley JE. Obesity in elderly endocrinology. In: Feingold KR, Ahmed SF, Anawalt B (Eds). South Dartmouth (MA): MDText.com, Inc.; 2000.
5. Australian Diabetes Society. (2024). Australian obesity management algorithm. [online] Available from https://www.diabetessociety.com.au/guideline/obesity/. [Last accessed May, 2025].
6. Samper-Ternent R, Al Snih S. Obesity in older adults: epidemiology and implications for disability and disease. Rev Clin Gerontol. 2012;22(1):10-34.
7. Jin X, Qiu T, Li L, Yu R, Chen X, Li C, et al. Pathophysiology of obesity and its associated diseases. Acta Pharm Sin B. 2023;13(6):2403-24.
8. Fonseca-Pérez D, Arteaga-Pazmiño C, Maza-Moscoso CP, Flores-Madrid S, Álvarez-Córdova L. Food insecurity as a risk factor of sarcopenic obesity. Front Nutr. 2022;9:1040089.
9. Collins KH, Herzog W, MacDonald GZ, Reimer RA, Rios JL, Smith IC, et al. Obesity, metabolic syndrome, and musculoskeletal disease: common inflammatory pathways suggest a central role for loss of muscle integrity. Front Physiol. 2018;9:112.
10. Wei S, Nguyen TT, Zhang Y. Ryu D, Gariani K. Sarcopenic obesity: epidemiology, pathophysiology, cardiovascular disease, mortality, and management. Front Endocrinol (Lausanne). 2023;14:1185221.

CHAPTER 27

Mobility Issue

Ruchika Madan, Anoop Aggarwal

CASE VIGNETTE

Personal information: Mr Rakesh Kumar, a 67-year-old male, autorickshaw driver.

Medical history: Type 2 diabetes, hypertension, mild arthritis in both knees, recent history of a minor stroke (6 months ago), and right middle cerebral artery (MCA) infarct.

Social history: Lives with wife, two daughters, and one son, uses public transport, previously active but now experiencing decreased mobility.

Presenting complaint: Mr Rakesh Kumar reports increasing difficulty walking, particularly after his stroke. He notes weakness on his left side and joint pain in his knees, which worsens after activity. He also had a few falls recently due to balance issues, making him anxious about moving around.

Assessment

- *Physical examination*:
  - *Muscle strength*: Reduced on the left side
  - *Joint pain*: Worse in the knees
  - *Range of motion*: Limited knee flexibility, slight stiffness in hip joints
  - *Balance and gait*: Unsteady gait, with a tendency to lean left; requires support when walking
- *Functional assessment*:
  - *Activities of daily living (ADLs)*: Struggles with standing up from a seated position, dressing, and walking for >5 minutes
  - *Fall risk assessment*: High risk of falls due to balance issues and previous falls
  - *Berg Balance score*: 37/56
  - *Mobility aids*: None currently used, although a walker or cane may be beneficial
- *Psychological assessment*:
  - Reports feeling anxious about walking alone
  - Has expressed fear of falling again, affecting his confidence and motivation to stay active

Diagnosis

- Poststroke hemiparesis (mild left-sided weakness)
- Osteoarthritis in both knees
- Fall risk due to unsteady gait and balance issues

Intervention Plan

- *Physiotherapy: Short-term goals (0–3 months)*
- *Pain reduction and management*:
  - *Goal*: Decrease knee pain and joint stiffness through targeted stretching and strengthening exercises
  - Electrotherapy modalities such as interferential therapy (IFT) over both knees for pain relief
  - *Measurement*: Reduced pain scores on a standardized pain scale (e.g., Numeric Pain Rating Scale 0–10) after physiotherapy sessions
  - *Expected outcome*: Patient reports at least a 30–40% reduction in pain by the end of 1 month
- *Improved balance and stability*:
  - *Goal*: Enhance stability and reduce risk of fall by working on balance exercises, weight shifting, and functional movement training
- *Increased lower limb strength*:
  - *Goal*: Strengthen muscles around the knees, hips, and lower legs to support joint function and gait stability

  - *Expected outcome*: Patient achieves at least a grade 4 muscle strength rating in lower limb muscles (e.g., quadriceps, hamstrings).
- *Safe use of mobility aids*:
  - *Goal*: Teach Mr Rakesh to safely and confidently use a walker to improve his independence and reduce anxiety about falls
  - *Measurement*: Observational assessment of gait and use of the walker, with minimal need for corrections
  - *Expected outcome*: Patient can walk with a walker safely, showing decreased reliance on therapist support.

Long-term Goals (3–12 Months)

- *Enhanced functional mobility and independence*: Enable Mr Rakesh to perform ADLs independently, such as standing up from a seated position, dressing, and walking longer distances
- *Gait improvement and balance recovery*: Achieve a more stable, symmetrical gait pattern with reduced unsteadiness and improved coordination on the left side
- *Increased physical activity tolerance*:
  - *Goal*: Build endurance to increase physical activity tolerance, allowing Mr Rakesh to walk for at least 15–20 minutes continuously with minimal fatigue
  - *Measurement*: Distance walked during the 6-minute walk test (6MWT)
- *Fall prevention and confidence in mobility*:
  - *Goal*: Increase confidence and reduce fear of falling through fall prevention training and progressive balance exercises
  - *Measurement*: Self-reported confidence level and anxiety reduction, assessed with tools such as the Falls Efficacy Scale (FES)
  - Functional training to practice ADLs and build confidence in movement
- *Occupational therapy*: Strategies for safe mobility within the home, such as improving room layout, adding grab bars, and using nonslip mats

INTRODUCTION

Advances in medical technology have led to an increase in life expectancy. It is projected that in 2050, about 25.1% of the total population will be over 65 years old. As the aging population is increasing worldwide, the concept of healthy aging should become an integral part of every individual's life. Mobility is fundamental to active and healthy aging and is directly linked to health status and quality of life.

The prevalence of mobility impairments among elders is significant and increases with age. According to research studies and surveys, around 35% of adults aged 65 years and older in the United States report mobility limitations. Among individuals aged 85 years and older, the prevalence of mobility impairments rises to approxiately 50%. Early identification and focused preventive strategic management of mobility-related issues are important to reduce the prevalence of disability in the elderly.

MOBILITY AND ITS IMPORTANCE

The capacity to move oneself (e.g., by walking, using assistive technology, or using transportation) throughout community contexts that extend from one's house to one's neighborhood and to areas beyond is known as mobility. Mobility is considered to be an essential key to quality of life (QOL), improved mental health, heart health, resistance to injury, and better confidence.

There are several factors that contribute to mobility impairment among elders **(Box 1)** and subsequent

BOX 1 **Risk factors for mobility impairment among elders.**

- Age-related physiological changes
- Sedentary behavior
- Age-related changes such as decreased muscle strength, reduced joint flexibility, and impaired balance
- Chronic health conditions such as stroke, Parkinson's disease, arthritic conditions, neurological conditions, and hip fractures
- Impact of chronic conditions such as difficulties with movement and navigating stairs
- Restricted or limited walking
- Obesity
- Cardiovascular disease, poor pulmonary reserves, and reduced vision
- Depression
- Advanced age
- Female gender
- Poor nutritional status
- Psychological fear of movement
- Fear of falling
- Limitations in activities of daily living (ADLs): ADLs and instrumental ADLs (IADLs)
- Slow gait speed
- Polypharmacy
- Painful joints
- Poor static and/or dynamic balance
- Decreased muscle strength
- Environmental barriers
- Inaccessible transportation difficulties

physical deconditioning, which has a huge impact on the functioning of physiological system reserves in older adults over the years. Potential deconditioning factors included frequent sleep disruption, frightening sounds, painful stimuli, mobility restrictions, and poor nutrition.

AGE-RELATED PHYSIOLOGICAL CHANGES IN ELDERLY

Age-related Changes in Muscle Mass, Strength, and Power

- *Muscle mass*: Muscle performance is linked to muscle mass, muscle strength, and muscle power which declines with age.
- *Muscle strength*: It is the ability to generate maximal muscle force, whereas muscle power refers to the product of force and velocity of the muscle contraction. The earliest such sign may include a decline in chair rise or stair-climbing performance.

Age-related Neuromuscular Changes Associated with Mobility

Some common changes observed in the neuromuscular system of body with aging include change in muscle fiber sizes, reduction in fast-twitch fibers, motor unit (MU) hypofunctioning-related sarcopenia, and a greater variability in MU discharge causing the reduction in isometric muscle strength; reduced neural activation of skeletal muscle is a key component for muscle weakness causing sarcopenia.

Age-related Physical Changes Associated with Mobility

Postural control includes two domains: (1) Static, and (2) dynamic components. In the static component, the center of mass remains between the base of support, whereas in dynamic component, the center of mass as well as the base of support shifts. Both types of balance are influenced by the visual, sensory, and vestibular systems, and, therefore, any decline in the visual, sensory, or vestibular system functioning may have an adverse effect on the static and dynamic balance abilities. Age-related declines in the functioning of the sensory system, especially for vision and hearing, cause balance impairments and compromise mobility and quality of life in older persons.

Gait Changes with Aging

Gait is a highly complex process that is influenced by the central/peripheral nervous system, muscular skeletal changes, and brain changes. The temporal or spatial gait changes occur with aging in the form of reduced step length and step time as well as increase in stance. Changes in gait parameters are also considered as an indicator for impaired physical function, as a predictor for falls, and even mortality.

Slow gait speed has 89% chance of increased risk of mortality. With aging, fast gait speed seems to decline earlier than normal walking speed. Fast gait speed (which is needed to catch a train/bus or to cross safely at the green signal lights) is needed in daily life.

Age-related Changes in Cognition Associated with Mobility

Processing speed is an important element for mobility, as the information from sensory input needs to be processed before the motor control system can adequately start. Apart from processing speed, attention, executive functions, and memory abilities also decline with advancing age. Executive functioning is vital to allow an older person to successfully engage in independent, appropriate, and goal-oriented behavior such as problem-solving abilities, planning, and organizing actions; such actions are cognitive elementary abilities with regard to mobility.

Sedentary Lifestyle

A sedentary way of living is "any waking activity characterized by an energy expenditure = 1.5 metabolic equivalents while being in a sitting, reclining, or lying posture" is the definition of sedentary behavior. Elevated levels of sedentary behavior have been linked to reduced motor system response to movement, weariness, and sleep deficit in addition to limitations in mobility. A lack of physical activity may give rise to weak muscles and poor balance, which may increase the risk of fractures and falls; increased risk of dementia in older persons; and cognitive decline and chronic diseases such as diabetes, heart disease, and stroke.

Nutritional Status

Nutritional status is a factor that is independently and favorably linked with mobility impairment and disability. Older adults who are obese or low weight have an increased chance of having mobility issues. Individuals who are underweight and malnourished have severe mobility impairments.

Mobility and Chronic Diseases

Literature has proved a significant association between chronic diseases and mobility limitations. Mobility limitation as defined by a walking speed of 0.8 m/s has been significantly associated with neurological diseases such as dementia or mild cognitive impairments.

Psychological Risk Factors for Mobility Limitation

Presence of depressive symptoms predicts an increased mobility limitations and functional impairment. Approximately 55% of older people have fall-related psychological concerns, with women experiencing this concern more frequently than men. As a consequence, they engage in fewer physical activities to prevent falls or because they feel embarrassed to ask for assistance in overcoming obstacles in their immediate surroundings, which causes their mobility to rapidly decline. Environmental barriers to mobility are another complex risk factor.

ADVERSE IMPACT OF MOBILITY IMPAIRMENTS

Immobility can impact multiple systems of the body which can be detrimental to older adult health.

- *Cardiovascular system deconditioning*: About 3 weeks of bed rest can lead to cardiovascular system deconditioning similar to that of 40 years of age. This is due to the structural changes that are undergone during stages of immobility, such as the reduction of venous return, increased heart rate, and cardiovascular deconditioning.
- *Respiratory system*: Changes in lung volumes and respiratory system difficulties may be caused by immobility. An extended period spent in the supine posture might impair ribcage movement, diminish lung volume, and even result in lung collapse.
- *Musculoskeletal deconditioning*: Immobility also leads to musculoskeletal deconditioning and contractures, resulting in a decline in physical health with associated sarcopenia, muscle weakness, and joint stiffness, further resulting in functional decline.
- *Vascular system*: Reduced mobility and medicine or illness-related dehydration result in fluid and electrolyte imbalance, increased blood viscosity, which increases the risk of deep vein thrombosis/pulmonary embolism (DVT/PE) development, constipation, urinary tract stasis, and infection.
- *Social isolation*: Reduced self-esteem, deconditioning, increased weariness, and confidence loss can all result from immobility. This can worsen their quality of life by raising their risk of falls, fractures, head injuries, and other major consequences; it can also reduce their independence in doing basic and instrumental activities of daily living (BADLs and IADLs), and it can lead to the formation of pressure ulcers.
- *Psychological impact*: Social isolation and challenge to participate in social activities, leading to feelings of loneliness and isolation. These problems combined with progressive mental health issues of depression, anxiety, and other psychological issues lead to a rapid decline in further health, seeking frequent medical visits, rehabilitation services, and assistance with activities of daily living, leading to higher healthcare costs and utilization. It may also lead to a higher risk of frequent and prolonged institutionalization.

ASSESSMENT OF MOBILITY IMPAIRMENTS IN ELDERS

Assessing and recognizing the existing mobility impairment among older adults is a crucial aspect of geriatric care as it helps to identify the extent of limitations.

The comprehensive and appropriate assessment typically involves a combination of clinical evaluations, medical report parameters, scores of subjective and objective functional tests, and self-reported measures. It also involves the carefully crafted and progressed questioning of the patients and their caregivers to understand the extent of mobility impairment in their home environment, community-dwelling challenges, extent of psychological impact, and cognitive influence. The appropriate assessment helps to set the baseline for planning the appropriate interventions and designing targeted interventions to improve mobility, progress tracking, patient inspiration, and enhanced interaction between the therapist and caregivers as well as the patient. It is crucial to regularly reevaluate and adjust care plans as necessary.

Box 2 summarizes the key components for the assessment of mobility impairment among elders.

During mobility impairment, the geriatric person is not to be considered in isolated context but should also considered with involvement of the environment and family members into the assessment and treatment procedure.

CHALLENGES RELATED TO THE MANAGEMENT OF MOBILITY IMPAIRMENT AMONG ELDERS

Managing mobility impairment in the elderly requires a multifaceted approach that considers medical, social, financial, and systemic factors. A multidisciplinary team, including physicians, physiotherapists, social workers, occupational therapists, and nutritionists, is essential for effective care. Polypharmacy, a common issue in the

BOX 2 Key components for assessment of mobility impairment among elders.

- *Current and past medical history*: Review of past and current medical conditions, medications, surgeries, and lifestyle factors that might affect mobility
- *Physical examination*: Assessment of strength (of key muscles of body, grip strength, knee and hip muscle strength, ankle muscle strength), balance, joint pain and joint malalignments, coordination, and range of motion. This includes checking for any pain, swelling, or deformities in joints and muscles
- *Functional assessment of basic activities of daily living (ADLs)*: Evaluation of basic self-care tasks such as bathing, dressing, eating, and toileting. It should also evaluate mobility in bed, ability to rise to a sitting position, ability to transfer from bed to chair and in and out of a bathtub, balance, ambulation, and gait
- *Functional assessment of instrumental activities of daily living (IADLs)*: Assessment of more complex activities necessary for independent living, such as managing finances, transportation, shopping, telephonic communication, device operating, and meal preparation
- *Gait speed test*: Evaluates walking speed over a short distance, typically 4 m. Slow gait speed is a strong predictor of future mobility issues. Gait symmetry, gait endurance, adaptability of gait, dual-task performance during gait, and self-reported confidence during gait are also evaluated
- *Mobility test*: Disability in the mobility domain results in both decreased independence and lower levels of life satisfaction. It includes timed up and go (TUG) test, 5 times sit-to-stand (5TSTS) test, backward walking (BW), and Short Physical Performance Battery (SPPB):
  - *TUG test*: TUG assesses functional mobility and fall risk in older adults. The patient starts in a seated position and stands up upon the therapist's command, walks 3 m, turns around, walks back to the chair, and sits down. The time stops when the patient is seated. In a prospective study conducted by Alexandre et al., a time of > 12.47 seconds on the TUG was found to be predictive of falls in community-dwelling older adults
  - *The 5TSTS test* requires patients to stand up from a chair five times as quickly as possible without the use of hand support. The time to complete the task is recorded in seconds, which can then be used to predict future mobility disability and disability in ADLs and IADLs in older adults. Regarding outcomes, results indicate that a time to complete of >13.7 seconds is predictive of future mobility disability
  - *BW* has been proposed as an additional measurement for assessing mobility in older adults. A study by Fritz et al. observed BW speed to be a more accurate identifier of fallers than forward walking speed in older individuals. Results from this study suggest that a BW speed of <0.6 m/s is indicative of fall risk in this population
  - *The SPPB* is a valid, reliable, and responsive measure of physical function and mobility in community-dwelling older adults. The measure is comprised of a self-selected walking speed test, a hierarchical balance test (feet side by side, semitandem stance, then tandem stance), and a 5TSTS test. Each of the included tests is scored on a 0–4 scale, making 12 the maximum possible total score. Low scores on the SPPB are predictive of mobility disability
- *Balance*: Berg Balance Scale (BBS), Performance-Oriented Mobility Assessment, Dynamic Gait Index, and Falls Efficacy Scale International are commonly used measures to test balance in geriatric population
- *6-minute walk test (6MWT)*: Measures the distance walked in 6 minutes to evaluate endurance and aerobic capacity
- *Assessment of cognitive function*: Tests such as the Mini–Mental State Examination (MMSE) or the Montreal Cognitive Assessment (MoCA) can identify cognitive impairments that may affect mobility
- *Assessment of depression and anxiety*: Psychological factors can significantly impact mobility. Screening tools such as the Geriatric Depression Scale (GDS) can be used
- *Evaluation of home environment*: Assessment of the living space for hazards that could contribute to falls or impede mobility, such as poor lighting, loose rugs, slippery floor, inappropriate working/toileting station, or narrow/high/twisted stairs without handrails
- *Social support*: Evaluation of the support system available to the elder, including family, friends, and community resources; accessible support during need and emergency
- *Evaluation of currently used assistive devices (if any)*: Assessment of the appropriateness (stability, height, weight-bearing portions, sharp edges) and condition of any mobility aids currently used (e.g., canes, walkers, wheelchairs)
- *Recommendation for appropriate new assistive devices*: Based on the assessment, recommendations for new or additional assistive devices might be made. A walking frame with sitting surface may be recommended for a person who gets frequent fatigue while walking; a walker with rolling wheels and a braking system may be recommended for person having difficulty in lifting and progressing the walker forward during ambulation, etc
- *Cardiovascular limitations* as related to immobility must be considered within practical existing limitations
- *The role of pulmonary limitation* on the mobility status must be considered too
- The nutritional status, dehydration, fluid and electrolyte imbalance, increased blood viscosity, risk of DVT/PE, constipation, urinary tract infection, incontinence, etc., may also lead to impaired mobility

(DVT: deep vein thrombosis; PE: pulmonary embolism)

elderly, can lead to adverse drug interactions and side effects. Therefore, careful medication management is crucial, with communication between team members, particularly nurses and physiotherapists, being vital to identify and address potential issues. Chronic pain, another frequent problem, can significantly impact mobility. Physiotherapists play a crucial role in pain management and rehabilitation, utilizing various modalities such as thermal agents, ultrasound, and manual therapies. Early mobilization is key to reducing complications associated with immobility, leading to shorter hospital stays and improved patient outcomes. Educating caregivers and the community on mobility aids, fall prevention strategies, and creating a safe environment for elders with mobility impairments are also essential.

MANAGEMENT OF MOBILITY IMPAIRMENT AMONG ELDERS

Fortunately, there are interventions and support systems available to help improve mobility and maintain independence for elders with mobility impairments. These may include physical therapy, assistive devices such as canes or walkers, home modifications for accessibility, and caregiver assistance when needed.

Studies have shown that regular exercise improves mobility. Exercise can readjust activities from a biomechanical perspective and the body's muscular strength to ensure safe movement and function in the elderly.

Exercises can effectively prevent chronic noncommunicable diseases such as diabetes, cardiovascular disease, and dementia. The World Health Organization (WHO) has defined physical activity as "any bodily movement produced by skeletal muscles that requires energy expenditure." It improves both cognitive health and physical mobility, intrinsic functions that are essential for functional ability and robust indicators of overall health.

Current guidelines stress the importance of multimodal exercise for elderly, including strengthening exercises, cardiovascular, flexibility, and balance training. The resistance training is required to be progressive in nature (progressive resistance training), defined as involving an increase in load across the training period. Aerobic training could include any exercise involving movement of large muscle groups for a period of time, including walking, cycling, and rowing. Balance/stability training includes any training that sought increases in the subject's ability to maintain balance in the face of a threat to stability and may have included specific balance exercises. The three modes of training need to be conducted concurrently.

Assessment of Mobility Impairment Among Elders

Based on available published evidence and published literature, the following aspects are important for the rehabilitation of mobility impairment among elders. To manage mobility impairments in the elderly, a comprehensive approach involving assessment, individualized exercise programs, and environmental modifications is crucial:

- *Assessment and goal setting*: A healthcare professional conducts a thorough evaluation to determine the extent of impairment and establish personalized mobility goals. This helps frame short-term and long-term rehabilitation objectives.
- *Individualized exercise programs*: Customized exercise plans are designed to improve strength, flexibility, and endurance. These programs target specific areas such as legs, shoulders, core, and upper body, considering individual abilities and limitations. Gradual progression is implemented based on the elder's capacity and response.
- Skills, knowledge, and experience of physiotherapists play the most crucial role to design an effective, safe, and feasible individual-specific person exercise protocol.
- *Balance and coordination training*: Exercises that enhance balance and coordination increase safety and confidence in daily tasks. Progressive balance training includes activities such as standing on one leg, walking heel-to-toe, and using balance boards. The program also incorporates functional tasks that challenge balance, such as stepping over obstacles or walking on uneven surfaces.
- *Environmental modifications*: Removing environmental hazards such as loose rugs, cluttered walkways, and inadequate lighting is essential. Modifications also include addressing low seats and ensuring appropriately heighted grab bars and handrails for support and stability.
- *Footwear assessment and changes*: Proper footwear with good fit, support, and nonslip soles is crucial for stability and fall prevention.
- *Assistive devices*: Canes, walkers, and walking sticks are recommended to improve balance and reduce fall risk. It is essential to ensure proper fitting, safe usage, and regular maintenance of these devices.
- *Gait training*: Improving the elder's walking pattern through exercises that focus on stride length, pace, and foot placement is important. Walking aids can be used if necessary, ensuring they are safe and properly fitted.
- *Education and lifestyle modifications*: Educating elders and caregivers about safe mobility techniques

and fall prevention strategies is crucial. Encouraging lifestyle modifications such as regular physical activity, a healthy diet, and adequate hydration supports overall health and mobility.

- *Monitoring and progress evaluation*: Regular monitoring of progress allows for adjustments to the rehabilitation program as needed. Periodic assessments help document improvement or deterioration and modify goals accordingly.
- *Community integration and social engagement*: Promoting participation in community activities fosters social interaction and maintains motivation. Local groups, fitness classes, and senior centers can facilitate community integration.
- *Fall prevention strategies*: Implementing strategies such as removing home hazards, improving lighting, and using appropriate footwear minimizes fall risk. Teaching techniques for safe recovery from falls is also essential.
- *Medication management*: Reviewing medications and routine timely follow-ups to identify any that may affect balance or mobility are important. The timing of medication should not interfere with mobility training sessions.
- *Maintenance plan*: Developing and implementing a long-term maintenance plan helps sustain gains achieved through rehabilitation. Guidance on maintaining an active lifestyle and continuing exercises preserves mobility and independence.
- *Nutrition and hydration*: A balanced diet rich in nutrients for bone health and muscle function is essential. Adequate hydration is crucial as dehydration can contribute to dizziness and affect balance. Addressing any nutritional concerns related to dyspnea or dental issues is important.

These interventions aim to improve mobility, reduce fall risk, enhance safety, and promote the overall well-being of elderly individuals with mobility impairments.

Exercise-based Rehabilitation for Mobility Impairment

Classification of recommendations by the American College of Cardiology/American Heart Association (ACC/AHA) and the methodology manual for ACC/AHA guideline summarize the detailed guidelines for the regular preventive physical activities.

They recommend regular physical activity, including aerobic activity, flexibility exercises, and muscle-strengthening activity, for healthy aging along with specific recommendations that specify how older adults, by engaging in each recommended type of physical activity, can reduce the risk of chronic disease, premature mortality, functional limitations, and disability. The summary of these guidelines is described below:

- *Endurance and cardiovascular conditioning* include activities such as walking, cycling, or water aerobics with gradually increasing duration and intensity to improve endurance over time.
- They should perform *moderate-intensity aerobic* (endurance) physical activity for a minimum of 30 minutes on 5 days each week or vigorous-intensity aerobic activity for a minimum of 20 minutes on 3 days each week.
- On Borg scale, the moderate-intensity aerobic activity involves a moderate level of effort relative to an individual's aerobic fitness. On a 10-point scale, where sitting is 0 and all-out effort is 10, moderate-intensity activity is a 5 or 6 and produces noticeable increases in heart rate and breathing.
- On the same scale, vigorous-intensity activity is a 7 or 8 and produces large increase in heart rate and breathing. For example, given the heterogeneity of fitness levels in older adults, for some older adults, a moderate-intensity walk is a slow walk, and for others, it is a brisk walk.
- *Muscle-strengthening exercise and resistance training*: In addition, at least twice each week, older adults should perform *muscle strengthening activities* using the major key muscles (of hip, spine, core, lower and upper extremity) of the body that maintain or increase muscular strength and endurance for 8–10 exercises be performed on at least 2 nonconsecutive days per week using the major muscle groups. To maximize strength development, a resistance (weight) should be used that allows 10–15 repetitions for each exercise. The level of effort for muscle-strengthening activities should be moderate to high. *Strength training must incorporate* resistance exercises using body weight, resistance bands, weight cuff, or light weights to strengthen muscles.
- *Flexibility exercise*: Older adults should perform activities that maintain or increase flexibility on at least 2 days each week for at least 10 minutes each day.
- *Balance exercises* help to reduce risk of injury from falls, community-dwelling older adults with a substantial risk of falls. Practice balance exercises such as standing on one leg, heel-to-toe walking, or balance board exercises include coordination drills that challenge the elder's ability to control movements and maintain balance.

- Sedentary older adults should always gradually increase the intensity of exercise to enhance physical activity over time. These people should not hurry up to increase the intensity of exercises and must continue at lower intensity levels for months or weeks before any progression in the intensity is done. Older adults must be educated and sensitized to monitor their physical activities and also the careful monitoring of their health status.
- *Gait training*: It implements exercises to improve walking pattern (gait), including heel-to-toe walking, marching in place, or practicing turns and direction changes. Use assistive devices as needed to support safe and effective gait training. Gait training focuses on improving stability, coordination, walking efficiency, and the ability to recover from a stumble, thereby reducing the risk of falls. It helps in maintaining independence in daily activities and essential tasks and participating in social activities. It boosts the elder's quality of life and confidence, as being able to move around safely, independently, and confidently will reduce fears of falling, boost self-confidence, and promote a sense of well-being.

Any increase in physical activity must be gradual and careful to minimize risk of overuse injury. Exercise in group and pleasant manner may be incorporated to provide positive reinforcement for achieving the desired laid goals. Adequate instructions, hydration, interset rests, and practice of any activity or exercises help to gain experience, fitness, and self-confidence.

Rehabilitation for Cognitive Impairments

The WHO recommended rehabilitation as a core recommendation in the global action plan on the public health response to dementia, with an aim to maximize independence and community participation in dementia care. Regular physical exercise in older adults improves physical health, reduces frailty, decreases the risk of depression, and improves cognitive function, and this lessens the risk of Alzheimer's disease by slowing the onset or progression. The recommended exercise program for dementia includes aerobic exercise, resistance training, balance, and flexibility training.

CONCLUSION

Mobility is one of the vital indicators of healthy aging and is affected by age related physiological, psychological, cognitive changes along with overall life style. Mobility impairment is a significant issue for older adults due to its high prevalence, impacts on managing ADL independently and higher risk of adverse health events.

Geriatrician needs to play proactive role along with physiotherapist in early assessment using standardized tools and a multidisciplinary intervention as per the need—including physical therapy, assistive devices, environmental modification, and caregiver education.

Every older adults should be recommended regular physical activities (aerobic, strengthening, flexibility, and balance training) with an individualized goal as per their health status to improve mobility, reduce fall risks, and foster social engagement.

Self-Assessment Questionnaire

Q1. What are the most common age-related physiological changes that contribute to mobility impairment in older adults?

Q2. How does muscle mass, strength, and power decline affect gait, balance, and fall risk among the elderly?

Q3. What are the major psychosocial and environmental factors that can exacerbate mobility limitations?

Q4. Which standardized tools are commonly used to assess mobility and balance in elderly individuals, and what do they measure?

Q5. How can multidisciplinary care help to improve mobility outcomes?

Q6. How can regular physical activity and progressive resistance training prevent or delay disability in older adults?

Q7. What modifications at home and in the community can promote safe and independent mobility among elders?

FURTHER READINGS

1. Wamble DE, Ciarametaro M, Dubois R. The effect of medical technology innovations on patient outcomes, 1990-2015: results of a physician survey. J Manag Care Spec Pharm. 2019;25(1).
2. Freiberger E, Sieber CC, Kob R. Mobility in older community-dwelling persons: a narrative review. Front Physiol. 2020;11.
3. Tremblay MS, Aubert S, Barnes JD, Saunders TJ, Carson V, Latimer-Cheung AE, et al. Sedentary Behavior Research Network (SBRN)—Terminology Consensus Project process and outcome. Int J Behav Nutr Phys Act. 2017;14(1).
4. Ehlers MM, Nielsen CV, Bjerrum MB. Experiences of older adults after hip fracture: an integrative review. Rehab Nur. 2018;43.
5. Chen Y, Almirall-Sánchez A, Mockler D, Adrion E, Domínguez-Vivero C, Romero-Ortuño R. Hospital-associated deconditioning: not only physical, but also cognitive. Int J Geriatric Psych. 2022;37.
6. Duan-Porter W, Vo TN, Ullman K, Langsetmo L, Strotmeyer ES, Taylor BC, et al. Hospitalization-associated change in gait speed and risk of functional limitations for older adults. J Gerontol. 2019;74(10).
7. Torres-de Araújo JR, Tomaz-de Lima RR, Ferreira-Bendassolli IM, Costa-de Lima K. Functional, nutritional and social factors associated with mobility limitations in the elderly: a systematic review. Salud Publica Mex. 2018;60(5).
8. Satariano WA, Guralnik JM, Jackson RJ, Marottoli RA, Phelan EA, Prohaska TR. Mobility and aging: new directions for public health action. Am J Public Health. 2012;102(8).
9. Maresova P, Krejcar O, Maskuriy R, Bakar NAA, Selamat A, Truhlarova Z, et al. Challenges and opportunity in mobility among older adults – key determinant identification. BMC Geriatr. 2023;23(1).
10. Brady AO, Straight CR, Evans EM. Body composition, muscle capacity, and physical function in older adults: an integrated conceptual model. J Aging Phys Act. 2014;22(3).
11. Corona LP, Pereira De Brito TR, Nunes DP, Da Silva Alexandre T, Ferreira Santos JL, De Oliveira Duarte YA, et al. Nutritional status and risk for disability in instrumental activities of daily living in older Brazilians. Public Health Nutr. 2014;17(2).
12. Doherty TJ. The influence of aging and sex on skeletal muscle mass and strength. Curr Opin Clin Nutr Metab Care. 2001;4(6).
13. Goodpaster BH, Park SW, Harris TB, Kritchevsky SB, Nevitt M, Schwartz AV, et al. The loss of skeletal muscle strength, mass, and quality in older adults: the health, aging and body composition study. J Gerontol. 2006;61(10).
14. Keller K, Engelhardt M. Strength and muscle mass loss with aging process. Age and strength loss. Muscles Ligaments Tendons J. 2013;3(4).
15. Reid KF, Fielding RA. Skeletal muscle power: a critical determinant of physical functioning in older adults. Exerc Sport Sci Rev. 2012;40(1).
16. Bell KE, von Allmen MT, Devries MC, Phillips SM. Muscle Disuse as a pivotal problem in sarcopenia-related muscle loss and dysfunction. J Frailty Aging. 2016;5.
17. Drey M, Krieger B, Sieber CC, Bauer JM, Hettwer S, Bertsch T. Motoneuron loss is associated with sarcopenia. J Am Med Dir Assoc. 2014;15(6).
18. Osoba MY, Rao AK, Agrawal SK, Lalwani AK. Balance and gait in the elderly: a contemporary review. Laryngoscope Investig Otolaryngol. 2019;4.
19. Lassale C, Liljas AEM, Jones A, Cadar D, Steptoe A. Association of multisensory impairment with quality of life and depression in english older adults. JAMA Otolaryngol Head Neck Surg. 2020;146(3).
20. Ruas CV, Pinto MD, Brown LE, Minozzo F, Mil-Homens P, Pinto RS. The association between conventional and dynamic control knee strength ratios in elite soccer players. Isokinet Exerc Sci. 2015;23(1):1-12.
21. Herssens N, Verbecque E, Hallemans A, Vereeck L, Van Rompaey V, Saeys W. Do spatiotemporal parameters and gait variability differ across the lifespan of healthy adults? A systematic review. Gait Posture. 2018;64.
22. Montero-Odasso M, Muir SW, Speechley M. Dual-task complexity affects gait in people with mild cognitive impairment: the interplay between gait variability, dual tasking, and risk of falls. Arch Phys Med Rehabil. 2012;93(2).
23. Tieland M, Trouwborst I, Clark BC. Skeletal muscle performance and ageing. J Cachexia, Sarcopenia Muscle. 2018;9.
24. Wennie Huang WN, Perera S, Vanswearingen J, Studenski S. Performance measures predict onset of activity of daily living difficulty in community-dwelling older adults. J Am Geriatr Soc. 2010;58(5):844-52.
25. Liu B, Hu X, Zhang Q, Fan Y, Li J, Zou R, et al. Usual walking speed and all-cause mortality risk in older people: A systematic review and meta-analysis. Gait Posture. 2016;44.
26. Callisaya ML, Launay CP, Srikanth VK, Verghese J, Allali G, Beauchet O. Cognitive status, fast walking speed and walking speed reserve—the Gait and Alzheimer Interactions Tracking (GAIT) study. Geroscience. 2017;39(2).
27. Donoghue OA, Dooley C, Kenny RA. Usual and dual-task walking speed: implications for pedestrians crossing the road. J Aging Health. 2016;28(5).
28. Eggenberger P, Tomovic S, Münzer T, De Bruin ED. Older adults must hurry at pedestrian lights! A cross-sectional analysis of preferred and fast walking speed under single- and dual-task conditions. PLoS One. 2017;12(7).
29. Salthouse TA. Trajectories of normal cognitive aging. Psychol Aging. 2019;34(1).
30. Harada CN, Natelson Love MC, Triebel KL. Normal cognitive aging. Clin Geriatric Med. 2013;29.
31. Kujala UM, Hautasaari P, Vähä-Ypyä H, Waller K, Lindgren N, Iso-Markku P, et al. Chronic diseases and objectively monitored physical activity profile among aged individuals–a cross-sectional twin cohort study. Ann Med. 2019;51(1).
32. Welmer AK, Angleman S, Rydwik E, Fratiglioni L, Qiu C. Association of cardiovascular burden with mobility limitation among elderly people: a population-based study. PLoS One. 2013;8(5).
33. Demnitz N, Zsoldos E, Mahmood A, Mackay CE, Kivimäki M, Singh-Manoux A, et al. Associations between mobility, cognition, and brain structure in healthy older adults. Front Aging Neurosci. 2017;9.
34. Hybels CF, Pieper CF, Blazer DG. The complex relationship between depressive symptoms and functional limitations in community-dwelling older adults: the impact of subthreshold depression. Psychol Med. 2009;39(10).
35. Pauelsen M, Nyberg L, Röijezon U, Vikman I. Both psychological factors and physical performance are associated with fall-related concerns. Aging Clin Exp Res. 2018;30(9).
36. Hinrichs T, Keskinen KE, Pavelka B, Eronen J, Schmidt-Trucksäss A, Rantanen T, et al. Perception of parks and trails as mobility facilitators and transportation walking in older adults: a study using digital geographical maps. Aging Clin Exp Res. 2019;31(5).
37. Brown CJ, Flood KL. Mobility limitation in the older patient: a clinical review. JAMA. 2013;310.

38. Mezuk B, Rebok GW. Social integration and social support among older adults following driving cessation. J Gerontol. 2008; 63(5).
39. Lee IM, Buchner DM. The importance of walking to public health. Med Sci Sports Exerc. 2008;40(7 Suppl 1).
40. Guralnik JM, Ferrucci L, Balfour JL, Volpato S, Iorio A Di. Progressive versus catastrophic loss of the ability to walk: implications for the prevention of mobility loss. J Am Geriatr Soc. 2001;49(11).
41. Alexandre TS, Meira DM, Rico NC, Mizuta SK. Accuracy of timed up and go test for screening risk of falls among community-dwelling elderly. Braz J Phys Ther. 2012;16(5).
42. Wang CY, Yeh CJ, Hu MH. Mobility-related performance tests to predict mobility disability at 2-year follow-up in community-dwelling older adults. Arch Gerontol Geriatr. 2011;52(1).
43. Zhang F, Ferrucci L, Culham E, Metter EJ, Guralnik J, Deshpande N. Performance on five times sit-to-stand task as a predictor of subsequent falls and disability in older persons. J Aging Health. 2013;25(3).
44. Deshpande N, Metter EJ, Guralnik J, Bandinelli S, Ferrucci L. Predicting 3-year incident mobility disability in middle-aged and older adults using physical performance tests. Arch Phys Med Rehabil. 2013;94(5).
45. Fritz NE, Worstell AM, Kloos AD, Siles AB, White SE, Kegelmeyer DA. Backward walking measures are sensitive to age-related changes in mobility and balance. Gait Posture. 2013;37(4).
46. Guralnik JM, Ferrucci L, Pieper CF, Leveille SG, Markides KS, Ostir GV, et al. Lower extremity function and subsequent disability: consistency across studies, predictive models, and value of gait speed alone compared with the short physical performance battery. J Gerontol. 2000;55(4).
47. Penninx BW, Ferrucci L, Leveille SG, Rantanen T, Pahor M, Guralnik JM. Lower extremity performance in nondisabled older persons as a predictor of subsequent hospitalization. J Gerontol. 2000;55(11).
48. Meyer MRU, Janke MC, Beaujean AA. Predictors of older adults personal and community mobility: using a comprehensive theoretical mobility framework. Gerontologist. 2014;54(3).
49. Norton S, Matthews FE, Barnes DE, Yaffe K, Brayne C. Potential for primary prevention of Alzheimer's disease: an analysis of population-based data. Lancet Neurol. 2014;13(8).
50. WHO. Global Recommendations on Physical Activity for Health. Geneva: World Health Organization Publications; 2010.
51. Baker MK, Atlantis E, Fiatarone Singh MA. Multi-modal exercise programs for older adults. Age Ageing. 2007;36.
52. Nelson ME, Rejeski WJ, Blair SN, Duncan PW, Judge JO, King AC, et al. Physical activity and public health in older adults: recommendation from the American College of Sports Medicine and the American Heart Association. Med Sci Sport Exer. 2007;39.
53. Poole JL, Gallegos M, O'Linc S. Recommendations for the medical management of osteoarthritis of the hip and knee: 2000 update. Arthritis Rheumatism. 2000;43.
54. Ravn MB, Petersen KS, Thuesen J. Rehabilitation for people living with dementia: a scoping review of processes and outcomes. J Aging Res. 2019;2019.
55. Langhammer B, Bergland A, Rydwik E. The importance of physical activity exercise among older people. BioMed Res Int. 2018;2018.
56. Tolppanen AM, Solomon A, Kulmala J, Kåreholt I, Ngandu T, Rusanen M, et al. Leisure-time physical activity from mid- to late life, body mass index, and risk of dementia. Alzheimers Dement. 2015;11(4).
57. Gupta A, Prakash NB, Sannyasi G. Rehabilitation in dementia. Indian J Psychol Med. 2021;43(5 Suppl).

CHAPTER 28

Osteoarthritis and Other Degenerative Joint Diseases

Mangala Suresh Borkar

CASE VIGNETTE

A 65-year-old obese lady with controlled diabetes presented with complaints of pain in both knees for last 1 year, which was initially related to exertion and walking. Now, it is present at rest also; she feels stiff while getting out of bed or after a long journey and is unable to stand or walk for a few minutes. She gets relief after flexing and extending her knees for a short time and then can resume her activities, though with pain. On examination, the right knee joint is swollen and has crepitus and generalized tenderness on movement. She has difficulty in getting up from a squatting posture and is unable to walk for a longer distance. The pain is aggravated by climbing up- or downstairs and when she tries to get up from a low seat. That is crepitus on the knee joint, and the X-ray of the knee shows loss of joint space and osteophytes. She has been advised to reduce her weight, do regular exercises, particularly of the quadriceps, and take hot fomentations and paracetamol SOS. She has mild relief with this treatment and is willing to continue this. The orthopedic surgeon has counseled her that she may be able to avoid a knee replacement if she takes sufficient efforts and advised her to follow up after 3 months.

INTRODUCTION

Osteoarthritis (OA) is the most common form of arthritis and the most common cause of disability among the elderly. The prevalence is increasing, mainly due to an increase in life expectancy and obesity.

Osteoarthritis significantly increases with age and is more common in women.

Almost 75% of older adults suffer from OA or other joint problems after the age of 70 years. Pain due to OA leads to muscle loss, limitations in activities of daily living, weakness, sleep disturbance, and poor quality of life. Sometimes, the elderly suffer from more than one type of arthritis, e.g., knee OA, frozen shoulder, and pain in the lower back. Since there are more than hundred different musculoskeletal conditions, a good history and examination are critical for diagnosing the possible cause of arthritis.

ANATOMY

Anatomy of the knee ***(Figs. 1A and B)***: The knee is a hinge joint that connects the femur above to the tibia below, and its main actions are flexion and extension, though a little lateral movement also can take place.

The medial and lateral menisci are shock absorbers that protect the cartilage from day-to-day impact and friction during movement. They do not regenerate on their own and are easily prone to sports injury.

The anterior and posterior cruciate ligaments stabilize the knee during flexion and extension. The medial and lateral collateral ligaments protect the knee from buckling sideway.

The articular cartilage coats the lower end of the femur, i.e., the condyles, the upper part of the tibia, and the inside of the patella. The menisci lie in between the femoral and tibial cartilage.

Anatomy of the hip joint ***(Figs. 2A and B)***: It is a ball-and-socket joint that connects the acetabulum of the pelvis to the femoral condyle. This type of joint provides a wide range of movement, bears weight, and stabilizes the lower limb. Flexion, extension, circumduction, and lateral movements are possible in this joint.

Cartilage covers the femoral head and the acetabulum.

The synovial membrane covers the joint and secretes the lubricating synovial fluid.

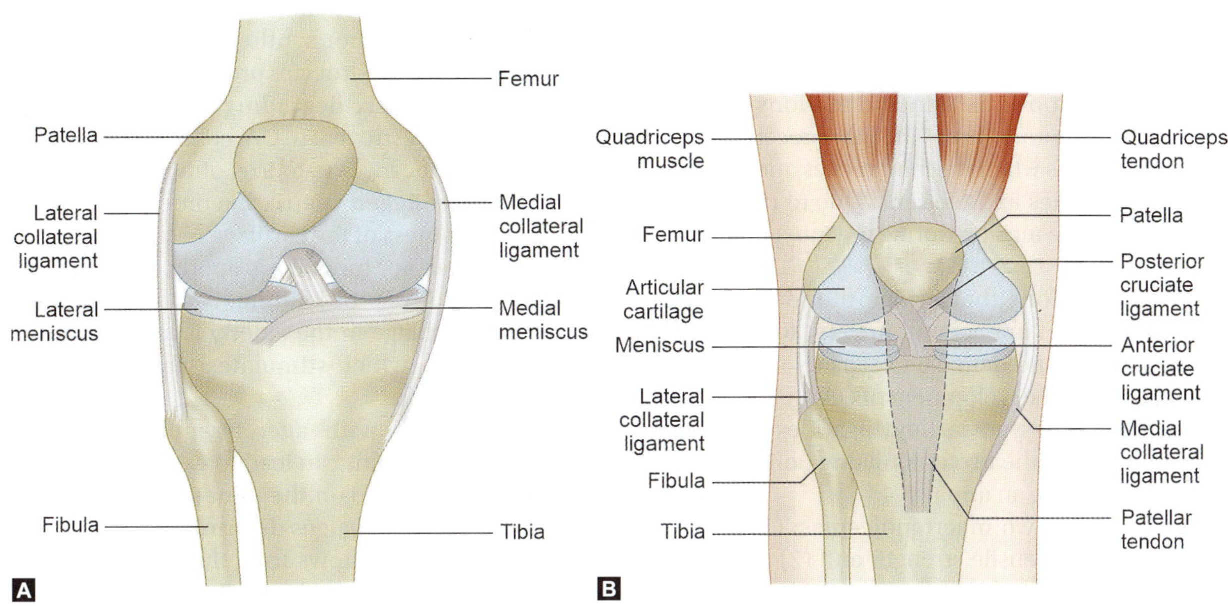

FIGS. 1A AND B: (A) Structure of human knee. (B) Anatomy of knee.

Source: Shutterstock. (2025). Knee anatomy. [online] Available from https://www.shutterstock.com/image-illustration/anatomy-human-knee-joint-structure-diagram-2347312467. [Last accessed May, 2025].

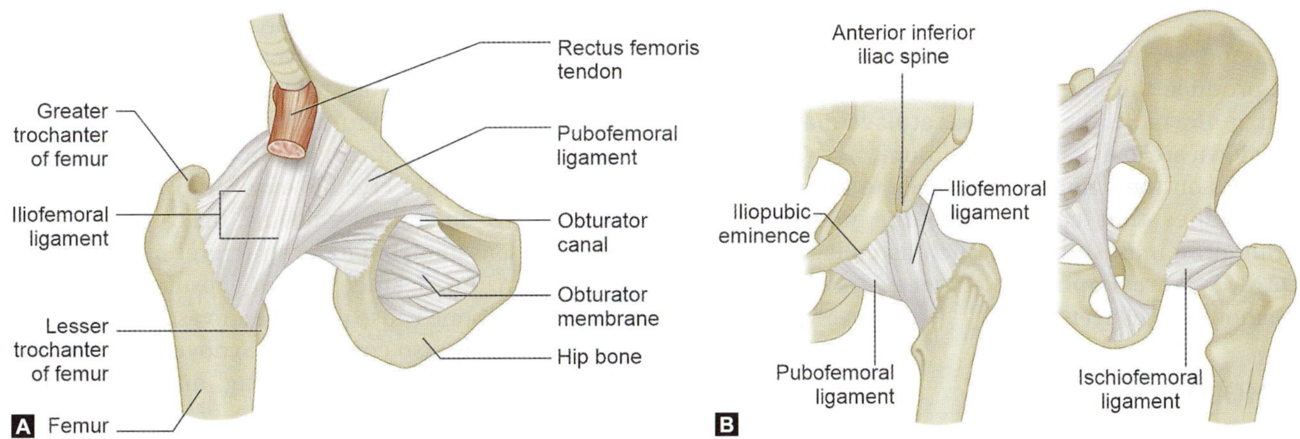

FIGS. 2A AND B: Structure of the Hip.

The muscles of the hip are the gluteal, quadriceps, iliopsoas, adductors, and hamstrings.

The capsular ligaments are the iliofemoral (Y ligament of Bigelow), pubofemoral, and ischiofemoral ligaments. The iliofemoral ligament is the strongest ligament in the body. It attaches the anterior inferior iliac spine to the intertrochanteric crest of the femur.

The dense, strong hip joint capsule is attached above to the acetabular margin, in front to the outer labral aspect and, near the acetabular notch, to the transverse acetabular ligament and the adjacent rim of the obturator foramen. It surrounds the femoral neck.

The capsule is thicker anterosuperiorly, where maximal stress occurs. It is thin and loosely attached posteroinferiorly. It has two sets of fibers: (1) Circular and (2) longitudinal.

PHYSIOLOGY

Joint protective mechanisms: The joint capsule and ligaments protect the joint by limiting the range of movement.

Synovial fluid decreases friction and cartilage wear and tear. The lubricating function depends on hyaluronic acid and lubricin (which is a mucinous glycoprotein, secreted by fibroblasts). This decreases if there is an injury or inflammation of the joint.

The ligaments that overlie skin and tendons contain sensory mechanoreceptors. These mechanoreceptors fire at different frequencies when the joint moves and provide feedback to the muscles and tendons. Due to this, these assume an appropriate tension during the movement and protect the joint.

Muscles and tendons that bridge the joint ensure uniform distribution of impact and prevent focal stress. Rupture of ligaments and damage to sensory nerves of a joint can lead to a rapid development of OA.

Cartilage, along with synovial fluid, provides a frictionless surface in between the two articulating bones. It also has the role of absorbing an impact.

Cartilage contains two macromolecules: (1) Type 2 collagen that provides tensile strength and (2) aggrecan, a proteoglycan linked with hyaluronic acid. Aggrecan consists of highly negatively charged glycosaminoglycans. Type 2 collagen is tightly woven, with the aggrecan molecules in the interstices, closely bound together. The cartilage gets its compressive stiffness due to the negatively charged aggrecan molecules that repel electrostatic charge.

Chondrocytes are cells within this avascular matrix that produce the matrix, as well as enzymes that can break it down. Synthesis of the cartilage matrix and its breakdown are in dynamic equilibrium.

Stress on the chondrocytes leads to the production of cytokines that can damage the matrix. Matrix metalloproteinases (MMPs) such as collagenases and ADAMTS-5 are important enzymes involved in the breakdown of collagen.

PATHOLOGY

Loss of cartilage, osteophytes, weakening of the muscles around the joint, sclerosis of the bony end plate, thickening of the capsule, and meniscal damage (in case of the knee) are some of the pathological changes that occur in OA.

An injury may start the process. Loss of protective mechanisms is the main propagating factor.

Local inflammation increases the development of OA and leads to pain. Mechanoinflammation is that which is caused by mechanical stimuli.

Cytokines, chemokines, and complement activation factor act on chondrocyte surface receptors. Fragments of matrix are released from cartilage and stimulate synovitis. Tumor necrosis factor induces chondrocytes to synthesize prostaglandin E2 and nitric oxide. Normal cartilage is avascular. Invasion of blood vessels into cartilage occurs in disease from underlying bone. This occurs due to vascular endothelial growth factor synthesis in the cartilage and bone. With aging, chondrocytes produce proinflammatory mediators and matrix-degrading enzymes. Thus, the cartilage is easily destroyed. In OA, collagen shows gradual depletion of aggrecan. Due to loss of type 2 collagen, the tightly bound collagen matrix becomes loose and the compressive stiffness of the cartilage is decreased.

If a joint does not function properly, OA can develop with minimum levels of loading. An important aspect in OA is that cartilage in the elderly is less responsive to dynamic loading, which stimulates matrix synthesis in younger individuals.

Cartilage thins with age. Irregular thinning of cartilage across the joint can lead to OA due to the wrong distribution of pressure on the joint surface, medially or laterally (as in varus or valgus deformity).

Initially, cartilage shows irregularity. Focal erosions develop and extend to the bone. A larger proportion of the joint surface is involved, though OA is basically a focal disease and the loss of cartilage is nonuniform.

After an injury to the cartilage, clusters of chondrocytes gather. Proteoglycan depletion occurs due to the greater catabolic activity. The collagen matrix becomes damaged, and cartilage swells due to the ionic attraction of the negative charges of proteoglycans to water molecules. Cartilage does not bounce back after loading as it used to when healthy. The subdural bone becomes thicker. The capsule stretches and can become fibrotic. Phosphate and pyrophosphate crystals enter into the joint space from cartilage and trigger synovitis. The cartilage does not have pain sensation, but inner structures in the joint such as the synovium, ligaments, joint capsule, muscles, and subchondral bone cause pain. Neurovascular invasion in later stages may also contribute. Synovial inflammation, joint effusions, capsule stretching, and bone marrow edema may lead to pain.

The subchondral bone has an important role in OA. The active osteocytes express inflammatory cytokines and proteins in response to mechanical stress. Bone formation becomes predominant, which results in thick and stiff bone. New blood vessels and nerves infiltrate damaged cartilage to facilitate new bone formation within the cartilage, and these create osteophytes. This causes cartilage thinning. Redistribution of joint forces occurs which is abnormal.

Muscles become weaker, sensory nervous input decreases, and feedback to make new receptors becomes less. Ligaments stretch and become less able to absorb impacts. Older women are at a higher risk of OA, especially after they reach their sixth decade. Hormone loss is one of the factors.

Inflammation is common secondary to bone and cartilage pathology. Cartilage breakdown products are released into the synovial fluid and lead to inflammation of the synovial membrane. The inflammatory cytokines aggravate the destructive process.

Pathology of Pain

Initially, the pain in OA occurs because nociceptors in the joint are stimulated when weight-bearing activities are carried out. Afterward, the pain tends to become chronic and constant and may be present at rest. Changes in nervous system signaling may occur, peripheral nociceptors can become more responsive to sensory input, and central nociceptive signaling may also increase. Insufficient descending inhibitory modulation to pain may also occur.

Adipokines produced by adipose tissue can act on the nervous system to enhance pain sensitivity. Hence, obesity increases the severity of pain.

The pain that is initially episodic becomes continuous, more at night, and disturbs the person's sleep. Depression can set in.

CAUSES

Heredity: Fifty percent of OA of the hand and hip is related to inheritance; however, <30% of knee OA is related to heredity.

Injuries: Major injuries to a joint make it susceptible to OA. Avascular necrosis of the joint also leads to OA. Tear of the meniscus can lead to premature OA. Weakness of the quadriceps can lead to painful OA in the knee.

Those with increased bone density have a higher risk of osteophytes at the joint margin.

Obesity is a high-risk factor for developing OA, especially of the knees, and this risk is higher in women. Weight loss lowers the risk and also the pain.

Occupational use of a joint repeatedly can lead to arthritis, e.g., hip OA in farmers, knee OA in miners, or those carrying heavy weights.

Exercise is indicated to maintain muscle mass. However, OA may be precipitated, especially of the knees, in those who have injured joints.

CLINICAL PRESENTATION

The commonly affected joints are the knee, hip, first metatarsophalangeal, cervical, and lumbar vertebrae. Interphalangeal joints and the base of thumb may be affected too.

The wrist, elbow, and ankle joints are usually spared. The ankles may be spared because their cartilage is resistant to loading stresses. On the other hand, the evolutionary upright position adapted by human beings places stress on the knees and hips.

Symptomatic OA of the knees is nearly three times as common as OA of the hip.

Activity-related pain in the early stages and chronic pain later on are the most important symptoms. Initially, it comes during or just after the use of the joint and gradually resolves. Later, chronic pain may set in. Stiffness of the affected joint may occur which is relieved to some extent with movement. Morning stiffness is common but lasts for <10 minutes and usually decreases with movement. Prolonged periods of disuse due to prolonged sitting, as during travel or at work, cause stiffness. It is useful to gently move the joint every few minutes to prevent this.

Buckling of the knees, catching, and locking can occur due to internal derangement, such as anterior cruciate ligament or meniscus tear.

In inflammatory arthritis or gout, mechanical joint pains worsen with prolonged use or weight bearing. If a joint is swollen, painful, and there is a change in the color of the overlying skin, it is more likely to be gout or a septic arthritis. Along with history related to the joint swelling, one should find out if there are any systemic symptoms, and the family history also may be useful.

Knee pain can be associated with a sensation of giving way, which may result in falls and affect the individual's confidence.

Examination

There is tenderness, crepitus, bony enlargement, effusion, misalignment, and reduction in the range of motion. OA leads to muscle loss. Hence, routine activities become difficult to perform.

Tenderness is generalized in OA, but pain of Anserine bursitis is medial and distal to the knee. It is a common cause of chronic knee pain that may respond to local steroid injection.

Crepitus may be present when you place your hand on the knee and extend it. Hip OA gives rise to the loss of internal rotation on passive movement. Pain which is isolated lateral to the hip joint is usually due to trochanteric bursitis.

Varus, or sometimes valgus deformity of the knee, Heberden's nodes may be seen. Difficulty in getting up from a chair or bed or squatting develops. Grip strength, or a slow straight leg raise, can give a good indication of muscle strength.

INVESTIGATIONS

An X-ray or CT scan may show a decrease in joint space, osteophytes, or damage to the ligaments. MRI may pick up even minor changes and injuries and usually does not warrant a change in therapy.

Plain X-ray shows loss of joint space, subchondral sclerosis, and osteophytes. However, overreliance on the X-ray for clinical decision making should be avoided. There is no specific laboratory test for OA. If there is an effusion, then synovial fluid may be examined by arthrocentesis.

Occasionally, synovial fluid examination may help in the diagnosis. If the synovial fluid white cell count is >1,000/mm^3, inflammatory arthritis, gout, or pseudogout is likely to occur.

Magnetic resonance imaging has shown bone lesions, fibrosis, necrosis, and bone marrow edema in many patients with symptomatic OA. These lesions cause pain. Also, these are indicated before the transplant.

There are no sufficient blood tests, and it is mainly clinical diagnosis assisted with X-ray radiographic changes.

DIAGNOSIS

The diagnosis of OA is based on symptoms and structural changes that are apparent clinically and by radiology.

As a person ages, radiological evidence of OA is almost universal, in the form of loss of cartilage (loss of joint space) and osteophytes. However, pain and disability are what really matter.

MANAGEMENT

The goal of the treatment of OA is to alleviate pain and decrease the loss of function.

Therapeutic goals involve minimizing pain and disability and maximizing function and quality of life. Patient education, exercise programs, and weight-loss strategies form an important aspect of treatment. Management plans need to be individualized. Drug toxicity has to be kept in mind, especially in older adults with comorbidities, which are common.

Comprehensive therapy includes physical modalities and pharmacological treatment. In mild cases, symptomatic management of pain, weight loss, exercise, and preventing activities with high impact which may damage the joint helps.

The mainstay of treatment of OA consists of:

- Altering loading across the painful joint
- Improving the function of joint protectors

Avoid painful activities as they usually overload the joint.

Improve the strength and conditioning of the muscles that bridge the joint. A brace, splint, cane, crutch, or holding side rails of stairs can help to unload the joint. Avoid running and climbing to heights. Climbing down the stairs, jumping, and squatting increase the stress on the knees.

Weight loss is very helpful in decreasing pain.

Optimal use of a quadripod stick of a proper height can help and is useful for preventing falls too.

Osteoarthritis leads to decreased physical activity, with negative consequences on the health of the heart and other parts of the body. Muscles may weaken due to age and limited mobility due to pain, causing disuse atrophy. Painful OA makes the patients alter their gait to lessen the loading across the joint, which further decreases the use of the muscles. A swollen and painful joint may inhibit the contraction of muscles around it by a nerve afferent feedback loop. This prevents the attainment of voluntary maximum strength. Weakness in the muscle that bridges the joint makes the joint more susceptible to further damage. The degree of weakness correlates strongly with the severity of pain and limitation of movement; hence, a very important aspect of treatment is to improve the strength and function of the muscles that surround the joint, especially the quadriceps.

Exercise performed correctly actually lessens pain and improves physical functions. Aerobic exercises and resistance training which focus on strengthening the muscles across the joints are most effective. Low-impact exercise, such as water aerobics, is better tolerated. Avoid running or treadmill exercises. Cycling may be helpful, provided the height of the cycle is optimal and the person does not have to hop and jump. Tai chi may also help in knee OA. Exercise has to be performed regularly, lifelong, modifying it as needed and preventing falls. Consistency with exercise and weight loss are the key to decrease pain.

Biomechanical factors can be corrected with the help of a stick, hand, splint, suitable footwear, knee brace, hot, or cold packs to the joint can benefit.

Varus valgus malalignment may be corrected with braces or surgically. Braces should be of the proper size, and correctly fitting shoes with proper soles also help.

Paracetamol should be the first-line oral therapy.

Nonsteroidal anti-inflammatory drugs (NSAIDs) can be administered, topically or orally, in minimum doses. As far as possible, paracetamol should be used. Diclofenac should be avoided in the elderly, especially if the person is a diabetic or has renal impairment.

Anti-inflammatory treatments administered into the joint may control the pain for up to 3 months. Synovitis may especially respond to this. Repeated injections may cause minor amounts of cartilage loss. Hyaluronic acid injections are used, but the effect is more likely to be that of a placebo.

Opioids may be useful when there is a strong psychological element to the pain, but glucosamine or chondroitin are not shown to be useful in large trials. They can cause confusion, falls, and constipation.

There is a risk of overuse of NSAIDs, often due to self-prescription, and dangerous side effects can occur to the kidneys in patients who are not counseled properly.

Surgery: Arthroscopic meniscectomies in meniscal tears do not improve long-term function or symptoms, though they may help in individual cases; if knee OA is isolated to the medial compartment, operations to lessen medial loading can relieve pain, e.g., high TBL osteotomy. Partial knee replacement can help. If the patient's quality of life is affected, then total knee or hip arthroplasty may be performed, which relieves pain and improves function in the majority of patients. Too much delay in performing knee or hip replacement may not improve the functional status much.

Chondrocyte transplantation has not been found to be efficacious because multiple reasons cause the symptoms in OA. Also, these procedures do not correct the misalignment and other mechanical changes that develop in OA.

Topical use of NSAIDs and capsaicin can help reduce symptoms.

For patients with OA of the knee and hip, the following instructions can help manage symptoms and improve quality of life:

- *Exercise*:
    - *Low-impact exercises*: Engage in activities such as walking, swimming, or cycling that do not strain the joints.
    - *Strengthening exercises*: Focus on strengthening the muscles around the knee and hip, such as quadriceps, hamstrings, and gluteal muscles.
    - *Flexibility exercises*: Incorporate stretching to maintain joint flexibility.
    - *Physical therapy*: A physical therapist can guide personalized exercises and proper techniques to avoid injury.
- *Weight management*:
    - *Maintain a healthy weight*: Reducing weight can decrease stress on the knee and hip joints, alleviating pain and slowing progression.
    - *Balanced diet*: Follow a diet rich in fruits, vegetables, whole grains, lean proteins, and healthy fats.
- *Pain management*:
    - *Medications*: NSAIDs or acetaminophen can help relieve pain. Topical pain relievers such as creams or gels may also be useful.
    - *Hot/cold therapy*: Apply heat to relax muscles and improve blood flow; use cold packs to reduce swelling and sharp pain.
- *Joint protection*:
    - *Assistive devices*: Use canes, walkers, or braces as recommended to reduce stress on the joints.
    - *Proper footwear*: Wear shoes with good arch support and cushioning to minimize impact on the joints.
    - *Modify activities*: Avoid high-impact activities that strain the knee and hip, such as running or jumping.
- *Lifestyle modifications*:
    - *Pacing one's activities*: Alternate periods of activity with rest to avoid overloading the joints.
    - *Ergonomics*: Ensure your home and work environments are set up to minimize joint strain (e.g., using supportive chairs, avoiding low seating).
    - Quitting addictions.
- *Treatment:*
    - *Injections*: Corticosteroid injections may provide temporary relief from inflammation, especially bursitis.
    - *Surgery*: In severe cases, joint replacement surgery may be recommended if other treatments are ineffective.
- *Education and support*:
    - *Patient education*: Learn about OA to better manage symptoms and understand treatment options.
    - *Support groups*: Joining a support group can provide emotional support and practical advice from others with similar experiences.
- *Follow-up*: Regular follow-up with your healthcare provider is crucial to monitor the condition, adjust treatment plans, and address any complications early.

CONCLUSION

Osteoarthritis remains a leading cause of disability among the older adults, underscoring the importance of early identification and individualized care strategies.

Patient education, regular exercise, achieving and maintaining a healthy weight can preserve mobility in early stage of the disease.

In diagnosed case of OA needs multidisciplinary care, lifestyle modifications, optimum pain management along with permissible exercise as per the expert and timely surgery can keep the older adults independent and improve quality of life.

Self-Assessment Questionnaire

Q1. What are the key anatomical structures that help stabilize and protect the knee joint from injury?

Q2. Describe the pathogenesis of osteoarthritis.

Q3. Why are elderly women more prone to osteoarthritis compared to men?

Q4. What are the typical clinical features and symptoms that help differentiate osteoarthritis from inflammatory arthritis?

Q5. How does obesity contribute to both the development and worsening of osteoarthritis pain?

Q6. What are the radiological features typically seen in a knee X-ray of a patient with osteoarthritis?

Q7. Outline the main nonpharmacological strategies for managing osteoarthritis in elderly patients.

Q8. When should surgical intervention, such as knee or hip replacement be considered in osteoarthritis management?

FURTHER READINGS

1. Halter JB, Ouslander JG, Studenski S, High KP, Asthana S, Supiano MA, Ritchie CS, Schmader K. Hazzard's Geriatric Medicine and Gerontology, 8th edition. New Delhi: McGraw Hill; 2022. pp. 813-24.
2. Jameson JL, Fauci AS, Kasper DL, Hauser SL, Longo DL, Loscalzo J (Eds). Harrison's Principles of Internal Medicine, 20th edition. New York: McGraw-Hill Education; 2018. pp. 10397-426.
3. Fillit HM, Rockwood K, Young JB. Brocklehurst's Textbook of Geriatric Medicine and Gerontology, 8th edition. Elsevier; 2016. pp. 552-6.

CHAPTER 29

Osteoporosis

Nidhi Soni

CASE VIGNETTE

Patient information: Mrs Rani, a 68-year-old female with a history of hypertension, bronchial asthma, and chronic heart failure. She had her menopause at the age of 55 years.

Living situation: Lives with her son and daughter-in-law in a joint family.

Primary care physician: Dr Kavya Verma.

Presenting complaint: Mrs Rani, a 68-year-old retired school principal, visits the outpatient clinic with right wrist pain and swelling following a fall on her outstretched hand in the bathroom.

History of present illness: Mrs Rani had a history of a fall in the bathroom in the morning. Since then, she is having pain and swelling in her wrist. She does not have any complaints of orthopnea, weakness, chest pain, palpitations, paroxysmal nocturnal dyspnea, or excessive bleeding.

Medical history: She is currently taking lisinopril for decreasing afterload, furosemide for reducing edema, atorvastatin for hypercholesterolemia, metoprolol for decreasing heart rate, omeprazole for stomach acidity, and prednisolone for her asthma. She also complains of reduced height over the years.

Social history: Mrs Rani lives with her son, her husband, and their two children in a joint family setup. She plays an active role in household activities, including helping to care for her grandchildren. She smokes one pack of cigarettes every day and occasionally takes alcohol. She does no exercise and is fully mobile with no disabilities.

Physical examination: During the physical examination, the patient is in acute distress and is oriented to time, place, and person. The patient weighs 60 kg and her blood pressure is 138/82 mm Hg and her heart rate is 78 beats/min. Examination reveals a slightly curved spine.

Other system examination: Respiratory system and cardiovascular examination did not reveal any significant abnormality. The right wrist is swollen and hurts to move. No edema was present anywhere else. All the peripheral pulses were palpable.

Investigations: Patient was sent for an X-ray, which reveals Colles fracture (distal radius) of the right hand. The patient was advised cast. Her blood investigations were normal except for low vitamin D. Her dual-energy X-ray absorptiometry (DEXA) scan revealed a T-score of –2.9. She was advised for X-ray of the thoracolumbar spine which showed multiple level vertebral collapse. She was started on bisphosphonates and vitamin D supplementation. She was advised for regular resistance exercises and eat a healthy diet.

INTRODUCTION

Osteoporosis is defined as a systemic skeletal disease characterized by low bone mineral density (BMD) and microarchitectural deterioration of bone tissue which leads to increased bone fragility and susceptibility to fractures. Diagnostic criteria by the World Health Organization (WHO) used standard deviation (SD) scores of BMD relative to peak bone mass in healthy young women, with osteoporosis being defined when BMD is ≤–2.5 SD and osteopenia being defined when T-score is between –1 and –2.5. The utility of BMD as a clinical indicator of osteoporosis is limited, as low BMD is one of the various risk factors for the fragility fracture. Osteoporosis-related/fragility fractures are fractures occurring in the setting of trauma less than or equal to a fall from a standing height, without major trauma such as a motor vehicle accident. Clinical diagnosis of osteoporosis can be made by the history of fragility fracture (particularly at spine, hip, wrist, humerus, and pelvis) without measuring BMD or calculating 10-year fracture risk by the fracture risk assessment tool (FRAX) algorithm. More than 50% of fractures among postmenopausal females occur in patients with osteopenia, as a proportion of this population is much more than patients with osteoporosis. Non-BMD factors contributing to fracture risk are falls, frailty, and poor bone quality. These fractures lead to increased psychosocial symptoms (depression, loss of self-esteem) as patients suffer from pain, physical limitations, and loss of independence.

EPIDEMIOLOGY

Fractures from osteoporosis are common in women >55 years and in men >65 years. This results in significant bone-related morbidities, mortalities, and healthcare costs. Approximately 30% of postmenopausal females have osteoporosis in the United States and Europe. One in three women over the age of 50 years and one in five men over the age of 50 years experience fragility fractures in their lifetime. In 2015, India had approximately 230 million people over the age of 50 years, of which 20% were osteoporotic women. Most of the data from India come from small studies. Prevalence of osteoporosis ranges from 8 to 62% in Indian women of different age groups and 8.5 to 24.6% in men. The peak incidence of osteoporosis occurs 10–20 years earlier in India than in Western countries, having a significant impact on health and economic resources. The Delhi Vertebral Osteoporosis Study (DeVOS) study reported a prevalence of 17.1% of vertebral fractures. Osteoporosis is a disease which is underdiagnosed and undertreated despite the availability of effective interventions and the poor consequences of fractures. As many as 80–95% of patients with hip fractures are discharged following surgical intervention with no management plan for osteoporosis. Timely intervention offers the opportunity to prevent the cycle of recurrent fractures, disability, and premature death in patients.

RISK FACTORS

All postmenopausal women and men >50 years should be evaluated for osteoporosis risk to determine the need for BMD testing and/or vertebral imaging. The more the number of risk factors, the higher the risk of fractures. Primary osteoporosis is osteoporosis because of aging or postmenopausal status. In patients suspected of having osteoporosis, evaluation is required to rule out secondary causes **(Box 1)**.

BOX 1 Nonmodifiable and modifiable risk factors for osteoporosis.

Nonmodifiable risk factors:
- Age
- Gender
- Peak bone mineral density
- Genetics
- Ethnicity

Modifiable risk factors:
- Lifestyle habits:
  - Sedentary lifestyle
  - Low physical activity
  - Decreased sunlight exposure (increased indoor living, traditional clothing use)
  - Smoking
  - Excessive alcohol
  - Excessive thinness (body weight <60 kg increases the risk of osteoporosis)
- Poor nutrition such as low calcium and vitamin D intake
- Hypogonadal states (estrogen deficiency due to premature menopause, androgen insensitivity)
- Medications:
  - Long-term steroids use
  - Proton-pump inhibitors
  - Anticonvulsants
  - Thiazolidinediones

Other risk factors are given as follows:
- Endocrine disorders such as diabetes mellitus (type 1 and type 2), Cushing's syndrome, hyperparathyroidism, thyrotoxicosis, and adrenal insufficiency
- *Gastrointestinal disorders*: Celiac disease, malabsorption, and gastrointestinal surgery
- *Hematologic disorders*: Multiple myeloma, leukemia, and lymphoma
- Rheumatologic diseases

Risk factors of osteoporotic fractures:
- Prior history of fractures
- Recurrent falls
- Poor eyesight
- Parental history of osteoporotic fractures

EVALUATION

Osteoporosis can affect both males and females and is most often undiagnosed until the patient visits a clinic for a fracture caused by minimal trauma. It is considered secondary until proven otherwise. There is no consensus definition of very high fracture risk, but different situations may include T-score ≤ –2.5 plus fragility fractures, T-score

≤ –3.0 in the absence of fragility fractures, or history of multiple or severe fractures. The patient should be evaluated comprehensively with detailed assessment of individual fracture risk, history, physical examination, focused studies to rule out secondary causes, and vertebral imaging to detect prevalent fractures.

History

History should include inquiry of risk factors of osteoporosis such as past medical conditions, drug exposure, dietary history, history of fragility fractures in parents, prior history of fragility fractures in the patient, any addiction history (smoking), and height loss of >4 cm in postmenopausal women. Any fractures can cause chronic pain, reduced mobility, increased dependence on others, and mortality. For women, age at menarche and menstrual, obstetric, and menopausal histories, including use of hormones, should be sought.

Examination

On examination, the patient can present with loss of height (due to multiple vertebral compression fractures), dorsal kyphosis, chest deformity, restrictive lung disease (due to thoracic spine fractures), a protuberant abdomen, persistent back pain from altered biomechanics, and sciatica (due to lumbar spine fractures).

Evaluation and Investigations

Dual-energy X-ray absorptiometry is the preferred method for diagnosing osteoporosis by measuring BMD. The purpose of measuring BMD is to identify individuals at high risk of fractures so that preventive strategies can be used and to determine patients' response to therapy **(Box 2)**.

In patients with osteopenia, clinical diagnosis of osteoporosis is made when FRAX 10-year probability of major osteoporotic fracture (clinical vertebral, hip, forearm, or proximal humerus) is ≥20% or the 10-year probability of hip fracture is ≥3%. FRAX is an online tool and uses femoral neck BMD (g/cm^2) and clinical risk factors including age, gender, parental history of hip fracture, RA, alcohol intake (3 or more drinks/day), BMI (low body mass index, kg/m^2), oral glucocorticoid intake ≥ 5 mg/day of prednisone for >3 months (ever), prior history of osteoporotic fractures (including clinical and subclinical vertebral fractures), current smoking, and presence of secondary causes of osteoporosis for calculation of fracture probability. FRAX is validated for patients aged 40–90 years. It was tested in treatment-naïve patients but can be used to assess risk in previously treated patients, who have stopped bisphosphonate for 2 years or nonbisphosphonate therapy for 1 year. The FRAX tool has some potential limitations. Multiple other factors such as non-DXA bone density measurements, frailty, multiple comorbid conditions, polypharmacy, and presence of multiple fractures experienced in a short period of time are not included in the FRAX algorithm due to nonavailability of significant data. FRAX is not validated for use with lumbar spine BMD, which might underestimate risk in patients with low BMD at the lumbar spine while normal BMD at the femoral neck.

BOX 2 International policy frameworks on aging.

- Women aged 60 years and older and men aged 65 years and older, regardless of clinical risk factors
- Postmenopausal women younger than 60 years, women in the menopausal transition, and men aged 50–64 years when there are concerns for osteoporosis based on their clinical risk factor profile
- Individuals who have had a fragility fracture after the age of 50 years
- Individuals with a condition (e.g., rheumatoid arthritis, diabetes mellitus, malabsorption syndrome) or who are taking medication (e.g., glucocorticoids in a daily dose ≥5 mg prednisone or equivalent for ≥3 months, androgen deprivation therapy) associated with low bone mass or bone loss
- Any individual being considered for pharmacologic therapy for osteoporosis

(BMD: bone mineral density)

In patients with a history of fragility fractures, BMD measurement is not necessary for initiating treatment, but baseline measurement of BMD is helpful to assess the severity of osteoporosis and to monitor treatment response. Most of the vertebral fractures are either subclinical or clinically asymptomatic and may go unnoticed for many years. Most of the women with asymptomatic vertebral fractures may have BMD levels not warranting treatment. So, if vertebral fractures are diagnosed, it may change the patient's diagnostic classification and treatment decision **(Box 3)**.

The methods for identification of vertebral fractures are lateral thoracic or lumbar spine X-ray or DXA-assisted vertebral fracture assessment (DXA-VFA). Baseline DXA-VFA can also help in future comparison when BMD is reassessed or the patient develops new symptoms such as prospective height loss, new backache, or postural changes or when the patient is considered for a drug holiday (as patients with recent vertebral fractures are not advised for discontinuing antifracture therapy). Other technologies can also be used to assess BMD, bone structure, bone strength, and fracture risk. These include quantitative computed tomography (QCT) and quantitative ultrasound. Some technologies largely used in research are peripheral QCT (pQCT), high-resolution pQCT, and magnetic resonance imaging (MRI).

Quantitative ultrasound is not recommended for screening or initial decision-making regarding osteoporosis treatment.

Laboratory tests include evaluating the underlying cause of osteoporosis. Basic biochemical and hormonal profile includes calcium, phosphorus, total alkaline phosphatase, 25-hydroxyvitamin D, thyroid function tests, creatinine, complete blood count, liver function tests, and intact parathyroid hormone (iPTH) to rule out secondary causes of osteoporosis. If height loss is reported, imaging of the thoracic and lumbar spine should be performed to rule out vertebral compression fractures.

Specific tests to be done in suspected secondary osteoporosis:

- Erythrocyte sedimentation rate and serum electrophoresis to rule out multiple myeloma
- Serum testosterone and estradiol in males and females, respectively, in suspected hypogonadism
- Overnight dexamethasone suppression test for Cushing's syndrome
- Fasting blood sugar, postprandial blood glucose, and glycated hemoglobin for diabetes mellitus
- Immunoglobulin A (IgA) tissue-transglutaminase for suspected celiac disease

Bone Turnover Markers

Bone turnover markers (BTMs) are dynamic parameters reflecting short-term and acute changes in bone remodeling status not measured by BMD. They have no role in the diagnosis of osteoporosis but can be used for follow-up of patients who are on antiosteoporotic medications.

BOX 3 Indications for vertebral imaging [Bone Health and Osteoporosis Foundation (BHOF)].

- All women aged ≥ 65 years and all men aged 80 years and more if T-score at lumbar spine, total hip, or femoral neck is ≤–1.0
- Men aged 70–79 years if T-score at lumbar spine, total hip, or femoral neck is ≤–1.5
- Postmenopausal women and men ≥50 years with specific risk factors:
    - Fracture during adulthood (age ≥ 50 years)
    - Historical height loss of 1.5 inches (4 cm) or more (current height compared to peak height in young adulthood)
    - Prospective height loss of 0.8 inch (2 cm) or more (cumulative height loss measured during interval medical assessment)
    - Recent or ongoing long-term glucocorticoid treatment
    - Medical conditions associated with bone loss such as hyperparathyroidism

Note: If BMD testing is not available, vertebral imaging is considered on the basis of age alone.

(BMD: bone mineral density)

MANAGEMENT

The goal of management of osteoporosis is to prevent fractures. Several pharmacological agents are available with different mechanisms of action: Reducing bone resorption or stimulating bone formation. Since this is a chronic condition, it might require long term with sometimes lifelong management. A history of fragility fracture is an important risk factor for subsequent fracture and requires medical treatment **(Box 4)**. Pharmacologic therapy is also recommended in patients with osteoporosis based on BMD or high fracture risk on FRAX (done for high-risk postmenopausal women with T-score between –1.0 and –2.5). For patients with low bone mass (osteopenia) with no prior fragility fracture or low-to-moderate fracture risk on FRAX, pharmacologic therapy is not recommended. All patients should have normal serum calcium and 25-hydroxyvitamin D prior to starting pharmacotherapy. All antifracture therapeutics treat but do not cure the disease. No uniform recommendation applies to all patients, and treatment should be individualized. Patients found to have secondary causes of bone fragility may require no additional therapy once their underlying conditions are treated.

Lifestyle Measures to Reduce Bone Loss (Table 1)

All individuals should adopt lifestyle measures, including adequate intake of calcium and vitamin D, exercise, cessation of smoking and excessive alcohol intake, and avoiding drugs which increase bone loss (such as steroids).

Choice of Pharmacologic Therapy

The current Food and Drug Administration (FDA)-approved pharmacologic therapeutics for prevention and/or treatment of postmenopausal osteoporosis include

BOX 4 Indications for antiosteoporotic therapy.

- History of fragility fracture (vertebral or nonvertebral)
- In patients aged > 50 years with osteoporosis measured by DEXA
- In individuals with osteopenia and clinical risk factors or high fracture risk on FRAX tool

(DEXA: dual-energy X-ray absorptiometry; FRAX: fracture risk assessment tool)

bisphosphonates (oral and intravenous), estrogens (hormone therapy), estrogen agonist/antagonist (raloxifene), parathyroid hormone (teriparatide), analog of parathyroid hormone-related peptide (abaloparatide), RANKL inhibitor (denosumab), fully human monoclonal antibody to sclerostin (romosozumab), and calcitonin **(Table 2)**.

There is limited data on the efficacy of the drugs in patients with secondary osteoporosis or men diagnosed with osteoporosis (majority of the studies have been conducted in postmenopausal women). In general, therapy with effects on both vertebral and nonvertebral fractures (alendronate, risedronate, zoledronic acid, denosumab, teriparatide, abaloparatide, or romosozumab) should be preferred over drugs with limited efficacy (raloxifene, calcitonin, and ibandronate). The choice of medication depends on efficacy, cost, long-term safety, convenience, and the individual's fracture risk.

Bisphosphonates: Oral Bisphosphonates are the First-line Therapy

- *Efficacy*: Reduce fracture rates (vertebral by 50–70%, nonvertebral by 20–30%, and hip by 40%)
- *Administration*: Oral bisphosphonates must be taken on an empty stomach, first thing in the morning with

TABLE 1: Summary of lifestyle measures to prevent osteoporosis.

Calcium	Approximately 1,000 mg daily either from diet or calcium supplements
Vitamin D	• 1,000–2,000 IU/day to maintain optimum serum 25-hydroxyvitamin D ≥ 20 ng/mL (≥30 ng/mL in patients with known or suspected metabolic bone disease) • Higher doses if malabsorption or concomitant intake of antiseizure medications, etc.
Diet	Adequate caloric intake to avoid malnutrition and adequate protein intake (~0.8 g/kg body weight/day)
Exercise	Weight-bearing exercise 30 minutes on most days of the week, muscle-strengthening and balance exercise 2–3 days/week. Brisk walking is a safe weight-bearing exercise in patients with frailty or a history of vertebral fractures. No significant evidence of the impact of the intensity of exercise on bone health
Smoking	Smoking cessation is strongly recommended
Alcohol	• Excess alcohol intake is detrimental to skeletal health • Limit to not >2 units/day

TABLE 2: US FDA-approved drugs for osteoporosis.

Antiresorptive agents: • Target and block osteoclast activity to decrease bone resorption and BMD loss • Side effects: hypocalcemia, osteonecrosis of jaw (ONJ)*, and atypical femur fracture (AFF)**	*Anabolic agents:* • Stimulates PTH receptor to stimulate osteoblasts and bone formation and activate bone remodeling
Bisphosphonates: • Alendronate: 70 mg PO weekly • Risedronate: 35 mg PO weekly • Ibandronate: 150 mg PO monthly • Zoledronate: 5 mg IV annually	*Parathyroid hormone analogs:* • Teriparatide: 20 µg subcutaneously daily for a maximum of 2 years • Abaloparatide: 80 µg daily subcutaneous injection in the periumbilical area of the abdomen. Treatment duration not to exceed 24 months
RANK-ligand inhibitor: • Denosumab: 60 mg subcutaneously every 6 months	
Estrogen-related therapy: • Raloxifene: 60 mg orally daily	
Sclerostin inhibitor: • Romosozumab: 210 mg monthly subcutaneous injections for 1 year • Monoclonal antibody to sclerostin has both antiresorptive and anabolic properties	

*ONJ: rare side effect and associated with high-dose use or prolonged duration use. Good oral hygiene practices and regular dental care may be the optimal method to reduce the risk of drug-related ONJ.

**AFF: Rare side effect and high risk of AFF are associated with Asian ethnicity, lateral bowing of the femur, autoimmune disease, or glucocorticoid use. It is important to make patients understand that these side effects are rare, and the risk of fracture is much higher if not treated.

(BMD: bone mineral density; FDA: Food and Drug Administration; IV: intravenous; PTH: parathyroid hormone)

a full glass of plain water, and after taking medication, the patient must remain upright for at least 30–60 minutes before eating/drinking or taking any other medication. To reduce the likelihood of acute-phase reactions with zoledronate, the patient should be well hydrated by taking at least two glasses of water before infusion and pretreatment with acetaminophen.
- *Selection of oral bisphosphonates*: Alendronate is the preferred agent. Risedronate is a reasonable alternative.
- *Adverse effects of bisphosphonates*: Hypocalcemia, esophagitis, and acute-phase reaction with the first infusion of zoledronate occur in around 32% of patients and consist of fever, myalgia, and flu-like symptoms lasting 24–72 hours. Other rare side effects are atypical femur fracture (AFF), osteonecrosis of jaw (ONJ), and ocular inflammation (anterior uveitis and episcleritis).
- *Contraindications*: Oral bisphosphonates are not indicated in patients with esophageal disorders (achalasia, scleroderma involving esophagus, esophageal strictures), inability to follow dosing requirements (stay upright for at least 30–60 minutes), advanced chronic kidney disease (CKD) [estimated glomerular filtration rate (eGFR) < 30–35 mL/min/1.73 m^2], or in patients with history of bariatric surgery with gastrointestinal tract anastomosis.

If the patient has contraindications for oral bisphosphonates (except CKD), intravenous bisphosphonates (zoledronic acid) are recommended.

Recent fractures should not preclude use of bisphosphonates, which can be started after 2 weeks post fracture if the patient is able to sit upright for at least 30 minutes for oral bisphosphonates.

RANKL Inhibitor

Denosumab is an alternative medication for patients with contraindication or reluctance or unresponsive to bisphosphonates:
- *Mechanism of action (MOA)*: Monoclonal antibody against RANKL that potently inhibits osteoclast development and activity.
- *Indication*: Patients who have failed or are intolerant to other available therapies.
- *Drug efficacy*: Reduces incidence of vertebral fractures by about 68% at 1 year, hip fractures by 40%, and other nonvertebral fractures by 20% at 3 years
- *Precaution*: Antifracture effects of denosumab are similar to those of the bisphosphonates, but there is a pronounced loss of antiresorptive effect from 7 months after the last injection, which can result in clusters of rebound vertebral fractures. Therefore, the need for indefinite treatment should be discussed with patient, and if it has to be discontinued, administering an alternative therapy is advised to prevent rapid bone loss.
- *Adverse effects*: Hypocalcemia, musculoskeletal pain, hypersensitivity reactions, rare cases of AFF and ONJ

Estrogen-related Therapies

Raloxifene is an estrogen agonist/antagonist [selective estrogen receptor modulator (SERM)]:
- *Indication*: To prevent vertebral fractures in postmenopausal women with low risk of deep venous thrombosis for whom other drugs are not appropriate or in women with a history of/high risk of breast cancer.
- *Drug efficacy*: Reduce risk of vertebral fractures by 30–40% (if prior history of vertebral fracture) and 55% (no prior vertebral fracture). No efficacy on nonvertebral fractures
- *Side effects*: Deep venous thrombosis, hot flashes, and leg cramps

Parathyroid Hormone-1 Receptor Analog

It is an anabolic agent:
- *MOA*: Constant high exposure to PTH causes bone resorption, while intermittent exposure to exogenous recombinant PTH stimulates bone formation. Two FDA-approved agents are teriparatide and abaloparatide, respectively.
- *Indication*: This is the potential medication for patients with a very high fracture risk. Also indicated in patients with intolerance/poor response to bisphosphonates. This is not the initial therapy for most of the patients.
- *Efficacy*: Teriparatide reduces the risk of vertebral fractures by 65–77% and nonvertebral fractures by 35–53%, after an average of 18 months of therapy. Abaloparatide reduces the risk of new vertebral fractures by 86% and nonvertebral fractures by 43% in postmenopausal women with osteoporosis after 18 months of therapy.
- *Administration*: Teriparatide needs daily subcutaneous injection initially limited to 1.5–2 years, recently changed to open the possibility of longer treatment in high-risk patients (high risk is defined as history of osteoporotic fracture and/or multiple risk factors for fracture).
- *Side effects*: Transient orthostatic hypotension, leg cramps, nausea, transient hypercalcemia

- *Contraindication*: Previous history of radiation to skeleton, Paget's disease of the bone, history of bone metastasis or malignancies, and unexplained elevated alkaline phosphatase (prolonged use is seen to be associated with osteosarcoma in rodent studies)
- Anabolic agents have greater antifracture efficacy and cause a greater increase in BMD, but the efficacy is transient, so these drugs will require transition to antiresorptive drugs to preserve the gains in BMD.

Sclerostin Inhibitor

Romosozumab is an anabolic agent:

- *MOA*: Antisclerostin monoclonal antibody stimulates bone formation and inhibits bone resorption.
- *Indication*: Treatment of osteoporosis in post-menopausal women at high risk of fracture (approved for males in some countries)
- *Drug efficacy*: In the pivotal FRAME trial, 12 months of romosozumab reduces new vertebral fractures by 73% and clinical fractures by 36%.
- *Black box warning*: Increased risk of myocardial infarction, stroke, and cardiovascular death and should not be initiated in a patient with a history of cardiovascular event in the last 1 year

Specific Situations

- *Osteoporosis in CKD patients and those in hemodialysis*:
  - Bisphosphonates are contraindicated in stage 4 and 5 kidney disease (eGFR below 30–35 mL/min/1.73 m^2).
  - Denosumab is not cleared by the kidneys and, hence, can be used in these patients, but the risk of hypocalcemia is there. Hence, maintain an optimal intake of calcium and vitamin D before starting denosumab.
  - Major concern with antiresorptive therapy is dynamic bone disease and selected patients should undergo undecalcified iliac bone biopsy if facilities are available to guide correct decision-making for osteoporosis.
- *Use of hormone replacement therapy (HRT)*:
  - HRT is effective but not recommended for osteoporosis management due to high risk of side effects such as cardiac events and breast cancer. Nonestrogen treatment should be considered first.
  - Testosterone supplementation may be used in androgen-deficient men, if accompanied by signs or symptoms of androgen deficiency (low libido, loss of body hair, unexplained fatigue, hot flushes). If there is no benefit in 3–6 months, it should be discontinued, and alternative therapy should be considered.
- *Intranasal calcitonin*: It is no longer commonly used for osteoporosis. It is banned in a few places for its risk-benefit (rhinitis, epistaxis, allergic reactions, and high risk of malignancy) profile.
- *Combination therapies*: These have not shown additional benefit for fracture prevention as compared to monotherapies. There are variable results. Two antiresorptive therapies are not recommended. But sequential therapies, with anabolic agents followed by antiresorptive agents, are recommended.

Follow-up for Patients with Osteoporosis

Bisphosphonates are the first line and most preferred therapy for osteoporosis. But different studies have shown variable compliance with medications, thus requiring regular follow-up of the patients. Follow-up is also required to observe the efficacy and side effects of the medications. The diagnosis of osteoporosis persists even if subsequent DEXA T-scores are >–2.5.

Frequency of Follow-up

No consensus exists for the frequency of follow-up. The first follow-up can be planned after 3 months, then 3–6 monthly for the initial two to three visits, and then annually.

Clinical Follow-up

History

At each visit, the patient should be enquired about any new incident fracture, new onset/worsening of kyphosis, scoliosis, new onset or worsening of backache, and change in height. The history of falls is a predictor of future falls and should be specifically enquired. History suggestive of possible side effects of antiosteoporosis therapy such as jaw pain and thigh pain should be elicited.

Physical Examination

Physical examination includes examining height, spinal tenderness, kyphosis, scoliosis, and oral hygiene. If patients are on antiresorptive medications with poor oral hygiene, a dental opinion is required.

Biochemical Evaluation

Serum 25-hydroxyvitamin D is estimated every 6 months for the initial two to three visits, to ensure optimal levels of vitamin D of at least 20 ng/mL.

Teriparatide treatment sometimes causes hypercalcemia. Serum calcium should be monitored initially after 12 hours, and the dose of oral supplements is to be reduced or stopped if hypercalcemia exists or persists simultaneously.

Radiology

Radiograph of the spine may be ordered annually in patients with new-onset or worsening backache or kyphosis to rule out any incident vertebral fracture. This can guide for patients being considered for a bisphosphonate holiday, since discontinuing therapy would not be advisable in patients with recent vertebral fractures. Radiograph of the upper femur is advised when a patient presents with thigh pain to rule out atypical femoral fracture in patients on antiresorptive therapy. Computed tomography of the jaw is advised to rule out osteonecrosis of the jaw in patients on antiresorptive therapy.

Bone Mineral Density

Monitoring of BMD by DEXA scan is recommended every 1–2 years. This identifies individuals who do not adhere to the treatment or have a secondary cause of osteoporosis. If the BMD increases above the least significant change (LSC), the treatment response is considered good. Studies have shown that improvement in BMD has a good correlation with a reduction in fracture risk. Change in BMD of the lumbar spine is more robust, and change in hip BMD is less dramatic. Stable BMD is also acceptable, but a drop in BMD beyond LSC (at least 5% in lumbar spine, 4% in total hip, and 5% in femoral neck) over 2 years indicates treatment failure. A history of two or more incident fractures, especially vertebral fractures, also indicates treatment failure. In these patients with treatment failure, low compliance, inadequate dosing, vitamin D deficiency, and other secondary causes need to be considered. It is important to be aware of certain limitations of bone densitometry. Degenerative changes or a new fracture can falsely give the impression of BMD gain. For meaningful interpretations, serial scans should be performed on the same densitometry device at the same facility.

Bone Turnover Markers

BTMs reflect bone turnover status. These are dynamic parameters reflecting short-term/acute changes in bone which are often missed by BMD. Hence, they can reflect treatment response earlier than BMD and can be used to monitor compliance and adherence to medical treatment. Though both absolute values and degree of change can be used, but considering ethnic variations in BTMs, the degree of change is more reasonable. The recommended BTMs are serum type 1 collagen C-telopeptide (CTx) and serum procollagen type 1 N-propeptide (PINP). CTx and PINP can be measured at baseline and then repeated at 3, 6, and 12 months after starting treatment with antiresorptive medications to evaluate patient adherence and drug effectiveness. PINP can be used for evaluating adherence to anabolic agents, with measurements at baseline, 3, 6, and 12 months. A decrease in CTx by at least 30% or 100 ng/mL from pretreatment value is expected in patients on antiresorptive therapy, while a threshold of 20% or >10 μg/mL from baseline for PINP is considered clinically significant.

Fall Prevention

Most fractures are associated with a fall. Falls occur in more than one third of the population, >65 years of age, with risk increasing with age. The risk of falls is higher in patients with a previous history of falls. A comprehensive evaluation should be done for these patients, and they should be educated about fall prevention. Modifiable risk factors associated with falls such as medications (sedating/hypnotic), polypharmacy, hypotension, gait and balance disorders, or visual impairment should be identified and addressed. Physical therapy and exercise regimens have been effective in reducing fall risk. In community-dwelling patients, at-home fall hazard evaluation should be done, followed by remediation.

CONCLUSION

Osteoporosis is a common but underdiagnosed condition in older adults, with significant health impacts due to fractures and associated loss of independence. Early diagnosis through standardised tools like DEXA scans is critical for timely intervention and reduction of fracture risk.

Geriatrician must be vigilant to screen for osteoporosis. A combination of lifestyle modifications, along with weight-bearing exercise can help to prevent bone loss and fractures. A multidisciplinary approach involving geriatricians, primary care physician, and orthopedician, physiotherapist would be the best approach in confirmed cases with due consideration on comorbidities and fall risk.

Self-Assessment Questionnaire

Q1. What is osteoporosis and epidemiology of osteoporosis?

Q2. What is the prevalence of osteoporosis and fragility fractures in older patients in India?

Q3. Who should undergo a bone density test?

Q4. How is a diagnosis of osteoporosis established?

Q5. How to evaluate a patient with osteoporosis?

Q6. Who should be treated for osteoporosis?

Q7. How should patients be monitored for response to therapy?

Q8. For how long should patients be treated? What is a drug holiday and which patients should be considered for it?

Q9. What is the role of a geriatric physician in the management of osteoporosis?

FURTHER READINGS

1. Bhadada SK, Chadha M, Sriram U, Pal R, Paul TV, Khadgawat R, et al. The Indian Society for Bone and Mineral Research (ISBMR) position statement for the diagnosis and treatment of osteoporosis in adults. Arch Osteoporos. 2021;16(1):102.
2. Sabri SA, Chavarria JC, Ackert-Bicknell C, Swanson C, Burger E. Osteoporosis: an update on screening, diagnosis, evaluation, and treatment. orthopedics. 2023;46(1):e20-6.
3. LeBoff MS, Greenspan SL, Insogna KL, Lewiecki EM, Saag KG, Singer AJ, et al. The clinician's guide to prevention and treatment of osteoporosis. Osteoporos Int. 2022;33(10):2049-102.

CHAPTER 30

Psychiatric Disorders in Older Population: Depression, Anxiety Disorder, Somatoform Disorder and Schizophrenia

Preethy Kathiresan, Raja Babu Ramawat

CASE VIGNETTES

Case Vignette 1

Ms X, a 75-year-old widow, presented with a history of low mood, decreased energy, and death wishes for the past 1 month. Around 1 month back, her son who was staying with her had to shift to another place due to transfer in his job. Following that, she started to have low mood, which initially was present only when she thought about her son but gradually increased throughout the day. The low mood would be present throughout the day and would not improve even when she watched her favorite TV shows or talked to her grandson, which earlier used to give her happiness. She would be often found crying in her room. She would also report that she does not find pleasure in listening to *bhajans* which she used to enjoy previously. Waking up in the morning and doing daily chores would appear as a burden to her, and she would keep on lying on the bed for most of the time. She reduced her interaction with other family members and started to avoid meeting relatives or friends who used to come to visit her. She would feel that she has become a burden on her family as she is not able to help in any household chores. She believed that her condition would never become better, and no one would be able to help her. She also complained of increased forgetfulness and would not be able to remember where she kept her glasses or her walking stick. Her sleep reduced to 1–2 h/day, her appetite also reduced significantly, and she ate only one to two *rotis* in the whole day. She would express that it would be better if she died and would pray to God to take her life. However, she denied any suicidal ideas. She stays on bed the whole day and does not talk to anyone.

Other relevant history: Ms X has comorbid diabetes, which is under control with medications for the past 10 years. There are no other medical comorbidities or substance use. There has been past history of three similar depressive episodes—around 10 years back, 5 years back, and 3 years back; all three lasted for around 3–4 months and improved with medications. There is a family history of depression in her brother who died by suicide.

Physical examination and investigations: No abnormality has been detected.

Mental status examination: Decreased psychomotor activity; affect—depressed; speech—increased reaction time; thought content—death wishes; decreased self-confidence; ideas of hopelessness, helplessness, and worthlessness; pessimistic views of future; attention and concentration—aroused but ill sustained; and partial insight.

Impression: Recurrent Depressive Disorder, Current Episode—Severe without Psychotic Symptoms

The above case vignette has shown the presence of the following criteria which enable us to diagnose depression—"persistent and pervasive sadness of mood"—sadness which is present for most part of the day (persistent) and present even when exposed to happy situations (pervasive); "anhedonia," i.e., finding reduced pleasure in activities which gave her pleasure in the past such as listening to *bhajans*; "fatigue," i.e., feeling even simple tasks as burden and having low energy, having "reduced verbal interaction," *ideas of hopelessness* (feeling that her condition will never become better), *ideas of helplessness* (thought that no one can help her), *ideas of worthlessness* (she has become a burden on her family), *reduced attention and concentration* (may present as forgetfulness), *disturbance in sleep, disturbance in appetite, and death wishes*. Due to the significant dysfunction caused by the disorder, the depression is considered to be severe. Since there have been past episodes of depression, the diagnosis is recurrent depressive disorder.

Case Vignette 2 (Anxiety Disorder)

Mrs M, a 69-year-old female, a retired librarian with a history of type 2 diabetes and hypertension for the past 20 years (well controlled with medications), living in a joint family of middle socioeconomic status, was maintaining well till around 3 years back. Around 3 years back, during the COVID-19 pandemic, she started to feel anxious, whenever her family used to go out or someone used to knock the door, and had the fear that someone or the other might catch COVID. This used to last only for 5–10 minutes at that time. However, gradually the anxiety started to increase in duration and started to occur for around 6–7 hours daily over the next 6 months. Even when the COVID lockdown lifted, and the incidence of COVID cases reduced, her symptoms did not reduce. She started to have feelings of anxiety, feeling keyed up or on edge, and feeling of worry about some or the other trivial day-to-day work of household such as cooking food on time or closing the door properly. Whenever her family would go out, she would have constant worry and repeatedly call them to ensure whether they are safe. She also started to complain of feelings of palpitations (*gabrahat*), sweating, trembling of hands and legs, feeling of tingling sensation in her legs, sometimes associated with nausea or abdominal distress, for the past 1.5 years, which initially used to last for 15–20 minutes for two to three times in a day. However, these symptoms also gradually increased and are present for most time of the day for the past 2 months. She also complains of increased frequency of nightmares for the past 1 month.

Other relevant history: No past history or family history of any psychiatric illness.

Physical examination and laboratory investigations: No abnormality detected.

Mental status examination: Increased psychomotor activity (fidgeting and restless), affect—anxious, thought content—anxious ruminations, and attention and concentration—aroused but ill sustained.

Impression: Generalized Anxiety Disorder

In the patient in the above case vignette, even though the symptoms initially started with normal fear related to COVID, these symptoms gradually increased in both intensity and duration. The anxiety in her case is free-floating anxiety and is not specific to any particular situation or object. She has cognitive symptoms of anxiety (anxious ruminations, excessive worries about trivial issues) as well as physiological/physical symptoms (palpitations, sweating, tremors, feeling on tingling sensation, nausea, and abdominal distress) and behavioral symptoms (repeatedly calling family to ensure that they are safe). In all cases of anxiety symptoms in the elderly, the first and foremost step is to rule out organic causes for the same. Since in this case vignette, the medical comorbidities are well under control, the patient is diagnosed to have generalized anxiety disorder based on the history.

Case Vignette 3 (Psychotic Spectrum Disorder)

Mr Ramesh Singh, a 66-year-old male with a history of type 2 diabetes, hypertension, and benign prostatic hypertrophy living in a joint family, was brought to the hospital by his family members, with no complaints from the patient's side. The son of the patient reported that there has been a change in the patient's behavior for the past 6–8 months, such that the patient would appear fearful and would tell that someone is behind him and wants to kill him; however, there would be no such person in actuality. Also, in some instances, the patient would report hearing voices of a few people which would only be heard by the patient. The patient would report these voices to be discussing about him in their conversation. Even when the family deny any such voices in the vicinity, the patient would not believe them and check various places in his home to find where they were hiding. The patient would often be found talking or muttering to self. He would also be found spitting on his hand and scanning the garbage repeatedly and would not give any explanation for the same. His sleep had reduced to around 1–2 h/day and he would take bath only once in 2–3 days. His appetite remained normal.

Medical and psychiatric history: Mr Singh has a history of type 2 diabetes, managed with oral medication, and hypertension, for which he takes antihypertensive medications. For benign prostatic hypertrophy, the patient would regularly be taking medications. He was apparently maintained well on her regular medications on both the medical comorbidities. There have not been any recent changes in medication or dosages. There is no past history of any psychiatric illness.

Family history: There has been a family history of psychiatric illness in his younger brother, with complaints suggestive of schizophrenia.

Physical examination and laboratory findings: No abnormality detected.

Impression: Schizophrenia

The above case vignette shows the presence of "delusion of persecution," "auditory hallucinations," *disorganized behavior* (spitting on hand, scanning garbage repeatedly), *reduced self-care, and reduced sleep*, which show the presence of psychotic symptoms in the patient.

Case Vignette 4 (Somatoform Disorder)

Mrs K, a 66-year-old female, presented with a history of chronic headache, backache, nausea, bloating sensation, chest pain, and episodes of dizziness for the past 5 years with no improvement on treatment from multiple doctors. She had been evaluated by gastroenterologist, cardiologist, neurologist, and ENT specialist, and all the relevant investigations done have revealed no major pathology which can lead to persistence of these symptoms. The patient reports an increase in distress due to these symptoms and repeatedly requests for relief from her symptoms. She denies any depressive or anxiety symptoms. Although her physical examinations and tests consistently yield normal results, Mrs K remains unconvinced. She expresses frustration and distrust toward medical professionals, often asking for repeat investigations or second opinions. She has stopped doing any household activities which she used to do previously, as well as avoids going to family functions or other social gatherings (where she used to go previously), believing that her symptoms might worsen. Despite reassurances, Mrs K remains fixated on her belief that something is seriously wrong with her health and that the doctors are not able to find the cause. However, she does not believe to have any particular disorder. On further exploration, it is found that there had been frequent conflicts in her family, between her two sons, with respect to the property issues for the past 5 years. However, the patient denies any excessive worries related to the same and reports that she is more concerned about her physical symptoms as it is very distressing for her.

Impression: Bodily Distress Disorder (International Classification of Diseases 11th Revision)

The above case vignette demonstrates the presence of multiple somatic complaints in different systems of the body (nervous system—headache, dizziness; gastrointestinal system—nausea, abdominal distress; orthopedics—backache); and cardiovascular system—chest pain, dizziness) which cannot be explained by any physical illness, or based on any laboratory investigations. Also, the patient has significant preoccupation with the symptoms leading to significant dysfunction in her life (stopped all her household activities, reduced social interaction). The symptoms are persisting despite repeated reassurances by doctors and family. Also, there is a presence of continuous stress in the form of conflicts between the sons. All these points toward the presence of somatoform disorder.

INTRODUCTION

With the advancement of medical research and technology in the current century, the mortality rate is significantly decreasing, and life expectancies are increasing, which is leading to an increase in the geriatric population across the world, including India. With the significant rise in the geriatric population, there has been an increasing need for a special focus on the unique psychological needs and issues faced by this group.

Multiple factors unique to the elderly make them more vulnerable to psychological issues, such as increased prevalence of medical or physical comorbidities, mobility issues secondary to physical problems, financial constraints, social neglect, role transition (retirement, etc.), bereavement due to loss of loved ones, etc. Among the various psychiatric disorders, the most common disorders among the elderly are depression, anxiety disorders, and dementia. Severe mental disorders, namely schizophrenia and bipolar disorder, also cause significant dysfunction and impair the quality of life.

As a medical practitioner, it is necessary to screen, diagnose, and manage psychiatric disorders due to multiple reasons: (1) There is a huge prevalence of psychiatric disorders in the elderly, which is often undiagnosed and leads to reduction in quality of life; (2) Psychiatric disorders can affect the compliance to medications as well as lifestyle modifications required to control medical disorders, affecting the prognosis (e.g., self-neglect, changes in appetite, decreased physical activity, secondary to psychiatric disorders, can increase risk of malnutrition or obesity); (3) Psychiatric disorders per se can increase the risk of medical disorders; (4) Medical disorders as well as medications used for medical disorders can increase the risk of psychiatric disorders; and (5) Management of psychiatric disorder can improve the outcome of both medical and psychiatric disorders.

Hence, assessment and management of psychiatric comorbidities in the elderly should be a part of the holistic care for the elderly. This chapter aims to provide a comprehensive overview of the common psychiatric disorders in the elderly, namely depression, anxiety disorder, and somatoform disorder, as well as severe mental disorders in the elderly, namely schizophrenia and bipolar disorder, their clinical signs and symptoms, screening and assessment, prevention, and management aspects.

EPIDEMIOLOGY OF PSYCHIATRIC DISORDERS AMONG ELDERLY

More than 20% of adults over the age of 60 years suffer from a mental or neurological disorder, contributing to 6.6% of all disabilities in this age group and is one of the significant contributors to the disease burden of the elderly.

As per the Longitudinal Aging Study in India (LASI), the prevalence of depression among the elderly aged 60 years and above in India is 8.3%. However, the self-reported prevalence of depression was just 0.8%, which shows the high prevalence of undiagnosed depression among elderly in India. Another systematic review and meta-analysis of 51 studies from 16 states in India found the prevalence of depression among elderly in India to be around 34.4% [95% confidence interval (CI) 29.3–39.7]. Depression has been found to be more common among females, those with lower literacy and from rural background, those with a larger number of medical comorbidities, poor self-perceived health, and poor coping skills.

The next most common mental disorder among the elderly is anxiety disorders. *A meta-analysis of 23 studies in India found the prevalence of anxiety disorders among elderly to be around 8.7% (95% CI 2.4–38.8).* The most common anxiety disorder seen in the clinical practice among elderly is *generalized anxiety disorder (GAD) (7.3%), followed by* phobias (3.1%), panic disorder (1%), and obsessive–compulsive disorder (OCD) (0.6%). Anxiety disorders are more common among females or those who had lower income, had less social contact frequency, did not have children, or had negative or traumatic life events.

The prevalence of somatoform disorders among the elderly varies widely between 1.5 and 13%. Schizophrenia affects approximately 0.1–0.5% of older adults, which is very less than the overall lifetime prevalence of schizophrenia in general population (which is around 1%). This reduced prevalence in older adults can be attributed to the higher rate of premature mortality (from various causes) among individuals with schizophrenia. Very late-onset schizophrenia (onset after 60 years of age) is more common among females and frequently has comorbid cognitive impairment.

CLINICAL HISTORY OF PSYCHIATRIC DISORDERS

A detailed history forms an important part of psychiatric evaluation. In case of elderly, as cognitive impairment is common, history often needs to be taken from the family members or caregivers along with the patient. Also, medical records form an important part of history, especially to find the past psychiatric history as well as response to treatment in the past, which in turn helps in formulating the management plan for the patient.

Depressive Disorders

Depressive disorders are one of the most common mental disorders among the elderly. These are characterized by a persistent low mood (such as sadness, irritability, or emptiness) or a loss of pleasure, along with other cognitive, behavioral, or neurovegetative symptoms that significantly impair an individual's functioning.

According to the International Classification of Diseases 11th Revision (ICD-11), for the diagnosis of depression, there should be clinical presentation in the form of the presence of at least five of the following characteristic symptoms occurring for most of the day, nearly every day, during a period lasting at least 2 weeks. Out of these five symptoms, at least one of the symptoms should be from the affective cluster.

Affective Cluster

- *Depressed mood* as reported by the individual (e.g., feeling down, sad) or as observed (e.g., tearful, defeated appearance): Depressed mood refers to the presence of low mood which is persistent (present for most part of the day) and pervasive (present across various situations and not confined to a particular situation). However, elderly may often report fewer emotional symptoms compared to younger adults with depression. They may also present with irritability rather than low mood.
- *Markedly diminished interest or pleasure in activities,* especially those normally found to be enjoyable to the individual:
- Elderly may restrict various activities due to medical problems or change in priorities. For example, a person with osteoarthritis in knees may stop going to park often which he/she used to enjoy previously. A person might have changed his interests from drawing to engaging in more religious activities. Hence, it is necessary to find whether the person is able to get pleasure in activities/has change of interest to other activities.

Cognitive–behavioral Cluster

- *Reduced ability to concentrate and sustain attention* on tasks or marked indecisiveness: This may manifest most commonly as forgetfulness in elderly. Hence, it is necessary to treat depression before assessing the extent of cognitive impairment in patients with comorbid depression.
- *Beliefs of low self-worth* or excessive and inappropriate guilt that may be manifestly delusional
- *Hopelessness* about the future
- *Recurrent thoughts of death* (not just fear of dying), *recurrent suicidal ideation* (with or without a specific plan), or *evidence of attempted suicide*: As older adults with depression have a higher risk of completed suicide, any expression of wish to die or suicidal ideas should not be ignored.

Neurovegetative Cluster

- *Significantly disrupted sleep* or excessive sleep
- *Significant change in appetite* or significant weight change
- *Psychomotor agitation or retardation*
- *Reduced energy, fatigue*, or marked tiredness following the expenditure of only a minimum of effort

Please note: Among elderly, more often, there are fewer emotional symptoms and somatization is more common. Also, cognitive symptoms in the form of memory or concentration difficulties are more common. Reduction in energy and loss of interest in activities (anhedonia) in the absence of a clear-cut depressed mood are also common which is labeled as "depression without sadness." Also note that the diagnosis of depressive disorder should not be made in individuals who have ever had a manic, mixed, or hypomanic episode, as this would suggest the presence of bipolar disorder.

Major types of depressive disorders as per the World Health Organization (WHO) ICD-11 are given as follows:
- 6A70—single-episode depressive disorder: When the current depressive episode has occurred for the first time and there has been no previous mood episodes
- 6A71—recurrent depressive disorder: When the patient is currently suffering from a depressive episode and has had one or more depressive episodes in the past
- 6A72—dysthymic disorder: When the patient never had/has symptoms fulfilling the criteria for a depressive episode but has persistent depressive mood for most part of the day, lasting for 2 years or more
- 6A73—mixed depressive and anxiety disorder: When the patient has prominent anxiety as well as depressive symptoms; however, the symptoms do not fulfill the criteria for either depressive episode or anxiety disorder

Psychotic symptoms in depression: Some patients with severe depression may also manifest psychotic symptoms in the form of delusions, hallucinations, or catatonic symptoms. Further details about these symptoms are given in the section on schizophrenia.

Anxiety Disorder

Anxiety is another very common psychological symptom among the elderly. Subsyndromal anxiety symptoms are more prevalent than anxiety disorders. Anxiety disorders are characterized by excessive fear or anxiety with associated behaviors. The symptoms of anxiety disorder should be intense enough to cause significant distress or functional impairment. The different types of anxiety disorders are primarily distinguished by the source of apprehension, or the situations and stimuli that trigger fear or anxiety. For instance, in specific phobia, the focus is specific to a particular stimulus (e.g., spider) or situation (e.g., height in acrophobia), whereas in GAD, it encompasses a broader range of situations. Anxiety disorders typically have three types of symptoms: (1) Cognitive symptoms, (2) physiological symptoms, and (3) behavioral symptoms. The symptoms should have been persistent for several months for the diagnosis to be made.

Cognitive Symptoms

Cognitive component refers to the anxious ruminations, excessive worries, the cognitive distortions in interpretation of the stimulus, as well as impairment in attention and concentration and memory disturbances. Thoughts in anxiety disorders are generally focused on the risk of being harmed.

Physiological Symptoms

Physiological component refers to the associated autonomic or somatic sensations in anxiety disorder, for example, palpitations, breathlessness, sweating, tremors, feeling of numbness or tingling sensation in hands or legs, headache, nausea, abdominal discomfort, increased urinary frequency, and diarrhea. These symptoms are excessive, either in duration, intensity, or both, for the particular situation or stimulus.

Behavioral Symptoms

Behavioral component refers to the actions taken to prevent exposure or reduce anxiety associated with exposure, for example, avoiding heights in acrophobia or repeated reassurance seeking in GAD.

The different types of anxiety disorder are usually identified by the distinct thought patterns that clarify the focus of the apprehension, as shown in **Table 1**.

Somatoform Disorder

Somatoform disorder, also called "bodily distress disorder" in ICD-11, refers to the mental disorder in which patients present with persistent physical symptoms that cause significant distress to the patient leading to excessive focus on the same, often resulting in frequent visits to healthcare providers. Even when another medical condition is present, the attention given to the symptoms is disproportionate to the condition's severity and progression. This heightened concern does not reduce even after repeated medical examinations, investigations, or reassurance.

Patients typically present with multiple somatic complaints, often involving multiple systems of the body. The symptoms are present most part of the day for several months. The symptoms may change, may fluctuate, or vary in intensity over time. In some patients, however, a single symptom may dominate the picture, especially pain or fatigue. The patient would typically have preoccupation with these symptoms and would have stopped their routine activities, as well as leisure activities. Often, there would be visits to multiple specialists or multiple doctors. The symptoms typically cause a significant negative impact not only on the individual's daily functioning or work performance, but also causes strain in relationship with friends and family.

Please note: The preoccupation in somatoform disorder or bodily distress disorder is the "symptoms," unlike hypochondriasis, where the preoccupation is with an "illness or disease or disorder." In hypochondriasis, the patient believes that he has some serious or major illness, such as cancer, which the doctors are not able to identify, while in somatoform disorder, the patient is more concerned about the symptoms which he is experiencing.

Schizophrenia

Schizophrenia and other primary psychotic disorders are a group of disorders characterized by significant impairments in reality testing and alterations in behavior. It has

TABLE 1: Anxiety disorders.

Domain	Phobias	Agoraphobia	Generalized anxiety disorder	Panic disorder	PTSD
Perception	Specific objects/events/ situations are perceived as threatening	Situations where escape might be difficult	The whole environment is perceived as threatening	Recurrence of panic attack is seen as threatening	Cues that remind trauma are perceived as threatening
Cognition	Contact with the phobic object or situation will lead to catastrophe	Fear of being overwhelmed by anxiety, where help is not available	Catastrophizing about many daily things	Panic attacks may lead to death/ serious injury	Recurrent memories of traumatic event occur
Affect	Intense fear/anger if contact with the feared object/situation occurs/anticipated	Intense fear of specific situations (e.g., public transport, open spaces)	Continual moderately high fear: "Free-floating anxiety"	During panic attacks, intense fear; between attacks: moderate fear of recurrence of attacks	Background of hyperarousal; periodic intrusive episodes of intense fear, horror, or anger. Emotional blunting can occur
Behavior	The phobic object or situation is avoided/ endured with great distress	The phobic situation is avoided/ endured with great distress	As worrying intensifies, social activities become restricted	May avoid public places to avoid panic attacks outside home	More focus on physical symptoms; may use drugs; more panicky or clingy
Interpersonal adjustment	• Simple phobias—problems confined to phobic situations • Agoraphobia—may lead to social situations	Social isolation may occur	Relationships may deteriorate	If agoraphobia develops secondary to panic attacks, social isolation may result	• Complete social isolation if trauma was solitary • If trauma was shared, confined interactions to group who shared the trauma

(PTSD: post-traumatic stress disorder)

three main types of symptoms: (1) Positive symptoms, (2) negative symptoms, and (3) cognitive symptoms.

Positive symptoms refer to delusions, hallucinations, formal thought disorder, and disorganized behavior, which are "added" to normal mental functions. These are the most prominent and easily recognizable symptoms of schizophrenia.

Negative symptoms refer to "loss or diminution of normal functions", e.g., flat affect (reduced emotional expression), lack of motivation (avolition), social withdrawal, and difficulty experiencing pleasure (anhedonia).

Cognitive symptoms refer to difficulty in concentration, problems with executive functioning, and memory disturbances that can occur in patients with schizophrenia.

Please note: Elderly with very late-onset schizophrenia (onset after 60 years of age) tend to have fewer formal thought disorders and fewer negative symptoms; however, they have higher prevalence of delusions (especially persecutory delusions, partition delusions, etc.) and hallucinations (more visual, olfactory, tactile, and auditory hallucinations). Also, cognitive symptoms are more common in the elderly. Family history is less common in very late-onset schizophrenia (indicating less role of genetics as a risk factor in late-onset schizophrenia). Also, the prevalence of early childhood trauma is very less among patients with very less-onset schizophrenia. These patients are more sensitive to the effects as well as side effects of antipsychotics. They have a higher propensity for tardive dyskinesia.

Positive Symptoms of Schizophrenia

- *Delusion*: It refers to a fixed false belief that is held in contrary to evidence or logical reasoning. It is easily recognizable when it is out of keeping with the person's educational and cultural background. In schizophrenia or other psychotic illnesses, patients may have one or more delusions. Delusions can occur in mood disorders (severe depression with psychotic symptoms, mania with psychotic symptoms) or in schizoaffective disorders. Some of the commonly seen delusions in clinical settings have been listed below:
  - *Delusion of persecution*: This is the most common type of delusion seen in clinical settings. The patient believes they are being mistreated, overlooked, or targeted by others. The perceived persecutor can be animate or inanimate, such as people, machines, systems, organizations, or institutions.
  - *Delusion of reference*: The patient believes that ordinary events, objects, or behaviors of others have a particular and unusual significance specifically for them. For example, a patient may think that people on television are speaking directly to him/her or that newspaper articles contain hidden messages meant for him/her.
  - *Delusion of infidelity*: The individual irrationally believes that their partner is unfaithful.
  - *Delusional misidentification*: This involves a group of complex, monothematic delusions where the person believes that the identity of a familiar person, object, location, or even themselves has been altered or replaced.
  - *Partition delusion*: In this, the patient believes that people, objects, or radiation can pass through usually nonpermeable barriers (e.g., wall).
  - *Delusion of guilt*: The patient believes that they have committed a terrible sin or crime or that they are responsible for a catastrophic event, even in the absence of any real wrongdoing. This is commonly found in severe depression.
  - *Nihilistic delusion*: The patient believes that either they or their body parts or the whole world no longer exists or are coming to an end soon. This type of delusion is often associated with severe depression.
  - *Delusion of grandiosity*: The patient has an inflated sense of self-worth, power, knowledge, or identity. They may believe that they have exceptional talents, have made significant discoveries, or have a special relationship with a famous person or deity.
  - *Hypochondriacal delusion*: The individual has an exaggerated concern about their health, interpreting minor or nonexistent physical symptoms as signs of a serious illness. They have an unreasonable fear of developing a serious medical condition.
- *Hallucinations*: Hallucinations are false perceptions that occur without any stimulus, but they have the same quality and characteristics as those of a true perception. The type of hallucinations is based on the involved sensory modality:
  - *Visual hallucinations*: Seeing objects, people, animals, etc., which are not present. Visual hallucinations are more common in organic conditions.
  - *Auditory hallucinations*: Hearing sounds or voices that are not present/real. The most common hallucination that occurs in schizophrenia is auditory hallucination.
  - *Tactile hallucinations*: Feeling sensations on the skin that are not real. The most common tactile hallucination is the feeling that some insect is crawling under the skin (delusional parasitosis).

  - *Olfactory hallucinations*: Smelling odors that are not present
  - *Gustatory hallucinations*: Tasting flavors that are not present
- *Formal thought disorder (FTD)*: This refers to a disturbance in the organization and expression of thought, which is manifested via a patient's speech. Some examples for formal thought disorders are tangentiality (patient deviates from the question that has been asked), loosening of associations (there is no connection between the lines), and word salad (incoherent, jumbled speech).
- *Disorganized behavior*: It refers to unpredictable, inappropriate, or erratic behaviors of a person that disrupt normal functioning. This can include aimless or unfocused behavior, inappropriate postures, inappropriate emotional reactions, etc.
- *Catatonic symptoms* are a distinct set of motor, affective, and cognitive-behavioral signs that can occur in some patients with schizophrenia, affective disorders with psychotic symptoms, or even with organic conditions. Some of the symptoms of catatonia are rigidity, stupor, mutism, staring, maintaining odd postures for long time, ambivalence, echolalia, echopraxia, etc.

Negative Symptoms of Schizophrenia

While negative symptoms are less common in very late-onset psychosis, it can occur, especially in those with schizophrenia with early onset, which is continuing in old age also. Some of the negative symptoms found in schizophrenia are as follows:

- *Blunted affect*: Reduction in the range of emotions
- *Alogia*: Reduction in the amount of speech
- *Avolition*: Reduction in the initiation as well as persistence of goal-directed activities
- *Asociality*: Reduction in social interactions
- *Anhedonia*: Reduction in the pleasure experienced out of activities which the person used to enjoy previously or in activities which people usually enjoy
- *Apathy*: Reduced motivation or drive

The major classification of schizophrenia and other primary psychotic disorders according to ICD-11 is as follows:

- *6A20: Schizophrenia*: In this, at least two of the following symptoms must be present for most of the time for at least 1 month:
  a. Persistent delusions
  b. Persistent hallucinations
  c. Disorganized thinking (formal thought disorder)
  d. Experiences of influence, passivity, or control (i.e., the experience that one's feelings, impulses, actions, or thoughts are not generated by oneself; are being placed in one's mind or withdrawn from one's mind by others; or one's thoughts are being broadcast to others)
  e. Negative symptoms such as affective flattening, alogia or paucity of speech, avolition, asociality, and anhedonia
  f. Grossly disorganized behavior that impedes goal-directed activity
  g. Psychomotor disturbances such as catatonic restlessness or agitation, posturing, waxy flexibility, negativism, mutism, or stupor

Of these, at least one symptom should be from (a) to (d).

- *6A21: Schizoaffective disorder*: Schizoaffective disorder is an episodic disorder in which the diagnostic requirements of both schizophrenia and a mood disorder (manic, mixed, or moderate or severe depressive episode) are met within the same episode for at least 1 month.
- *6A23: Acute and transient psychotic disorder*: It is characterized by acute onset of psychotic symptoms (within 2 weeks). Symptoms often fluctuate rapidly in both type and severity, varying from day to day or even within the same day. The episode typically lasts no longer than 3 months, with most cases ranging from a few days to 1 month.
- *6A24: Delusional disorder*: Delusional disorder is characterized by the presence of one or more delusions, typically lasting at least 3 months, without the presence of a mood episode. Other hallmark symptoms of schizophrenia—such as persistent hallucinations, negative symptoms, disorganized thinking, or experiences of influence, passivity, or control—are absent. However, perceptual disturbances such as hallucinations, illusions, or misidentifications related to the delusion can occur and are consistent with the diagnosis. Aside from behaviors or attitudes directly related to the delusion, the person's affect, speech, and behavior are generally unaffected.

Please note: Psychotic symptoms can also occur in mood disorders. When mood disorders preceded the onset of psychotic symptoms, we diagnose the person to have a mood episode along with psychotic symptoms (e.g., moderate depressive episode with psychotic symptoms, severe depressive episode with psychotic symptoms, or manic episode with psychotic symptoms).

Also, people with organic conditions such as dementia and Parkinson's disease can have psychotic symptoms. In such cases, organic psychosis is always considered to be the first differential diagnosis.

ASSESSMENT AND INVESTIGATIONS

Assessment of psychiatric disorder involves detailed history taking, followed by meticulous physical examination as well as mental status examination.

Psychiatric disorders can be either a continuation of the mental disorders with onset at a younger age or those which had onset at a late age. In all patients, but more specifically in those who had onset at late age, it is always mandatory to look for organic causes of psychiatric symptoms, as most often it is secondary to organic causes in such a scenario.

History

A detailed interview is needed to assess the various aspects of an individual's life history. Among elderly, due to cognitive impairment, it is often necessary to gather information from multiple sources—family members, caregivers, and medical records. Also, since organic causes for psychiatric illness are common, it is necessary to rule out if there has been either any change in medications or psychoactive substances before the onset of psychiatric symptoms or has it led to any change in the course of psychiatric symptoms. Also, explore whether there has been any new onset of any medical illness or exacerbation of already known medical illness and its relation to psychiatric symptoms. History taking usually includes the following steps:

1. Assessment of the chief and presenting psychiatric complaints of the patient: Start by asking the patient about their current concerns and symptoms. Use open-ended questions like "*Can you tell me what brought you here today?*"
2. Assessment of the onset, duration, frequency, and progression of each of the presenting symptoms
3. Assessment of the various associated psychiatric symptoms
4. Always look for mood symptoms, changes in behavior (hallucinatory behavior, withdrawn behavior, agitation, etc.), and cognitive symptoms (which may include ruminations, obsessions, delusions, formal thought disorder, etc.)
5. Also, assess the relation of these symptoms to the various life events, medical illness, medications, psychoactive substance use, trauma, etc.
6. Assess the risk of harm to self (suicidal ideas, plan, attempts) in all patients
7. Special attention to cognitive changes/impairment needs to be given
8. Assessment of the dysfunction in various domains of the person's life—self-care, biological domain, social domain, financial aspects, familial problems, occupational and legal complications, etc.
9. Assessment of treatment history for the current psychiatric symptoms (assess whether the dose of medications given was adequate, whether medications have been tried for adequate duration, whether compliance to the medications was good, what were the effects and side effects of medications taken by the patient, reason for discontinuation of medications)
10. Assessment of past psychiatric history and past treatment history
11. Also take into account medical history and current status of the same (whether controlled or uncontrolled). Specifically, look for any sensory impairment.
12. Assessment of family history, occupational history, substance-use history, marital history, menstrual history (in case of females), and premorbid personality is also done. Any major events in the birth and developmental history and childhood history is also noted (if appropriate informants or medical records are available).
13. Assessment of ability of the patient to perform basic and instrumental activities of daily living
14. Assessment of the social support for the patient

Examination

Examination forms an important component of psychiatric assessment and includes both general physical and mental status examination. As mentioned earlier, since elderly have a higher prevalence of medical comorbidities, and in those with late onset of psychiatric symptoms, organic causes for the symptoms are more likely, it is necessary to do a meticulous general physical examination.

General Physical Examination

A head-to-toe examination is to be done, including pallor, icterus, clubbing, cyanosis, lymphadenopathy, pedal edema, or any other abnormal finding. Height, weight, body mass index, and vitals (temperature, blood pressure, pulse rate, respiratory rate, and SpO_2) should also be assessed. Look for any sensory impairment.

Systemic Examination

A thorough systemic examination of the nervous system (both central and peripheral), respiratory system, cardiovascular system, abdomen, and musculoskeletal system should be done.

Mental Status Examination

Mental status examination (MSE) forms an important part of psychiatric evaluation. It is a structured way of observing and describing a patient's current state of mind. MSE involves assessment in the following domains:

- *General appearance and behavior*: In this, the patient's general appearance and behavior are assessed. Assess the patient's general appearance (whether the patient appears to be of stated age or is older or younger than the stated age—gives clue about self-care as well as some medical conditions), patient's gait (this gives clue about organic causes, if any), whether the patient is appropriately dressed and appropriately groomed (this gives clue about self-care), any abnormal movements or behavior during interview (patients with psychosis may exhibit hallucinatory behavior, patients with anxiety disorder may appear restless or fidgety), and whether the patient is able to make eye-to-eye contact with the interviewer (patients with depression or social anxiety disorder may not be comfortable in making eye-to-eye contact). Also, overall rapport with the patient is also noted.
- *Psychomotor activity*: In this, overall psychomotor activity of the patient during the interview is noted. It may be decreased in persons with depression, while it may be increased in patients who are agitated. (Also, rule out organic causes—patients with encephalopathy or delirium may also have changes in psychomotor activity.)
- *Speech*: In this, the speech of the patient is assessed to check whether it is spontaneous, relevant to the question asked, coherent, and goal directed or not. The rate, tone, volume, productivity, and reaction time (time taken to respond to interview questions) are also noted.
- *Affect*: It is the cross-sectional emotional state of the person. Both subjective perception of the affect, as reported by the patient, and objective state of the affect, as assessed by the interviewer, are noted. Whether the patient is able to react to the situations and experience the full range of the affect is assessed. (In mood disorders, the patient's affect may be restricted to one end of the spectrum. For example, affect may be restricted to sadness in depression.) We also observe whether the affect is appropriate to the situation being described and whether there is any lability of mood observed during the interview. (Lability of mood is observed in some organic conditions such as epilepsy.)
- *Thought*: In this, the form, flow, possession, and content of the thought are assessed. Form refers to the way in which a person puts together the ideas and associations. Formal thought disorders are mostly found in mania and schizophrenia. Flow refers to the uninterrupted sequence of thoughts. In thought content, the thoughts expressed by the person are noted. It may include a person's ideas, beliefs, or preoccupations. Under possession, we assess whether the person believes the thoughts to be his own or is someone else's (as occurs in some patients with schizophrenia).
- *Perception*: Any perceptual abnormality (i.e., hallucinations, illusions) is noted here.

Neurocognitive Assessment

- *Orientation*: Orientation of the patient with regard to time, place, and person is assessed.
- *Attention and concentration*: This domain is assessed by below-mentioned tests:
  - *Digit span test*
  - *Digit forward test*: In the forward test, the patient would be told a few digits of mathematics (i.e., 5, 3, 8, 2), in an interval of 1 second. The immediate correct or incorrect response is noted. The appropriate response would be a minimum of 5 digits correct.
  - *Digit backward test*: In this test, the process is similar to digit forward test, but the patient would be asked to tell the sequence in backward direction (i.e., given word 3, 8, 2, correct response should be 2, 8, 3). The appropriate response would be a minimum of 3 digits correct.
  - *Serial subtraction test*: Increasing difficulty task is given.
    - *20-1*: 20 to 0 (reversed counting) in 15 seconds
    - *40-3*: 40, 37, 34, etc., in 60 seconds
    - *100-7*: 93, 86, 79, etc., in 120 seconds
- *Memory*: Assessment of immediate, recent, and remote memory
  - *Immediate memory*: In this, registration and recall of the patient are tested. To test for registration, three unrelated words are given, and the patient is asked to repeat immediately. To test for recall, the patient is asked to repeat the three words after few seconds. Digit span test is also another way of testing immediate memory.
  - *Recent memory*: In this, memory is assessed by asking events of past few hours, usually of events that have occurred in the past 24 hours.
  - *Remote memory*: In this, memory of events of the past is assessed by asking about information of important life events, name of school where one studied, etc.
- *Intelligence*: It includes assessment in the areas of general information (e.g., name of Prime Minister, name of Chief Minister of state, five rivers, five cities), comprehension (i.e., giving a few hypothetical situations and noting down the patient's response), and arithmetic calculation (both simple and complex arithmetic problems are given).

- *Abstraction*: It refers to the ability to grasp the essentials of a whole, to break the whole into its parts, and to discern the common properties. This is assessed by asking the person to tell the meaning of the proverbs (i.e., slow and steady wins the race), as well as similarities and differences between two objects (i.e., orange and banana).
- *Judgment*: It refers to the ability to compare and evaluate choices for the purpose of deciding a course of action. It is assessed in the following domains:
    - *Personal judgment*: Ask questions related to his/her future plans, in personal domain
    - *Social judgment*: Judged by assessing behavior during interview
    - *Test judgment*: Patient will be given three hypothetical questions and his response noted (i.e., fire situation—fire in the house and you are in the house, what would you do now?).
- *Insight*: It refers to the conscious awareness and understanding of one's own psychological state, attribution of current symptoms to an underlying mental health condition, understanding the need for treatment, and acceptance of the same. The insight is rated on a Likert scale from 1 to 5.

Investigations

In all patients, routine investigations (complete hemogram, blood sugar, kidney and liver function tests) are done. Also, investigations should be done to rule out organic causes of the psychiatric symptoms (thyroid profile, serum electrolytes, vitamin B12, folate, vitamin D levels, neuroimaging), depending on the clinical history and examination.

Scales that can be used for psychiatric symptoms in elderly are:

- *Depression*:
    - Geriatric Depression Scale (GDS)
    - Patient Health Questionnaire-9 (PHQ-9)
    - Evans Liverpool Depression Rating Scale (ELDRS)
    - Hamilton Rating Scale for Depression (HAM-D)
    - Beck Depression Inventory (BDI)
    - Cornell Scale for Depression in Dementia (CSDD)

    Among these scales, GDS is the most validated scale to be used in elderly patients with intact cognitive function, while CSDD is useful in patients with dementia.
- *Anxiety disorder*:
    - Geriatric Anxiety Inventory
    - Hamilton Anxiety Rating Scale (HAM-A)
    - Beck Anxiety Inventory
    - State-Trait Anxiety Inventory
    - Geriatric Anxiety Inventory is the most commonly used scale to assess the anxiety disorder in elderly patients.
- *Psychotic disorder*:
    - Brief Psychiatric Rating Scale (BPRS)
    - Positive and Negative Syndrome Scale (PANSS)
    - Scale for the Assessment of Positive Symptoms (SAPS)
    - Scale for the Assessment of Negative Symptoms (SANS)

Brief Psychiatric Rating Scale is most commonly used scale for the assessment of psychosis in elderly.

MANAGEMENT

Management of psychiatric disorder in elderly includes both pharmacological measures and nonpharmacological measures.

Depression and Anxiety Disorders

- The main neurochemicals implicated in the etiology of depression as well as anxiety disorder are serotonin of a reduced level and, to some extent, norepinephrine of a reduced level.
- Antidepressants inhibit the reuptake of serotonin and norepinephrine, thereby increasing the level of serotonin and norepinephrine in the brain.
- The main classes of drugs used in depression include:
    - Selective serotonin reuptake inhibitor (SSRI)
    - Serotonin-norepinephrine reuptake inhibitor (SNRI)
    - Tricyclic antidepressants (TCAs)
    - Newer antidepressants
- TCAs, even though very effective, are not first line due to their poor tolerability profile; especially anticholinergic side effects are more pronounced in the elderly.
- SSRI and SNRIs are usually preferred medications. The selection of medication within each class is further decided by patient-specific and drug-specific factors.
- The Central Government has included escitalopram, fluoxetine, and amitriptyline in the National Essential Drug List.
- Escitalopram and fluoxetine belong to the SSRI class of drugs, and amitriptyline belongs to the TCA class of drugs.
- In the case of elderly people, "start low and go slow" is the basic principle that needs to be followed for medications, due to higher propensity of development of side effects due to age-related changes in pharmacokinetics and pharmacodynamics.

- If compliances with medications are ensured, the dosage of antidepressants can be increased if there is no response in the initial 3 week's period time. In the case of partial response to the treatment, the clinician can wait for at least 2 more weeks to get further effect. If at least a moderate response is also not achieved in 4–8 weeks of duration, then a plan to increase to the maximum dose or switch the antidepressant medication (after a full trial of initial medication) can be considered.
- In case of partial response, augmentation can be planned with other antidepressants **(Table 2)**, psychotherapy, or electroconvulsive therapy.

Medication Management of Depression/Anxiety Disorder (Flowchart 1)

- *Always rule out past history of mania/hypomania in all patients before starting antidepressants*: If past history of mania/hypomania is present, mood stabilizers are given along with antidepressants **(Table 3)**.
- *Always inform the patient about the following before prescribing medications*:
  - Illness and its management
  - Common side effects of SSRI (GI symptoms, sedation/insomnia, etc., can occur with SSRI, especially in the initial few days—these are usually transient and can be managed symptomatically)
  - The antidepressants take at least 2 weeks to show their effect. The medications have to be continued on a daily basis for the effect to occur.
  - Medications should be continued till prescribed by the doctor.
  - Medications should never be stopped abruptly. They need to be only tapered and stopped in order to prevent discomfort (serotonin discontinuation syndrome can occur on sudden stopping of SSRI).
- Medications are usually prescribed at least for 1 year in case of the first episode of depression or anxiety disorder.

- Always rule out past history of mania/hypomania in all patients before starting antidepressants
- If past history present, please add mood stabilizers (lithium/valproate/atypical antipsychotic) along with antidepressants

↓

Start antidepressant at the lowest dose and call patient for review after 1/2 weeks

↓

During follow-up:
- *Ask for improvement in symptoms—see next step in flowchart*
- *Ask for side effects due to medications:*
  - Common side effects—manage symptomatically
  - Serious/major side effects—stop medication and manage the side effects; consider another antidepressant or nonpharmacological measures when the patient is medically stable
- *Look for emergence of manic/hypomanic symptoms:* If present, stop antidepressant and start a mood stabilizer

↓

Good improvement in symptoms
Continue same dose
Minimal improvement in symptoms
Increase the antidepressant dose gradually monitoring the symptoms
No improvement in symptoms after 4 weeks of adequate dose
Shift to another antidepressant

↓

If no improvement with two antidepressants/symptoms are severe/worsening: Refer to psychiatrist
(Plan for nonpharmacological measures/other medications)

FLOWCHART 1: Stepwise approach to antidepressant initiation, titration and follow-up management.

TABLE 2: Common antidepressants used in depression and anxiety disorders.

Medication	Adult dose (mg/day)		Side effects
	Acute dose	Maintenance dose	
Escitalopram	5–20	Same as acute dose	Common—gastritis (self-limited), sexual side effects, hyponatremia in elderly
Fluoxetine	20–40	Same as the acute dose	• Sexual side effects • Insomnia
Sertraline	25–200	Same as the acute dose	• Common—gastritis (self-limited) • Sexual side effects, hyponatremia in elderly
Venlafaxine	37.5–225	Same as the acute dose	Risk of increase in blood pressure and pulse rate; gastrointestinal symptoms
Duloxetine	20–60	Same as the acute dose	Risk of increase in blood pressure and pulse rate; gastrointestinal symptoms
Amitriptyline	Start with 25–50 mg (can be increased up to 200 mg/day according to tolerability and response)	Same as acute dose	Anticholinergic side effects (dryness of mouth, constipation) and orthostatic hypotensionCan worsen cognitive performance in dementia

TABLE 3: Recommended dose ranges and titration schedule for common antidepressants.

SSRI	Starting dose (mg)	Minimum effective dose (mg)	Maximum dose for elderly (mg)	How much dose can be increased at a time*
Escitalopram	5	10	20	Increased by 5 mg once in 2–4 weeks
Fluoxetine	20	20	60	Increased by 20 mg once in 2–4 weeks
Sertraline	12.5	50	150	Increased by 25 mg once in 2–4 weeks
Venlafaxine	37.5	37.5	225	Increased by 37.5 mg once in 2–4 weeks
Duloxetine	30	30	120	Increased by 30 mg once in 2–4 weeks

*Dose of medication is to be increased only if there is no/minimal improvement in symptoms; the dose need not be increased if there is good improvement at a lower dose itself.

- Medications are usually prescribed for longer duration for recurrent depressive disorder and obsessive-compulsive disorder. Also, in some cases of anxiety disorder, medications are prescribed for longer duration.

An example illustrating management of a patient suffering from depression with Escitalopram medication has been given below:

- Escitalopram and sertraline have relatively less drug interactions with other medications and, hence, are preferred.
- The minimum effective dose of escitalopram is 10 mg and the maximum dose that can be prescribed is 20 mg.
- Start tablet escitalopram 5 mg once daily for 1 week.
- Call the patient for review after 1 week
  - *Ask for any improvement in symptoms*: If there is no improvement, reassure the patient that the effect of medications takes at least 2 weeks or more to produce effect.
  - *Look for any side effects after the start of medications*: If common and minor side effects are present, manage symptomatically **(Table 4)**.
  - If there are any major side effects: Excessive bleeding/seizures/serotonin syndrome—stop medications immediately and refer to higher center.
  - *Look for any emergence of manic/hypomanic symptoms*: If manic/hypomanic symptoms present, stop escitalopram immediately and refer to psychiatrist or start a mood stabilizer.
  - *Increase dose of tablet escitalopram to 10 mg (minimum effective dose) in the first follow-up (1 week after start of tablet escitalopram 5 mg) if the following conditions are met:*
    - No manic/hypomanic symptoms emerged.
    - No major side effects of medications (increase in bleeding/seizures/anaphylaxis) occurred.

TABLE 4: Common side effects of antidepressants and their management.

Common side effect	Management
Nausea/vomiting	Antiemetics
Gastritis	Ranitidine/proton-pump inhibitors
Increased sedation	Shift medication to night dose only
Insomnia	• Shift medication to morning dose • Give tablet clonazepam 0.25 or 0.5 mg at night time for 1 week
Increase in anxiety symptoms	• Give capsule propranolol 20 mg once daily (if no contraindication for the same) • If propranolol is contraindicated/not available, tablet clonazepam 0.25 mg may be added, preferably at night

- *Call the patient for review/follow-up after 2 weeks of increase in dose to 10 mg*:
  - *Ask for any change in symptoms of mental illness:*
    - Good improvement in symptoms:
      - Continue the medication in same dose till the decision to taper and stop is made.
    - Minimal improvement in symptoms:
      - Continue the medication in same dose for the next 1–2 weeks and review the patient again.
    - No improvement in symptoms:
      - If the patient is able to tolerate the medications, increase the dose of medication to tablet escitalopram 15 mg and review the patient again after 2 weeks
      - If the patient is having side effects but no improvement, manage the side effects and wait for 2 more weeks in the same dose and review the patient.

   - *Any side effects of medications*:
     - *Common and minor side effects:* Manage symptomatically
     - *Major side effects*: Excessive bleeding/seizures/serotonin syndrome—stop medications immediately and manage the same
   - *Any emergence of manic/hypomanic symptoms*:
     - Stop the antidepressant immediately and refer to a psychiatrist or start mood stabilizer.
- *In the next follow-up*:
  - *Again ask for change in symptoms of mental illness, side effects of medications and look for emergence of manic/hypomanic symptoms*
  - Good improvement in symptoms: Continue the same dose
  - Minimal improvement: Increase dose gradually if tolerated
  - *If no improvement/very minimal improvement after 4 weeks of adequate dose of medications (adequate dose is any dose at or above the minimum effective dose mentioned)*:
    - Consider shifting to another antidepressant
    - If no improvement with trials of two antidepressants/the symptoms are severe or worsening:
      - Refer the patient to a nearby psychiatrist who will plan further management.
      - Ask the patient to continue the medication in the same dose till they meet the psychiatrist and not to stop the same abruptly.

Somatization Disorders

In somatization disorder, psychotherapy or nonpharmacological interventions are the mainstay of treatment.

Selective serotonin reuptake inhibitors and SNRIs have been shown to reduce the pain threshold. However, these patients are also more prone to adverse effects, and, hence, lower doses are usually preferred.

Psychotic Disorders

- All types of psychosis will require antipsychotics as the first-line treatment.
- Second-generation antipsychotics are preferred over first-generation antipsychotics in the elderly due to the side-effect profile.
- The most common antipsychotics that are used and their doses have been mentioned in **Table 5**.
- Follow-up to be done after 2–4 weeks after the start of medications
- *In follow-up, assess the following*:
  - Compliance to medications
  - Any improvement/worsening of symptoms
  - Side effects of the medication
- *At the end of first month*:
  - If improvement is <50%, consider increasing the dosage to the next level.
  - If improvement is >50%, observe for a period of another month before deciding on dose titration, and if the improvement remains <50% even after 2 months, then consider increasing the dosage to the next level.
- Once treatment has been initiated with antipsychotics, if there is no improvement within 2 weeks, then refer to a psychiatrist.
- Follow-up is to be continued.

Extrapyramidal Side Effects of Antipsychotics

The common side effect of antipsychotic medications is a group of symptoms called extrapyramidal side effects.

- *Dystonia*: It is the first side effect that can appear after giving antipsychotic medication, typically within a few hours of receiving the first dose of antipsychotic. It is characterized by sudden, sustained contraction of a muscle group, thereby leading to twisting of arms, head turning to one side, or uprolling of eyeballs. When this side effect appears, injection phenergan 25 mg

TABLE 5: Common antipsychotics used for psychotic disorders.

Drug	Starting dose (mg)	Usual maintenance dose (mg)	Maximum dose (mg)	Common side effects	Remarks
Risperidone	1	1–2.5	4	EPS, sexual side effects	
Olanzapine	2.5	5–10	15	Sedation, weight gain, metabolic syndrome	Avoid in those with high BMI
Quetiapine	12.5–25	75–125	200–300	Sedation, weight gain, metabolic syndrome, QTc prolongation	Avoid in those with high BMI, those with cardiac disorders
Aripiprazole	5	5–15	20	Akathisia	

(EPS: extrapyramidal symptoms; BMI: body mass index)

intramuscular should be given, and as a prophylaxis to prevent further such episodes, trihexyphenidyl 2 mg/day should be added to the ongoing prescription.

- *Akathisia*: This is characterized by an inner feeling of restlessness, because of which the patient will not be able to sit at one place and will be roaming around constantly. This generally appears in the first week after the antipsychotics have been started. For treating this, we can either give propranolol in the dosage range of 20 or 40 mg/day or alternatively we can also treat it with clonazepam 0.25 mg in the morning.
- *Pseudo-Parkinson's syndrome*: This is characterized by symptoms such as Parkinson's disease. The symptoms are rigidity of arms, tremors, slowness in activities, and drooling of saliva. The treatment of this should be done by giving trihexyphenidyl, the dosage of which can be from 2 to 6 mg/day, depending upon the severity of EPS.

Nonpharmacological Management of Psychiatric Disorders

- Psychoeducation (educating patient and family about illness, medication compliance, and follow-ups): Explain about the nature of the illness, duration of treatment, important side effects, the need for regular follow-ups, setting realistic expectations from treatment, and practical tips to handle stressors
- Address family burnout by using supportive counseling
- *Psychotherapeutic intervention*: There are various psychotherapies done for common mental disorders, i.e., cognitive-behavioral therapy, interpersonal psychotherapy, exposure and response prevention, relaxation therapy (deep breathing exercise, Jacobson's progressive muscle relaxation), and social skills training. The therapy sessions are individualized as per the individual need of the patient.
- *Lifestyle modifications*: There are various lifestyle modifications that will help the patient to reach early remission and to maintain the remission. Activity scheduling, exercise, yoga meditation, healthy diet, sleep hygiene, avoidance of substances, etc., are the main lifestyle modifications, which should be advised to all the elderly patients irrespective of their primary diagnosis
- *Neuromodulation methods*: Neuromodulation methods such as modified electroconvulsive therapy, repetitive transcranial magnetic stimulation, and transcranial direct current stimulation are also used, especially in those with treatment resistance.

CONCLUSION

In this chapter, we discussed the common psychiatric disorders seen in the elderly—depression, anxiety disorders, somatoform disorders, and schizophrenia. With advancing age, multiple biological, psychological, and social factors contribute to increased vulnerability to these conditions. The presentation of psychiatric disorders in older adults may differ from that in younger individuals, often with predominant somatic or cognitive symptoms, making diagnosis challenging.

It is, therefore, important for clinicians to be aware of the characteristic features, assessment methods, and management strategies specific to this age group. Early identification and appropriate treatment can significantly improve quality of life and functional outcomes for both older adults and their caregivers. A comprehensive and compassionate approach remains essential for effective geriatric mental healthcare.

Self-Assessment Questionnaire

Q1. What is mental health?

Q2. What are the common psychological issues in elderly?

Q3. What are the risk factors of psychiatric disorders in elderly?

Q4. When to suspect a comorbid psychiatric disorder in a person coming for treatment of physical illness?

Q5. What is the consequence of not taking treatment for psychiatric disorder?

Q6. What can be done to prevent psychological issues in the elderly?

Q7. What is the role of a geriatrician in patients with psychological disorders?

FURTHER READINGS

1. Nobles J, Frankenberg E, Thomas D. The effects of mortality on fertility: population dynamics after a natural disaster. Demography. 2015;52(1):15-38.
2. Thakur U, Varma AR, Varma A. Psychological problem diagnosis and management in the geriatric age group. Cureus. 2023;15(4).
3. Petrova NN, Khvostikova DA. Prevalence, structure, and risk factors for mental disorders in older adults. Adv Gerontol. 2021;34(1):152-9.
4. Prince MJ, Wu F, Guo Y, Gutierrez Robledo LM, O'Donnell M, Sullivan R, et al. The burden of disease in older people and implications for health policy and practice. The Lancet. 2015;385(9967):549-62.
5. Srivastava S, Sulaiman K, Drishti D, Muhammad T. Factors associated with psychiatric disorders and treatment-seeking behaviour among older adults in India. Scientific Rep. 2021;11(1):24085.
6. Pilania M, Yadav V, Bairwa M, Behera P, Gupta SD, Khurana H, et al. Prevalence of depression among the elderly (60 years and above) population in India, 1997-2016: a systematic review and meta-analysis. BMC Public Health. 2019;19(1):832
7. Vink D, Aartsen MJ, Schoevers RA. Risk factors for anxiety and depression in the elderly: a review. J Affect Dis. 2008;106(1):29-44.
8. Patel M, Mantri N, Joshi N, Jain Y, Goel AD, Gupta M, et al. Is anxiety a public health problem among older adults in India: results from a systematic review and meta-analysis. J Family Med Prim Care. 2024;13(7):2545-54.
9. Subramanyam AA, Kedare J, Singh O, Pinto C. Clinical practice guidelines for geriatric anxiety disorders. Indian J Psych. 2018;60(Suppl 3):S371-82.
10. Hilderink PH, Collard R, Rosmalen JGM, Oude Voshaar RC. Prevalence of somatoform disorders and medically unexplained symptoms in old age populations in comparison with younger age groups: a systematic review. Ageing Res Rev. 2013;12(1): 151-6.
11. Tampi RR, Young J, Hoq R, Resnick K, Tampi DJ. Psychotic disorders in late life: a narrative review. Ther Adv Psychopharmacol. 2019;9:2045125319882798.
12. Oyebode F. Sims' Symptoms in the Mind: Textbook of Descriptive Psychopathology. London: Elsevier Health Sciences; 2022.
13. Klein CA, Hirachan S. The masks of identities: who's who? Delusional misidentification syndromes. J Am Acad Psych Law Online. 2014;42(3):369-78.
14. Taylor DM, Barnes TR, Young AH. The Maudsley Prescribing Guidelines in Psychiatry. United States: John Wiley & Sons; 2021
15. Sadock BJ, Sadock VA, Ruiz P. Kaplan and Sadock's Comprehensive Textbook of Psychiatry. United States: Wolters Kluwer Health; 2017.
16. Lertxundi U, Medrano J, Hernández R. (Eds.). Psychopharmacological Issues in Geriatrics. Sharjah: Bentham Books; 2017.
17. Steffens DC, Zdanys KF. (Eds.). The American Psychiatric Association Publishing Textbook of Geriatric Psychiatry. Washington, DC: American Psychiatric Publishing; 2022.

CHAPTER 31

Hearing Impairment in Elderly

Kapil Sikka, Pragya Tyagi

CASE VIGNETTE

Patient information: Mr Bala Krishnan, a 75-year-old male, with a history of hypertension.

Living situation: Lives with his wife in a nuclear family.

Primary care physician: Dr Richa Singh

Presenting complaint: Mr Bala Krishnan, a 75-year-old retired bank officer, visits the nearby ENT clinic with the complaint of reduced hearing in both ears since a month. He reported of being unable to communicate through phone and difficulty in listening to television with increased reliability on the visual subtitles than auditory information. He feels disturbed due to his inability to effectively communicate in day-to-day life and increased feeling of handicap.

History of present illness: Mr Krishnan defines his hearing impairment to be more pronounced when the speaker is speaking from behind or from a distance. He reports of often missing certain sounds or words in a speech and often relying on the lip movement of the speaker to understand the entire message. The condition has increased significantly over time with family members often complaining of not being able to communicate well with him along with several repetitions of the message intended to be communicated.

Medical history: Mr Krishnan has a history of hypertension and is on antihypertensive medications for the same. He does not complain of any ear discharge or ear pain. He reports of ringing sensation in the left ear 1 year back which subsided with medication for tinnitus. There has been no episode since then.

Social history: Mr Krishnan lives with his wife in a nuclear family with a son and a daughter settled in another city. He goes to a yoga class every alternate day in the nearby park and has an active social circle with his bank colleagues residing nearby. He likes to keep himself abreast with recent developments and spends a significant amount of time watching television and cell phone. He does not have a history of alcohol or tobacco use.

Review of systems: No other systematic condition or symptoms were reported by the patient.

Physical examination: In physical examination, his blood pressure was 132/89 mm Hg and heart rate was 75 beats/min. Otoscopic examination revealed bilateral tympanic membrane (TM) intact in both ears. Rinne test was positive with Weber test suggestive of lateralization toward a better ear. The audiological evaluation revealed bilateral moderate-to-severe sloping sensorineural hearing loss with "A" type tympanogram and absent auditory reflexes.

INTRODUCTION

The age-related hearing loss commonly known as presbycusis is often evident beyond the age of 60 years. It is a complex condition resulting in progressive and symmetrical hearing loss, characterized by impaired neural ability to understand high-frequency components of speech and nonspeech sounds initially. The peripheral loss of sensory hair cells in the inner ear affects the neural coding of sound waves propagated through the external and middle ear. This further results in speech discrimination and central auditory processing difficulties.

Presbycusis, being the third most common chronic condition after hypertension and arthritis, is among the major sociomedical problems in older adults. It results in a hidden disability that impacts the overall well-being of an individual and significantly interferes with daily activities and social communication. With the increase in elderly population in India, the management of age-related hearing loss necessitates an active combating strategy and a multidisciplinary task force. A comprehensive test battery for the assessment and suitable hearing assistive devices catering to the individual's hearing loss configuration is crucial for effective management of hearing loss in elderly population.

EPIDEMIOLOGY

The epidemiological analysis of age-related hearing loss is important in understanding the probable risk factors associated with hearing impairment in older adults and methods to minimize its effects. It will help in identifying the distribution pattern of presbycusis across different regions with respect to Indian and global perspectives.

Prevalence and Global Perspective

With the increase in life expectancy, the prevalence of presbycusis has increased immensely. It is reported to affect more than half of older adults by age 75 years and nearly all adults over age 90 years. The World Health Organization (WHO) estimated that by the year 2025, more than 500 million individuals aged 60 years and above will have significant age-related hearing loss. In a cross-sectional National Health and Nutrition Examination Survey (NHANES) on noninstitutionalized Americans, the reported prevalence of hearing impairment approximately doubled with each subsequent decade from age 12 to 79 years.

In a developing country such as India, hearing impairment can significantly affect the social and economic productivity of an individual. This can consequently burden the society. Often, this is evident due to limited healthcare services and their accessibility. The rural and urban slum areas of the country having limited availability of tertiary healthcare are reported to have a considerably higher prevalence of hearing loss. In an Indian study, the prevalence of disabling hearing loss was reported to be half in those aged >60 years; that is, almost 50% of individuals aged 60 years and above have a hearing impairment.

ETIOLOGY

Age-related hearing loss can be accounted to multiple factors. Other than the physiological and anatomic changes due to natural degeneration, presbycusis can also be attributed to factors, including noise exposure, ototoxicity, history of ear infection, hormones, presence of certain systemic diseases, and genetics.

Noise Exposure

A sustained long-term exposure to high intensity of noise at a younger age can result in noise-induced hearing loss followed by a more severe degeneration. Noise exposure anatomically has been found to affect auditory neurons and lead to loss of spiral ganglion. This can subsequently develop into severe and early presbycusis.

Ototoxicity

Several medications have been known to cause ototoxicity such as salicylates, loop diuretics, aminoglycosides, and certain chemotherapeutic agents. Alongside, exposure to certain chemicals, including lead, toluene, carbon monoxide, styrene, and mercury, has also been reported to contribute significantly to ototoxicity. Limiting the exposure to these agents can be effective in delaying or reducing the severity of presbycusis.

Hormonal Factors

Melanin is primarily associated with the development of metabolic presbycusis. It is produced by intermediate cells in the vascular stria and is reported to bind metal ions such as calcium ions to the inactivate oxygen free radicals. Melanin is absorbed by the central basal cells when secreted in extracellular space and is further transported to lysosomes. As marginal cells responsible for maintaining stria vascularis function also express the transporters, multiple ion channels, and sodium-potassium ATPase, they are vulnerable to damage due to oxidative stress. Also, prolonged corticosterone levels and loss of nuclear factor kappa B have been reported to cause increased spiral ganglion neuron damage. Alongside, the combination of hormone replacement therapy in postmenopausal women and the use of progestin has been known to result in a higher incidence of hearing impairment.

Genetic Factors

Several genetic factors are responsible for causing hearing loss with gene expression beyond 60 years of age. Specifically, differences in mitochondrial DNA expression genes have been reported to be associated with oxidative stress in patients with presbycusis **(Flowchart 1)**.

CLINICAL PRESENTATION

A thorough understanding of the clinical presentation of hearing impairment is of utmost importance, as it helps in identifying hearing loss at an early stage in this high-risk population. It facilitates timely and

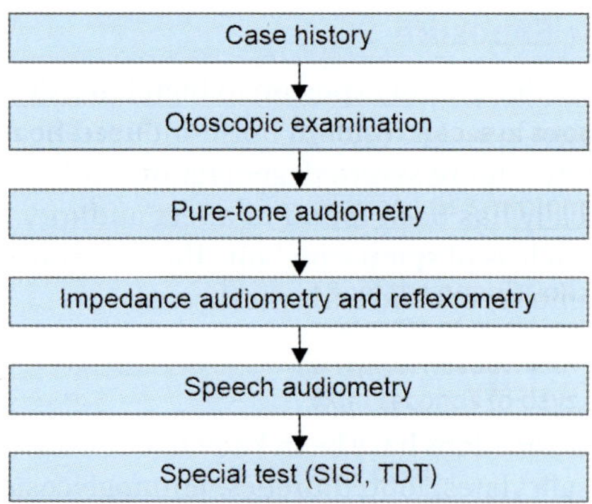

FLOWCHART 1: Illustration of diagnostic protocol for presbycusis. (SISI: Short Increment Sensitivity Index; TDT: tone decay test)

appropriate intervention with suitable hearing assistive devices.

- *History of hearing loss*: A detailed medical history is crucial. The description of a patient's experience with hearing loss (duration, degree, unilateral/bilateral) is essential. The associated symptoms such as tinnitus and vertigo should also be investigated and documented.
- *Symptoms and complaints*: Probing the various difficulties such as missing out on conversations, difficulty in attending telephone, inability to listen to television, and failure to follow the conversation without any visual cues or lip reading is helpful in giving crucial insight into difficulties encountered by an individual with hearing impairment. It will help us to understand the configuration of hearing loss and correlate it clinically.
- *Medication review*: Reviewing the patient's medication list is essential; any ototoxic drugs such as aminoglycoside antibiotics, macrolide antibiotics, salicylates, chemotherapeutic agents, or loop diuretics if included in routine prescription should be noted as they can potentially increase the risk of hearing loss.
- *Coexisting medical conditions*: Assessment of the coexisting medical conditions such as diabetes, cardiovascular diseases, hypertension, and balance issues that can worsen the condition should be recorded.
- *Functional assessment*: Evaluation of patient's frailty and functional status, including mobility, balance, and activities of daily living, can have a profound impact on the patient's daily living when coexisting with hearing impairment and, therefore, should be assessed to evaluate the functional manifestation of hearing loss.
- *Environmental factors*: Consideration of individuals living environmental and essentially the noise exposure if present should be assessed as it can contribute significantly to the degree of hearing loss.

EVALUATION

The clinical investigation comprising ear examination by an ENT surgeon and administration of a comprehensive audiological test battery are necessary to investigate the degree and nature of hearing loss in elderly population. These will help to further determine the line of treatment and management strategies to be tailored according to one's need.

- *Ear examination*:
    - *Outer ear examination*: To assess for any structural abnormality in outer ear such as pinna
    - *Otoscopic evaluation*: To visualize the ear canal and look for the presence of cerumen, discharge, or any blockage. Also, it helps to assess the tympanic membrane structure.
- *Audiological evaluation*:
    - *Pure-tone audiometry (PTA)*: The test gives a threshold at a hearing frequency range of 250 Hz to 8 kHz necessary for the perception of speech and environmental sounds. A graph plot is attained with hearing threshold points of the patient known as an audiogram for both ears. It also helps to determine the site of lesion, i.e., conductive, sensorineural, or mixed hearing loss, and degree of hearing impairment such as mild, moderate, moderately severe, severe, and profound. PTA is a gold standard test to assess hearing impairment in adults.
    - *Tympanometry and reflexometry*: Tympanometry helps to subjectively evaluate the middle ear function and nature of conductive problem if any, i.e., mass dominant or stiffness dominant pathology, presence of middle ear effusion, and eustachian tube dysfunction. It also helps in differentiating between cochlear and retrocochlear disorders and correlates with PTA findings. Reflexometry is used to evaluate the acoustic reflex pathways that include cranial nerves VII and VIII.
    - *Speech audiometry*: Speech audiometry tests such as speech recognition threshold (SRT) and speech identification scores (SIS) are used to assess the audibility and processing of connected speech, including words and sentences.
    - *Electrophysiological tests*: In difficult-to-test conditions such as outer ear malformation, inconclusive PTA response, functional hearing loss, and malingering the electrophysiological evaluations such as auditory brainstem responses (ABRs),

otoacoustic emissions (OAEs), and higher cortical potentials can be recorded. These objective evaluations give a clearer picture of the condition and help to correlate clinically.

- *Special tests*: Various other special tests such as tone decay test (TDT) and Short Increment Sensitivity Index (SISI) can be performed to differentiate between cochlear and retrocochlear pathology. They can be done as and when required and are often not part of a standard test battery.

MANAGEMENT

The management of hearing loss in elderly is based on the diagnostic conclusion. It will depend on the type of loss and its severity. In the case of conductive hearing loss (not very common), drugs are prescribed as the primary line of treatment targeting the existing pathological conditions such as otitis media and otomycosis. Surgical intervention may also be required in conditions such as otosclerosis.

In sensorineural hearing loss, the condition is mostly irreversible and is managed and rehabilitated with suitable assistive listening devices. Depending on the degree of hearing impairment and configuration of the audiogram, various types of hearing aid devices, bone-anchored hearing aids (BAHAs), and cochlear implants (in case of postlingual deafness) can be fitted. Currently, different types of hearing aids such as behind-the-ear (BTE), in-the-canal (ITC), and receiver-in-canal (RIC) are quite beneficial in the process of rehabilitation of patients **(Figs. 1A to D)**.

The selection of appropriate hearing aids and post-fitting hearing aid rehabilitation is crucial for the desired prognosis. Posthearing aid selection the software programming of digital hearing aids to suit a patient's hearing loss configuration is necessary to ensure overall benefit and acceptance. Other necessary features such as ear molds can be recommended in certain cases such as in severe or profound degree of hearing loss. One of the decisive steps in hearing aid fitting is patient counseling. The acceptance of foreign devices can be challenging for the patient, especially at old age. Proper counseling and follow-up sessions as and when required are an absolute necessity of an effective aural rehabilitation program.

PREVENTION OF PRESBYCUSIS

Age-related hearing loss can be delayed if not completely preventable by taking the following precautions:

- Improving general health condition
- Avoiding exposure to high-intensity sounds
- Avoiding self-medication with over-the-counter drugs causing ototoxicity
- Avoiding the use of earbuds and insertion of foreign body in the ear canal

NEEDS AND PROBLEMS FACED IN PRESBYCUSIS

Communication Needs

In the presence of hearing loss, an individual may face difficulty in communication that may significantly affect his/her interaction with family members, spouse, and children. They may fail to attend to important information during the discussions. Older adults have more difficulty in understanding speech in noisy environments, when people speak quickly in reverberant conditions, when there are multiple speakers, when the message is complex, or when the contextual information is limited.

Economic Needs

Longer lifespan and forced retirement have resulted in greater numbers of older persons living in poverty. While giving management options, one should consider economic status of hearing impaired. Decisions with monaural versus binaural amplification or selective assistive listening devices may be influenced by a patient's financial resources, cost of devices, and related services.

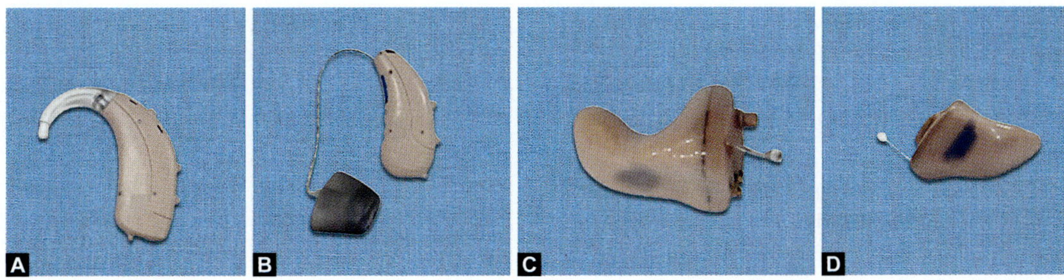

FIGS. 1A TO D: Types of hearing aids commercially available. (A) Behind-the-ear (BTE); (B) Receiver-in-canal (RIC); (C) In-the-canal (ITC); (D) Completely-in-the-canal (CIC).

Social Needs

Also, the details of a patient's communication partners and where the individual resides are important when designing an aural rehabilitation program. Information on whether the patient resides alone or with a family member and is socially active or inactive can also be helpful.

Psychological Needs

It is not unusual for older people who have hearing loss to experience depression, isolation, anger, insecurity, and loneliness. Sometimes, an individual feels ashamed either from a sense of incompleteness or from a sense of being a burden on family, friends, and coworkers. Some older individuals may attempt to hide their hearing loss from people whose help they need in facilitating communication considering it to be a social taboo. These kinds of emotions and frustration may lead older adults to undergo lifestyle changes and experience a diminished quality of life.

ROLE OF A GERIATRICIAN IN MANAGEMENT

Neurodegenerative disorders such as dementia are a chronic complex condition with long-term effects on several domains of a patient's day-to-day life. A geriatrician plays a crucial role in identifying signs and symptoms at an early stage and initiates multidisciplinary care along with psychologist, psychiatrist, neurologist, physiotherapist for further assessment and treatment. Patient's and caregiver's timely counseling and suitable pharmaceutical intervention are also a decisive factor for a favorable prognosis primarily managed by the geriatrician. Simultaneously, hearing loss is a multifactorial condition affecting several domains and significantly affecting overall well-being. Along with ENT consultants and audiologists who are at the forefront of hearing loss management, the geriatrician can play a vital role by addressing the hearing loss complaint by the patient or identifying it while communicating and giving timely referral. Also, they can play a vital role in counseling the patient and family members during the course of intervention and aural rehabilitation.

CONCLUSION

Age-related hearing loss (presbycusis) is a widespread, multifactorial condition impacting the well-being of older adults and necessitates a multidisciplinary approach for effective management.

Presbycusis is not only affects communication, it has significant impact on psychological health, and impaired social functioning leading to reduced quality of life.

Tailored audiological assessments by specialist team and the appropriate hearing assistive devices as per the need is critical for rehabilitation and ensuring better outcomes. However, compliance to the device is a major challenge in older adults.

Prevention strategies, such as avoiding ototoxic medications and excessive noise exposure, can delay the progression of hearing loss. Geriatricians needs to screen all their clients for hearing impairment, and counsel for appropriate intervention as hearing impairment has significant impact on cognition and overall QOL.

Self-Assessment Questionnaire

Q1. What are the characteristic audiological features of presbycusis, and how does it differ from conductive hearing loss?

Q2. List the common etiological factors contributing to age-related hearing loss.

Q3. Why is noise exposure during younger years considered a risk factor for severe presbycusis later in life?

Q4. What classes of ototoxic medications are essential to review in elderly patients presenting with new-onset hearing loss?

Q5. What are the key components of a comprehensive audiological evaluation in older adults with suspected presbycusis?

Q6. Discuss the rehabilitative options available for sensorineural hearing loss in elderly patients and factors influencing hearing-aid acceptance.

Q7. Enumerate the psychosocial and communication challenges faced by older adults with hearing impairment.

Q8. Outline the preventive strategies to delay the onset or progression of presbycusis.

Q9. What is the role of a geriatrician in the multidisciplinary management and counseling of elderly patients with hearing.

FURTHER READINGS

1. Heidari A, Moossavi A, Yadegari F, Bakhshi E, Ahadi M. Effects of age on speech-in-noise identification: subjective ratings of hearing difficulties and encoding of fundamental frequency in older adults. J Audiol Otol. 2018;22(3):134-9.
2. Wattamwar K, Qian ZJ, Otter J, Leskowitz MJ, Caruana FF, Siedlecki B, et al. Increases in the rate of age-related hearing loss in the older old. JAMA Otolaryngol Head Neck Surg. 2017;143(1):41-5.
3. Sprinzl GM, Riechelmann H. Current trends in treating hearing loss in elderly people: a review of the technology and treatment options—a mini-review. Gerontology. 2010;56(3):351-8.
4. Lin FR, Niparko JK, Ferrucci L. Hearing loss prevalence in the United States. Arch Intern Med. 2011;171(20):1851-2.
5. Verma RR, Konkimalla A, Thakar A, Sikka K, Singh AC, Khanna T. Prevalence of hearing loss in India. Natl Med J India. 2021;34(4):216-22.
6. Kidd Iii AR, Bao J. Recent advances in the study of age-related hearing loss: a mini-review. Gerontology. 2012;58(6):490-6.
7. Bielefeld EC, Tanaka C, Chen GD, Henderson D. Age-related hearing loss: is it a preventable condition? Hear Res. 2010;264(1-2):98-107.
8. Ruan Q, Ma C, Zhang R, Yu Z. Current status of auditory aging and anti-aging research. Geriatr Gerontol Int. 2014;14(1):40-53.
9. Falah M, Farhadi M, Kamrava SK, Mahmoudian S, Daneshi A, Balali M, et al. Association of genetic variations in the mitochondrial DNA control region with presbycusis. Clin Interv Aging. 2017;12:459-65.
10. Martin JS, Jerger JF. Some effects of aging on central auditory processing. J Rehabil Res Dev. 2005;42:25-44.
11. Wingfield A, McCoy SL, Peelle JE, Tun PA, Cox CL. Effects of adult aging and hearing loss on comprehension of rapid speech varying in syntactic complexity. J Am Acad Audiol. 2006;17(7):487-97.
12. Heine C, Browning CJ. The communication and psychosocial perceptions of older adults with sensory loss: a qualitative study. Ageing Soc. 2004;24(1):113-30.

CHAPTER 32

Vertigo in Elderly

Sankha Shubra Chakrabarti, Sumit Jaiswal

CASE VIGNETTE

Patient information: Mrs Gulabi Devi, a 60-year-old female homemaker, with type 2 diabetes mellitus, ischemic cardiomyopathy with a left ventricular ejection fraction of 30%, and bilateral knee osteoarthritis presented with vertigo.

Living situation: Lives in a joint family that includes 16 members.

Presenting complaint: The patient presented to us with vertigo and vomiting for the last 7 days.

History of present illness: Mrs Gulabi Devi describes her vertigo as multiple episodes of whirling sensation for the past 7 days which occurs at all times and is not related to her posture or whether she is lying or standing or sitting. She also complains of experiencing nausea and a few episodes of nonbilious vomiting over this period of 7 days. There are no aggravating or relieving factors of vertigo. She had just recovered from a bout of common cold (which she calls a viral fever) around 10 days back, which resolved without any medications apart from paracetamol and some multivitamins with supportive measures.

Medical history: Mrs Gulabi Devi has a history of type 2 diabetes, which is well controlled with oral metformin. She also has ischemic cardiomyopathy for which, she is taking ramipril, bisoprolol, spironolactone, and a combination of aspirin and rosuvastatin. She is in good compliance with her earlier prescription.

Social history: She lives in a joint family which includes her husband, her daughter, four sons, three daughters-in-law, and six grandchildren. She does not have any history of using tobacco, alcohol, or any other habit-forming substance.

Review of systems: Apart from whirling sensation and associated nausea/vomiting episodes, Mrs Gulabi Devi denies other significant symptoms, including recent-onset chest pain, palpitations, shortness of breath, blackening of vision (presyncope), tremors or any other neurological complaints, hearing difficulty, fullness of the ears or headache.

Physical examination: During the physical examination, her blood pressure is 122/78 mm Hg in the right arm (supine position) and her heart rate is 95 beats/min with regular pulse and all peripheral pulses palpable. There is no orthostatic hypotension and carotid bruit. The HINTS examination is benign (positive head impulse test with direction-fixed horizontal nystagmus with no skew deviation). Neurological examination does not reveal any focal deficits.

INTRODUCTION

Of all the geriatric syndromes, none is probably as puzzling as the syndrome labeled "vertigo." Besides being a source of morbidity for the patients, it is frustrating for the geriatrician due to the high inaccuracy of differential diagnoses, the often-inadequate response to therapy, and the propensity for recurrence. Much of the confusion lies in defining vertigo in the first place. A casual evaluation of postgraduate trainees of geriatrics or associated specialties in the country would reveal how the words "vertigo" and "dizziness" are often used interchangeably by them, and without ascribing any definite meaning to them as such. When the beginning of the history-taking process is on such shaky grounds, it is quite natural that arriving at a proper final diagnosis and management protocol would be difficult.

DEFINING VERTIGO AND DIZZINESS AND DIFFERENTIATING BETWEEN THE TWO

Vertigo and dizziness are variously defined. There is little consensus between international bodies in this regard, and in fact, till 2009, no attempt was made to define these entities separately. The Barany Society set in process the first comprehensive classification of vestibular disorders which was published in detail in 2015. The classification system defines vertigo as a "false sense of motion of spinning or nonspinning quality" and dizziness as "disturbed spatial orientation without a false sense of motion." It also created a separate category of vestibulovisual symptoms which include external vertigo or "false sensations of motion in the visual surround." Simply put, patients often complain of their surroundings spinning. The fourth category introduced is known as "postural balance symptoms" which include the common old-age complaint of unsteadiness of gait, resulting from diverse etiologies such as posterior column dysfunction, vestibular pathologies, and others. Interestingly, while the definition of vertigo is straightforward, dizziness has been defined as something quite different from what most neurologists and geriatricians normally understand. In most of the English-speaking world, dizziness is an umbrella term for conditions ranging from vertigo to presyncope to unsteadiness. The international classification, hence, is yet to find general acceptance among most clinicians and raises the important question: How do you mention presyncope in patient's terms while taking a history—what do you call it? It would be fair to say that the authors of this chapter, in their routine practice, use "vertigo" to describe all sensations of spinning around and use "dizziness" to denote all presyncopal tendencies. After all, these are the two broad groups of pathologies that we as geriatricians are trying to diagnose, and examinations and investigative protocols are confined to these two discrete arms.

SIGNIFICANCE AND EPIDEMIOLOGY OF BALANCE DISORDERS IN ELDERLY

Vertigo and dizziness are of paramount importance in the elderly owing to a high prevalence of 30% or more in those aged > 60 years. While evaluating an elderly patient with any of these symptoms, the main aim remains not to miss potentially life-threatening conditions but also to provide adequate reassurance in cases of benign diagnoses. Preventing the overuse of medications, especially in conditions where they have questionable therapeutic benefits, is another concern. The close association of vertigo/dizziness with another notorious geriatric syndrome—"falls"—makes the evaluation of these symptoms even more important.

The prevalence of vertigo and related disorders has been scantily explored among the elderly in India. Hence, we have to depend mostly on world literature. Nearly one third of the elderly complained of dizziness and vertigo in an elderly urban population in Sweden. Overall, benign paroxysmal positional vertigo (BPPV), Meniere's disease, and vestibular neuronitis remain the most common causes of vertigo in the elderly.

BALANCE APPARATUS IN THE ELDERLY

Balance and the feeling of steadiness are maintained by the concerted effort of the peripheral vestibular apparatus, the eyes, the postural muscles, the somatic nerves sending inputs to the brain about posture and joint position, the brainstem, the cerebellum, and the cortex. Blood perfusion of the brain is maintained by the heart, the bilateral carotid arteries, the vertebrobasilar system, and the intracranial circulatory network. Various sensory structures such as the carotid body baroreceptors and neural feedback loops are also involved in the regulation of blood flow to the brain and the vestibular structures. It is common sense that pathologies in any of these structures may result in balance disorders. While a detailed description of these structures is beyond the scope of this chapter, a brief description of the peripheral vestibular system is warranted. The anatomy of the peripheral vestibular system located in the inner ear is depicted in **Figure 1**. It comprises a bony and membranous labyrinth enclosed in the otic capsule in the petrous temporal bone. The bony labyrinth is constituted by the cochlea—the hearing apparatus, the vestibule, and the semicircular canals. The bony labyrinth is filled by perilymph which is similar in composition to cerebrospinal fluid. The membranous labyrinth is suspended in the perilymph and within it is located the vestibular apparatus. The vestibular apparatus in turn is made of the utricle, saccule, lateral, posterior, and superior semicircular ducts. The macula and the crista ampullaris are the two primary sensory neuroepithelia of the vestibular apparatus. Separate maculae serve the utricle and saccule which both sense the orientation of the head in space and respond to linear acceleration, gravitational forces, and tilting of the head. The macula of the utricle senses motion in the horizontal plane, while that of the saccule senses motion in the vertical plane. The semicircular ducts, which are oriented at right angles to each other, sense angular acceleration or rotation of the head. They are served by the sensory neuroepithelium called the crista ampullaris. Both the neuroepithelia—the macula and the crista ampullaris—contain hair

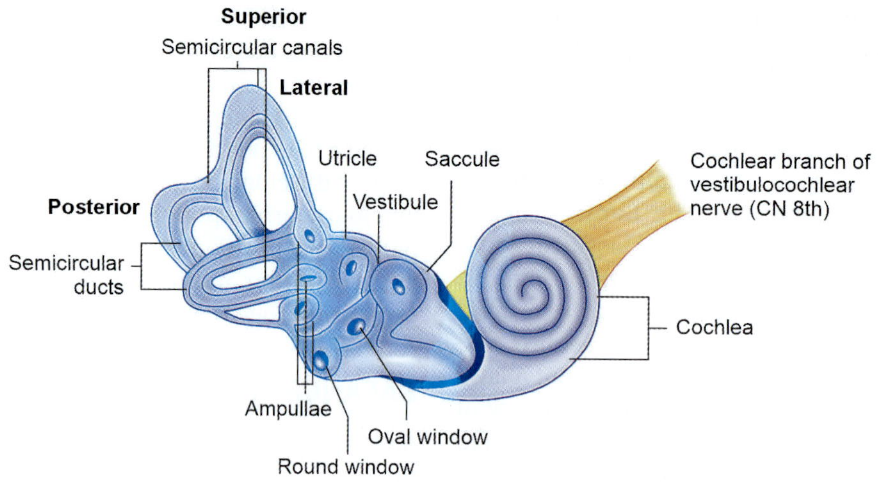

FIG. 1: Anatomy of the peripheral vestibular system located in the inner ear.
Courtesy: Dr Amandeep Kaur, Indian Institute of Technology, Jodhpur, Rajasthan, India.

cells which are rod-shaped sensory mechanoreceptors. Depolarization and hyperpolarization of the hair cells in various patterns are responsible for the generation of nerve impulses which send information regarding position and balance to the central vestibular system. While the hair cells in the maculae project through the gelatinous otolithic membrane with embedded calcium carbonate crystals (otoconia or otoliths), those in the crista ampullaris are embedded in the cupula which is devoid of otoliths. The vestibular or Scarpa's ganglion is composed of bipolar cell bodies that receive afferent impulses from the hair cells of both the macula and the crista ampullaris. It is divided into a superior and an inferior division. The superior division serves the crista ampullaris of the superior and lateral semicircular ducts and the macula of the utricle. The macula of the saccule and the crista ampullaris of the posterior semicircular duct are served by the inferior section of the vestibular ganglion. Axons from the superior and inferior divisions merge to form the vestibular nerve which combines with the cochlear nerve to become the vestibulocochlear (8th cranial) nerve. This nerve travels with the facial nerve, nervus intermedius, and labyrinthine artery through the internal auditory canal, to reach the posterior fossa. The vestibular nerve fibers mainly project to the vestibular nuclear complex in the pons and the flocculonodular lobe of the cerebellum.

PATHOPHYSIOLOGY OF VERTIGO IN THE ELDERLY

The pathogenesis of vertigo in the elderly is more complex. Balance generation is a composite of inputs from the visual, somatosensory, and vestibular systems. While an age-related decline in the first two is well known in the form of cataracts, presbyopia, and age-related neuropathy, the vestibular system also undergoes what is now known as presbystasis. The hair cell density decreases and so do the vestibular and cerebellar neuronal numbers. The most significant decline occurs in the semicircular canals. Whereas one would expect typical rotatory vertigo to occur with such a decline, the age-related decline in canal function in the elderly is quite slow and due to natural bodily compensation, the resultant symptom is more often gait instability. However, in pathologies such as BPPV where the defect is more acute in onset, typical rotatory vertigo may manifest. Compensation of vestibular deficit by other sensory inputs or central structures also declines with age. However, there is a large variation in the pathology observed in individual patients and their symptom magnitudes, thus raising pertinent queries on the validity of the entity of presbystasis. Another interesting finding may be that in conditions such as bilateral vestibulopathy, vertigo may not be a feature as the balance systems of both sides are affected and the neural inputs are balanced. Similarly, symptoms may be minimal in cases of slow-growing tumors of the cerebellopontine angle where adequate time for compensation is present.

Risk Factors for Vertigo

It has been suggested that females may be more prone to developing vertigo compared to males. This could be due to hormonal differences, structural differences in the inner ear, or other factors. However, the exact reasons for this disparity may vary and are still being researched. Recent studies suggest several comorbidities too that could increase the risk of developing vertigo. These include hypertension (by affecting blood flow to the inner ear), type 2 diabetes mellitus (through cupular deposits and free-floating debris in the semicircular canals probably due to variation in plasma glucose and insulin level), hyperlipidemia/hypercholesterolemia (through vascular issues, potentially affecting blood flow to the inner ear), and osteoporosis (through changes in the structure of the bony inner ear). Previous head trauma has also been reported to increase the likelihood of experiencing vertigo by damaging structures related to balance, such as the inner ear or the vestibular nerve. Another factor that has been linked to various health issues, including musculoskeletal problems and possibly vertigo, is vitamin D deficiency. However, it is essential to note that vertigo can have multifactorial etiology, and individual cases may require thorough evaluation to determine the underlying factors contributing to the symptoms.

Clinical Approach to a Case of Vertigo

The approach to a case of vertigo is depicted in **Flowchart 1**. The starting point is usually to differentiate between the two main sets of pathologies: (1) those resulting in vertigo and (2) those causing a presyncope-like sensation. Frank syncope should always be considered if loss of consciousness occurs with a fall, if there is an unexplained nonaccidental fall, or if there are recurrent falls despite a multifactorial management program. Through a series of questions regarding the duration and nature of symptoms and associated symptoms such as hearing loss, tinnitus, falls, and seizure-like activity, the provisional diagnosis is narrowed down. Further confirmation may require the entire range from basic bedside tests to advanced investigations.

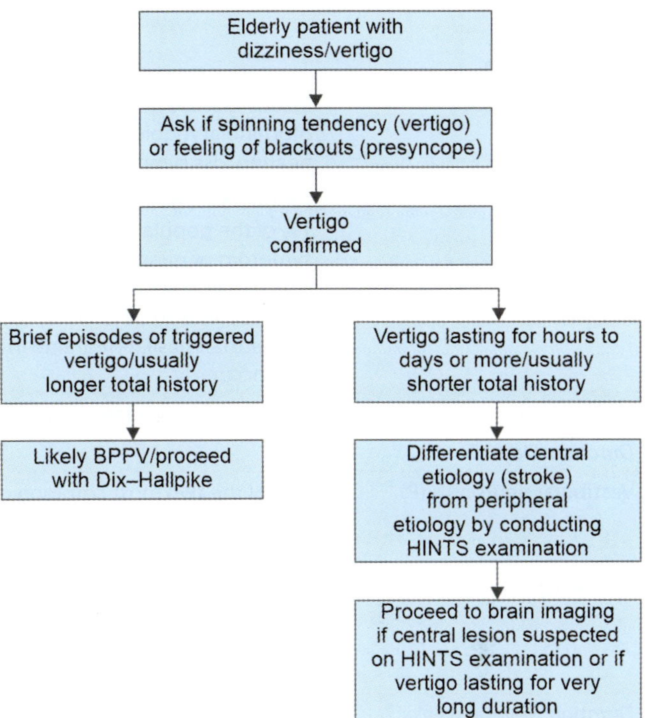

FLOWCHART 1: Approach to vertigo.
(BPPV: benign paroxysmal positional vertigo; HINTS: head impulse, nystagmus, test of skew)

The differential diagnoses of vertigo with relevant clinical features and examination findings are presented in **Table 1**, and the salient features of BPPV are elaborated in **Table 2**. A life-threatening condition resulting in vertigo is a stroke of the posterior circulation territories. Needless to say, neither the common nor the life-threatening etiologies should be missed in geriatric practice.

TABLE 1: Differential diagnoses of vertigo: History and examination.

Duration of attack: Few seconds	
Late stages of acute vestibular Neuronitis (P)	
Unilateral loss of vestibular function (P)	Diagnosed by caloric testing
Duration: Several seconds to few minutes	
Benign paroxysmal positional vertigo (BPPV) (P)	Nearly half of all peripheral vertigo cases. Females are affected twice more often. More of a disease of the elderly and with a possible link to previous episodes of labyrinthitis. Occurs due to the displacement of otoconia. Very good therapeutic response to repositioning maneuvers
Duration: Several minutes to few hours	
Transient ischemic attack (posterior circulation/brainstem) (C)	Acute cerebellar infarcts are the most common cause of central vascular vertigo. Small infarcts of the cerebellum or brainstem may result in only vertigo and no other symptoms. Sometimes Meniere's-like symptoms may be the prodrome of a frank stroke. Differentiated from peripheral causes of vertigo by the HINTS examination

Continued

Continued

Duration: Hours	
Meniere's disease (P)	Mostly disease of middle age. A significant minority, however, occurs in the elderly. Presents in otorhinolaryngology service usually rather than to a geriatrician, due to prominent ear fullness and hearing loss symptoms
Migraine (C)	Around 50% patients of with migraine also have vertigo, but pure vestibular migraine affects 1% of the population. Females are more affected. Family history may be positive. Vertigo as a symptom of migraine is more common later in life and after a long gap of years from the onset of a typical headache of migraine. Mostly duration is minutes to hours, but variations are possible from seconds to days. Many cases may be acephalgic, lacking any headache. Vestibular migraine is milder than basilar migraine in which headache is usually present and frank brainstem symptoms may occur
Panic attacks	Often, other psychiatric features may coexist
Duration: Days	
Vestibular neuronitis (P)	One of the two most common causes of vertigo in the elderly. Usually follows or occurs with an acute viral infection of the ear or upper respiratory tract. If associated with hearing loss, it is called labyrinthitis, and this is less common. Symptoms may continue up to >2 weeks
Stroke (C)	May or may not follow transient ischemic attacks in a patient with other vascular risk factors. May be ischemic or hemorrhagic. The prognosis varies, as for other types of strokes. Other brainstem signs may be found on examination. HINTS helps in differentiating from peripheral etiologies of vertigo
Duration: Several weeks	
Psychogenic	Often other psychiatric features may coexist. It may be a diagnosis of exclusion. Vestibular neuronitis or stroke symptoms may sometimes last for long durations, and this may be confused with psychogenic vertigo

Notes: P in parentheses (P) represents peripheral etiology, while (C) represents central etiology. Vertigo in Meniere's disease, vertebrobasilar TIA, vestibular neuronitis, panic attacks, and vestibular migraine usually occur spontaneously, while vertigo in BPPV is triggered by specific head movements.
(BPPV: benign paroxysmal positional vertigo; HINTS: head impulse, nystagmus, test of skew; TIA: transient ischemic attack)

TABLE 2: Benign paroxysmal positional vertigo.

Posterior canal	Horizontal/lateral canal	Anterior/superior canal
The most common and classic form of BPPV. *Typical symptom*: Brief vertigo episodes specifically while turning in bed or getting up from a lying position or lying from a sitting position	Atypical BPPV symptoms. Vertigo while turning head left or right while upright	The rarest type of BPPV but with typical symptoms such as posterior canal type
Dix–Hallpike test used for diagnosis	Supine head roll test used for diagnosis	Dix–Hallpike test used for diagnosis
Nystagmus on Dix–Hallpike testing is usually unilateral and when the head turned toward the affected side	Nystagmus is usually bilateral. The side where it is more intense should be taken as the affected side in most cases	Nystagmus is usually bilateral. Side determination is not necessary as management is by common maneuver
Vertical (up-beating) nystagmus with torsion. Torsion is counterclockwise for the right-side lesion and clockwise for the left side	Horizontal nystagmus toward the ground (geotropic) or away from the ground (apogeotropic)	Vertical (down-beating) nystagmus with torsion
Treated by Epley maneuver (best), Semont maneuver, or others	Treated by Gufoni maneuver	Treated by deep head hanging maneuver

Note: Self-explanatory videos by Dr Peter Johns may be accessed freely on YouTube concerning both BPPV types and diagnoses and the HINTS examination.
(BPPV: benign paroxysmal positional vertigo)

BEDSIDE TESTS FOR DISORDERS OF VERTIGO, DIZZINESS, AND IMBALANCE

The techniques for diagnosing disorders of balance are diverse and the sheer number of tests may overwhelm the uninitiated geriatrician, especially the postgraduate trainee. It is prudent to develop one's own outpatient and in-patient protocol for the evaluation of a patient with dizziness or vertigo. A sample of the main tests with standard techniques for performing them and their interpretation is provided in **Table 3**. These may be categorized into five groups: (1) Test of orthostatic hypotension (which helps in differentiating vertigo from presyncope), (2) tests of gait and balance concerning somatosensory systems, (3) tests to differentiate cerebrovascular events causing vertigo from peripheral etiologies of vertigo, (4) tests for nystagmus, and (5) specialized tests for individual organs/conditions. They usually need to be performed on a case-by-case basis, and not every test is essential for every patient. **Flowchart 1** may be followed for guidance.

TABLE 3: Clinical examination—tests in vertigo.

Test of orthostatic hypotension	Blood pressure is measured using the standard technique in the supine position and then after 1 and 3 minutes of standing erect. The cuff is kept wrapped throughout the procedure
Tests of gait and balance concerning somatosensory systems	
General observation of gait	Type of gait may give clues regarding the affected organ/system
Romberg's test	Patient is made to stand with his feet close together, arms by the side and eyes open. The patient is then asked to close his eyes. Romberg's test is considered positive if there is a significant imbalance with the eyes closed or if the imbalance significantly worsens upon closing the eyes. A positive test indicates posterior column dysfunction
Brief neurological screen including sensory/motor and reflex domains	Mostly performed when unsteadiness is the main complaint
Tandem gait	The patient is asked to walk along a straight line touching the heel of one foot to the toes of the other with each subsequent step. Impaired in cerebellar disease, vestibular disease, and also some peripheral neuropathies
Tests to differentiate cerebrovascular events from peripheral etiologies of vertigo	
HINTS protocol	Most commonly used to differentiate vestibular neuronitis (peripheral) from stroke (central). Hence, performed in patients with hours to a few days of vertigo. It has three components: 1. *Head impulse test*: The patient is asked to relax his/her head and maintain his/her gaze on the examiner's nose. The patient's head is gently moved back and forth to right and left a few times and then rapidly moved back to the neutral position. The head impulse test is positive (consistent with peripheral vertigo) if there is a significant lag with corrective saccades, which is visible to the examiner. The corrective saccade is observed when the head is turned rapidly toward the affected side (For example, in right-sided pathology, saccades would be observed when the head is rapidly turned from left to neutral). The test is negative in central pathologies 2. *Nystagmus*: Nystagmus is checked at the neutral position of gaze (mostly absent) and at eccentric gaze. Vertical nystagmus is mostly central in origin. Bidirectional nystagmus (e.g., fast phase toward left while gazing toward left and toward right while gazing toward the right) is indicative of central pathology. Unidirectional nystagmus with a fast component beating toward the healthy side and increasing in intensity in the direction of the fast component is indicative of a peripheral lesion (For example, in a patient with right vestibular neuronitis, nystagmus beats toward the left in rightward gaze and beats more strongly toward the left in leftward gaze) 3. *Skew deviation*: This is a vertical misalignment of the visual axes which is explained in **Figure 2A**. Skew deviation is positive in central pathologies All three components need to give similar results, i.e., unidirectional nystagmus, positive head impulse test (abnormal head impulse test result), and negative skew for diagnosing a peripheral pathology
Tests for nystagmus	
Vertical nystagmus	Usually, central pathology/is also seen in BPPV
Nystagmus in the setting of the Dix–Hallpike test	BPPV

Continued

Continued

Spontaneous unidirectional nystagmus	As discussed above in the HINTS examination. This is usually suppressed by visual fixation and, hence, may not be observed in the neutral position unless using Frenzel glasses. Usually indicative of peripheral pathology
Gaze-evoked nystagmus	Only occurs on eccentric gaze. It is indicative of central pathologies or alcohol/drug intoxication. The fast phase is always in the direction of gaze, which is also the side of the lesion if nystagmus is unilateral. It may be confused with spontaneous nystagmus when the latter is evident only in eccentric gaze. Frenzel glasses differentiate gaze-evoked from spontaneous unidirectional nystagmus
Perverted head shaking nystagmus	Following vigorous horizontal head shaking around 20 times with 30° forward tilt, three or more vertical beats may indicate a cerebellar or brainstem lesion
Specialized tests for individual organs/conditions	
Dix–Hallpike test	Diagnostic of posterior and anterior column BPPV, as demonstrated in **Figure 2B**
Head impulse test	As described above as part of HINTS. Test of the vestibulo-ocular reflex
Cerebellar tests	Finger–nose test, heel shin test, and test for dysdiadochokinesia
Subjective visual vertical bucket test	Description beyond the scope of the chapter. Test of utricle and saccule
(BPPV: benign paroxysmal positional vertigo; HINTS: head impulse, nystagmus, test of skew)	

INVESTIGATIVE PROTOCOL

After ruling out presyncope clinically, evaluation of vertigo should be done. Examination of the ear canal and eardrum may be performed using an otoscope. The otoscope is a handheld instrument with a light and a magnifying lens that allows healthcare providers to see inside the ear. During otoscopy, the healthcare provider looks for abnormalities such as inflammation, fluid buildup, earwax blockage, or perforation of the tympanic membrane (eardrum). In contrast to dizziness/presyncope where investigations are of paramount importance, probably the only major investigation employed in the differential diagnosis of vertigo is magnetic resonance imaging of the brain, which aids in evaluating the posterior fossa and ruling out potentially threatening conditions such as stroke of the brainstem. Specialized testing such as computerized subjective visual vertical test, vestibular evoked myogenic potential testing, and electrocochleography/dynamic computerized posturography are rarely available even in the best centers unless research in vestibular dysfunction is being actively pursued. A detailed description of these tests is beyond the scope of this chapter, but certain representative examples are described in brief in **Table 4**.

TABLE 4: Examples of specialized investigations in the evaluation of vertigo.

Caloric testing	Cold or warm water is introduced into the external ear canal using a syringe. Cold water induces nystagmus with fast components toward opposite sides, whereas the response to warm water is the opposite. This will be absent in the affected side in cases of unilateral vestibular dysfunction
Vestibular-evoked myogenic potentials	A short latency electromyographic potential is evoked in response to high-level acoustic stimuli and allows the testing of otolith and vestibular nerve function. It is recorded from the sternocleidomastoid and extraocular muscles
Computerized dynamic posturography	A quantitative test of measuring postural sway by using a foot platform. It has the same basis as Romberg's test and focuses on the vestibulospinal reflex

RARER ENTITIES CAUSING VERTIGO

Apart from the common entities discussed in the previous sections, a few rare causes of vertigo that affect the elderly deserve mention. These include paroxysmal brainstem attacks caused by multiple sclerosis, space-occupying lesions of the brainstem or cerebellopontine angle, rotational vertebral artery occlusion syndrome, perilymphatic fistula, and superior canal dehiscence syndrome. Two especially relevant entities are vestibular paroxysmia which is highly responsive to carbamazepine and vestibular epileptic spells. In fact, in the absence of another definite diagnosis, a trial of antiepileptics is often used in patients with recurrent spells of syncope and possibly vertigo. Cervicogenic dizziness, i.e., vertigo attributed to cervical spondylosis which is quite a popular diagnosis among the lay public and even many physicians, has not been proven in experimental models conclusively and remains a dubious entity. The relief occurring with cervical collar use may actually result from not moving the head at all and not from any benefit rendered to cervical vertebral disease.

THERAPY OF VERTIGO IN THE ELDERLY

As is evident from the diversity of etiologies of vertigo and dizziness, the management of individual conditions is highly specific and highly personalized.

Management of posterior canal BPPV: The Epley maneuver is commonly performed in the clinic as well as advised to patients at home after a definite diagnosis of posterior canal BPPV. While a single sitting may be curative, repeat efforts are required in refractory cases. The first step is the same as the Dix–Hallpike maneuver for the affected side **(Fig. 2B)**, and the head is held in that position for 30–120 seconds. Following this, the patient's head is turned 90° to the other side, keeping both shoulders still on the bed (again for 30–120 seconds). The third step involves turning both the body and the head through 90° more so that one shoulder touches the bed, and the head looks 45° downward toward the unaffected side (30–120 seconds). The patient is then made to sit up straight facing the unaffected side, completing the curative maneuver.

Management of vestibular neuronitis: Antihistaminics such as promethazine and meclizine may be used, the former being preferred at our center. Though the dose of promethazine recommended is 25 mg QID, significantly lower doses such as 10 mg OD or BID suffice in many elderly patients. Antiemetics such as metoclopramide and prochlorperazine are the drugs of choice in the young but as neither is used at our center in geriatric practice due to its high adverse effect profile, symptomatic benefit is instead rendered by ondansetron. Benzodiazepines may also be used for symptom alleviation, while the role of oral steroids and antivirals is controversial. Vestibular rehabilitation may be useful.

Role of betahistine: The histamine analog, H1 receptor agonist, betahistine remains one of the most overused medications in India for practically all forms of vertigo, and surprisingly, it seems to do well. While approved in most countries for Meniere's disease alone, it is routinely prescribed for all other forms of vertigo including BPPV. A Cochrane review seems to support such off-label uses. The exact mechanism of how betahistine helps or probably helps in these conditions is unclear. Benefits may be obtained with as little as a single dose or sometimes with months of treatment. Some of the

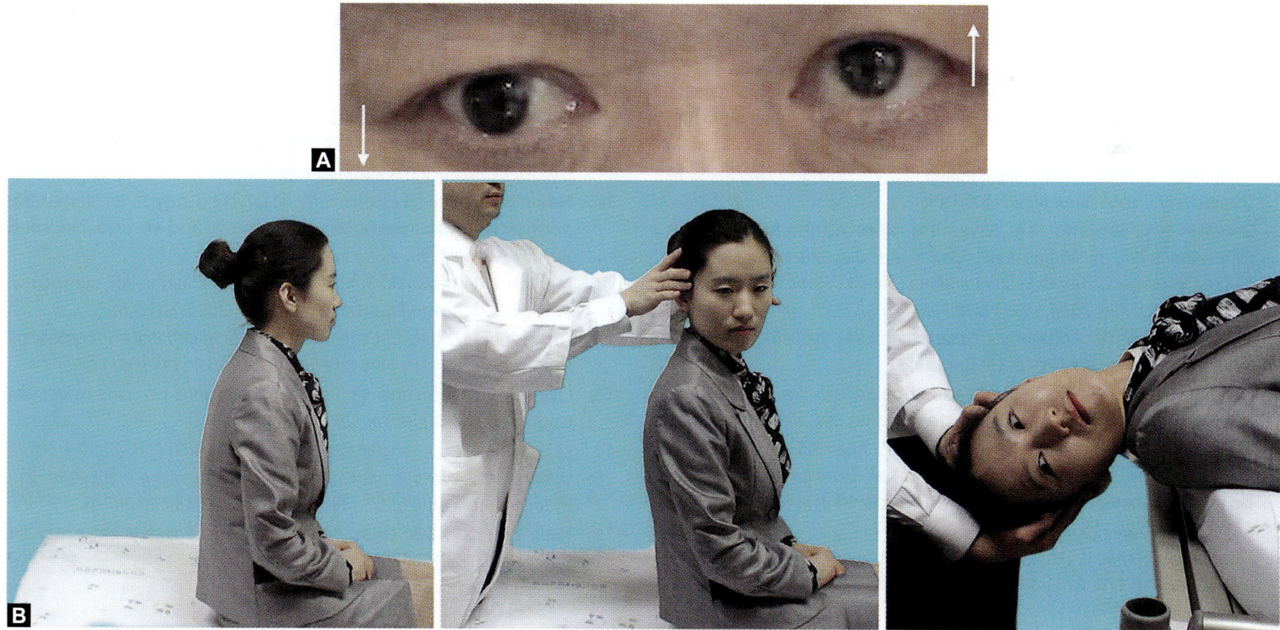

FIGS. 2A AND B: (A) Skew deviation (part of HINTS examination); (B) Dix–Hallpike test.

(HINTS: head impulse, nystagmus, test of skew)

Source: Reproduced with permission from Professor Ji Soo Kim, Department of Neurology, Seoul National University College of Medicine, Seoul, South Korea.

Note: In Figure 2A, the eyes are covered alternately one after the other. As soon as one eye is uncovered, observe for vertical gaze correction which if present indicates a central lesion as a cause of vertigo. In Figure 2B, in Dix–Hallpike testing, if the right ear is thought to be affected by BPPV, the patient's head is turned 45° to the right while in a sitting position. Then, the patient is brought to a supine position with the head turned as before and hanging by 20° from the edge of the bed. Nystagmus usually starts after a latent period of around 20 seconds and may show fatigue.

cases that respond may be actually undiagnosed cases of Meniere's disease. The preference for this drug in geriatric practice also stems from its evidently low side-effect profile and the probability of parkinsonian symptoms with the other oft-used vestibular suppressant cinnarizine.

The management of vertigo due to stroke, transient ischemic attacks, and epileptic vertigo are as per existing treatment protocols for these conditions in the absence of vertigo. Topiramate and lamotrigine are especially useful in vestibular migraine although standard therapeutic options for migraine may also be employed with success. Meniere's disease benefits from diuretics, vestibular suppressants, etc., whereas antidepressants and anxiolytics are often helpful in psychiatric causes of vertigo and dizziness.

CONCLUSION

The syndrome of vertigo in the elderly remains an intriguing condition. However, following a stepwise and logical approach to such cases may result in more accurate diagnoses and better treatment results.

What is best to remember?

- Vertigo and presyncope have diverse etiologies and need to be differentiated at the onset of history taking, as diagnostic and therapeutic pathways for the two conditions are different.
- BPPV and vestibular neuronitis are the most common etiologies of vertigo in the elderly.
- One should promptly exclude probable life-threatening etiologies of vertigo such as stroke, while not overlooking common etiologies.

Self-Assessment Questionnaire

Q1. What do you think is the clinical diagnosis of Gulabi Devi?

Q2. Which specific physical examination will be relevant in this case?

Q3. Is there a role of Dix–Hallpike maneuver in this case?

Q4. Will you do any special investigation for this patient?

Q5. What may be a good treatment option for this patient?

FURTHER READINGS

1. Bisdorff AR, Staab JP, Newman-Toker DE. Overview of the international classification of vestibular disorders. Neurol Clin. 2015;33(3):541-50.
2. Fernández L, Breinbauer HA, Delano PH. Vertigo and dizziness in the elderly. Front Neurol. 2015;6:144.
3. Sanders NA, Supiano MA. Assessing older adults for syncope following a fall. In: Williams BA, Chang A (Eds). Current Diagnosis & Treatment—Geriatrics, 2nd edition. New York: McGraw-Hill Education Lange; 2014. pp. 443-6.
4. Khan S, Chang R. Anatomy of the vestibular system: a review. Neuro Rehabilitation. 2013;32(3):437-43.
5. Iwasaki S, Yamasoba T. Dizziness and imbalance in the elderly: age-related decline in the vestibular system. Aging Dis. 2015;6(1):38-47.
6. Balatsouras DG, Koukoutsis G, Ganelis P, Korres GS, Kaberos A. Diagnosis of single- or multiple-canal benign paroxysmal positional vertigo according to the type of nystagmus. Int J Otolaryngol. 2011;2011:1-13.
7. Muncie HL, Sirmans SM, James E. Dizziness: approach to evaluation and management. Am Fam Physician. 2017;95(3):154-62.
8. Lui F, Foris LA, Tadi P. Central Vertigo. Treasure Island, FL: StatPearls Publishing; 2025.
9. Baumgartner B, Taylor RS. Peripheral Vertigo (Archived). Treasure Island, FL: StatPearls Publishing; 2025.
10. Newman-Toker DE, Edlow JA. TiTrATE: a novel, evidence-based approach to diagnosing acute dizziness and vertigo. Neurol Clin. 2015;33(3):577-99.
11. Murdin L, Hussain K, Schilder AGM. Betahistine for symptoms of vertigo. Cochrane Database Syst Rev. 2013;2013(8).
12. Arnold AC, Shibao C. Current concepts in orthostatic hypotension management. Curr Hypertens Rep. 2013;15(4):304-12.
13. Obermann M, Strupp M. Current treatment options in vestibular migraine. Front Neurol. 2014;5:257.
14. Lee H. Isolated vascular vertigo. J Stroke. 2014;16(3):124-30.
15. Vibert D, Caversaccio M, Häusler R. Meniere's disease in the elderly. Otolaryngol Clin North Am. 2010;43(5):1041-6.
16. Huh Y-E, Kim J-S. Bedside evaluation of dizzy patients. J Clin Neurol. 2013;9(4):203-13.

CHAPTER 33

Sexuality in Older Age

Sudeep Mathew George, Vasu Digra

INTRODUCTION

Aging is a natural process that causes various physiological changes throughout the human body. One significant area affected by aging is the reproductive system. As individuals grow older, the reproductive organs undergo various alterations, leading to a decline in reproductive function. The reproductive-cell cycle theory posits that the hormones that regulate reproduction act in an antagonistic pleiotropic manner to control aging via cell cycle signaling, promoting growth and development early in life in order to achieve reproduction, but later in life, in a futile attempt to maintain reproduction, become dysregulated and drive senescence.

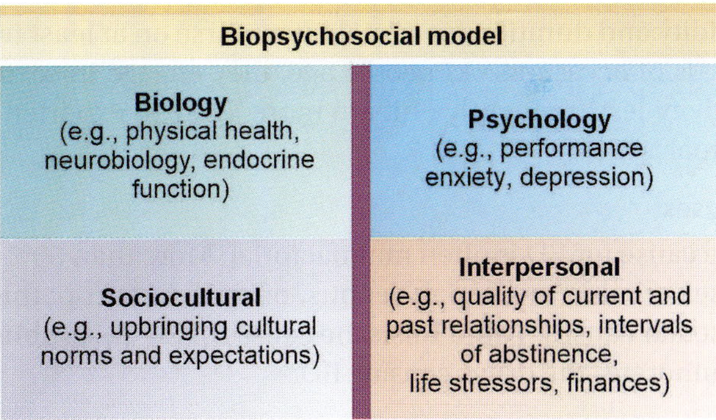

FIG. 1: Biopsychosocial model.

Source: Thomas HN, Thurston RC. A biopsychosocial approach to women's sexual function and dysfunction at midlife: a narrative review. Maturitas. 2016;87:49-60.

INTERACTIVE BIOPSYCHOSOCIAL MODEL

An understanding of the reciprocal relationship between health and sexuality throughout life can be gained by utilizing the interactive biopsychosocial model (IBM) to the degree that medicine attends to matters of sexuality, and the orientation is largely negative. The perspective of the medical model on sexuality emphasizes sexual dysfunction as a negative outcome of aging, illness, or therapy **(Fig. 1)**.

Although the IBM recognizes the correlation between sexuality and health, it also takes into account the potential benefits that sexuality may have on one's health and the potential benefits that aging or illness may have on one's sexual life.

The definition of sexual activity is "any mutually voluntary activity involving sexual contact with another person, whether or not intercourse or orgasm occurs."

The population patterns of sexual activity are projected by sexually active life expectancy, which calculates the number of years of expected future sexual activity for any given age.

SEXUALITY AND OLDER MALES

Physiological Aspects of Aging and Sexuality in Males

Sexual excitement may not always follow desire as one age. The catalysts for arousing sexual desire become increasingly particular and may ask for close physical touch as well as manual stimulation. A male may experience a decrease in the intensity of his sexual desires, take longer to acquire an erection, and require more time after ejaculation before experiencing an erection.

Masters and Johnson have described the physiology of coitus as having four components: (1) Excitement, (2) plateau, (3) orgasm, and (4) resolution, all of which show age-related changes.

Changes in the sexual response cycle with age include:

- *Excitement phase*: Delay in erection, decreased tensing of the scrotal sac, and loss of testicular elevation.
- *Plateau phase*: Prolonged time in phase and reduced pre-ejaculatory secretion.
- Orgasm is reduced in intensity and duration.
- Refractory period between erections is prolonged.

Types of Male Sexual Dysfunction

Male sexual dysfunction is of the following types:

- Erectile dysfunction (ED)
- Decreased libido
- Ejaculatory disorders

Erectile Dysfunction

Erectile dysfunction is defined as the consistent or recurrent inability to acquire or sustain an erection of sufficient rigidity and duration for sexual intercourse on at least two thirds of occasions. As people age, they engage in sexual activity less frequently and are more likely to experience sexual issues.

Causes

The cause for ED is often multifactorial. More than 50% of cases are due to arterial, venous, or mixed neuropathic/vascular causes. **Table 1** lists the causes of ED and **Table 2** enumerates the drugs causing ED.

TABLE 1: Causes of erectile dysfunction.

Causes	Associated findings/risk factors
Vascular	Cardiovascular disease, hypertension, diabetes mellitus, hyperlipidemia, smoking, major surgery (radical prostatectomy), or radiotherapy (pelvis or retroperitoneum)
Neurologic	Spinal cord and brain injuries, Parkinson's disease, Alzheimer's disease, multiple sclerosis, stroke, major surgery (radical prostatectomy), or radiotherapy of the prostate
Local penile (cavernous) factors	Peyronie's disease, cavernous fibrosis, and penile fracture
Hormonal	Hypogonadism, hyperprolactinemia, hyper- and hypothyroidism, and hyper- and hypocortisolism
Drug induced	Antihypertensives, antidepressants, antipsychotics, antiandrogens, recreational drugs, and alcohol
Psychogenic	Performance-related anxiety, traumatic past experiences, relationship problems, anxiety, depression, and stress

In cases of suspected drug-induced sexual dysfunction, improvement after drug withdrawal provides the best evidence for the adverse effect.

Decreased Libido

Libido declines with age in sexually active men. Low libido is linked to low levels of overall happiness as well as low levels of emotional and physical sexual fulfillment. Low testosterone, stress, interpersonal problems, depression, systemic illness, polypharmacy, and use of recreational substances are associated with decreased libido. There is a strong association between low libido in men with lower urinary tract symptoms (LUTS) and other sexual and voiding disorders.

Causes

The major causes of low libido include:

- Medications [selective serotonin reuptake inhibitors (SSRIs), antiandrogens, 5-alpha reductase inhibitors, and opioid analgesics]
- Alcoholism
- Depression
- Fatigue
- Hypoactive sexual disorder
- Recreational drugs
- Relationship problems
- Other sexual dysfunction (fear of humiliation)
- Sexual aversion disorder
- Systemic illness
- Testosterone deficiency and other hormonal abnormalities

Since most of these conditions have the potential to be treated, it is critical to get a thorough medical history, conduct a thorough examination, and acquire pertinent laboratory investigations to identify any potential conditions.

TABLE 2: Drugs that cause erectile dysfunction.

Drug class	Examples
Diuretics	Thiazides and spironolactone
Antihypertensives	CCB, beta-blockers, methyldopa, clonidine, reserpine, and guanethidine
Cardiac	Digoxin, gemfibrozil, and clofibrate
Antidepressants	SSRI, TCA, lithium, and MAOI
Tranquilizers	Butyrophenones and phenothiazines
H2 antagonists	Ranitidine and cimetidine
Hormones	Progesterone, estrogens, and corticosteroids

(CCB: calcium channel blocker; MAOI: monoamine oxidase inhibitor; SSRI: selective serotonin reuptake inhibitor; TCA: tricyclic antidepressant)

Hypogonadism

Age-related declines in testosterone have multiple causes. Older male hypogonadal has slightly higher amounts of luteinizing hormone, although they are rarely abnormal. Because of this, it is thought that these men have secondary hypogonadism (hypothalamic-pituitary hypogonadism). The major cause of this is due to erratic release of gonadotropin-releasing hormone from hypothalamus. Additionally, there is a rise in the pituitary gland's negative feedback of testosterone. Older men have a reduction in their testosterone response to human chorionic gonadotropin. The number of Leydig cells is declining.

With aging, there is an increase in sex hormone-binding globulin (SHBG), leading to less testosterone being available to the tissues.

Ejaculatory Disorders

Ejaculatory disorders are a heterogeneous group of disorders that include premature, delayed, and retrograde ejaculation and anorgasmia.

SEXUALITY AND OLDER FEMALES

Physiological Aspects of Aging and Sexuality in Females

The phases of the sexual response cycle—excitement, plateau, orgasm, and resolution—remain generally the same, but the timing, intensity, and duration of each phase can change with age. Changes in the sexual response cycle are given as follows:

- *Excitement phase*:
  - *Hormonal changes*: With age, there may be alterations in hormone levels, such as decreased production of estrogen. Arousal levels generally, genital responses, and sexual desire can all be impacted by these hormonal shifts.
  - *Slower arousal*: Compared to younger adults, older adults may need more time or more stimulation to become sexually aroused. This could be brought on by variations in blood flow, genital sensitivity, or psychological elements such as stress or distraction.
- *Plateau phase*:
  - *Longer plateau phase*: An extended period of increased arousal preceding an orgasm may be experienced by older adults. This could be explained by altered genital lubrication and blood flow or by slower physiological reactions.
  - *Increased need for stimulation*: Due to aging-related changes in arousal or genital sensation, older adults may need to engage in longer or more intense sexual stimulation sessions in order to sustain arousal during the plateau phase.
- *Orgasm phase*:
  - *Absence, delayed onset, or altered intensity of orgasms*: Aging-related alterations in physiological arousal or psychological factors such as relationship problems, stress, or anxiety can cause some older adults to have trouble experiencing orgasms. With age, females may also notice changes in the length or intensity of their orgasms.
- *Resolution phase*:
  - *Longer recovery time*: Older adults may experience a longer resolution phase following orgasm, with a slower return to baseline levels of arousal and longer refractory periods. This could be brought on by aging-related changes in hormone levels, muscle recovery, or cardiovascular function.
  - *Enhanced satisfaction*: The quality of relationships, emotional intimacy, and communication are some of the factors that may contribute to older adults reporting higher levels of sexual intimacy and satisfaction despite changes in the sexual response cycle.

Changes in Female Reproductive Organs

Menopause marks the end of a woman's reproductive years and is characterized by a cessation of menstruation, typically occurring between the ages of 45 and 55 years. Numerous anatomical, physiological, and psychological changes are linked to this transition and can have an effect on a woman's quality of life, emotional stability, and physical health.

Anatomical Changes

- *Ovaries*: There are notable alterations to the ovaries during menopause. The quantity and functionality of ovarian follicles, which house immature eggs, decline with time, which lowers the production of progesterone and estrogen. The onset of menopausal symptoms and the end of menstruation are both influenced by this drop in hormone levels.
- *Uterus*: During menopause, the uterus may also experience anatomical changes. The reduction in estrogen levels may cause the endometrium, or inner lining of the uterus, to thin and become less vascularized. Consequently, before menstruation completely stops, women may notice changes in their menstrual flow or irregular bleeding.

Other Anatomical Changes

- Narrowing and shortening of vaginal barrel
- Atrophy of vaginal mucosa
- Decreased elasticity of mucosa

- Loss of vaginal folds
- Increased friability/fragility/fissures
- Loss of labia minora
- Uterine/vaginal prolapse

Types of Female Sexual Dysfunction

Based on the International Classification of Diseases 11th Revision (ICD-11) diagnostic guidelines, sexual dysfunctions are classified into four primary groups:

1. Sexual desire and arousal dysfunctions
2. Orgasmic dysfunctions
3. Ejaculatory dysfunctions
4. Other specified sexual dysfunctions

Desire and arousal disorders in older females refer to difficulties in experiencing or maintaining sexual arousal during sexual activity, leading to distress or impairment in sexual function and satisfaction. These conditions can show up as psychological or physiological difficulties that affect a woman's capacity to arouse sexually or to remain aroused during close relationships.

Diagnostic Criteria

- *A*: Lack of, or significantly reduced, sexual interest or arousal as manifested by at least three of the following:
  - i. Absent or reduced interest in sexual activity
  - ii. Absent/reduced sexual/erotic thoughts or fantasies
  - iii. No/reduced sexual initiation of sexual activity and typically unreceptive to a partner's attempt to initiate
  - iv. Absent/reduced excitement/pleasure during sexual activity in almost all or all (approximately 75–100%) sexual encounters (in identified situational contexts or if generalized in all contexts)
  - v. Absent/reduced sexual interest/arousal in response to any internal or external sexual/erotic cues (e.g., written, verbal, visual)
  - vi. Absent/reduced genital or nongenital sensations during sexual activity in almost all or all (approximately 75–100%) sexual encounters (in identified situational contexts or if generalized in all contexts)
- *B*: The symptoms in criterion A have persisted for a minimum duration of approximately 6 months.
- *C*: The symptoms in criterion A cause clinically significant distress in the individual.
- *D*: The sexual dysfunction is not better explained by a nonsexual mental disorder or as a consequence of severe relationship distress or other significant stressors and is not attributed to the effects of a substance/medication or other medical disorders.

Also, specify whether this problem has been lifelong or acquired, generalized, or situational and the severity—mild, moderate, and severe.

- *Hypoactive sexual desire disorder (HSDD)*: Although the main symptom of HSDD is an absence or lack of sexual desire, in certain situations, it can also affect sexual arousal. A decline in libido or interest in sexual activity is a common occurrence in older women.
- *Female sexual arousal disorder (FSAD)*: FSAD is characterized by problems achieving physical arousal during intercourse, such as inadequate lubrication, genital engorgement, or arousal sensations. These disorders are the result of both physiological and psychological alterations.
- *Situational arousal disorder*: In the absence of general arousal issues, situational arousal disorder is defined as the inability to become sexually aroused in situations or contexts. Anxiety, relationship problems, environmental distractions, or discomfort with aging-related changes in sexual function or appearance can all contribute to situational arousal difficulties experienced by older females.
- *Medication-induced arousal disorders*: Several drugs, including hormone therapies, antidepressants, and antihypertensives, are frequently prescribed to older adults. However, some of these drugs have side effects that affect arousal and function during sexual activity. Changes in blood flow regulation, neurotransmitter levels, or hormonal balance can all contribute to medication-induced arousal disorders in older females.

Treatment of Arousal Disorders

There is evidence for modified Masters and Johnson treatment, behavioral sex therapy, cognitive behavioral therapy, and mindfulness-based approaches.

When relationship factors are contributing to low sexual desire, counseling the patient about changes the couple can make in their sexual relationship can lead to improvement. Discuss with the patient that sexual interest typically decreases with relationship duration, so encourage interventions that increase novelty. These may include spending a night away from home, trying a new sexual position, incorporating a device, or having sex in an unusual location or at a different time of day. Establishing a regular "date night" often improves sexual satisfaction, as couples that enjoy time together outside of the bedroom often have more pleasure in the bedroom.

Androgen treatments that increase serum concentrations to supraphysiologic levels in the low male range may significantly increase sexual desire and frequency in females but are not advised due to potential risks and side effects.

Orgasmic disorders in elderly females refer to difficulties or challenges related to achieving orgasm during sexual activity. These conditions may show up as absent, weakened, or delayed orgasms, which can cause discomfort or impair sexual pleasure and function.

Diagnostic Criteria

- *A*: Presence of either of the following symptoms and experienced on almost all or all (approximately 75–100%) occasions of sexual activity (in identified situational contexts or if generalized in all contexts):
  - Marked delay in, marked infrequency of, or absence of orgasm
  - Marked reduced intensity of orgasmic sensations
- *B*: The symptoms in criterion A have persisted for a minimum duration of approximately 6 months.
- *C*: The symptoms in criterion A cause clinically significant distress in the individual.
- *D*: The sexual dysfunction is not better explained by a nonsexual mental disorder or as a consequence of severe relationship distress or other significant stressors and is not attributed to the effects of a substance/medication or other medical disorder.

Also, specify whether this problem has been lifelong or acquired, generalized, or situational and the severity—mild, moderate, and severe.

- *Delayed orgasm*: Despite sufficient sexual stimulation, delayed orgasm refers to a continuous delay or difficulty in experiencing orgasm. Delay in orgasm in older females can be brought on by hormonal fluctuations, drug side effects, illnesses that impair blood flow or nerve function, or psychological problems such as depression, anxiety, or relationship problems. Delayed orgasm may also be caused by age-related changes in sexual response, such as a decrease in genital sensitivity or arousal.
- *Diminished orgasm*: Diminished orgasm involves experiencing weaker, less intense, or unsatisfying orgasms compared to previous experiences. As they age, older women may experience changes in the length or intensity of orgasms, which can be caused by hormonal fluctuations, modifications to genital sensation, or adjustments to the tone of the pelvic floor muscles. Psychological variables such as stress, exhaustion, or unfavorable sexual beliefs may also be connected to diminished orgasm.
- *Anorgasmia*: Anorgasmia is the term for the ongoing incapacity to experience an orgasm even in the presence of sufficient sexual stimulation and arousal. Anorgasmia in older women can be primary (lifelong) or secondary (acquired), and it can be brought on by a number of medical conditions that impair blood flow or nerve function (e.g., diabetes, cardiovascular disease), hormonal imbalances (e.g., menopause), adverse drug reactions (e.g., antidepressants), psychological factors (anxiety, depression, trauma from the past), or interpersonal problems.
- *Age-related changes in sexual response*: For older females, orgasmic difficulties may be exacerbated by age-related changes in sexual response, such as increased time to orgasm, slower arousal, and decreased genital sensitivity. The genital sensation and lubrication can be affected by menopausal hormonal changes, such as decreased estrogen levels and dry vagina, which can hinder the ability to experience an orgasm. Moreover, variations in the tone of the pelvic floor muscles or nerve activity may impact the orgasmic response.

Treatment of Orgasmic Disorders

Management depends heavily on whether the disorder is lifelong or acquired and situational or generalized.

Acquired situational orgasmic disorder is most common and occurs in the setting of decreased libido and/or relational strain. Treatment primarily focuses on instruction in masturbation, also known as "sexual skills training."

Encouragement to self-stimulate either manually or with a vibrator must take into account the woman's experience with and attitudes about masturbation.

Psychotherapy to assess psychological issues and attitudes regarding orgasm and to complement physical interventions may be necessary. Education about vulvar anatomy, the role of the clitoris in orgasm, and variations in female orgasm may be therapeutic for some women. Women with arousal disorders also commonly have difficulty experiencing orgasm, so evaluation of arousal should be included in women with this complaint. Sleep dysfunction is a common comorbidity in women with libido, arousal, and orgasm disorders.

Penetrative disorders in elderly females refer to difficulties or challenges related to vaginal penetration during sexual activity. Sexual function and satisfaction may be compromised or discomfort may arise from these disorders as a result of physical pain, discomfort, or an inability to have penetrating sex. Although sexual function can alter as people age, penetrative disorders are not a normal aspect of aging and should be evaluated and treated to address underlying issues and enhance sexual health.

Diagnostic Criteria

- *A*: Persistent or recurrent difficulties with one (or more) of the following:
  i. Vaginal penetration during intercourse
  ii. Marked vulvovaginal or pelvic pain during vaginal intercourse or penetration attempts
  iii. Marked fear or anxiety about vulvovaginal or pelvic pain in anticipation of, during, or as a result of vaginal penetration
  iv. Marked tensing or tightening of pelvic floor muscles during attempted vaginal penetration
- *B*: The symptoms in criterion A have persisted for a minimum duration of approximately 6 months.
- *C*: The symptoms in criterion A cause clinically significant distress in the individual.
- *D*: The sexual dysfunction is not better explained by a nonsexual mental disorder or as a consequence of severe relationship distress or other significant stressors and is not attributed to the effects of a substance/medication or other medical disorder.

Also, specify whether this problem has been lifelong or acquired, generalized, or situational and the severity—mild, moderate, and severe.

- *Dyspareunia*: Dyspareunia refers to persistent or recurrent genital pain experienced before, during, or after sexual intercourse. Several conditions, such as vulvodynia, endometriosis, or pelvic inflammatory disease, as well as decreased lubrication, thinning of the vaginal tissue (vaginal atrophy), pelvic floor dysfunction, and other factors, can cause dyspareunia in aging females. Dyspareunia can also be caused by psychological variables such as anxiety, depression, or traumatic experiences in the past.
- *Vaginismus*: Vaginismus is a condition characterized by involuntary muscle spasms in the pelvic floor muscles, which can make vaginal penetration painful or impossible. Alterations in the tone or sensitivity of the pelvic floor, hormonal imbalances, traumatic past experiences, or anxiety about the changing sexual function of aging may all contribute to vaginismus in older females. Vaginismus can have a substantial negative influence on sexual intimacy and may be treated with medical or psychological therapies.
- *Pelvic organ prolapse (POP)*: POP occurs when the pelvic organs, such as the uterus, bladder, or rectum, descend into the vaginal canal due to weakened pelvic floor muscles or connective tissue. POP can lead to discomfort, pressure, or pain during sexual intercourse, particularly with deep penetration. Older women may be at an increased risk of POP due to factors such as childbirth, hormonal changes, obesity, or connective tissue disorders.
- *Vulvar vestibulitis syndrome (VVS)*: VVS is a condition characterized by pain or discomfort in the vestibule, the area surrounding the vaginal opening. Women with VVS may experience burning, stinging, or irritation with touch, including penetration during intercourse. VVS can be caused by inflammation, infection, hormonal changes, or hypersensitivity of the vulvar tissues. In elderly females, VVS may be exacerbated by hormonal changes associated with menopause or age-related thinning of vaginal tissue.
- *Scar tissue or surgical adhesions*: Older women who have undergone pelvic surgery, such as hysterectomy, may experience scar tissue formation or adhesions that can interfere with vaginal penetration and cause discomfort or pain during intercourse. Scar tissue or adhesions may restrict vaginal mobility, alter vaginal anatomy, or increase sensitivity to pressure or friction.

Treatment of Penetrative Disorders

Management involves treatment of the underlying condition. Lubricants are typically used to reduce friction during vaginal or anal penetration in women with dyspareunia and are also available in hundreds of variations over the counter.

Both moisturizers and lubricants may be used in conjunction with hormone therapy.

Pelvic physical therapy is an effective modality for treating dyspareunia when there is a pelvic, abdominal, and/or low-back component to the dyspareunia and when vaginismus is present.

Vaginal dilation with graded dilators or other devices and behavioral, sex, or couples' therapy are additional modalities that benefit many women with sexual pain disorders. Kegel exercises for sphincter strengthening are also recommended.

Genitourinary syndrome of menopause (GSM) is a common condition that affects many elderly females during and after menopause. Formerly known as vulvovaginal atrophy or atrophic vaginitis, GSM is defined as a collection of symptoms and signs caused by hypoestrogenic changes to the labia majora/minora, clitoris, vestibule/introitus, vagina, urethra, and bladder that occur in menopausal patients. The syndrome may include, but is not limited to, genital symptoms of dryness, burning, and irritation; sexual symptoms of lack of lubrication, discomfort or pain, and impaired function; and urinary symptoms of urgency, dysuria, and recurrent urinary tract infections. Patients may present with some or all the signs and symptoms, which must be bothersome and should not be better accounted for by another diagnosis. The spectrum of adverse consequences requires long-term treatment in many patients.

The term GSM was first introduced in 2014 and has since replaced the term vaginal atrophy. However, there remains controversy over the term GSM as it includes normal age-related changes and symptoms not necessarily attributable to menopause.

A Core Outcome Set, developed by the Core OutcoMes in MenopAuse (COMMA) consortium and based on an international consensus approach across 21 countries of individuals with lived experience of menopause and their healthcare providers, identifies measures to be used in clinical trials of treatments for genitourinary symptoms. It has since been adopted by the National Institute for Health and Care Excellence and the American Urological Society.

Eight outcomes of core interest include:

1. Pain with sex
2. Vulvovaginal dryness
3. Vulvovaginal discomfort or irritation
4. Discomfort or pain when urinating
5. Change in most bothersome symptom
6. Distress, bother, or interference with genitourinary symptoms
7. Satisfaction with treatment
8. Side effects of treatment

Not included in this outcome set are anatomic and histopathologic appearance of the genitals, vaginal pH, superficial cell appearance, and clinician report of genital appearance.

Symptoms

- Vulvovaginal dryness
- Decreased vaginal lubrication during sexual activity
- Dyspareunia, including vulvar or vaginal pain (at the introitus or within the vagina)
- Vulvar or vaginal bleeding (e.g., postcoital bleeding, labial fissures)
- Decreased arousal, orgasm, or sexual desire
- Vulvovaginal burning, irritation, or itching
- Vaginal discharge (leukorrhea or yellow and malodorous)
- Levator spasm
- Urinary tract symptoms (e.g., urinary frequency, urinary urgency, dysuria, urethral discomfort, hematuria, recurrent urinary tract infections)
- Urethral prolapse/caruncle, etc.

Causes

Hypoestrogenemia, aging, certain medications, medical conditions (e.g., diabetes, autoimmune disorders), and lifestyle factors (e.g., smoking, inadequate hydration) can exacerbate symptoms of GSM or contribute to vaginal and urinary discomfort in elderly females.

Diagnosis

Diagnosis of GSM is typically based on a thorough medical history, physical examination, and assessment of symptoms.

Examination

Labia minora resorption or fusion, tissue fragility/fissures/petechiae, introital retraction, loss of hymenal remnants, prominence of urethral meatus, urethral eversion or prolapse, vulvovaginal pallor/erythema, loss of vaginal rugae, decreased vulvovaginal secretions/lubrication, decreased elasticity, abnormal discharge, and spasm of levator muscles on palpation of the posterior vagina.

Labs

- *Vaginal pH testing*: Vaginal pH may reach levels of 5.5–6.8 or higher in postmenopausal patients, especially those who are not on estrogen therapy. Thus, a pH of ≥5 in the absence of other causes (e.g., infection, semen in setting of recent intercourse) can be an indicator of vaginal atrophy due to estrogen deficiency.
- *Maturation index*: The maturation index is the proportion of parabasal, intermediate, and superficial cells in each 100 cells counted on a smear of the upper two thirds of the vagina. It is used to quantify the proportions of cell types of the vaginal epithelium. In patients with vaginal atrophy, an increase in parabasal cells and a decrease in superficial cells are observed. Patients in early menopause typically have a maturation index of 65 parabasal cells, 30 intermediate cells, and 5 superficial cells. As patients age, parabasal cells will continue to increase, and the maturation index may eventually consist entirely of parabasal cells.
- Urine analysis

Treatment

- *General measures*:
  - *Lifestyle modifications*: Maintaining proper genital and urinary hygiene, staying hydrated, and avoiding irritants such as perfumed soaps or douches can help alleviate symptoms of GSM.
  - *Pelvic floor exercises*: Kegel exercises and pelvic floor physical therapy may help strengthen pelvic floor muscles and improve urinary control in women with GSM-related urinary symptoms.
  - *Regular follow-up*: Women with GSM should have regular follow-up appointments with their healthcare providers to monitor symptoms, adjust treatment as needed, and address any concerns or complications.

- *Pharmacotherapy*:
    - Estradiol ring intravaginally, to change every 90 days
    - Estradiol vaginal tablet 4–10 μg/day
    - Estradiol cream 0.5–4 g/day intravaginally × 2 weeks and then every 2–3 days
    - Dehydroepiandrosterone (DHEA) 6.5 mg/day intravaginally

Overall, GSM is a common and treatable condition that affects many elderly females during and after menopause. Open communication with healthcare providers and a comprehensive approach to care are essential for addressing the complex needs of women with GSM.

PSYCHOLOGICAL CHANGES REGARDING SEX IN OLD AGE

People's attitudes, desires, and experiences with sex often change significantly as they get older.

- *Reevaluating priorities and views on sexuality*: As women age, their perspectives on sexuality may change. A more comprehensive understanding of intimacy and connection in relationships may replace the pursuit of sexual activity for the sake of reproduction or social pressures as people get older. Emotional closeness, camaraderie, and reciprocal regard are frequently more important to older women than the purely physical components of sexual engagement. In addition, how older women view themselves sexually can be influenced by societal attitudes regarding aging and sex. The idea that older women are less desirable sexually or that sexual desire decreases with age is potentially supported by ageist stereotypes and cultural norms. These ideas may cause older women to feel invisible, doubtful of themselves, or ashamed of their sexuality. Nonetheless, it is critical to acknowledge that many older women still view sexuality as a significant part of their lives and that their preferences and needs are varied and legitimate.
- *Biological and health factors*: Aging-related biological changes can also affect the psychological experiences of older women with sex. Menopause can affect a woman's desire and satisfaction with her sexual life. It is marked by hormonal changes and physical symptoms such as dryness or discomfort in the vagina. Furthermore, medications, physical function changes, and long-term health issues can all have an impact on the confidence and sexual function of older women.
- *Relationship dynamics and psychological well-being*: Mental health issues such as anxiety, depression, or body image issues can affect a person's ability to feel and want sexually. In addition, maintaining sexual satisfaction and intimacy into old age depends heavily on the quality of the relationship as well as on communication and mutual understanding between partners.
- *Embracing and adjusting to physical changes*: Older women can experience a smoother transition in their sexual lives by being open with their partners, experimenting with new forms of intimacy, and adjusting to physical changes. Getting assistance from medical professionals, therapists, or support groups can also offer helpful direction and materials for dealing with sexual issues as one age.
- *Mood swings*: For some women, menopausal hormone fluctuations can have an adverse effect on mood regulation, resulting in mood swings, irritability, anxiety, and depression. Additional factors such as sleep disturbances and identity and self-image changes may make these psychological symptoms worse.
- *Self-image and identity*: For many women, menopause marks the end of fertility and the beginning of a new phase of life, marking a significant life transition. Emotions as complex as loss, grief, or liberation may be evoked by this shift. It is possible for women to struggle with shifting ideas about who they are, how they age, and how society views them during this period.

Ageist conceptions of sex are the stereotypes, attitudes, and beliefs that the general public has about older people and sex. One common misconception is that as people get older, they become less interested in having sex. This idea perpetuates the myth that older people are less sexually active or interested in closeness by implying that sexual desire decreases with age. These presumptions ignore the range of experiences that older adults have and the significance of sexuality in their lives even today. Media representations often reinforce ageist stereotypes about sex and aging. Older adults are often portrayed as unattractive or asexual. These portrayals contribute to the marginalization of older adults in discussions about sex and reinforce ageist attitudes in society. Compared to older men, older women may experience more stigma and discrimination for expressing their sexuality due to gender stereotypes and double standards. If they seek sexual relationships or express desires that defy social norms, they might be called "cougars" or "old maids." This double standard is a reflection of long-standing ideas about the sexuality and aging of women.

Age-related prejudice in healthcare occurs when senior citizens seek medical advice or treatment for sexually transmitted illnesses. Healthcare providers may minimize or pathologize older patients' sexual problems, attributing them only to aging rather than treating underlying medical, psychological, or interpersonal issues.

Ageist thinking can contribute to the neglect of sexual health and education initiatives targeted at older adults. Since sexuality is frequently seen as a taboo subject in conversations about aging, older people who need information or help with sexual health issues have fewer resources and support available to them. This neglect impedes efforts to support sexual well-being in later life and perpetuates ageist stereotypes.

It is necessary to question stereotypes, advance inclusivity, and encourage candid conversations about sexuality throughout the lifespan to combat ageist views on sex. It is imperative to acknowledge and honor the varied experiences and aspirations of elderly individuals to counteract ageism and encourage sexual empowerment and fulfillment in later life. Society can foster a more welcoming and encouraging atmosphere for people of all ages to explore by opposing ageist beliefs and encouraging positive portrayals of sexuality in later life.

CONCLUSION

Elderly sexuality and issues related to it have long been neglected not only from the treatment aspect but also from a research point of view. The common misconception is that the elderly are asexual individuals, and sexual activity is meant only for the young. Sexuality in older individuals cannot be seen through the lenses of the youth, primarily focusing on performance and erectile capacity, while overlooking psychological and interpersonal dimensions. In conclusion, the evaluation of sexual dysfunction in older adults requires a comprehensive and individualized approach that considers the unique physiological, psychological, and sociocultural factors associated with aging. By conducting a thorough assessment of medical, psychosocial, and sexual history, healthcare providers can identify underlying causes and develop tailored treatment plans aimed at improving sexual function, enhancing satisfaction, and promoting overall well-being in older adults. Effective management of female sexual dysfunction (FSD) often involves a combination of medical interventions, psychotherapy, lifestyle modifications, and sexual counseling tailored to address the specific needs and concerns of this population.

Self-Assessment Questionnaire

Q1. How does the interactive biopsychosocial model (IBM) help explain the relationship between health, illness, and sexuality in older adults?

Q2. What are the main physiological changes in the sexual response cycle observed in older males and females?

Q3. Which medical and psychological factors commonly contribute to erectile dysfunction and decreased libido in elderly men?

Q4. How does hypogonadism develop in older males, and what hormonal changes are typically observed?

Q5. What are the diagnostic criteria for female sexual dysfunction as per ICD-11, and how can these disorders be categorized?

Q6. Describe the major features and management principles of genitourinary syndrome of menopause (GSM) in elderly women.

Q7. How do psychological and sociocultural factors—such as self-image, ageism, and societal attitudes—impact sexual health and satisfaction in older adults?

Q8. In what ways can relationship counseling and behavioral interventions enhance sexual satisfaction among elderly couples?

FURTHER READINGS

1. Thomas HN, Thurston RC. A biopsychosocial approach to women's sexual function and dysfunction at midlife: A narrative review. Maturitas. 2016;87:49-60.
2. Brecher EM. Review of Human Sexual Inadequacy by Masters WH, Johnson VE. J Sex Res. 1970;6(3):247-50.
3. Avasthi A, Grover S, Sathyanarayana Rao TS. Clinical Practice Guidelines for Management of Sexual Dysfunction. Indian J Psychiatry. 2017;59(Suppl 1):S91-S115.
4. Feldman HA, Goldstein I, Hatzichristou DG, Krane RJ, McKinlay JB. Impotence and its medical and psychosocial correlates: results of the Massachusetts Male Aging Study. J Urol. 1994;151(1): 54-61.
5. Montorsi F, Adaikan G, Becher E, Giuliano F, Khoury S, Lue TF, et al. Summary of the recommendations on sexual dysfunctions in men. J Sex Med. 2010;7(11):3572-88.
6. Lue TF. Erectile dysfunction. N Engl J Med. 2000;342(24):1802-13.

7. Miner MM, Seftel AD. Testosterone and ageing: what have we learned since the Institute of Medicine report and what lies ahead? Int J Clin Pract. 2007;61(4):622-32.
8. Rajfer J, Magee T, Gonzalez-Cadavid N. Future strategies for treating erectile dysfunction. Rev Urol. 2002;4 Suppl 3(Suppl 3): S48-53.
9. Vasconcelos P, Gomez Ponce de Leon R, Serruya SJ, Carneiro B, Nóbrega C, Pereira R, et al. A systematic review on psychological interventions for sexual health in older age. Int J Sex Health. 2023;35(3):399-413.
10. Burnett AL, Nehra A, Breau RH, Culkin DJ, Faraday MM, Hakim LS, et al. Erectile Dysfunction: AUA Guideline. J Urol. 2018;200(3): 633-41.
11. Kloner RA, Goldstein I, Kirby MG, Parker JD, Sadovsky R. Cardiovascular Safety of Phosphodiesterase Type 5 Inhibitors After Nearly 2 Decades on the Market. Sex Med Rev. 2018;6(4): 583-94.
12. Bhasin S, Brito JP, Cunningham GR, Hayes FJ, Hodis HN, Matsumoto AM, et al. Testosterone Therapy in Men With Hypogonadism: An Endocrine Society Clinical Practice Guideline. J Clin Endocrinol Metab. 2018;103(5):1715-44.
13. Yeap BB, Tran C, Douglass CM, McNeil JJ. Testosterone Therapy in Older Men: Present and Future Considerations. Drugs Aging. 2025;42(6):501-12.
14. Kim S, Cho MC, Cho SY, Chung H, Rajasekaran MR. Novel Emerging Therapies for Erectile Dysfunction. World J Mens Health. 2021;39(1):48-64.
15. Frydman V, Pinar U, Abdessater M, Akakpo W, Grande P, Audouin M, et al. Long-term outcomes after penile prosthesis placement for the Management of Erectile Dysfunction: a single-Centre experience. Basic Clin Androl. 2021;31(1):4.
16. Segraves RT. Sexual dysfunction associated with antidepressant therapy. Urol Clin North Am. 2007;34(4):575-9, vii.
17. Brotto LA, Chivers ML, Millman RD, Albert A. Mindfulness-Based Sex Therapy Improves Genital-Subjective Arousal Concordance in Women With Sexual Desire/Arousal Difficulties. Arch Sex Behav. 2016;45(8):1907-21.
18. Raveendran AV, Agarwal A. Premature ejaculation-current concepts in the management: A narrative review. Int J Reprod Biomed. 2021;19(1):5-22.
19. Abdel-Hamid IA, Ali OI. Delayed Ejaculation: Pathophysiology, Diagnosis, and Treatment. World J Mens Health. 2018;36(1): 22-40.
20. Konstantinidis C, Zachariou A, Evgeni E, Çayan S, Boeri L, Agarwal A. Recent Advances in the Diagnosis and Management of Retrograde Ejaculation: A Narrative Review. Diagnostics (Basel). 2025;15(6):726.
21. Myers C, Smith M. Pelvic floor muscle training improves erectile dysfunction and premature ejaculation: a systematic review. Physiotherapy. 2019;105(2):235-43.
22. Simopoulos EF, Trinidad AC. Male erectile dysfunction: integrating psychopharmacology and psychotherapy. Gen Hosp Psychiatry. 2013;35(1):33-8.
23. Fisher JS, Rezk A, Nwefo E, Masterson J, Ramasamy R. Sexual Health in the Elderly Population. Curr Sex Health Rep. 2020;12(4): 381-8.
24. Binder RL, Freedman MA, Sharma KB, Farage MA, Wang Y, Combs C, et al. Histological and Gene Expression Analysis of the Effects of Menopause Status and Hormone Therapy on the Vaginal Introitus and Labia Majora. J Clin Med Res. 2019;11(11):745-59.
25. Dennerstein L, Randolph J, Taffe J, Dudley E, Burger H. Hormones, mood, sexuality, and the menopausal transition. Fertil Steril. 2002;77 Suppl 4:S42-8.
26. Rosen R, Brown C, Heiman J, Leiblum S, Meston C, Shabsigh R, et al. The Female Sexual Function Index (FSFI): a multidimensional self-report instrument for the assessment of female sexual function. J Sex Marital Ther. 2000;26(2):191-208.
27. Lensen S, Archer D, Bell RJ, Carpenter JS, Christmas M, Davis SR, et al. A core outcome set for vasomotor symptoms associated with menopause: the COMMA (Core Outcomes in Menopause) global initiative. Menopause. 2021;28(8):852-8.
28. DeLamater J. Sexual expression in later life: a review and synthesis. J Sex Res. 2012;49(2-3):125-41.
29. Fileborn B, Thorpe R, Hawkes G, Minichiello V, Pitts M, Dune T. Sex, desire and pleasure: considering the experiences of older Australian women. Sex Relation Ther. 2015;30(1):117-30.
30. Hinchliff S, Lewis R, Wellings K, Datta J, Mitchell K. Pathways to help-seeking for sexual difficulties in older adults: qualitative findings from the third National Survey of Sexual Attitudes and Lifestyles (Natsal-3). Age Ageing. 2021;50(2):546-53.

CHAPTER 34

Spirituality in Older Adults

Lt Col Pritam Priyansu Purohit, Rasika Panwar

CASE VIGNETTE

Mr Akshay, a retired government official, is 64 years old and recently diagnosed with *type 2 diabetes mellitus*. He often expresses feelings of *frustration*, perceiving his life's circumstances as unfair. Despite devoutly practicing religious rituals, he believes that he has been given a *disproportionate burden*. His son, unemployed and financially dependent, lives with him, adding further stress, especially in light of his recent diabetes diagnosis and the lifelong medications now required. Mr Akshay also expresses resentment that his *wife, who suffers from rheumatoid arthritis (RA)*, requires regular care.

In contrast, his wife, *Mrs Kamla*, who shares similar life challenges, perceives their circumstances differently. She sees her *son's presence as a blessing*, viewing their *pension as a fortunate provision* and *appreciating the supportive neighbors* around them. Despite her RA diagnosis, she is *grateful for the available treatment options* and views her illness with acceptance, believing that *spiritual fulfillment comes from kindness and humanity*. Her perspective enables her to maintain a resilient and positive outlook.

This vignette highlights the *profound influence of spirituality on perception and coping in older adults, showcasing how deeply rooted beliefs shape responses to similar life situations.*

INTRODUCTION

Spirituality is broadly understood as a journey toward *personal fulfillment, encompassing a spectrum of beliefs, practices, and existential questions*. At its essence, spirituality involves *seeking a deeper connection, whether with a higher power, nature, or one's inner self*. This pursuit of purpose, meaning, and peace is uniquely individual, varying widely among individuals. While often linked with organized religion, spirituality is inherently distinct and may be separate from any specific tradition, *grounded instead in introspection, meditation, or even service to others.*

For many older adults, spirituality becomes increasingly central as they face the transitions and reflections characteristic of aging. Spirituality can provide a critical framework, *offering comfort, community, and resilience, which are essential for navigating life's physical, emotional, and existential challenges*. In geriatric care, recognizing the role of spirituality is essential to providing holistic support that respects and incorporates the patient's beliefs and values.

SPIRITUALITY ACROSS LIFE STAGES

The significance and manifestation of spirituality evolve over different life stages, reflecting changing priorities and experiences.

Childhood and Adolescence

- *Formation of beliefs*: Spiritual beliefs often start forming during childhood and adolescence, influenced by family traditions, cultural norms, and personal experiences. Early exposure to rituals, values, and community activities provides a foundation for lifelong spiritual development.
- *Exploration and questioning*: Adolescence is a period of curiosity, exploration, and questioning, with young individuals often beginning to grapple with questions of faith, purpose, and identity. This stage may include experimenting with different spiritual traditions, encountering doubts, and shaping a more personal set of beliefs.

- *Participation in rituals and traditions*: Children and adolescents may take part in family or community rituals, religious ceremonies, and rites of passage that create a shared sense of spirituality and tradition.

Young Adulthood

- *Identity formation*: Young adulthood is marked by identity exploration, including spiritual identity. Individuals continue to refine and integrate their beliefs with other aspects of life, such as career and relationships, aligning spirituality with emerging life goals.
- *Transition and independence*: Major life transitions, such as leaving home, beginning higher education, or starting a career, prompt young adults to seek spiritual guidance and support, often as a source of stability during these significant changes.
- *Community engagement and service*: Many young adults engage actively in spiritual or religious communities, participating in worship, service projects, and social justice activities that resonate with their values.

Adulthood

- *Integration of beliefs*: In adulthood, individuals often weave their spiritual beliefs into everyday life, grounding them in relationships, work, and decision-making. Spirituality may offer meaning, purpose, and resilience during challenges such as career pressures, family responsibilities, or personal growth.
- *Family and parenthood*: Parenthood often prompts a reconsideration of values and beliefs, particularly as parents introduce children to family traditions and spiritual beliefs. Discussions about spirituality may deepen, and rituals become a way to instill values in the younger generation.
- *Crisis and growth*: Life events such as marriage, childbirth, career changes, and bereavement prompt reflection, with spirituality often offering comfort and guidance in these moments. For many, it provides a perspective that helps cope with uncertainty and grief.

Later Life and Aging

- *Reflection and legacy*: In later life, spirituality may take on heightened significance as individuals engage in self-reflection, contemplating legacy, values, and mortality. Older adults often draw on spirituality to reconcile past experiences and find peace with the life they have lived.
- *Community and connection*: Many older adults find support and companionship in religious or spiritual communities, participating in fellowship activities and service. For some, these connections reduce feelings of isolation and create a sense of belonging.
- *Preparation for death*: Spirituality becomes especially salient as individuals approach the end of life, offering comfort in contemplating mortality. Many older adults find solace in their beliefs, which help them face death with a sense of meaning, forgiveness, and readiness.

ROLE OF SPIRITUALITY IN GERIATRIC CARE

Spirituality profoundly impacts various aspects of health and coping in older adults given as follows:

- *Coping with aging and illness*: As individuals age, they may encounter physical, emotional, and existential challenges such as chronic illness, disability, and the deaths of loved ones. Spirituality can be a source of resilience, providing meaning, comfort, and strength amid these life transitions.
- *Sense of meaning and purpose*: Older adults may grapple with questions about meaning, purpose, and legacy. Spiritual beliefs often provide a framework for exploring these existential concerns, offering a sense of fulfillment and peace.
- *Mental and emotional well-being*: Spirituality supports mental health by alleviating feelings of isolation, grief, and existential distress. Practices such as meditation, prayer, and community participation foster a sense of connection, hope, and inner peace, particularly valuable for individuals who experience loneliness or depression.
- *Coping with grief and loss*: The experience of bereavement becomes more common in later life, as individuals confront the loss of spouses, friends, and family members. Spirituality often aids in the grieving process, providing rituals, beliefs, and community ties that offer solace and help individuals process loss.
- *End-of-life and palliative care*: Spirituality frequently becomes an essential component of end-of-life care. It shapes care preferences, influences decisions regarding medical interventions, and provides comfort. Palliative care teams often incorporate spiritual care, addressing the patient's needs holistically and supporting both patients and their families.
- *Social support and community engagement*: For many older adults, participation in religious or spiritual communities offers critical social support, reducing isolation and enhancing overall well-being. These communities provide companionship, caregiving

assistance, and opportunities for involvement, supporting a sense of purpose.

- *Forgiveness and reconciliation*: As individuals approach the end of life, they often reflect on relationships and past experiences. Spiritual beliefs may encourage forgiveness, reconciliation, and healing, fostering a sense of closure for both the individual and their loved ones.
- *Legacy and remembrance*: Spirituality shapes thoughts around legacy, with many older adults engaging in activities such as writing memoirs or sharing life lessons with loved ones. This legacy can offer peace and continuity, often creating a bridge of connection for family members.
- *Transcendence and connection*: Many individuals experience moments of spiritual transcendence as they approach death, feeling a sense of unity or oneness with something greater than themselves. These experiences often bring reassurance and affirmation, underscoring the spiritual dimensions of life and death.

SPIRITUAL HISTORY TAKING IN GERIATRIC PATIENTS

When working with older adults, taking a spiritual history can offer valuable insight into how their beliefs and practices influence health, coping mechanisms, and end-of-life considerations. The key steps are given as follows:

- *Building rapport*: Establishing trust is critical. Engage the patient empathetically, creating a safe environment that invites open discussion about spirituality. Show genuine interest in the patient's beliefs to help develop a comfortable and respectful space for this sensitive dialogue.
- *Open-ended questions*: Begin with broad questions, such as "Can you tell me about your spiritual or religious beliefs?" or "How do you find meaning in life?" Open-ended questions encourage patients to share freely and explore their unique perspectives.
- *Exploring beliefs and practices*: Inquire about specific spiritual practices, such as prayer, meditation, or community involvement, and ask how these practices influence their daily life and approach to health. Delve into their beliefs regarding suffering, life, death, and the afterlife, as these can guide healthcare decisions and coping mechanisms.
- *Impact on health and well-being*: Assess how spiritual beliefs affect health, coping, and resilience. Explore whether spirituality provides the patient with strength, comfort, or inner peace and whether these beliefs influence their approach to illness and end-of-life care.
- *Cultural and contextual sensitivity*: Recognize the cultural context surrounding spirituality. Appreciate diverse spiritual beliefs within cultural backgrounds, ensuring a nonjudgmental approach that respects the individual's worldview.
- *Integration into care planning*: Integrate the patient's spiritual beliefs and preferences into a holistic care plan. Collaborate with the patient on ways to incorporate their beliefs into treatment strategies and support interventions, promoting an individualized, compassionate care approach.
- *Respect for autonomy*: Honor the patient's autonomy by acknowledging and respecting their beliefs without imposing personal views. Validate their spiritual perspectives, creating a supportive environment that fosters open, honest discussion.

BARRIERS TO SPIRITUAL CARE IN GERIATRICS

Implementing spiritual care in clinical practice can be challenging, and barriers may include the following:

- *Internal barriers*:
  - *Cognitive impairment*: Communication about spirituality can be challenging if a patient has cognitive decline or language barriers, limiting meaningful dialogue.
  - *Lack of provider training*: Healthcare providers may lack formal training in addressing spiritual issues, making it challenging to assess and meet spiritual needs effectively.
- *External barriers*:
  - *Time constraints*: Healthcare providers often work under time constraints, limiting the depth of discussion on spiritual matters.
  - *Lack of privacy*: Privacy in clinical settings may inhibit patients from sharing personal beliefs, particularly in settings where they feel exposed or rushed.
  - *Overworked healthcare providers*: High patient loads and administrative demands may make it difficult for healthcare providers to focus on spiritual care alongside physical health needs.

CLINICAL EXAMINATION AND SPIRITUAL ASSESSMENT

Assessing spirituality involves more than verbal inquiry; observing nonverbal cues and using structured tools can provide a fuller picture of a patient's spiritual health.

- *Observation and nonverbal cues:*
  - Pay attention to body language, facial expressions, and general demeanor. Signs of peace, distress,

agitation, or calmness can reflect spiritual well-being or distress.
    - Observe interactions with caregivers or healthcare providers, noting if any spiritual objects or symbols (e.g., religious books, jewelry) are present.
- *Assessment tools*:
    - *FICA Spiritual History Tool (FICA; Puchalski 1996)*: This tool assesses four domains: (1) Faith, (2) importance and influence, (3) community, and (4) address/action in care in clinical care, offering a structured approach to spiritual inquiry.
    - *Spiritual Well-Being Scale (SWB; Paloutzian and Ellison 1982)*: This validated tool measures religious and existential well-being, helping providers understand a patient's connection to faith and meaning in life.
    - *Brief Religious Coping Scale (Brief RCOPE Scale; Pargament et al. 1998)*: Used to assess religious coping strategies, the Brief RCOPE examines both positive and negative coping mechanisms, such as seeking support or struggling with spiritual beliefs.
    - *Spiritual distress assessment*: Recognize signs of existential suffering, such as feelings of hopelessness or loss of meaning. Address these concerns compassionately, offering support and appropriate referrals.

MANAGEMENT OF SPIRITUAL ISSUES IN GERIATRIC PATIENTS

Effectively managing spiritual issues in geriatric patients involves a patient-centered approach that respects and aligns with individual beliefs and values. Key strategies include the following:

- *Collaborative exploration*:
    - Collaborate with patients to identify how spirituality can be integrated into their care plan, addressing spiritual goals alongside medical and psychological needs.
    - Discuss potential resources or interventions, such as spiritual counseling, rituals, or community support, that could support the patient's well-being.
- *Validation and empowerment*:
    - Validate the patient's spiritual experiences and perspectives, recognizing spirituality as a legitimate aspect of health and wellness.
    - Empower patients to express their spiritual needs and preferences, encouraging self-advocacy in their healthcare journey.
- *Supportive interventions*:
    - Offer resources such as religious texts, meditation guides, or spiritual counseling tailored to the patient's beliefs. Help connect them with community or religious groups that resonate with their spirituality.
    - Facilitate access to spiritual care providers or chaplains who can offer additional support, especially during times of crisis or end-of-life care.
    - *Holistic care planning*: Integrate spirituality into a holistic care plan that addresses physical, emotional, social, and spiritual dimensions, creating a comprehensive approach to well-being.
    - *Crisis intervention and palliative care*: Offer compassionate, empathetic support during crises, addressing spiritual distress in conjunction with physical and emotional suffering. In palliative care settings, support patients' dignity and comfort, respecting their beliefs about death and dying.
    - *Education and training for healthcare providers*: Provide training on cultural competence and spiritual sensitivity, helping providers address spiritual needs with respect. Equip healthcare providers with practical tools for effective spiritual assessments.

PREVENTION OF SPIRITUAL DISTRESS

Preventive care for spiritual issues promotes resilience, well-being, and coping mechanisms, supporting quality of life in later years.

- *Early spiritual assessment*: Incorporate spiritual assessments into routine geriatric evaluations to identify needs, concerns, and resources that can guide future care.
- *Promotion of spiritual resilience*: Educate older adults on the value of spiritual resilience and coping strategies, such as engaging in meditation, prayer, or mindfulness practices, to navigate transitions, losses, and health challenges.
- *Integration into self-care practices*: Encourage patients to incorporate spiritual practices into daily routines, such as meditation, journaling, or gratitude exercises, which foster inner peace and stress reduction.
- *Supportive environments*: Create healthcare settings that respect and accommodate spiritual needs. Collaborate with religious or spiritual care providers to support patients' spiritual well-being.
- *Advance care planning and end-of-life care*: Engage patients in advance care planning discussions that include spiritual priorities and end-of-life preferences.

Support patients in identifying and communicating their spiritual goals and values, enhancing their comfort and autonomy.

- *Community engagement and social support*: Facilitate connections with religious or spiritual communities, peer support groups, and community organizations that promote spiritual well-being. Encourage older adults to participate in social activities and intergenerational programs that foster a sense of belonging.

CONCLUSION

Spirituality represents a profound dimension of the human experience, especially in the lives of older adults who often turn to it as a source of strength, resilience, and meaning. By integrating spirituality into geriatric care, healthcare providers can create a more holistic, compassionate approach that respects the diverse beliefs and values of their patients. Spiritual care in geriatric medicine offers comfort, connection, and dignity, particularly as individuals face aging, illness, and the end of life.

Incorporating spiritual care not only enriches clinical practice but also honors the deeply personal journeys that each patient undertakes. By addressing spirituality with empathy and respect, healthcare providers can play a vital role in promoting peace, resilience, and fulfillment in the later stages of life.

Self-Assessment Questionnaire

Q1. How does spirituality impact the health and well-being of older adults?

Q2. What are some common barriers to addressing spiritual needs in geriatric care?

Q3. How can healthcare providers incorporate spirituality into the care of older adults?

Q4. What is the role of spirituality in end-of-life care for older adults?

Q5. Why is it essential to consider cultural and contextual factors when addressing spirituality in geriatric patients?

Q6. What are some effective ways to assess spirituality in older adults?

FURTHER READINGS

1. Dhar N, Chaturvedi S, Nandan D. Spiritual health scale 2011: defining and measuring 4th dimension of health. Indian J Community Med. 2011;36:275-82.
2. Jackson D, Doyle C, Capon H, Pringle E. Spirituality, spiritual need, and spiritual care in aged care: what the literature says. J Religion Spiritual Aging. 2016;28(6):281-95.
3. Anandarajah G, Hight E. Spirituality and medical practice: using the HOPE questions as a practical tool for spiritual assessment. Am Fam Physician. 2001;63:81-9.
4. Puchalski CM. The FICA Spiritual History Tool #274. J Palliat Med. 2014;17(1):105-6.
5. Paloutzian RF, Ellison CW. Manual for the spiritual well-being scale. Westmont College; 1982.
6. Pargament K, Feuille M, Burdzy D. The Brief RCOPE: Current psychometric status of a short measure of religious coping. Religions. 2011;2:51-76.
7. Bredle JM, Salsman JM, Debb SM, Arnold BJ, Cella D. Spiritual well-being as a component of health-related quality of life: the functional assessment of chronic illness therapy—spiritual well-being scale (FACIT-Sp). Religions. 2011;2:77-94.

CHAPTER 35

Occupational Therapy for Older Adults

Prakash Kumar

CASE VIGNETTE

Background: Mrs A G is a 72-year-old woman who lives alone in a two-bedroom apartment in a metropolitan area. She is a retired school teacher with a strong friends and family support network. However, her daughter lives in another city. Mrs Gupta has a history of osteoarthritis, hypertension, and mild cognitive impairment, which has been progressively worsening over the past year. She is independent in her activities of daily living (ADLs), although she has started to struggle with certain tasks, particularly those requiring fine motor skills and mobility.

Presenting concerns: Mrs Gupta has recently experienced a fall in her home, resulting in a bruised hip. Following the incident, she became more fearful of falling again, leading to decreased engagement in her usual activities, including cooking, gardening, and attending community events. She expresses feelings of loneliness and frustration regarding her limitations. Her daughter is concerned about her safety at home and the risk of further falls.

Occupational therapy assessment: An occupational therapist (OT) is consulted to assess Mrs Gupta's functional abilities, home environment, and psychosocial needs. The assessment reveals the following:

- *Physical assessment*: Decreased range of motion in her knees and hands, moderate difficulty with tasks requiring fine motor skills (e.g., buttoning shirts, opening jars), and balance issues when standing for extended periods.
- *Cognitive assessment*: Mild cognitive impairment impacting her short-term memory and judgment, particularly when planning daily activities or managing medications.
- *Home environment*: The apartment has several hazards, including loose rugs, cluttered walkways, and inadequate lighting, which increase the risk of falls.

Intervention plan: The OT develops a comprehensive intervention plan, which includes the following:

- *Home modifications*: Recommendations for decluttering pathways, removing loose rugs, installing grab bars in the bathroom, and enhancing lighting in key areas.
- *Exercise program*: A tailored exercise program focusing on strength, balance, and flexibility to enhance her physical capabilities and reduce fall risk. This includes specific exercises to improve her fine motor skills.
- *Cognitive strategies*: Implementation of memory aids, such as a daily planner and pill organizer, to assist with medication management and daily planning.
- *Activity engagement*: Encouraging participation in adapted community activities, such as a gardening club or book group, to combat feelings of loneliness and foster social connections.
- *Education*: Providing education on fall prevention strategies and the importance of engaging in physical and social activities to maintain independence.

Outcome: After 6 weeks of occupational therapy, Mrs Gupta shows significant improvement. She reports increased confidence in her ability to move around her home and engage in activities she enjoys. The fear of falling has diminished, and she has rejoined her gardening club, enhancing her social interactions. Home modifications have made her environment safer, and her daughter notes that Mrs Gupta has become more independent in managing her daily routines.

INTRODUCTION

Geriatrics is a specialty dedicated to the health care of older adults and addressing the unique challenges associated with aging. It originated from the Greek word "Geron", an old man. There is no universal agreement or direction on what it means to be old, but the most used and relevant definition of the geriatric population is 65 years or older.

Increasing longevity and falling fertility have resulted in a dramatic increase in the population, entailing almost a tripling of adults aged 60 years and above (Government of India, 2011). As we know, elderly persons constitute one of the most vulnerable groups and have more chances of developing a chronic degenerative disease, infections, and subsequent disabilities. According to the 2011 Government of India (GoI) census, the population aged 60 years and older in India was 10.3 crore, accounting for 8.6% of the total population. Around 5% of the elderly population is affected by some form of disability, and the burden is predicted to increase substantially in the coming years. Disability increases the level of assistance (dependency), increases demands for healthcare services (hospitalization), and leads to premature death. In addition, higher morbidity and disability rates are directly associated with higher per capita health spending, out-of-pocket expenditure (OOPE), and catastrophic health expenditure (CHE). High OOPE is positively associated with catastrophic health spending (CHS) and reduced access to health services, increases untreated morbidity, and leads to long-term impoverishment. There is, therefore, an urgent need to scale up services for disability prevention, which has become a paramount public health concern. The National Health Policy 2017 has set an ambitious goal of raising public health spending to 2.5% from the existing 1.15% of gross domestic product (GDP) and reducing CHE by 25% by 2025. Further, the Ayushman Bharat Yojana, launched in September 2018, is a laudable effort to provide preventive, curative, and promotive healthcare.

OLDER ADULTS AND DISABILITY

In the older population, disability has been defined as the inability to perform or complete particular tasks or roles that previously could be accomplished without difficulty or the help of another person. Deterioration or reduction in physical, cognitive, and psychosocial ability over time is a characteristic of the aging population. The most important element in the discourse on disability is to assess who is a person with a disability. Disability is not a homogeneous concept, as it varies from person to person. The development of disability in old age relates to an individual's physiological, psychological, and medical conditions as well as socioeconomic status, cultural norms, and environment. In another way, disease or injuries (*pathology*) result in dysfunction of body systems (*impairments*), leading to the inability to carry out basic physical and cognitive functions (*functional limitations*) that alter the individual's capacity to meet the demands of their environment (*disability*). According to the World Health Organization (WHO) International Classification of Impairments, Disabilities and Handicaps and International Classification of Functioning, Disability and Health (ICIDH): 1980—replaced by International Classification of Functioning, Disability and Health (ICF) in 2001, *impairment* concerns physical aspects of health and *disability* is the functional consequence of the impairment in terms of altered functional capacity by the individuals. *Handicap* measures the social consequences of an impairment or disability in terms of disadvantages experienced by individuals in society. Individuals with knee arthritis are categorized as an impairment; being unable to walk is a disability, and limiting the social role of individuals is a handicap. Having difficulty performing a daily activity is understood as a functional limitation or disability in that activity area. "Activities of daily living" (ADLs) provide a basic framework to evaluate an older person's ability to live independently, require assistance, or be dependent. Deterioration in the ability to perform basic self-care activities [basic activities of daily living (BADLs)], such as bathing, dressing, toileting, transferring (e.g., in and out of bed), eating, and other independent living skills [instrumental activities of daily living (IADLs)], related to a person's ability to cope with their environment, and include such as household chores, shopping, cooking, use of transportation, managing medication, and telephone use is also regarded as a disability in old age. Disability in old age limits the autonomy of older people, is dependent on daily functioning, reduces the quality of life, and increases the risk of hospitalization and premature death. According to one of the WHO reports, 10% of the world population has some form of disability. According to a recent community-based study in India, the prevalence of all types of disability was 6.3%, out of which mental disability was found to be the most common type of disability at 36.37%. The disability prevalence also varied between age groups and urban-rural areas. It was also seen that the burden of disability is prevalent more in the older population, i.e., an age group of 60 years and above.

The ICF is a framework for describing functioning and disability in relation to health conditions, and it was approved by the World Health Assembly in 2001. ICF defines disability as an umbrella term that includes various types of disability, such as sensory impairments and physical, mental, and intellectual impairments. Many other chronic illnesses can influence the quality of life in the elderly population, increasing the risk of multiple comorbidities in the elderly population, thereby leading to disability. Other morbidity patterns such as hypertension, diabetes, arthritis, constipation, and hearing loss are also significant risk factors for disability seen in elderly populations. Moreover, the number of noncommunicable diseases and life expectancy has been rising in recent years, and the magnitude of this problem will rapidly increase in the future. The ICIDH provides indicators that allow a more structured approach to health disorders. In their definition, disability is the interaction between environmental and personal factors and a health condition. Multiple factors are associated with functional decline and disability in old age, varying between individuals and populations. At an individual's level, the health and behavioral factors contribute to disability in old age, including inappropriately treated diseases, a sedentary lifestyle, unhealthy dietary habits, insufficient social support, etc. Many studies suggest that socioeconomic status may also result in different disability patterns. Older adults with more material resources were being protected against unfavorable trajectories of change. Poverty can also lead to malnutrition and inadequate health services, and sanitation.

In addition to ICIDH and ICF, another school of thought, the *Disablement model* defined disability and related concepts **(Flowcharts 1 and 2)**. It has four central concepts: (1) Active pathology, (2) functional impairment, (3) functional limitation, and (4) disability. The *active pathology* interrupts normal cellular processes and can result from infections, trauma, metabolic imbalance, and degenerative disease processes such as decreased muscle strength, poor balance, and low oxygen consumption. *Functional impairment* is a loss or abnormality at the tissue, organ, and body systems level. At the individual level, *Nagi* uses *functional limitations* (e.g., slow walking speed and inability to grasp with hands). *Disability* is a limitation in performing socially defined roles and tasks expected of an individual within a sociocultural and physical environment (e.g., difficulties in mobility and self-care). Pathology (e.g., sarcopenia) in the Nagi pathway leads to impairment (e.g., lower extremity weakness). After a certain period, this weakness changes into a functional limitation (e.g., slow gait speed), and a person has a disability (e.g., difficulty or needing assistance for walking across the room).

To better understand disability complexity, ICIDH-2 **(Flowchart 3)** has created a framework that includes environmental factors, addresses dimensional overlaps, and proposes an association between dimensions. The framework identifies three levels of human functioning.

1. The first level, health conditions, designates functioning at the body or body parts level.
2. The second level designates functioning at the level of the whole person.
3. The third level designates the functioning of the whole person in the context of their complete environment.

Did You Know?

Disability defines as any limitation, restriction, or impairment which restricts everyday activities and has lasted, or is likely to last, for at least 6 months.

Within the person level, there are three dimensions of human functioning: (1) Body level, (2) individual level, and (3) societal level. These dimensions are named: (1) body functions and structure, (2) activities, and (3) participation. The second part of this framework is the contextual factors, including environmental and personal factors. Environmental factors include the physical, social, and attitudinal environments that influence an individual's functioning. It ranges from an individual's immediate environment to the general environment. Personal factors include age, race, gender, educational background, personality, fitness, lifestyle, habits, coping styles, and other characteristics, all of which may play a role in disability at any level. Through these models,

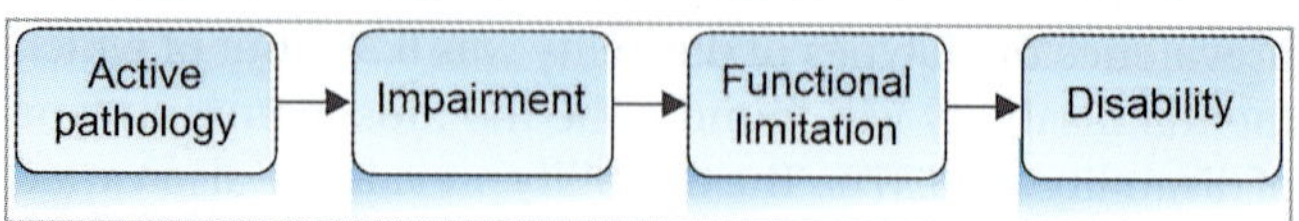

FLOWCHART 1: Theoretical pathway from disease to disability proposed by Nagi.

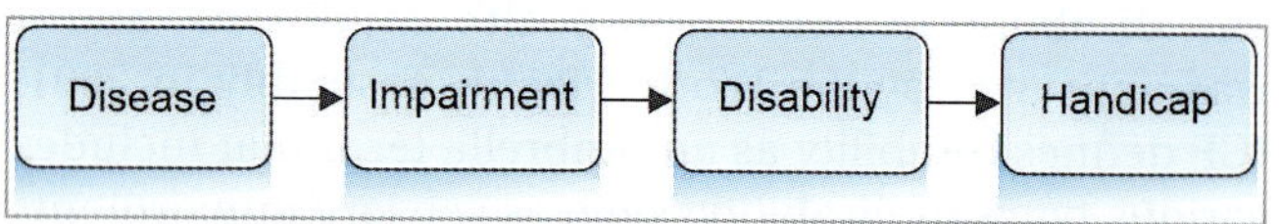

FLOWCHART 2: International Classification of Impairments, Disabilities, and Handicaps (ICIDH).

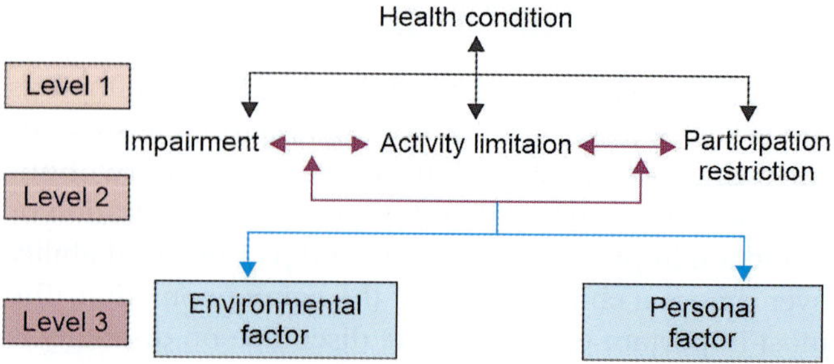

FLOWCHART 3: Current understanding of interactions between the dimensions of ICIDH-2.

(ICIDH-2: International Classification of Impairments, Disabilities and Handicaps-2)

interventions can be designed to modify impairments, activity limitations, or participation restrictions. For example, a treatment plan may be developed to improve strength (impairment level), but the significance of this intervention is due to its effect on physical mobility (activity) and, ultimately, the ability to return to social or physical roles (participation).

OLD AGE CONCEPT

Understanding old age is crucial, as it represents a significant stage in human life characterized by physical, mental, and social changes. As individuals grow older, they often experience a decline in physical abilities, an increase in mental health challenges, and shifts in social relationships, all of which require attention to enhance their quality of life.

Physical Changes

With aging, many physical abilities diminish. General mobility, balance, and muscle strength often decrease, leading to greater risks of falls and injury. Additionally, sensory capacities such as vision and hearing tend to deteriorate, making daily tasks more difficult. Chronic conditions such as Alzheimer's disease, arthritis, heart disease, and diabetes become more prevalent, impacting overall health and well-being.

Mental Changes

Alongside physical decline, mental health challenges are common. Older adults may face depression, anxiety, cognitive decline, and memory loss, which can be exacerbated by social isolation or chronic illness. Cognitive impairments such as dementia also pose significant challenges, affecting not only memory but also decision-making and emotional regulation. Sleep disorders and increased mental stress further contribute to diminished mental health in old age.

Social Changes

Old age can bring changes in social relationships. As social circles shrink due to the passing of peers or limited mobility, many older adults experience loneliness and social isolation. The depth of social interactions may also decrease, leaving elderly individuals feeling excluded from social groups. Such isolation can have a profound impact on both mental and physical health.

In conclusion, understanding the complexities of old age is essential for providing tailored support and care to the elderly. Addressing their physical, mental, and social needs through healthcare services, mental health care, and strong social support networks can significantly improve their quality of life, allowing them to age with dignity and well-being.

GERIATRIC REHABILITATION

Geriatric rehabilitation focuses on restoring and enhancing older adults' physical, mental, and social functioning. It involves conducting comprehensive geriatric assessments, using multidisciplinary teams, and employing resource-efficient practices to address impairments caused by illness, injury, or inactivity. It is essential for improving the ability impaired by acute illness or injury, or the physical, mental, or social disabilities associated with inactivity. Effective rehabilitation improves the elderly's chances of an independent and self-sufficient life. In recent years, this field has expanded to cover various levels of care, from home-based interventions to hospital rehabilitation units (Tilvis et al., 2016). Multidisciplinary teamwork, which includes professionals such as physical therapists, nurses, psychologists, and social workers, plays a critical role in successful rehabilitation. Occupational therapists (OTs), in particular, contribute by addressing functional limitations, helping improve mobility, cognitive functioning, and daily living skills. Their interventions holistically enhance the physical, mental, and social well-being of elderly patients, significantly improving their quality of life and independence.

OCCUPATIONAL THERAPY

Occupational therapy is a healthcare field focused on helping individuals maintain stability and independence in their mental and physical abilities. Its primary goal is to improve individual and social life despite challenges caused by disease, injury, or aging. It teaches skills to live independently and perform daily tasks efficiently and with less pain. The American Occupational Therapy Association (AOTA) describes occupational therapy as assisting people across their lifespan to participate in activities through the therapeutic use of everyday ADLs. OTs achieve this outcome by working with people and communities to enhance their ability to engage in the occupations they want to, need to, or are expected to do or by modifying the occupation of the environment to support their occupational engagement better. They help older adults experiencing physical and cognitive changes to adapt to those changes. As can be observed from this definition, the main focus of occupational therapy is "occupation." In public feeling, the common understanding of this word is that it is employment (paid or unpaid) or a vocation. However, for OTs, the term refers to a group of activities and tasks that an individual performs daily, given the values and meaning of these activities in their culture. Occupation is everything people do to occupy themselves, including looking after themselves (self-care), enjoying life (leisure), and contributing to their communities' social and economic fabric of their communities (productivity). From this background, it can be seen that OTs have two traditions: (1) impairment-based and (2) occupation-based. The selection of occupations depends on their meaning for older adults, and it will improve an individual's participation and engagement in meaningful occupations. OTs are healthcare providers who help people learn or regain daily living skills after experiencing changes in their abilities. OTs are often needed in cases where individuals require assistance managing daily activities. They work with older adults facing challenges in daily tasks such as bathing, dressing, walking, attending school, and working. Some OTs work in hospitals, clinics, or rehabilitation centers. Each patient is unique, so treatment plans depend on the patient's specific needs. For example, the occupational therapy needs of an older adult with Parkinson's disease will differ from those of a person recovering from a severe fall at home.

The core elements of occupational therapy are as follows:

- *Assessment*: The first step is to evaluate the patient's condition, which involves gathering detailed information about their situation.
- *Goal setting*: Clarify the patient's goals and needs to help create an effective therapy plan.
- *Intervention*: Provide supportive treatment according to the therapy plan, which may include exercises, the use of therapeutic devices, or mental health support.
- *Evaluation*: Assess the outcomes of the treatment to determine its effectiveness and make necessary adjustments.

IMPORTANCE OF OCCUPATIONAL THERAPY

Occupational therapy is extremely important for elderly individuals as its primary goal is to support their health and independence. It is a supportive and appropriate therapeutic approach that aids elderly individuals based on their specific characteristics, needs, and abilities. Some reasons why occupational therapy is vital for elderly individuals are as follows:

- *Preservation of independence*: Occupational therapy helps maintain the independence of elderly individuals, enabling them to perform daily tasks on their own and retain their autonomy.
- *Improvement in quality of life*: Occupational therapy improves the lifestyle quality of elderly individuals by providing modified approaches that help them lead active and healthy lives.
- *Personalized care plans*: Occupational therapy assists elderly individuals in creating personalized care plans based on their unique needs, ensuring more appropriate and effective health services.
- *Assistance with daily routines*: Occupational therapy provides solutions for daily activities, offering support that helps elderly individuals manage their daily lives independently.
- *Enhanced self-acceptance*: Occupational therapy helps elderly individuals accept and understand their health conditions, thereby enhancing their self-acceptance.

In this way, occupational therapy plays a crucial role in bringing positive changes to the lives of elderly individuals, supporting them in leading healthy and independent lives.

BENEFITS OF OCCUPATIONAL THERAPY

Overcoming Daily Challenges

For seniors recovering from illness or injury, performing daily activities can be challenging. This includes everything from bathing, dressing, grooming, eating, using the toilet, and managing the household. When seniors struggle with these daily tasks, it can leave them feeling frustrated, exhausted, and embarrassed. This can lead to social withdrawal and decreased enthusiasm for activities they once loved, resulting in feelings of sadness and loneliness. To help overcome these daily challenges, OTs assist patients in learning new skills and developing plans that make completing ADLs easier. These activities include walking, dressing, bathing, eating, and using the toilet. OTs help seniors improve their fundamental motor skills, strength, dexterity, mobility, and walking ability. By gradually enhancing these critical skills, patients will find it easier to complete everyday tasks and regain their independence safely.

Preventing Falls

One in four individuals over the age of 60 years experiences a fall each year. Approximately 3 million seniors annually receive treatment in emergency rooms due to fall-related injuries. Fall prevention has become a top priority for today's seniors. Falls pose significant health risks for older adults. Therapists can teach seniors specific techniques and exercises designed to improve their balance, strengthen their muscles, and prevent future falls. Patients will find walking and carrying out their daily activities easier as their balance and strength improve.

Improving Vision and Memory

It is estimated that one in three people over the age of 60 years experiences some form of vision loss or eye disease. Seniors with vision loss or eye diseases may struggle with daily activities, increasing their risk of mental health issues such as anxiety and depression. OTs can assist seniors with vision-related problems by providing activities designed to improve their vision. Specifically, therapists can recommend programs to enhance a patient's reactive vision, pattern recognition, and visual awareness. In addition to activities, therapists can suggest ways to make the patient's home safer to manage daily challenges associated with vision loss.

An OT might recommend the following:

- Removing clutter from the home to prevent falls or slips
- Color-coding household items and medications for easier identification
- Improving the lighting in the patient's home
- Using magnifiers for reading small print
- Labeling tools with bright-colored tape
- Painting walls in light colors and electrical outlets in dark colors to create visual contrast
- Applying brightly colored tape on stairs to prevent falls

Enhancing Memory

Some may be surprised to learn that occupational therapy improves a patient's physical and mental health. When therapists meet with their patients, they evaluate their cognitive abilities and then create personalized care plans based on their needs. Therapists can design plans that aim to maintain the patient's strengths and work on areas that need improvement. OTs play a crucial role in helping seniors regain the memory skills necessary for everyday life.

These techniques may include:

- Engaging in memory-enhancing activities, such as puzzles and matching games
- Labeling the front door with stop signs for patients who easily become confused and may wander off
- Educating caregivers on effective techniques for managing patients with severe personality changes
- *Simplifying techniques for memory aid*: Instructing caregivers on simple methods to help patients remember, such as limiting the number of items in the fridge or pantry.

Home Modifications

For many older adults, remaining in their homes and communities represents independence, dignity, and continuity of life. However, many conventional homes are not designed with the safety of elderly individuals in mind, often increasing the risk of accidents. As a result, features such as high thresholds, slippery floors, poor lighting, or inaccessible bathrooms can increase the risk of fall-related injuries and dependence in daily life. A home modification assessment begins with an on-site evaluation, during which an occupational therapist assesses a patient's home and nearby community to determine the necessary modifications to enhance safety and support independent living. The therapist identifies the needed area where assistance or modification is required and finally proposes individualized environmental solutions. These may include simple, low-cost changes to more complex technological solutions, depending on the client's physical and cognitive status.

Examples of common home modifications include:

Grab bars: Place grab bars in critical areas, such as bathrooms, near toilets, and along hallways, to provide physical support and reduce the risk of falls. Older adults with balance issues and lower limb weakness may benefit from these grab bars.

Power lift recliners and adjustable chairs: For individuals with limited lower-limb strength or arthritis, power lift recliners allow easier transitions between sitting and standing, reducing the strain on joints.

Slip-resistant flooring: Replacing or coating slippery surfaces with non-slip materials can prevent accidental falls, especially in high-risk areas such as kitchens and bathrooms.

Shower benches and handheld showers: Providing a sturdy shower bench enables older adults to bathe safely while seated, conserving energy and reducing fatigue. For example, a senior with Parkinson's disease may use a shower bench to maintain stability during grooming.

Wheelchair ramps: Building ramps to improve accessibility for those using wheelchairs or walkers. By making these modifications, OTs can help seniors maintain their independence and continue living safely in their own homes, which is particularly important for promoting their overall well-being and quality of life.

Modifying the home: Living independently at home is ideal for many healthy seniors. However, many homes are not designed to accommodate the needs of elderly individuals and may pose safety risks. OTs can assess a patient's home to determine necessary modifications. They can provide recommendations to improve safety and promote independent living.

Monitoring alert systems: Installing alert systems to monitor safety and notify caregivers or family members in emergencies

By implementing such home modifications, occupational therapists enable older adults to "age in place" that is, to live independently and safely within their familiar environment. This not only reduces healthcare costs and the burden on caregivers but also significantly contributes to the individual's sense of control, self-efficacy, and overall quality of life.

OCCUPATIONAL THERAPY TECHNIQUES

Occupational therapy techniques are specially designed to help elderly individuals lead independent and healthy lives.

Some important occupational therapy techniques are as follows:

- *Time management programs*: These programs help elderly individuals organize their daily activities. They may include scheduling, focusing strategies, and effective time management techniques.
- *Physical exercise programs*: These programs are tailored to meet the exercise needs of elderly individuals to keep them healthy and active. They can include exercise routines, yoga, and regular physical activities.
- *Cognitive stimulation*: These techniques assist elderly individuals in addressing mental challenges. They can include mental exercises, puzzles, recreational activities, and social interactions.
- *Mobility aids*: These aids are used to help elderly individuals with mobility. They can include canes, wheelchairs, walkers, and other assistive devices.
- *Environmental modifications*: These techniques involve modifying the surrounding environment to improve the condition of elderly individuals. They can include home structure adjustments, safety devices, and comfortable materials.

The importance of personalized treatment plans lies in their customization based on the individual's specific condition, needs, and health circumstances. This allows for appropriate support and helps improve the individual's condition. These techniques assist in living an independent and healthy life and provide support in a conducive environment.

CHALLENGES AND SOLUTIONS IN ELDERLY CARE SERVICES

Working in the field of elderly care services presents numerous challenges for OTs. These challenges can include managing individual needs, lack of access to services, addressing social and mental health issues, a shortage of expertise in occupational therapy, and adhering to various related regulations and procedures. OTs must strategically plan and implement effective solutions to overcome these challenges.

Managing individual needs: One of the primary challenges is catering to individual needs. Services for elderly individuals depend on their specific requirements, such as health conditions, social relationships, and independence in daily activities. To address this, the medical team must prepare personalized plans that help improve their quality of life.

Lack of access to services: Another challenge is the limited access to services. This issue is particularly significant for the elderly living in rural areas or long-term care institutions. Collaborating with local community organizations and utilizing digital technology can help bridge this gap.

Addressing social and mental health issues: Elderly individuals often face social and mental health problems, such as loneliness, depression, or anxiety. The medical team needs to recognize these issues and collaborate with mental health specialists to provide effective solutions.

Shortage of expertise in occupational therapy: A significant challenge is the lack of specialists in occupational therapy for elderly care services. To overcome this, the medical team should coordinate efforts with relevant institutions and experts for service acceptance and consultation.

Adhering to regulations and procedures: Understanding and following the regulations and procedures in occupational therapy can also be challenging. To address this, the medical team should be trained to provide services in compliance with regulations and work in coordination with authorized bodies. OTs must rely on their experience, knowledge, and capabilities to tackle these challenges. Collaborating with relevant institutions, communities, and experts, utilizing new technologies, and adhering to ethical standards are the keys to success in this field.

Collaboration with Other Health Services

In elderly care services, the importance of collaboration between OTs and other health service professionals is a broad and significant topic. This cooperation enhances the quality, accessibility, and effectiveness of services, ensuring that all patients receive excellent care. This chapter delves into the importance of such collaboration.

Professional Coordination and Joint Efforts

Collaboration between OTs and other health professionals increases the potential for joint efforts. They face shared challenges and work together in a problem-solving process. Mutual understanding benefits patients, providing them with precise and dedicated care.

Sharing Professional Knowledge and Experience

Patients receive a comprehensive medical approach by collaborating across various healthcare fields. Cooperation between doctors, medical, and therapy services ensures that patients benefit from the expertise needed to improve their health conditions.

Importance of Communication

Effective communication is crucial in collaboration. Good communication skills among health professionals ensure that patients receive accurate and timely information, improving their quality of care.

Utilization of Technology

Modern technology also enhances collaboration between OTs and health professionals. Patients receive more appropriate, comprehensive, and supportive services using digital services, telemedicine, and IT solutions.

Organizational collaboration: Collaboration can also occur between different health service organizations. This creates a robust service structure, ensuring that patients receive holistic care.

Education and Training

Through collaboration, professionals are introduced to the best practices and techniques in health services. This helps share new ideas, ensure better quality services, and achieve better patient outcomes.

CONCLUSION

The collaboration between OTs and other health service professionals is crucial for providing patients with comprehensive and excellent care. This cooperation plays a vital role in delivering effective services and improving healthcare quality.

Self-Assessment Questionnaire

Q1. What are the primary goals of occupational therapy (OT) in the care of older adults?

Q2. How does the International Classification of Functioning, Disability, and Health (ICF) framework define disability and its components?

Q3. Explain the difference between impairment, disability, and handicap using the ICIDH model.

Q4. What are some key home modifications that can enhance the safety and independence of older adults?

Q5. Discuss the importance of multidisciplinary collaboration in geriatric rehabilitation.

Q6. Using the case vignette of Mrs Gupta, identify the central occupational therapy interventions that contributed to her improved quality of life.

FURTHER READINGS

1. American Occupational Therapy Association. Occupational therapy practice framework: Domain and process. 4th ed. Am J Occup Ther. 2020;74(Suppl 2):7412410010p1–87.
2. Baum CM, Edwards DF. Occupational therapy practice for older adults: Promoting quality of life through occupation. Philadelphia: F.A. Davis; 2008.
3. Law M, Cooper B, Strong S, Stewart D, Rigby P, Letts L. The Person–Environment–Occupation model: A transactive approach to occupational performance. Can J Occup Ther. 1996;63(1):9-23.
4. Gitlin LN, Corcoran MA. Managing dementia at home: The role of home environmental modifications. Alzheimers Care Q. 2005;6(4):289-97.
5. Kielhofner G. Model of human occupation: Theory and application. 4th ed. Philadelphia: Lippincott Williams & Wilkins; 2008.
6. Lach HW, Reed AT, Armer JM, Miller JP. Fall prevention through environmental modification in the homes of older adults. J Geriatr Phys Ther. 2019;42(2):E23-31.
7. Lawton MP, Nahemow L. Ecology and the aging process. In: Eisdorfer C, Lawton MP, editors. The psychology of adult development and aging. Washington (DC): American Psychological Association; 1973;619-74.
8. World Health Organization. World report on ageing and health. Geneva: WHO Press; 2015. Available from: https://www.who.int/publications/i/item/9789241565042
9. Rodger S, Brown GT. Enhancing occupational performance in older adults through environmental adaptations and assistive technology. In: Creek J, Lougher L, editors. Occupational therapy and mental health. 5th ed. Edinburgh: Churchill Livingstone Elsevier; 2010;377-91.
10. Schell BAB, Gillen G, Scaffa ME, editors. Willard and Spackman's occupational therapy. 13th ed. Philadelphia: Wolters Kluwer; 2019.
11. Verghese J, Wang C, Lipton RB, Holtzer R. Mobility decline in older persons: Role of cognition and lifestyle activities. Ann Neurol. 2006;60(4):678-85.

CHAPTER 36

Geriatric Models of Care

Yogesh Poonia

CASE VIGNETTE

Mrs Sunita Rai, a 78-year-old woman, presents to the clinic with complaints of increasing difficulty in managing her daily activities. She has been experiencing memory lapses, reduced mobility, and frequent falls. Her daughter is concerned about Sunita's ability to live independently and seeks advice on how best to support her mother's health and well-being.

Background: Sunita has a history of hypertension, osteoarthritis, and mild cognitive impairment. Her living conditions are suboptimal, with several safety hazards around the home. She has also recently been discharged from the hospital after a fall that resulted in a hip fracture.

INTRODUCTION

Geriatric models of care are crucial in addressing the unique needs of the growing older adult population, leveraging evidence-based practices to enhance patient outcomes. These models utilize interdisciplinary approaches to manage complex health conditions, aiming to engage patients and families actively in their care. Key objectives include maintaining patients in the least restrictive care settings and implementing preventive strategies to improve functional status and quality of life. By focusing on specific populations, these models demonstrate how healthcare systems can fulfill their community missions. For successful implementation, geriatrics leaders must align these models with hospital priorities, engage stakeholders, and develop strategies to integrate and continually improve care.

EPIDEMIOLOGY

The aging population is growing rapidly. According to the World Health Organization (WHO), the global population aged 60 years and older is projected to reach 2.1 billion by 2050, and according to the United Nations Population Fund (UNFPA), India's population aged 60 years and older is projected to reach 347 million by 2050. This demographic shift presents significant challenges, including increased prevalence of chronic diseases, cognitive impairments, and functional disabilities. Over the past decade, new concepts and strategies have emerged globally and nationally to incorporate the unique needs of our aging population. The WHO introduced the "age-friendly systems and communities," a policy framework designed to address outdoor spaces and public buildings, transportation, housing, social participation, respect and social inclusion, civic participation and employment, communication and information, community support, and health services.

Key components to successful geriatric best practice models:

- Enable older adults to remain safely at home.
- Prevent functional disability.
- Preserve patient quality of life.
- Respect patient values, preferences, and goals.
- Consider patient safety.
- Address the needs of family caregivers.
- Appreciate and address patient's psychosocial needs.

GERIATRIC MODELS OF CARE

- *Hospital-based models of care*:
    - Acute Care for Elders (ACE)
    - Nurses Improving Care for Health System Elders (NICHE)

- American Geriatrics Society (AGS) CoCare: Hospital Elder Life Program (HELP)
  - Veterans Affairs (VA)-based Strategies to Reduce Injuries and Develop Confidence in Elders (STRIDE) Program
  - AGS CoCare Ortho
  - AGS Geriatric Surgery Verification Program
  - Duke Perioperative Optimization of Senior Health (POSH)
  - Stopping Elderly Accidents, Deaths, and Injuries (STEADI)
  - STRIDE Program
  - UCLA Dementia Care Program
  - Gerofit
- *Community-based models of care*:
  - Geriatric Resources for Assessment and Care of Elders (GRACE) Program
  - Program of All-inclusive Care for the Elderly (PACE)
- *Home-based models of care*:
  - Home-based Primary Care (HBPC)
  - Independence at Home
  - Community Aging in Place, Advancing Better Living for Elders (CAPABLE)

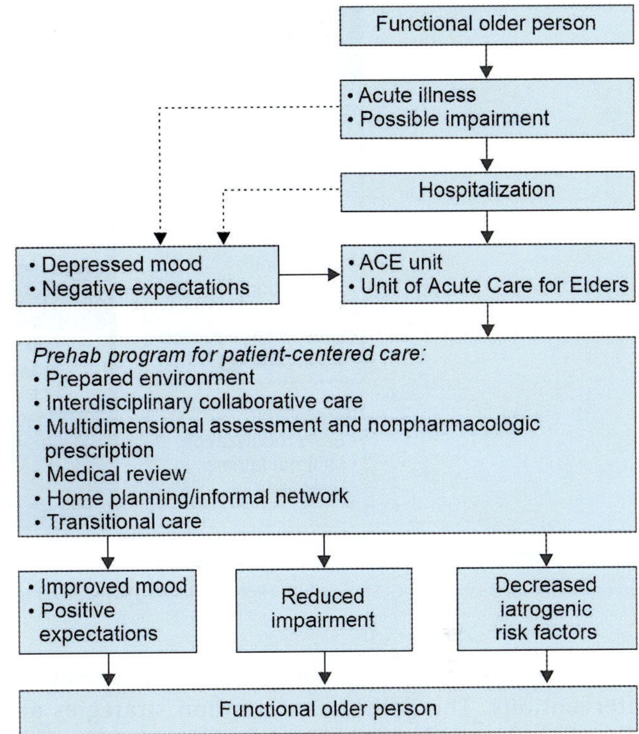

FLOWCHART 1: Acute Care for Elders (ACE).

Source: Halter JB, Ouslander JG, Studenski S, High KP. Hazzard's Geriatric Medicine and Gerontology, 8th edition. New Delhi: McGraw Hill; 2022.

Acute Care for Elders

The ACE model is designed to prevent functional decline and restore independent physical functioning in hospitalized, medically ill patients. The intervention merges principles of geriatric assessment with continuous quality improvement to prevent dysfunctional syndrome that results from hostile physical environments and processes of care and negative expectations of caregivers and patients **(Flowchart 1)**.

- *Goal*: Lessen the chance of functional decline for hospitalized older adults
- *Key components*:
  - Interdisciplinary team assessment and care
  - Prepared environment
  - Early planning to go home
  - Medical care review (using ACE tracker report)
- *Findings that support this intervention*:
  - Less disability
  - Decreased falls
  - Shorter hospital length of stay
  - Reduction in total hospital costs
  - Reduced mortality

AGS CoCare: Hospital Elder Life Program

The HELP is a multicomponent intervention designed to prevent incidents of delirium in hospitalized older patients. The intervention consists of six standardized protocols for reducing specific risk factors for delirium: (1) Cognitive impairment, (2) sleep deprivation, (3) immobility, (4) visual impairment, (5) hearing impairment, and (6) dehydration. The intervention is targeted at patients aged 70 years and older with at least one risk factor for delirium **(Flowchart 2)**.

- *Goal*: Lessen the chance of new development of delirium in hospital.
- *Key components*:
  - Screening of vulnerable older patients at risk for delirium
  - Trained and supervised volunteers deploying protocols
- *Findings that support this intervention*:
  - Decreased delirium
  - Decreased readmissions to hospital
  - Decreased rate of hospital falls
  - Decreased hospital length of stay
  - Decreased sitter use

The HELP intervention is conducted by an interdisciplinary HELP team. The team includes an advanced practice or geriatric-trained nurse, the Elder Life Specialist, a geriatrician, and a program coordinator—the Elder Life Nurse Specialist. The Elder

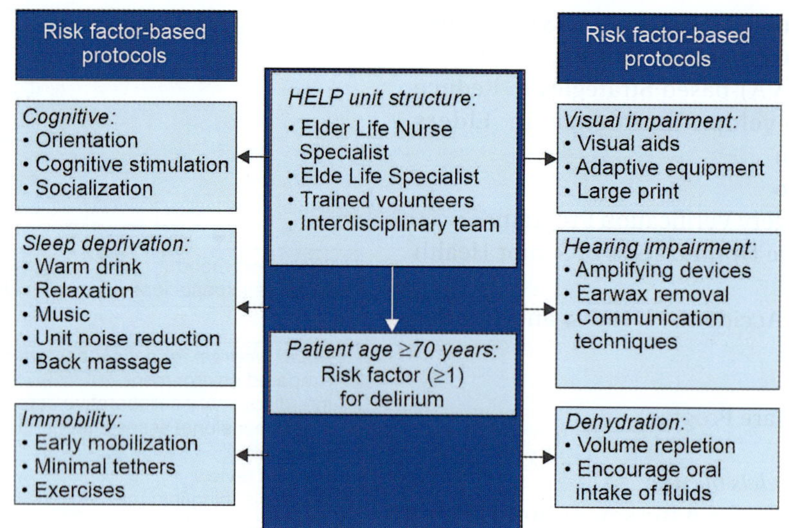

FLOWCHART 2: Hospital Elder Life Program (HELP).

Source: Halter JB, Ouslander JG, Studenski S, High KP. Hazzard's Geriatric Medicine and Gerontology, 8th edition. New Delhi: McGraw Hill; 2022.

Life Nurse Specialist trains volunteers and oversees the interventions. The delirium-prevention strategies are carried out by highly trained and supervised volunteers. The HELP team collaborates with a unit-based interdisciplinary team that includes nursing, medicine, physical therapy, occupational therapy, pharmacy, nutrition, and chaplaincy care.

PACE

PACE aims to keep nursing home-eligible patients living in the community as long as possible. PACE programs are fully capitated and operate out of "day health centers" and include an interdisciplinary team that provides coordination of care and effective communication to provide services necessary to care for complex patients in the community. Patients in PACE have been demonstrated to have lower rates of nursing home admission and hospitalization.

GRACE

GRACE is a patient-centered support team, consisting of an advanced practice nurse and a licensed master's-level social worker. The goal of the GRACE intervention is to improve functional status, decrease emergency department visits not resulting in hospitalization, and decrease the overall cost of care in community-dwelling older adults.

HBPC Model

Home-based primary care model targets homebound older adults with multiple chronic diseases in the ambulatory setting (home-based care). The main goal of HBPC is to provide long-term primary care and help at-risk patients to stay home and live independently and to avoid unwanted emergency department visits and hospital admissions.

HOMEMEDS is designed for agencies that provide home care for patients, and it specifically targets polypharmacy and appropriate medication use. A pharmacist works in conjunction with a patient's nurse or care manager to review medications with a particular focus on therapeutic duplication, cardiovascular medications and adverse effects, psychotropic medications, and nonsteroidal anti-inflammatory drugs (NSAIDs).

CLINICAL SETTING

Mrs Rai presents to a clinic where a decision is made to transition her care to an ACE unit to better address her complex needs and improve her overall health and safety.

IMPLEMENTATION OF THE ACE MODEL

- *Specialized geriatric unit*:
  - *Transition*: Mrs Rai is admitted to an ACE unit designed specifically for older adults. The unit features age-appropriate modifications such as low-height beds, grab bars, and nonslip floors to reduce fall risk and enhance safety.
  - *Environmental adjustments*: Her room is equipped with visual aids such as clocks and calendars to aid orientation and minimize confusion.

- *Interdisciplinary team*:
  - *Assessment*: An interdisciplinary team, including a geriatrician, nurse specialist, physical therapist, occupational therapist, and social worker, conducts a comprehensive assessment of Mrs Rai's medical, functional, and cognitive needs.
  - *Care planning*: The team develops a tailored care plan that addresses her hypertension, osteoarthritis, cognitive impairment, and fall risk.
- *Functional status maintenance*:
  - *Physical therapy*: Mrs Rai participates in daily physical therapy sessions aimed at improving strength, balance, and mobility. Exercises are customized to her condition to prevent further falls and enhance her functional capabilities.
  - *Occupational therapy*: The occupational therapist introduces adaptive devices and modifications to help Mrs Rai with daily living activities, such as using assistive devices for dressing and bathing.
- *Cognitive support*:
  - *Cognitive stimulation*: Structured activities and cognitive exercises are implemented to address Mrs Rai's memory lapses and support cognitive function.
  - *Routine*: A consistent daily routine helps Mrs Rai adapt better and reduces the risk of disorientation and confusion.
- *Family and home safety education*:
  - *Education*: Mrs Rai's daughter receives training on fall prevention, safe home modifications, and managing her mother's chronic conditions.
  - *Home safety*: Recommendations are provided for making Mrs Rai's home safer, including removing tripping hazards, installing grab bars, and ensuring adequate lighting.
- *Discharge planning and follow-up*:
  - *Comprehensive plan*: A detailed discharge plan is created, including home health services for continued physical therapy, follow-up visits with her primary care physician, and coordination with community support services.
  - *Support services*: The plan also includes arranging for a home safety assessment and potential modifications to her living environment to ensure a safe return home.

FINDINGS AND OUTCOMES

- *Functional improvement*: Throughout her stay in the ACE unit, Mrs Rai shows significant improvement in mobility and functional abilities. The targeted interventions help her regain strength and reduce her risk of falls.
- *Safety and independence*: The environmental modifications and home safety recommendations contribute to a safer living environment, enhancing Mrs Rai's ability to live independently and reducing her daughter's concerns.
- *Quality of care*: Mrs Rai's overall health improves with coordinated care from the interdisciplinary team, and her daughter reports greater confidence in managing her mother's needs postdischarge.

ROLE OF GERIATRICIANS

Geriatricians are medical doctors with specialized training in the care of older adults. Their role is crucial in managing the complex health needs of the elderly population. Key responsibilities include the following:

- *Coordinating care*: Integrate and manage care across different healthcare providers and settings.
- *Conducting comprehensive assessments*: Perform thorough evaluations to address medical, psychological, and functional aspects of aging.
- *Developing treatment plans*: Create individualized care plans that address multiple conditions and prioritize the patient's quality of life and functional independence.
- *Education and advocacy*: Educate patients, families, and caregivers about aging-related issues and advocate for appropriate resources and services.
- *Research and innovation*: Contribute to research aimed at improving care models and developing new interventions for aging-related conditions.

In summary, geriatric models of care are essential for meeting the diverse needs of older adults. By adopting a multidisciplinary, patient-centered approach, healthcare providers can enhance the well-being of elderly patients and support them in leading fulfilling, independent lives.

CONCLUSION

The ACE model effectively addresses Mrs Sunita Rai's complex needs by integrating specialized care and environmental modifications. By focusing on her functional, cognitive, and safety requirements, the ACE model helps improve her quality of life, facilitates a smoother transition home, and supports her ongoing well-being.

Self-Assessment Questionnaire

Q1. What are the primary objectives of geriatric models of care, and how do they differ from traditional medical models

Q2. List the key components of the acute care for elders (ACE) model and describe how each contributes to preventing functional decline.

Q3. Explain various protocols used to prevent delirium.

Q4. Describe how home-based primary care (HBPC) promotes independence and prevents unnecessary hospitalizations in frail older adults.

Q5. In Mrs Sunita Rai's case, what environmental and team-based strategies were implemented to enhance safety and independence?

Q6. How does interdisciplinary collaboration improve quality of care and outcomes in older adults within the ACE unit?

Q7. Discuss the role of family education and home-safety interventions in post-discharge continuity of care.

Q8. Summarize the major roles of geriatricians in coordinating, assessing, and advocating for elderly patients across care settings.

FURTHER READINGS

1. Ahmed NN, Pearce SE. Acute care for the elderly: a literature review. Popul Health Manag. 2010;13(4):219-25.
2. American Geriatrics Society CoCare®: HELP (Hospital Elder Life Program). (2022). AGS CoCare: HELP Group Coaching Call #20. [online] Available from https://help.agscocare.org/ [Last accessed May, 2025].
3. Morishita L, Kunz EM. Program of all-inclusive care (PACE) model. In: Malone ML, Capezuti EA, Palmer RM (Eds). Geriatrics Models of Care: Bringing "Best Practice" to an Aging America. Cham: Springer International Publishing; 2015. pp. 259-66.
4. Friedman SM, Steinwachs DM, Rathouz PJ, Burton LC, Mukamel DB. Characteristics predicting nursing home admission in the program of all-inclusive care for elderly people. Gerontologist. 2005;45(2):157-66.
5. Nadash P. Two models of managed long-term care: comparing PACE with a Medicaid-only plan. Gerontologist. 2004;44(5): 644-54.
6. Counsell SR, Callahan CM, Buttar AB, Clark DO, Frank KI. Geriatric resources for assessment and care of elders (GRACE): a new model of primary care for low-income seniors. J Am Geriatr Soc. 2006;54(7):1136-41.
7. Halter JB, Ouslander JG, Studenski S, High KP. Hazzard's Geriatric Medicine and Gerontology, 8th edition. New Delhi: McGraw Hill; 2022.

SECTION 3

Preventive and Social Geriatrics

CHAPTER 37

Social Geriatrics

Ashish Goel, Dhruvendra Lal, Baldeep Kaur

INTRODUCTION

The definition of health has evolved in parallel with societal and technological advancements. The traditional medical model of health merely equates health with the absence of disease, dysfunction, or injury. Instead, modern models such as Lindau et al.'s "interactive biopsychosocial model" go beyond this and recognize the intricate interplay of social, biophysical, and psychocognitive health within an individual's social milieu. This holistic approach underscores the interconnectedness of these dimensions, emphasizing that an individual's health is profoundly shaped by their environment, relationships, and personal experiences. This comprehensive concept applies to all demographics, thus also laying the foundations for our discussions in social geriatrics.

DEFINITION

Social geriatrics is a subfield of geriatrics that focuses on the social, psychological, and environmental factors affecting the health and well-being of older adults in their later life. According to the National Statistical Office's "Elderly in India 2021" report, these disciplines have grown more and more important since India's aging population is expected to increase by 41% over the next 10 years. By 2031, the number of people aged 60 years and above is predicted to reach 194 million, up from 138 million in 2021, while the general population is expected to rise at an 8.4% rate. This demographic shift is known as "population aging." When population age increases rapidly, this has significant implications for the socioeconomic and health status of the elderly **(Fig. 1)**.

The intricate relationship between social factors and aging is well-established in the scientific literature. In a recent systematic review, Mogic et al. explored how functional social support correlates with cognitive abilities in adults of middle and older age, highlighting the importance of social support in preserving mental health as one age. Another review article by Roy et al. discusses the negative health impacts of social isolation and loneliness on older adults, highlighting the need for evaluation and intervention to address these issues in the geriatric population.

Social geriatrics aims to enhance the quality of life for older adults by addressing the various social factors and ensuring that older persons have the necessary support to age with dignity and independence. A healthy social environment and strong social connections are nearly as crucial as medical interventions for healthy aging **(Fig. 2)**.

SOCIAL DETERMINANTS OF HEALTH IN OLDER ADULTS

Social determinants of health (SDOH) in older adults are a constellation of nonmedical factors that profoundly shape the health, functioning, and quality of life of individuals. They are the array of conditions in which people are born, grow, live, work, and age. These determinants span a broad spectrum of conditions, from the immediate family and community environments to broader socioeconomic, educational, and policy contexts at national and international levels. The significance of SDOH is evident from the fact that healthcare professionals often conduct a social history to evaluate a person's care needs and social support, which is also a testament to the importance of social factors in geriatric care.

For the elderly, SDOH can have a profound impact on their health and well-being. They exert a substantial influence on their susceptibility to and experience of illnesses. For example, older adults with limited income may struggle to afford medications, nutritious food, or

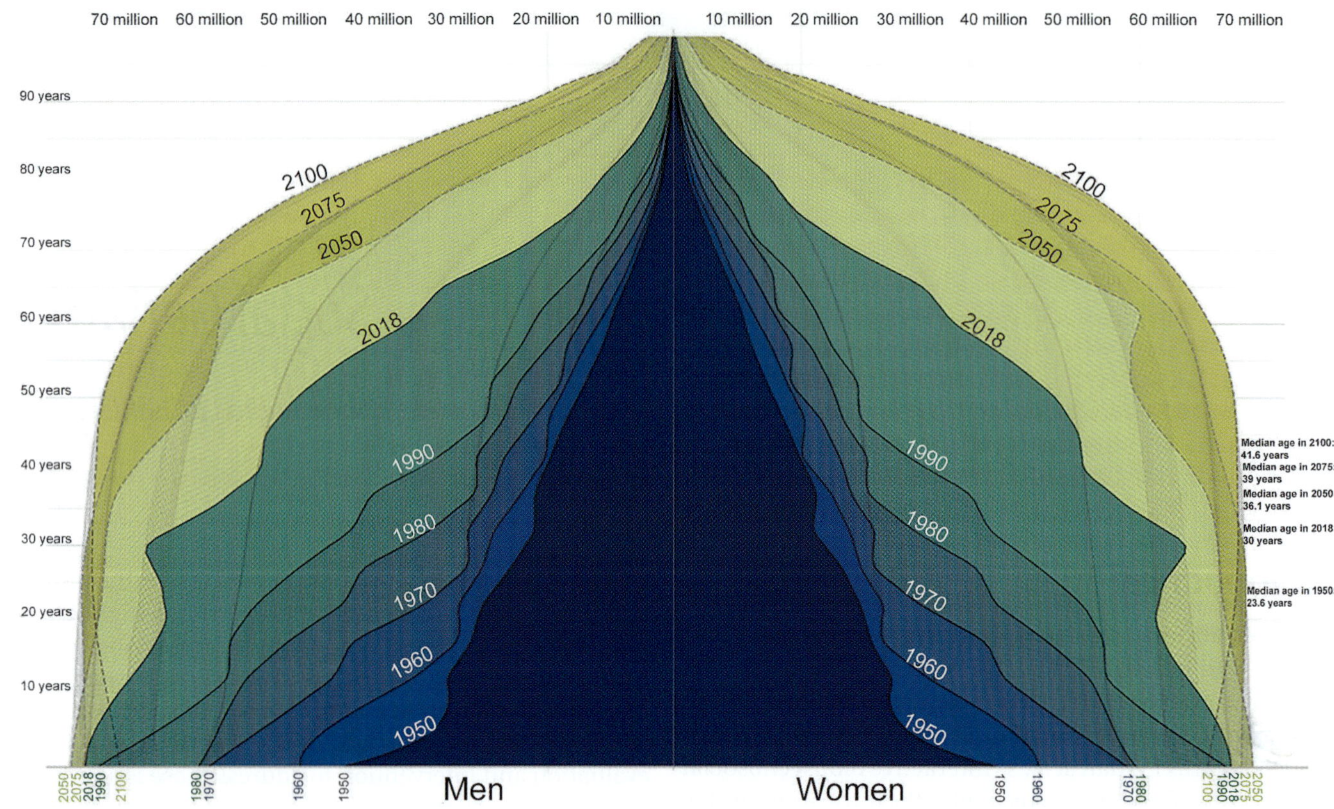

FIG. 1: World population pyramid (1950–2100).

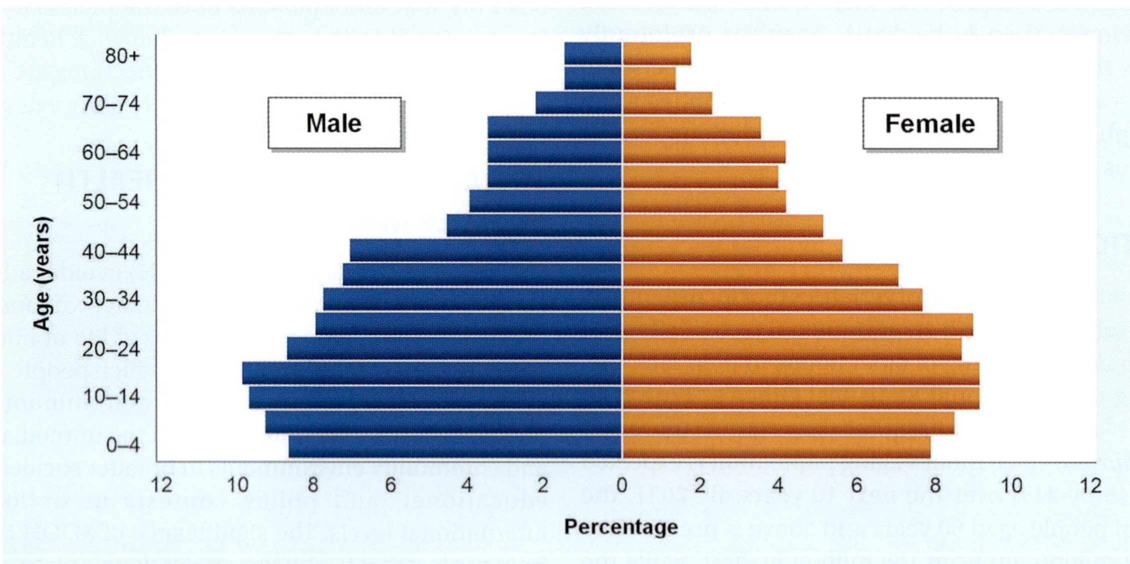

FIG. 2: Population pyramid, India, LASI Wave 1, 2017–2018.
(LASI: Longitudinal Aging Study in India)

safe housing, which can exacerbate health problems. Those with lower levels of education may have difficulty navigating the healthcare system or understanding medical advice, leading to poorer health outcomes. In contrast, strong social connections and support networks can enhance health and extend life expectancy by providing emotional support, practical assistance, and a sense of belonging in the community.

These examples highlight the pivotal role of social determinants in shaping the health and life quality of older adults. Healthcare systems must integrate these factors into their care planning and delivery processes. The subsequent sections will delve into the individual SDOH pertinent to the elderly, elucidating their impact in greater detail.

Family

Family plays an essential part in elderly care **(Fig. 3)**. Parent–child and intimate partner relationships are critical because they provide constant support and have a significant impact on the physical and mental health of the elderly. According to research, elderly men who live alone are twice as likely to have cognitive decline as those who live with others. In everyday life, family members provide hands-on physical help, assisting with personal care duties to maintain health and hygiene while lowering the danger of falling. They also guarantee that medical needs are satisfied and play an important role in drug management, identifying therapeutic advantages, and providing patients with clear information. As parents or grandparents, their emotional needs are better met within the family, helping the elderly feel loved, listened to, cared for, and accepted. Recognizing and incorporating elder family members into decision-making processes promote inclusivity while also honoring their important insights and experienced wisdom. Socially, families keep the elderly connected and enrich their lives through community interactions. They also provide financial help, which is especially important for low-income individuals **(Table 1)**. Overall, family involvement promotes holistic care and has a considerable impact on cognitive health, emotional well-being, and financial aspects of geriatric care **(Fig. 4)**.

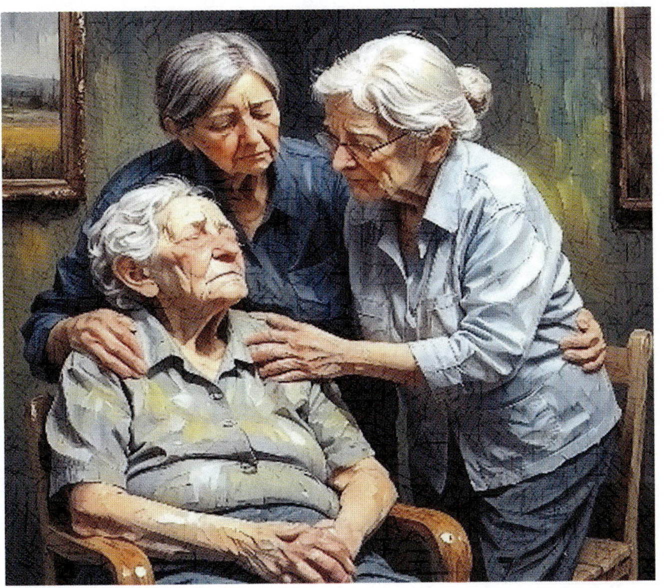

FIG. 3: Family.

Living Arrangements

The well-being of older adults is greatly affected by their living situation. In India, the traditional "joint family" system, based on the concept of "Dharma," prioritizes respecting and caring for elderly parents. Living with multiple generations can provide valuable support for the elderly in terms of both financial and nonfinancial help, including assistance during times of illness. Older adults who live in their communities as per their preferences rather than in nursing homes tend to report higher levels

TABLE 1: Family and social network indicators among elderly age 60 years and above by type of living arrangement, India, LASI Wave 1, 2017–2018.

	Age		Sex		Residence		
Individual-level key indicators	*45–59 years*	*60 years and above*	*Male*	*Female*	*Rural*	*Urban*	*Total*
Family and social network							
Current living arrangement							
Living alone (%)	1.4	5.7	1.8	4.5	3.9	2.3	3.4
Living with spouse and/or others (%)	12.2	20.3	19.3	13.5	16.8	14.0	15.9
Living with spouse and children (%)	74.2	40.6	67.1	52.7	58.4	59.7	58.8
Living with children and others (%)	9.4	27.6	8.6	24.4	16.9	19.6	17.7
Living with others only (%)	2.9	5.7	3.3	4.9	4.1	4.4	4.2
Satisfaction with current living arrangement							
Satisfied with current living arrangement (%)	79.7	74.8	78.3	76.9	76.0	80.9	77.5

Continued

Continued

		Age	Sex		Residence		
Shares most of the personal matters with (for age 60 years and above having spouse)							
Spouse partner (%)	NA	82.2	84.1	79.0	82.8	80.5	82.2
Children/grandchildren (%)	NA	31.9	30.3	34.7	32.2	31.4	31.9
Financial support received from or provided to family/friends during the past 12 months							
Received financial support (%)	12.3	15.2	12.5	14.5	14.9	10.9	13.6
Provided financial support (%)	8.2	5.9	9.9	5.2	6.8	8.0	7.2
Instrumental care							
Having family members who are unable to carry out basic daily activities (%)	2.9	2.4	2.4	2.8	2.8	2.4	2.7
Role in decision-making in[32]							
Marriage of son or daughter (%)	97.3	92.3	96.8	93.6	94.6	97.5	95.0
Buying and selling of property (%)	95.8	90.0	96.9	90.3	92.4	94.8	93.2
Education of family members (%)	94.7	83.7	93.3	87.3	88.5	93.0	89.9
Experience of ill-treatment during the last 1 year (for age 60 years and above only)[33]							
Experienced any ill-treatment (%)	NA	5.2	4.8	5.6	5.8	3.8	5.2
Perceived life satisfaction/social status							
Persons reporting satisfied with their own life (%)[34]	42.8	43.9	45.2	41.9	41.4	47.6	43.3
(LASI: Longitudinal Aging Study in India)							

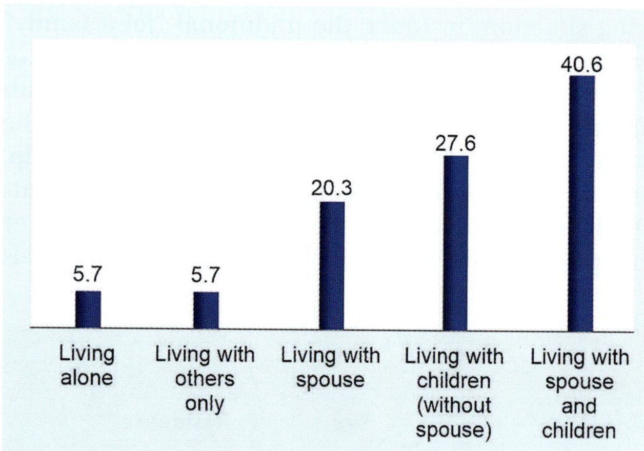

FIG. 4: Percent distribution of the elderly age 60 years and above by type of living arrangement, India, LASI Wave 1, 2017–2018.
(LASI: Longitudinal Aging Study in India)

of happiness, contentment, and overall life satisfaction. However, as urbanization, globalization, and evolving family structures result in fewer multigenerational households, providing support for older adults becomes more challenging. To support the well-being of older adults, especially those living alone, community-based programs should be established with regular check-ins by volunteers, providing essential amenities, transportation assistance, and access to healthcare resources. These initiatives will require a robust support network, enhancing their quality of life amidst changing family dynamics.

Education

Education has a tremendous impact on older individuals' well-being and quality of life. Lifelong learning improves cognitive function, lowering the risk of dementia as people age. Each year of education leads to a longer life expectancy, with primary education lowering death risk by 13%. Further, education improves socioeconomic position, resulting in better overall health outcomes. Education is essential for seniors navigating digital health resources such as websites, apps, and telehealth platforms. Strengthening digital health literacy also improves knowledge of medical information, from basic principles to sophisticated details, allowing for more informed decision-making. Educational meetings encourage social interaction, which helps to counteract emotions of loneliness and exclusion. Encouraging lifelong learning via exploring history, mastering new skills, or delving into the latest technology is paramount to promoting healthy aging. Accessible infrastructure for the same through community technology centers, free internet/wi-fi facilities will contribute to elderly education, thus promising a more fulfilling life in the later years.

Socioeconomic Status

The socioeconomic status (SES) of older people has a major impact on their health outcomes and quality of life. Individuals with a higher SES have better access to healthcare and lead healthier lives. Lower SES, on the other hand, is linked to an increased risk of chronic diseases and mortality. Key factors include economic stability, healthcare accessibility, and the quality of the living environment. Adequate income enables access to quality healthcare, nutritious food, and improved housing. Enhancing home environments—such as installing easy-access bathrooms, nonslip mats, and well-lit rooms—reduce the risk of falls. As mobility declines with age, accessible neighborhoods become crucial for active living. SES impacts an individual's social participation, access to social services, and resource allocation. People with higher economic resources tend to have broader social networks and engage in community activities and leisure pursuits. Addressing SES disparities is crucial for enhancing elderly well-being and reducing health inequalities, necessitating collaboration among healthcare providers, policymakers, and community organizations **(Fig. 5)**.

Healthcare Access and Equality

Access to healthcare and equality are critical for the elderly, who frequently suffer from chronic illnesses. Healthcare for the elderly should be available in all regions, regardless of geography, accessible to individuals with physical disabilities, affordable regardless of income, accommodating of various health needs, and acceptable in terms of cultural awareness and respect for diverse backgrounds. However, obstacles such as high expenses, limited facilities in remote regions, a lack of transportation for persons with physical limitations, and complicated insurance transitions impede progress. Health disparities by age, race, and income exacerbate the situation, with lower-income seniors incurring more disabilities and living shorter lives. Language obstacles and cultural conventions should not deter the elderly from seeking treatment. For the equal distribution of services, public investments in healthcare infrastructure are essential, particularly in rural areas. Given that an aging population will soon require more extensive healthcare services, addressing these challenges is essential to supporting healthy aging and improving older individuals' quality of life.

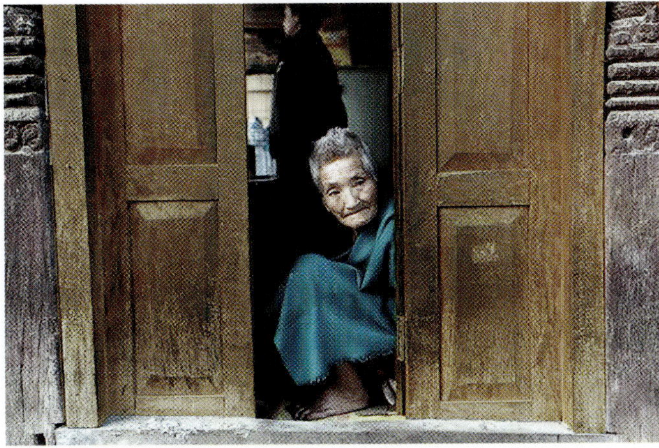

FIG. 5: Socioeconomic status.

Religion and Spirituality

Religion and spirituality (RS) are significant social determinants of older health, influencing mental well-being and social cohesiveness. An inverse connection between the prevalence of anxiety and depressive illnesses with RS participation has been frequently shown by observational research. In addition, people who participate in RS actively report being more satisfied with their lives, being more resilient psychologically, having a stronger sense of existential meaning, and having less dread of dying. Religion and spirituality are important sources of social support, meaningful relationships, and comfort, especially for individuals facing health issues. Thus, RS not only improves mental health in the elderly population but also plays a crucial role in their general well-being and social engagement throughout the complexities of aging.

Age-friendly Environment

A society that respects older people's empowerment and dignity must establish settings that are friendly and encouraging to them. Problems in old age such as delirium, immobility, falls, pressure ulcers, and malnourishment can be made worse by unfavorable environments at home and hospital. Age-friendly settings encourage independence and well-being in older people by being accessible, equitable, inclusive, safe, and secure. Examples at home include adding grab bars to the restroom, upgrading the lighting, and removing fall hazards. In the environment, well-lit streets, gated public spaces, convenient transportation, exercise parks, and public spaces for recreation and social interaction, along with neighborhood initiatives to stop elder abuse, form a part of an age-friendly environment. Cities such as Manchester and Hong Kong are commended for their initiatives to establish senior-friendly environments that adhere to the WHO framework and support the preservation of their abilities and independence, thereby enhancing their involvement and quality of life and are a good example of age-friendly cities. Finally, age-friendly settings have a major positive impact on senior citizens' health by enabling them to live longer, healthier lives with greater social connections **(Fig. 6)**.

Aging in Place

"Aging in place" is emphasized by social geriatrics as a means of preserving older individuals' autonomy and social networks within their own homes and communities. This method has been shown to enhance health outcomes, increase satisfaction, and reduce healthcare costs. It depends on a comprehensive network of health and social services, as well as proactive collaboration among families, community groups, healthcare providers, and policymakers. Preparation for potential changes in health status and mobility is essential in advance, including home modifications and service coordination. The aim is to provide seniors with options that promote their well-being and enable them to age healthily in their chosen setting. As the concept evolves, "aging in community" highlights the value of social connections in preventing isolation, "aging in the right place" adapts living arrangements to evolving health requirements, and "aging with grace" focuses on mental and emotional health, ensuring a dignified aging process. Collectively, these concepts foster a rewarding and flexible aging experience.

Social Isolation and Loneliness

Human are social creatures, and they need interactions and connections to be an essential part of their lives enabling them to thrive and survive. However, as individuals grow older, they frequently experience increased periods of solitude. This period can render older adults more susceptible to loneliness and social isolation, adversely impacting their health and overall quality of life **(Fig. 7)**.

Loneliness and social isolation are distinct yet interrelated. Loneliness refers to the distressing sensation of being alone or separated, whereas social isolation denotes a lack of social contacts and few regular interactions with others. One crucial scientific inquiry revolves around whether social isolation and loneliness operate

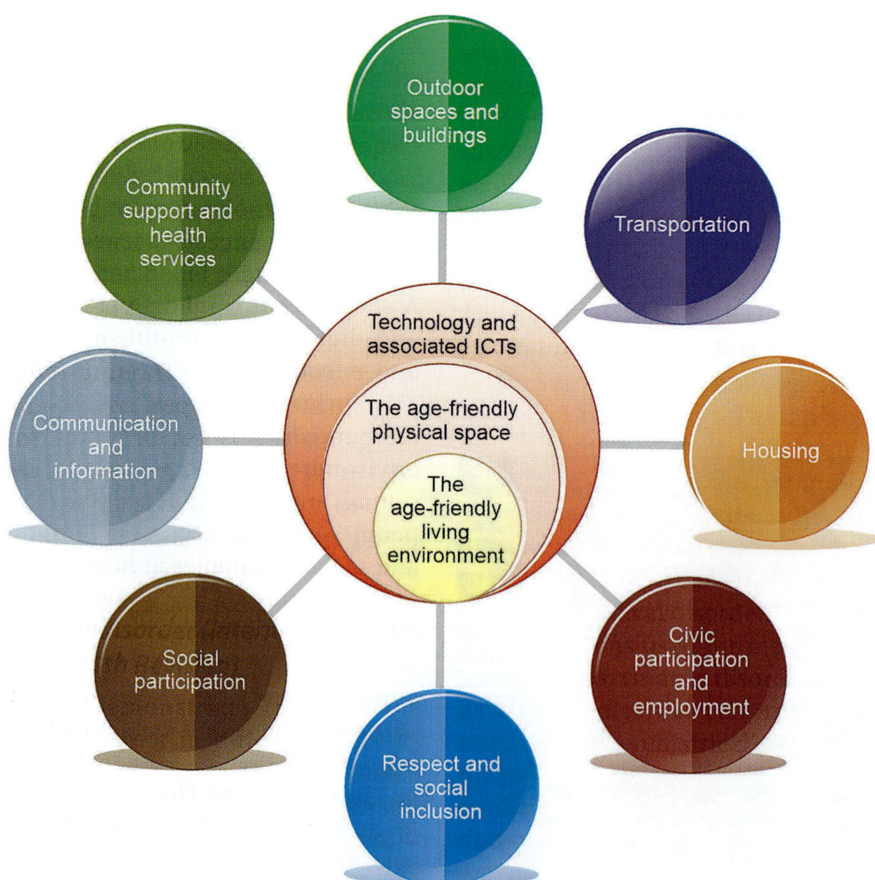

FIG. 6: The age-friendly ecosystem: A synthesis of age-friendly programs.
(ICTs: information and communication technologies)

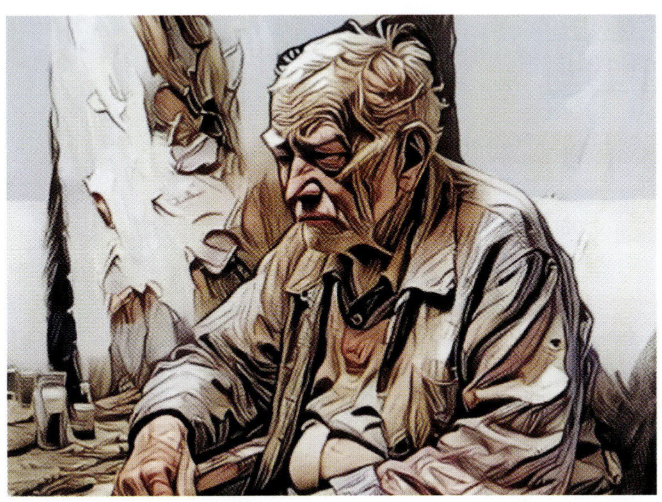

FIG. 7: Social isolation and loneliness.

as separate processes, each impacting health differently, or whether loneliness serves as a conduit through which social isolation influences health outcomes. The answer to this lies in the fact that loneliness is a subjective psychological discomfort individuals experience when their social network lacks sufficient quality or quantity. On the other hand, social isolation is an objective state of being alone or lacking social relationships, while social loneliness is a type of loneliness that arises when an individual lacks the sense of social integration or community involvement typically provided by a network of friends, neighbors, or coworkers.

The prevalence of loneliness is widespread among older adults. For instance, in 11 European countries, loneliness varied from 10% in France and Norway to over 30% in Bulgaria. Research utilizing data from the first wave (2017–2018) of the Longitudinal Aging Study in India (LASI) revealed that 20.5% of adults aged 45 years and older in India reported moderate loneliness, with 13.3% reporting severe loneliness. There exists a significant correlation between loneliness and major depressive disorder, potentially due to their high comorbidity with depression. Loneliness may manifest both consequently and as a risk factor for depressive symptoms. Social isolation significantly elevates the risk of premature death from all causes, a risk comparable to that posed by smoking, obesity, and physical inactivity, apart from a documented 50% increased risk of dementia. Poor social relationships, whether characterized by social isolation or loneliness, pose significant risks to health. Specifically, such inadequate social connections are associated with a 29% increased risk of heart disease and a 32% heightened risk of stroke. Moreover, loneliness has been closely linked to elevated rates of depression, anxiety, and suicide. Among individuals grappling with heart failure, loneliness emerges as a particularly concerning factor, with those experiencing loneliness facing nearly a fourfold increased risk of mortality, a 68% heightened risk of hospitalization, and a 57% increased likelihood of emergency department visits. These findings underscore the critical importance of addressing social isolation and loneliness in the promotion of overall health and well-being, especially in the elderly age group **(Figs. 8 and 9)**.

Ageism

Ageism, a pervasive form of discrimination fueled by inaccurate stereotypes, traps older adults in a box and limits their potential. We must challenge these biases to ensure a more equitable society for all ages. Ageism creates a generational blind spot. Younger adults operate within a social circle of similar experiences, while older adults might unintentionally filter the world through outdated perceptions. So, ageism is a complex web of stereotypes (how we think about age), prejudice (negative feelings based on age), and discrimination (unequal treatment based on age) that can be directed at others or even internalized by ourselves. Ageism is a double-edged sword. It not only diminishes our view of ourselves and weakens the bonds between generations but also hinders our ability to benefit from the strengths of both younger and older people. This prejudice has detrimental effects on our health, longevity, and overall well-being while also posing significant economic challenges.

Ageism is a widespread bias that manifests in both professional and personal settings. In the workplace, it can take the form of discriminatory hiring practices, unfair policies favoring specific age groups, and negative stereotypes about productivity or skills based on age. Similarly, personal relationships can be strained by ageism through dismissive attitudes, hurtful jokes, or disregard for someone's opinions solely due to their age. Ultimately, ageism exploits and undermines individuals across generations.

Combating ageism requires a multifaceted approach. Three key strategies stand out: (1) Policy and law, (2) educational activities, and (3) intergenerational interventions. *Policy and law* can provide a strong foundation by enacting antidiscrimination legislation and promoting policies that ensure equal opportunities for all ages. *Educational activities* can raise awareness and challenge stereotypes. Workshops on unconscious bias and the value of diverse perspectives can foster empathy and understanding across generations. Finally, *intergenerational interventions* bring people together to break down barriers. Mentorship programs pairing young and experienced professionals or volunteer initiatives where different generations collaborate can create positive connections and dismantle ageist assumptions **(Fig. 10)**.

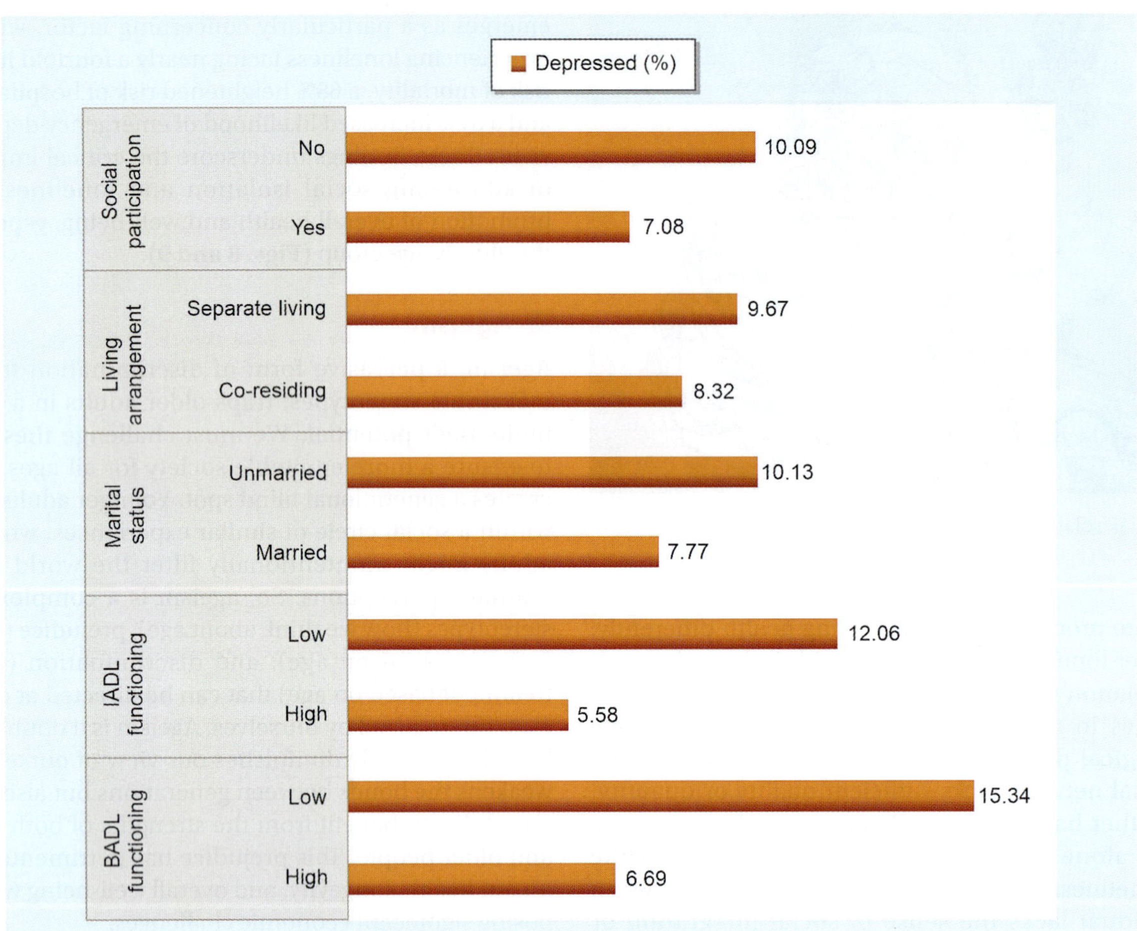

FIG. 8: Prevalence estimated of major depression with various variables.
(BADL: basic activities of daily living; IADL: instrumental activities of daily living)

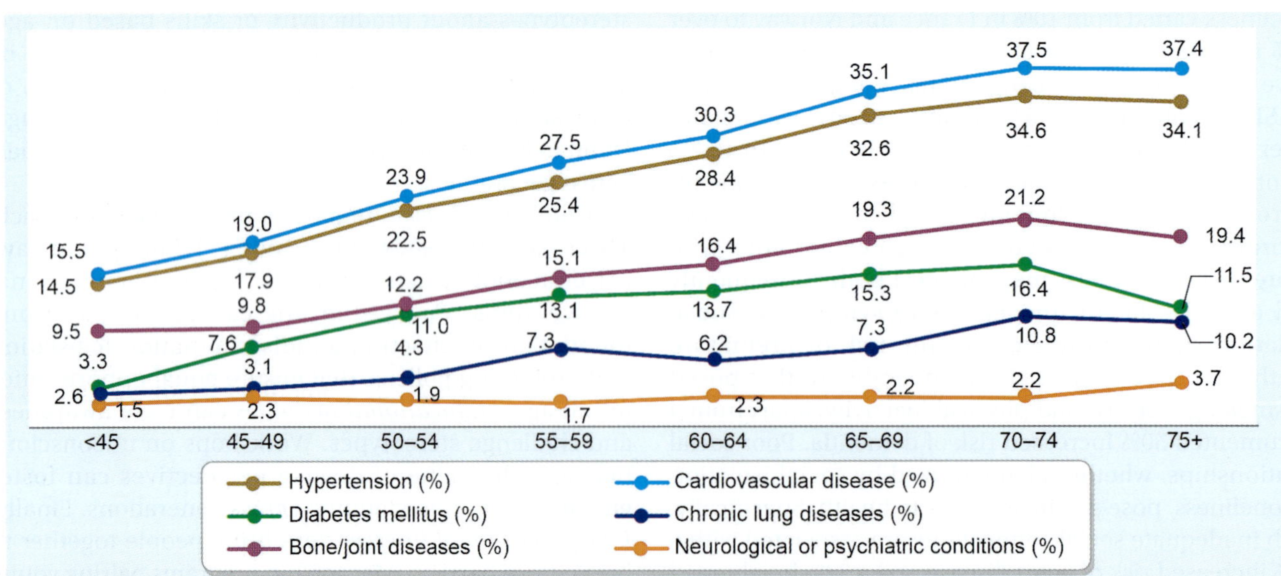

FIG. 9: Self-reported prevalence (%) of diagnosed major chronic health conditions among older adults by age, India, LASI Wave 1, 2017–2018.
(LASI: Longitudinal Aging Study in India)

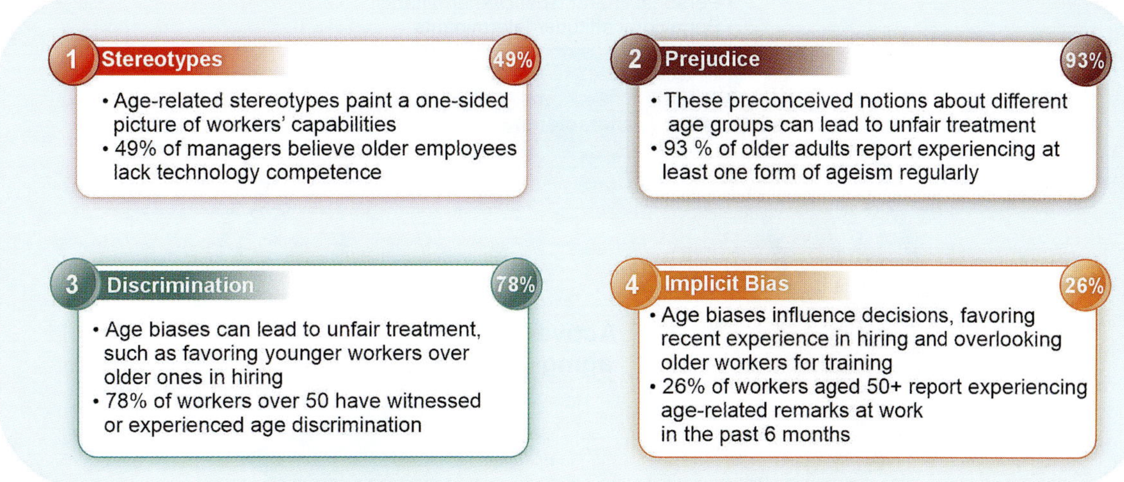

FIG. 10: Ageism in the modern workplace.

Healthy Ageing Collaborative

The Healthy Ageing Collaborative (HAC) brings together governments, businesses, NGOs, and academic institutions to foster healthy aging and advance the UN Decade of Healthy Ageing (2021–2030). The objectives of HAC include raising awareness of the UN Decade of Healthy Ageing (2021–2030) and its linkages with other agendas and mechanisms, including but not limited to the WHO Global Strategy and Action Plan on Ageing and Health 2016–2030, the Madrid International Plan of Action on Ageing, the 2030 Agenda for Sustainable Development Goals (SDGs), and Our Common Agenda; strengthening international coordination on healthy aging and promoting multisectoral engagement and cooperation; encouraging and supporting the national level implementation of the UN Decade of Healthy Ageing, including to reach people where they live; and recognizing the role of older persons, ensuring their meaningful engagement in the implementation of the decade, including through the applications of human-rights-related approaches.

The progress report on the UN Decade of Healthy Ageing, spanning from 2021 to 2030, offers a comprehensive overview of advancements made in the initial phase of implementation (2021 to mid-2023). It includes a comparative analysis of 10 national progress indicators for the decade, contrasting data from 2020 with that from 2022. This evaluation framework enables stakeholders to gauge the effectiveness of their efforts and identify areas requiring further attention. Ultimately, the report serves as a catalyst for scaling up interventions aimed at promoting healthy aging. By highlighting progress, identifying challenges, and emphasizing the collective responsibility of stakeholders, it seeks to galvanize ongoing efforts to ensure that older populations around the world can lead fulfilling and healthy lives. It involved four action areas which included (1) changing how we think, feel, and act toward age and aging; (2) ensuring that communities foster the abilities of older people; (3) delivering person-centered, integrated care and primary health services responsive to older people; and (4) providing access to long-term care for older people who need it **(Fig. 11)**.

SCHEMES FOR THE WELFARE OF SENIOR CITIZENS IN INDIA

The Government of India is actively executing an array of schemes and programs aimed at ensuring senior citizens lead lives that are not just healthy and happy but also empowered, dignified, and self-reliant, fostering robust social and intergenerational bonds. Recognizing the essential requirements of love, care, medical support, housing, and more for senior citizens, the government has instituted a multitude of schemes and programs dedicated to their welfare.

National Policy for Senior Citizens 2011: The Government of India introduced the National Policy on Older Persons in 1999, aligning with the UN General Assembly Resolution 47/5, which designated 1999 as the International Year of Older Persons. This initiative underscores the nation's commitment to upholding the rights and well-being of senior citizens, as enshrined in the Constitution under Article 41.

Currently, a range of support measures are being extended to older persons, including pensions, travel concessions, income tax relief, medical benefits, and

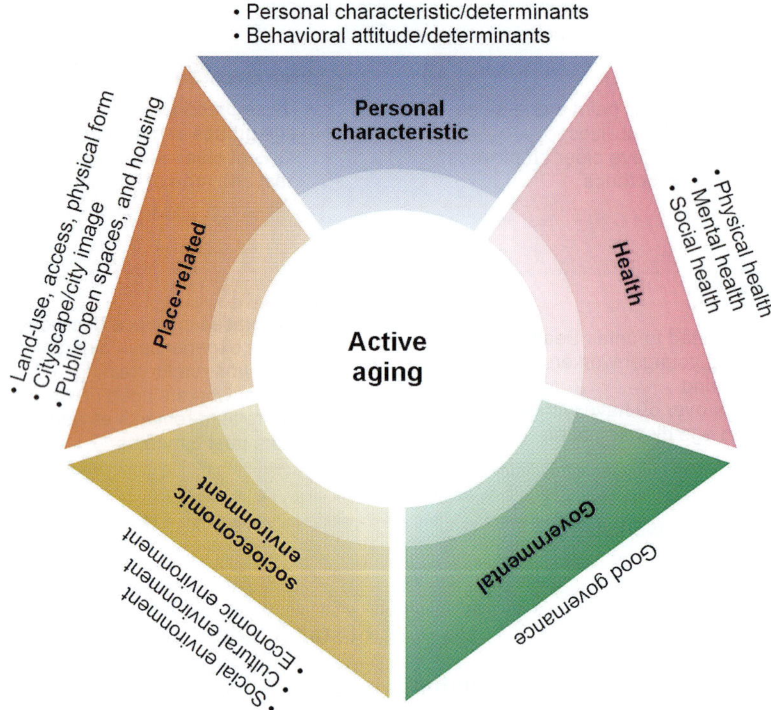

FIG. 11: Components of active and healthy aging.

additional interest on savings. The Ministry of Social Justice and Empowerment administers an integrated scheme aimed at ensuring the security of older persons, while financial assistance is allocated for facilities such as homes, daycare centers, medical vans, and helplines.

The new policy concerning senior citizens outlines several key objectives aimed at mainstreaming older individuals, particularly older women, into national development discussions and prioritizing the implementation of existing mechanisms supported by governments and civil society. It advocates for the promotion and establishment of senior citizens' associations, with a focus on empowering women in this regard. Additionally, the policy emphasizes the concept of "Aging in Place," which entails ensuring housing, income security, homecare services, old age pensions, and access to healthcare insurance schemes to maintain dignity in old age, with a preventive approach. Institutional care is regarded as a last resort, with an emphasis on family-based care supported by the community, government, and private sector. Furthermore, the policy aims to create an inclusive, barrier-free, and age-friendly society, in alignment with international agreements such as the Madrid Plan of Action and Barrier-Free Framework. It recognizes senior citizens as valuable resources and envisions equal opportunities, rights protection, and full societal participation for them, especially for those living below the poverty line, with measures to safeguard them from abuse and exploitation. The policy also advocates for the promotion of long-term saving instruments and credit activities, encouragement of postretirement employment, support for counseling and training services, and implementation of legislation to ensure the welfare of elderly parents and senior citizens. Additionally, it calls for the establishment of assisted living facilities for abandoned senior citizens in every district of the country, with adequate budgetary support from the states.

There are various schemes and programs which are being implemented by the Government of India in the care of senior citizens in India. A few of the schemes under the Department of Social Justice and Empowerment include the following:

- *Atal Vayo Abhyudaya Yojana (AVYAY)*: Umbrella scheme addressing financial security, food, healthcare, and dignity for senior citizens, including safety and general well-being through awareness and sensitization
- *Integrated Programme for Senior Citizens (IPSrC)*: Provides grants for running homes to offer basic amenities and improve the quality of life for indigent senior citizens
- *State Action Plan for Senior Citizens (SAPSrC)*: State-level plans for senior citizen welfare, considering local needs and implementing strategies for social security, healthcare, and shelter

- *Rashtriya Vayoshri Yojana (RVY)*: Offers free aids and assisted living devices to BPL senior citizens with age-related disabilities, enhancing mobility and quality of life
- *Senior Able Citizens for Re-Employment in Dignity (SACRED)*: Connects senior citizens with business enterprises for re-employment opportunities, utilizing their experience and stability
- *Action Groups Aimed at Social Reconstruction (AGRASR) groups*: Encourages senior citizens to form self-help groups for social and financial engagement, providing a constructive platform for interaction
- *Promoting silver economy*: Provides financial assistance to entrepreneurs developing innovative solutions for elderly care, fostering economic activities benefiting seniors
- *Channelizing CSR funds for elderly care*: Directs corporate social responsibility funds toward projects such as old age homes and daycare centers for senior citizens
- *Scheme for awareness generation and capacity building*: Includes the National Helpline for Senior Citizens, training, research, and awareness programs to address elderly issues and sensitize society
- *National Social Assistance Programme (NSAP)*: Financial assistance for BPL elderly, widows, and disabled, including old age pensions and lumpsum assistance upon the breadwinner's death
- *Indira Gandhi National Old Age Pension Scheme (IGNOAPS)*: Monthly pension for BPL elderly, increasing with age, to support their financial needs
- *Indira Gandhi National Disability Pension Scheme (IGNDPS)*: Monthly pension for BPL persons with severe disabilities, providing financial support for their living expenses
- *National Programme for the Health Care of Elderly (NPHCE)*: Comprehensive healthcare facilities for elderly at primary, secondary, and tertiary levels, including specialized geriatric services
- *Atal Pension Yojana (APY)*: Universal social security scheme providing guaranteed pensions for all citizens, especially targeting unorganized sector workers
- *Model Building Bye Laws, 2016*: Standards for elder-friendly, barrier-free environments in urban infrastructure, ensuring accessibility in buildings and public transport
- *Urban Bus Specification-II*: Emphasizes low-floor buses with ramps and wheelchair space, facilitating ease of travel for elderly and disabled passengers
- *Housing for All Mission/Pradhan Mantri Awas Yojana*: Prioritizes housing allocation for senior citizens, ensuring ground floor or lower floor accommodations for ease of access
- *Deendayal Antyodaya Yojana-National Urban Livelihoods Mission (DAY-NULM)*: Provides permanent shelters with essential services for urban homeless, including elderly, aiming to reduce urban poverty and vulnerability

FUTURE DIRECTIONS

The future of social geriatrics in India will significantly focus on integrating SDOH, addressing social isolation, enhancing mental health services, and promoting healthy aging, guided by robust policies and expanded schemes for the elderly. Incorporating SES, education, and social support into healthcare assessments will facilitate targeted interventions, particularly in underserved areas. Community programs and technological solutions can mitigate social isolation, providing elderly individuals with opportunities for social engagement and connection through social clubs, intergenerational activities, and digital communication tools. Enhanced availability of mental health services, including counseling, support groups, and psychiatric care tailored to the elderly, will address the growing psychological needs of this population.

Promoting healthy aging through regular health screenings, preventive healthcare measures, and lifestyle programs focused on diet, exercise, and wellness activities such as yoga and physiotherapy is crucial for maintaining the well-being of the elderly. Policies must be strengthened and effectively implemented to protect the rights and well-being of the elderly, complemented by expanding schemes such as the IGNOAPS to increase coverage and provide comprehensive support, including financial assistance, healthcare, housing, and social services.

Interdisciplinary collaboration among healthcare providers, social workers, policymakers, and community organizations will create a comprehensive support system for the elderly, while research and culturally inclusive approaches will ensure that the diverse needs of India's aging population are met. By focusing on these future directions, social geriatrics in India can evolve to better address the challenges faced by the elderly population, promoting their well-being and ensuring that they lead dignified and fulfilling lives.

CONCLUSION

The multifaceted concept of health has evolved significantly, moving beyond the simplistic absence of disease to embrace a holistic understanding of well-being that encompasses social, biophysical, and psychocognitive dimensions. Social geriatrics, as a subfield, highlights the crucial interplay of these factors in the lives of older adults. As India's aging population surges, the importance of addressing the SDOH becomes increasingly apparent. This chapter has illustrated how family dynamics, living arrangements, education, SES, healthcare access, religion, and age-friendly environments significantly impact the health and quality of life of the elderly.

The role of family and community is paramount, providing essential support systems that enhance physical, mental, and emotional well-being. Education and SES are pivotal in shaping health outcomes, with lifelong learning and economic stability offering protective benefits. Addressing healthcare access and equality, fostering age-friendly environments, and combating ageism are essential steps toward ensuring that older adults can lead dignified, independent lives.

Policy responses, at both the national and international levels, are critical in this endeavor. India's National Policy for Senior Citizens and initiatives such as the HAC emphasize the need for comprehensive, inclusive strategies that promote healthy aging. These efforts must be supported by robust public investments, community-based programs, and intergenerational initiatives that bridge gaps and foster a supportive environment for the elderly.

In conclusion, the well-being of older adults is intricately tied to their social environment. By recognizing and addressing the diverse SDOH, societies can create conditions that enable older individuals to age with dignity, independence, and a high quality of life. The insights from social geriatrics provide a roadmap for achieving this goal, underscoring the need for a concerted, holistic approach to elderly care in an aging world.

Self-Assessment Questionnaire

Q1. How does the interactive biopsychosocial model redefine the concept of health in the context of aging?

Q2. What are the major social determinants of health (SDOH) that influence the well-being of older adults?

Q3. How do living arrangements and the decline of the traditional joint family system affect the quality of life of the elderly in India?

Q4. How do religion and spirituality contribute to psychological resilience and mental well-being in older adults?

Q5. Define "age-friendly environment." What measures can be taken at home and in the community to create such environments?

Q6. Explain the differences between social isolation and loneliness, and discuss their health implications for older adults.

FURTHER READINGS

1. Flexner A. Medical Education in the United States and Canada. Washington, DC: Science and Health Publications; 1910.
2. Lindau ST, Laumann EO, Levinson W, Waite LJ. Synthesis of scientific disciplines in pursuit of health: the interactive biopsychosocial model. Perspect Biol Med. 2003;46(3 Suppl):S74-86.
3. National Statistical Office. (2021). National Statistical Office (NSO)'s Elderly in India. [online] Available from https://ruralindiaonline.org/hi/library/resource/elderly-in-india-2021. [Last accessed May, 2025].
4. Mogic L, Rutter EC, Tyas SL, Maxwell CJ, O'Connell ME, Oremus M. Functional social support and cognitive function in middle- and older-aged adults: a systematic review of cross-sectional and cohort studies. Syst Rev. 2023;12(1):86.
5. Roy K, Smilowitz S, Bhatt S, Conroy ML. Impact of social isolation and loneliness in older adults: current understanding and future directions. Curr Geri Rep. 2023;12:138-48.
6. Van Gelder BM, Tijhuis M, Kalmijn S, Giampaoli S, Nissinen A, Kromhout D. Marital status and living situation during a 5-year period are associated with a subsequent 10-year cognitive decline in older men: the FINE study. J Gerontol B Psychol Sci Soc Sci. 2006;61(4):P213-19.
7. Kasper JD, Wolff JL, Skehan M. Care arrangements of older adults: what they prefer, what they have, and implications for quality of life. Gerontologist. 2019;59(5):845-55.
8. Lövdén M, Fratiglioni L, Glymour MM, Lindenberger U, Tucker-Drob EM. Education and cognitive functioning across the life span. Psychol Sci Public Interest. 2020;21(1):6-41.
9. IHME-CHAIN Collaborators. Effects of education on adult mortality: a global systematic review and meta-analysis. Lancet Public Health. 2024;9(3):e155-65.
10. Coelho-Júnior HJ, Calvani R, Panza F, Allegri RF, Picca A, Marzetti E, et al. Religiosity/spirituality and mental health in older adults: a systematic review and meta-analysis of observational studies. Front Med (Lausanne). 2022;9:877213.
11. National Institute on Aging. (2024). Loneliness and Social Isolation—Tips for Staying Connected. [online] Available from https://www.nia.nih.gov/health/loneliness-and-social-isolation/loneliness-and-social-isolation-tips-staying-connected#:~:text=Older%20adults%20are%20at%20higher,loss%20of%20family%20and%20friends. [Last accessed May, 2025].
12. Peplau LA, Perlman D. Perspectives on loneliness. In: Peplau LA, Perlman D (Eds). Loneliness: A Sourcebook of Current Theory, Research and Therapy. New York, NY: John Wiley & Sons; 1982. pp. 1-18.
13. Hansen T, Slagsvold B. Late-life loneliness in 11 European countries: results from the generations and gender survey. Soc Indic Res. 2016;129:445-64.

14. Centers for Disease Control and Prevention. Loneliness and social isolation linked to serious health conditions [Internet]. 2021 [cited 2025 May]. Available from: https://www.cdc.gov/aging/publications/features/lonely-older-adults.html
15. Weir K. A new concept of aging: Ageism is one of the last socially acceptable prejudices. Psychologists are working to change that. Monitor on Psychology. 2023;54:36-43. Available from: https://www.apa.org/monitor/2023/03/cover-new-concept-of-aging
16. World Health Organization. Ageing: Ageism [Internet]. 2024 [cited 2025 May]. Available from: https://www.who.int/news-room/questions-and-answers/item/ageing-ageism
17. UN Decade of Healthy Ageing—The Platform. (2024). Healthy Ageing Collaborative. [online] Available from https://www.decadeofhealthyageing.org/about/join-us/collaborative. [Last accessed May, 2025].
18. World Health Organization. (2023). Progress report on the United Nations decade of healthy ageing, 2021–2023: executive summary. [online] Available from https://www.who.int/publications/i/item/9789240082120. [Last accessed May, 2025].
19. Ministry of Social Justice & Empowerment. (2022). Schemes for the welfare of senior citizens. [online] Available from https://pib.gov.in/PressReleasePage.aspx?PRID=1806506. [Last accessed May, 2025].
20. Giri M, Sabharwal MM, Gangadharan KR, Sreenivasan S, Mitra PP. National policy for senior citizens [Internet]. 2011 [cited 2025 May]. Available from: https://socialjustice.gov.in/writereaddata/UploadFile/dnpsc.pdf
21. Government of India, Rajya Sabha. National policy on senior citizen [Internet]. Unstarred Question No. 1733. 2023 [cited 2025 May]. Available from: https://sansad.in/getFile/annex/259/AU1733.pdf
22. Bhatt J, Verma R, Verma S. Social determinants of health and their impact on the elderly in India. J Geriatr Care. 2021;15(2):125-38.
23. Rajan SI. Social isolation and mental health among the elderly in India. Indian J Soc Work. 2020;81(3):259-72.
24. Gupta A. Policy framework for elderly care in India: analysis and recommendations. Policy Briefs Social Welf. 2019;9(4):45-59.
25. Soneja S. Interdisciplinary collaboration in geriatric care: a model for India. Health Aging. 2017;23(1):11-22.
26. Tiwari SC. Culturally inclusive approaches to elderly care in India. J Cross-Cult Gerontol. 2021;36(1):47-65.
27. Muhammad T, Maurya P. Social support moderates the association of functional difficulty with major depression among community-dwelling older adults: evidence from LASI, 2017-18. BMC Psychiatry. 2022;22(1):317.
28. Lak A, Rashidghalam P, Amiri SN, Myint PK, Baradaran HR. An ecological approach to the development of an active aging measurement in urban areas (AAMU). BMC Public Health. 2021; 21:4.
29. van Hoof J, Marston HR, Kazak JK, Buffel T. Ten questions concerning age-friendly cities and communities and the built environment. Build Environ. 2021;199:107922.
30. HR Vision. (2024). Ageism in the Modern Workplace—A Growing Challenge. [online] Available from https://www.hrvisionevent.com/content-hub/ageism-in-the-modern-workplace-a-growing-challenge/. [Last accessed May, 2025].
31. Roser M. (2019). The global population pyramid: how global demography has changed and what we can expect for the 21st Century. [online] Available from https://ourworldindata.org/global-population-pyramid. [Last accessed May, 2025].

CHAPTER 38

Vaccination in Elderly

Gaurav Sharma, Anup Singh

INTRODUCTION

With an increase in age, many physiological changes occur in the body, such as decreased physiological lung capacity, decreased cardiac contractility, loss of nephrons, and declining immune function. This declining immune function is also called immunosenescence.

Immunosenescence refers to the cumulative impact of aging on immune function, affecting all types of immune cells and many molecular pathways across the immune response. This leads to a general phenotype characterized by low-level inflammation but impaired innate and adaptive immune responses to acute stimuli. Responses to new antigens are often more affected than memory responses.

Age-related declines in the older population affect virtually all cell lineages of the immune system, including reductions in T-cell lymphopoiesis, naïve T cells, mitogen-associated proliferation signal transduction, diversity of the T-cell repertoire, expression of CD28 on CD8+ cells and B cells, antibody-secreting cells, class switch recombination, expression of activation-induced cytidine deaminase (AID), and diversity of B cells. This results in alterations in diverse innate immune responses mediating the earliest interactions of the immune system with pathogens or vaccines, as well as slower onset and highly specific adaptive immune responses in B and T cells.

These consequences of immunosenescence have important clinical consequences reflected in increased susceptibility to infectious diseases found in older adults as well as increased risk of development of reactivation of tuberculosis and varicella-zoster virus (VZV) infection. Several other host factors, such as gender, age-related alterations in body composition (like changes in adipose tissue), and related comorbidities or medication use, also play a role in diminishing immune responses and increasing the need for vaccination.

INFLUENZA VACCINE

Influenza viruses are enveloped viruses with RNA genomes comprising eight gene segments. Influenza A viruses are categorized into subtypes according to their primary surface glycoproteins, known as hemagglutinin (HA) and neuraminidase.

Mechanism

The typical flu vaccine is a trivalent or quadrivalent formula made of inactivated split virions, which are enriched with HA and neuraminidase. It is designed to contain 15 µg of HA from each virus strain included in the vaccine. The development of antibodies against HA is associated with protection against illness. Many factors cause decreased efficacy of the vaccine like antigenic match between the circulating strain and vaccine strain, adaptation mutations, and age.

Antigenic change is an associated term used with influenza virus. Antigenic drift is a continuous process where point mutations occur in proteins allowing the virus to evade neutralization of antibodies by previous infection or vaccination. Antigenic shift is a major antigenic change where a novel HA and/or neuraminidase is formed which is typically introduced from another species and results in transmission between humans, sometimes causing a pandemic. With this high mutation rate in the HA protein, the composition of viral strains in the vaccine is adjusted annually based on the surveillance of circulating strains. For the same reason, it is recommended to have an annual vaccination, especially for high-risk individuals.

The standard quadrivalent influenza vaccine contains four strains: Two influenza A strains (usually one H1N1 and one H3N2 subtype) and two B strains. Its efficacy is around 40% for preventing influenza-like illness and approximately 60% for confirmed influenza.

Vaccine efficacy as well as immunogenicity of the influenza vaccine is lower in older adults. Evidence for poor vaccine efficacy, combined with the demonstration of impaired antibody responses to vaccination reflected in decreased levels of antibody-producing cells following influenza immunization, has led to interest in alternative vaccine formats to improve response in older adults.

Thus, many techniques have been developed such as:

- Increasing the dose of the vaccine (high dose trivalent)
- Addition of an adjuvant vaccine (MF59)
- Changing the route of the vaccine (intradermal)

There is evidence that indicates better immunogenicity of high-dose vaccine Fluzone (60 µg of each HA); the study also suggested that a high-dose trivalent vaccine is more cost-effective and can prevent substantial influenza-related deaths. A high-dose trivalent influenza vaccine containing four times the dose of HA protein for each vaccine strain was approved for adults aged 65 years and older in 2009.

The recombinant hemagglutinin (rHA) vaccine contains 45 µg rHA per strain which is three times more than the standard vaccine; notably, it does not contain neuraminidase and egg protein. A systematic review indicated that enhanced vaccine in the form of either high dose or adjuvanted vaccine proved to induce higher antibody responses than standard-dose vaccine.

An additional approved vaccine for adults aged 65 years and older includes a standard-dose quadrivalent vaccine combined with MF59, an adjuvant derived from squalene. This adjuvant is believed to improve antigen presentation, potentially enhancing the vaccine's effectiveness.

In terms of vaccine safety, there have been limited trials directly comparing various vaccines. A study in Hong Kong suggested that while local reactions were more frequent with MF59 and high-dose influenza vaccines, systemic symptoms were similar across all vaccines.

Another strategy is changing the route to the vaccine as intradermal influenza vaccine that utilizes the immunologic milieu of the skin [which contains antigen-presenting cells (APCs) including Langerhans cells], i.e., bypassed by intramuscular vaccination; however, these are not approved for adults aged 65 years or older.

Future Directions

Efforts to enhance influenza vaccines continue, including the use of adjuvants that activate the innate immune system, such as toll-like receptor (TLR) agonists. Another focus is on developing a "universal" influenza vaccine that would eliminate the need for annual updates. However, ensuring the safety of enhanced vaccines requires conducting large trials before they can be recommended for widespread use.

Current Recommendations

Age 65 years or older: Any one of high-dose quadrivalent inactivated influenza vaccine (HD-IIV4), quadrivalent recombinant influenza vaccine (RIV4), or adjuvanted quadrivalent inactivated influenza vaccine (aIIV4) is preferred annually. If none of these three vaccines is available, then any other age-appropriate influenza vaccine should be used.

VARICELLA–ZOSTER VACCINE

Herpes zoster is the result of reactivation of VZV, frequently affecting older adults which is prevented or controlled as a subclinical infection or by VZV-specific T-cell-mediated immunity. When VZV-specific T-cell-mediated immunity falls below some critical threshold in the setting of immunosuppression or malignancy, this causes damage to neurons and causes ganglionitis resulting in neuropathic pain in the affected dermatome. This reactivation also travels to the affected sensory nerve causing pathognomonic dermatomal rash and nociceptive pain. The typical dermatomal herpes zoster rash remains for 7–10 days, but the pain preceding the rash is often severe.

Studies in immunosuppressed adults have established that defects in T-cell immunity, like those associated with aging, are essential in maintaining VZV in a state of latency in ganglia associated with peripheral and cranial nerves, although the precise mechanisms involved in maintaining VZV latency remain incompletely understood. Nondetectable or very low detectable CD4+ VZV responses can correlate with a potentially increased risk of older adults for zoster infection.

Vaccine

Live Attenuated Herpes Zoster Vaccine

The first-generation vaccine to develop is the live attenuated herpes zoster vaccine (ZVL).

Mechanism and Efficacy

Based on a large placebo-controlled efficacy trial enrolling over 38,000 adults aged 60 years and older, the vaccine reduced the incidence of zoster by 51%, but a substantial decrease in efficacy was seen as a function of age: Protection against zoster was estimated at 64% in individuals aged 60–69 years, 41% in those aged 70–79 years, and 18% in individuals over 80 years, demonstrating reduced morbidity from herpes zoster and postherpetic neuralgia among older adults.

Further long-term follow-up indicated a decline in efficacy after 4–8 years of vaccination. Various other studies followed similar data.

Efforts were undertaken to enhance the vaccine's effectiveness by:

- Increasing the concentration of the vaccine virus
- Administering two doses

However, despite being generally safe, these measures did not significantly enhance VZV-specific immunity. Further 10-year follow-up vaccine reported severe adverse effects in severely immunocompromised patients. Thus, another limitation of this vaccine is its contraindication for use in moderate-to-severe immunocompromised patients.

Recombinant Subunit Herpes Zoster Vaccine

The more effective second generation subunit herpes zoster vaccine (RZV)-Shingrix consists of recombinant varicella zoster virus glycoprotein (gE) and the AS01B adjuvant system.

Mechanism

VZV gE is combined with the AS01B adjuvant, which comprises monophosphoryl lipid A (an agonist for TLR4) complexed with a saponin derivative (QS-21) in the liposomal form. AS01B has been shown to induce specific CD4+ T cell and antibody responses in animal models.

Extensive studies were carried out to determine the effectiveness of recombinant zoster vaccine (RZV) in key clinical trials. The efficacy rates were found to be 97% in the ZOE-50 trial and 89% in the ZOE-70 trial. The efficacy against postherpetic neuralgia was observed to be 91.2%. However, RZV was associated with more injection sites and systemic reactions within 7 days of administration compared to most other vaccines. Grade 3 injection site reactions were reported in 8.5–9.5% of vaccine recipients. The risk of complications from herpes zoster is three times higher in individuals infected with HIV. In autologous stem cell transplantation, the efficacy of RZV against herpes zoster is 68 and against postherpetic neuralgia is 90%. In hematologic malignancies, the efficacy is 87%.

Future Directions

Research is ongoing to determine the efficacy and complications in less immunocompromised conditions, such as autoimmune diseases treated with biologics. Suggesting more direct comparisons between RZV and ZVL in different types of models would be a helpful research question.

Recommendations

Age 50 years or older: Two-dose series RZV (Shingrix) 2–6 months apart (minimum interval: 4 weeks; repeat dose if administered too soon), regardless of previous herpes zoster or history of intake of live attenuated herpes zoster vaccine (ZVL, Zostavax) vaccination.

PNEUMOCOCCAL VACCINE

Streptococcus pneumoniae is a gram-positive bacterium commonly carried in the nasopharynx that can extend to cause pneumonia, otitis media, and sinusitis, and on spreading to sterile sites, can lead to meningitis and septic arthritis.

Mechanism

The pneumococcal vaccine works through various mechanisms to combat the infection. One of these mechanisms involves the polysaccharide capsule, which hinders mucosal clearance, has antiphagocytic properties, and inhibits complement and immunoglobulin binding to host receptors. Adults 65 years and older and children aged 2 years are at the greatest risk for the development of invasive pneumococcal disease (IPD). There are over 90 capsular serotypes, each characterized by the molecular structure of its specific polysaccharide.

Vaccine

Pneumococcal Polysaccharide Vaccines

The first pneumococcal vaccine to be developed in 1970 remained unchanged until 1989.

There has been periodic decrement of vaccine serotype pneumonia over the years and studies have been going on to target no remaining pneumonia conjugates, as shown in **Figure 1**.

For decades, vaccination against *S. pneumoniae* utilized the 23-valent polysaccharide vaccine, which contains purified pneumococcal capsular polysaccharides from 23 (of at least 90) strains that are commonly associated with infection in the United States.

The major mechanism for the protection of this vaccine was the production of the polysaccharide vaccine which is generally considered to be a so-called T-independent vaccine, as the pneumococcal polysaccharides stimulate B cells directly, inducing activation and differentiation to antibody-secreting cells.

Pneumococcal Conjugate Vaccine

For this reason, a pneumococcal conjugate was developed where polysaccharides are conjugated to a carrier protein, CRM197—a nontoxic mutant of diphtheria toxin that increased the possibility of improved efficacy.

Initial studies were conducted for the PCV7 and then PCV13 vaccine which resulted in dramatic reductions

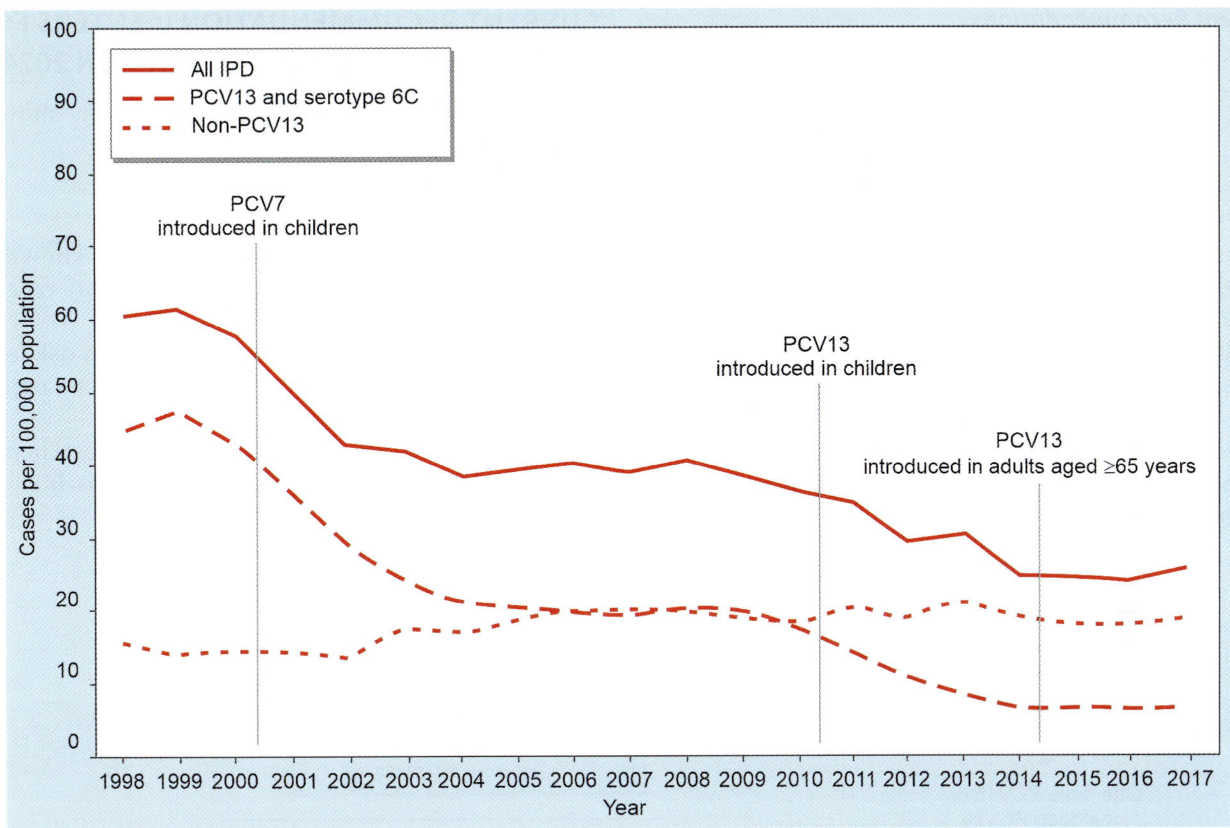

FIG. 1: Invasive pneumococcal disease (IPD) incidence among adults aged ≥ 65 years, by pneumococcal serotype in United States, 1998–2017. [PCV: pneumococcal conjugate vaccine; PCV7: 7-valent PCV (serotypes 4, 6B, 9V, 14, 18C, 19F, and 23F); PCV13: 13 valent PCV (PCV7 serotypes plus 1, 3, 5, 6A, 19A and 7F)]

Source: Matanock A, Lee G, Gierke R, et al. Use of PCV13 and PPSV23 among adults ≥65 years: updated ACIP recommendations. MMWR Morb Mortal Wkly Rep. 2019;68(46):1069-75.

in pneumococcal diseases caused by various vaccine serotype.

Immunogenicity

A systematic meta-analysis comparing the immunogenicity and safety profile found that in adults, a single dose of PCV13 induces a stronger immune response compared to PPV23 while maintaining a safety profile similar to that of PPV23. A large observational study conducted in the United Kingdom revealed that the effectiveness of 23vPPV declines in immunocompromised individuals, with rates ranging from 23 to 41% among immunocompetent individuals aged 65–84 years.

The CAPiTA study specifically evaluated the 13-valent conjugate pneumococcal vaccine in a randomized, placebo-controlled trial of more than 85,000 adults 65 years and older in the Netherlands who had never previously received a pneumococcal vaccine. However, PCV13 was effective with bacteremic, nonbacteremic, and vaccine-type pneumococcal diseases but did not prevent community-acquired pneumonia (CAP) from any cause.

This study did not incorporate data on infants previously vaccinated with PCV13. Reports suggest that vaccine effectiveness varied depending on the presence of comorbidities, showing lower effectiveness in lung disease and higher effectiveness in diabetes mellitus. After the US recommendations in 2014 regarding the PCV13 vaccine, a study was conducted that included individuals aged over 65 years. This study demonstrated a significant reduction in invasive pulmonary disease and vaccine-associated pneumonia compared to the CAPiTA study.

Future Directions

Efforts are underway to explore the coadministration of PCV13 with the first herpes zoster vaccine (ZVL). Initial reports suggested a reduction in the antibody response to ZVL, but more rigorous trials are required before this can be considered for recommendation.

Current Recommendations

The study revealed that direct use of PCV13 in older adults did not result in additional reductions in vaccine-type IPD, and there was limited evidence of reduced non-IPD CAP. Economic analyses conducted in the Netherlands, Australia, and the United Kingdom concluded that, in comparison, 23vPPV but not PCV13 met cost-effectiveness criteria for adults aged over 70 years.

With this presently, the 23-valent polysaccharide vaccine is the primary recommendation for preventing pneumococcal disease in older adults. For adults with compromised immune systems, a vaccination series with the 13-valent conjugate vaccine followed by the polysaccharide vaccine at least 8 weeks later is recommended.

CURRENT RECOMMENDATION (CENTERS FOR DISEASE CONTROL AND PREVENTION 2024)

The current recommendation for vaccine is shown in **Flowchart 1**.

Hepatitis B

- *Adults aged 60 years or older without* known risk factors for hepatitis B virus infection *may* receive a hepatitis B vaccine series.
- *Adults aged 60 years or older with* known risk factors for hepatitis B virus infection *should* receive a hepatitis B vaccine series.
- *Any adult aged 60 years or older* who requests hepatitis B vaccination should receive a hepatitis B vaccine series.

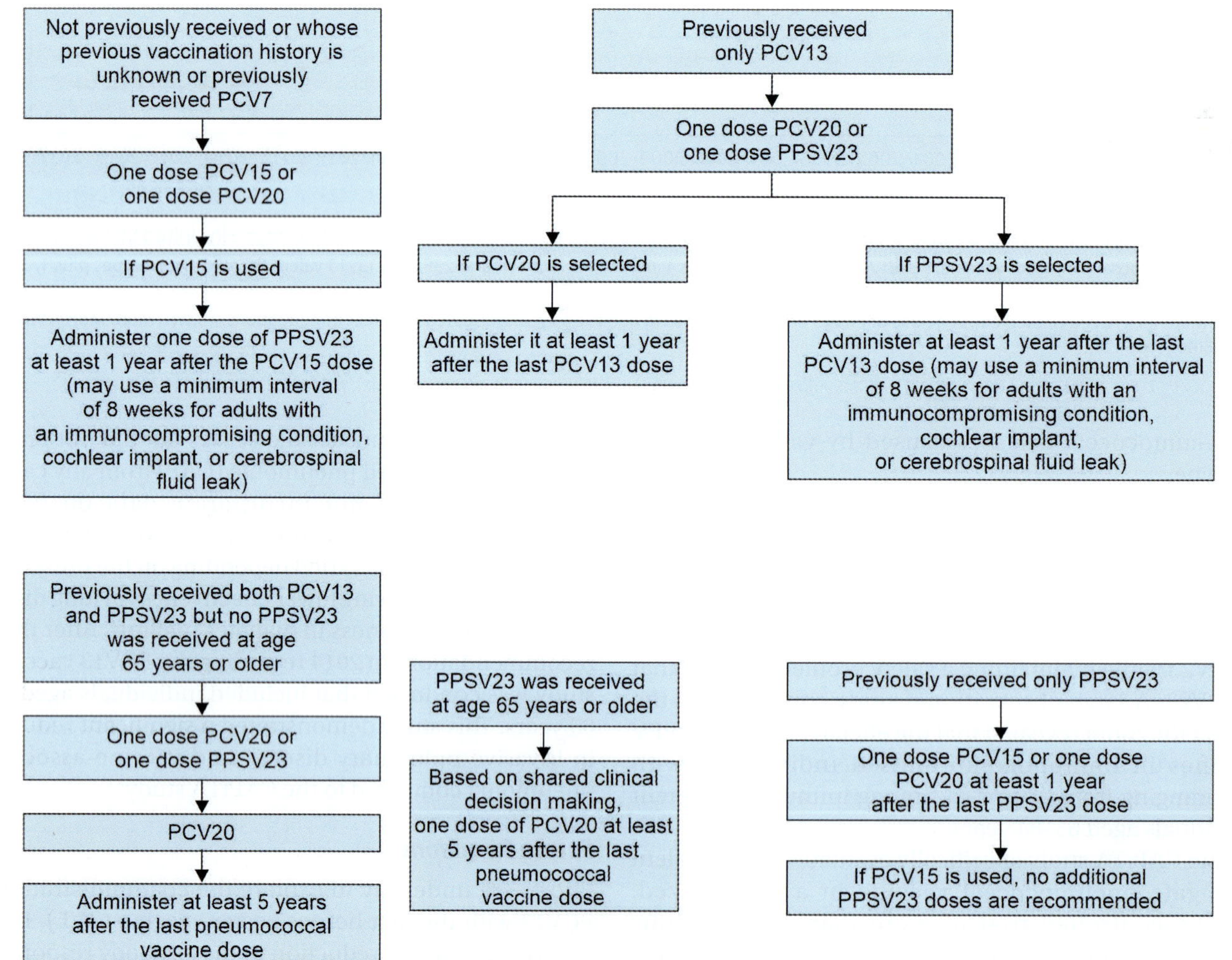

FLOWCHART 1: Current recommendation for pneumococcal vaccine based on CDC 2024.

TABLE 1: Efficacy of vaccines in older people.

Vaccine	Vaccine subtype	Vaccine efficacy	Country and reference
Influenza	Quadrivalent influenza vaccine (QIV)	2018–2019: 44% against H1N1, 9% against H3N2	United States (20)
Varicella	Live attenuated herpes zoster vaccine (ZVL)	Herpes zoster—51.3% Postherpetic neuralgia—66.5%	United States (9)
	Recombinant subunit herpes zoster vaccine (RZV)	ZOE-50 trial (15,411 participants): 97.2% ZOE-70 trial (13,900): 89% 91.2% against postherpetic neuralgia	18 countries (13) 18 countries (21)
Pneumococcal	Pneumococcal polysaccharide vaccines (PPVs)	PPV23: APSG-Japan 40.1% against vaccine-type community-acquired pneumonia (13v serotype)	Japan (22)
	Pneumococcal conjugate vaccine (PCV)	PCV13: CAPiTA: 45.6% against vaccine-type community-acquired pneumonia (13v serotypes) 14.3%: Against death PCV13: Adjusted VE 71.1–73% against vaccine-type community-acquired pneumonia	Netherlands (17) United States (19)

TABLE 2: CDC vaccination recommendation 2024.

Vaccine	Recommendation	Route
Influenza inactivated (IIV4) or influenza recombinant (RIV4)	One dose annually	Intramuscular
Respiratory syncytial virus (RSV)	One dose	Intramuscular
Tetanus, diphtheria, and pertussis (Tdap or Td)	• One dose Td/Tdap for wound management • One dose Tdap, then Td or Tdap booster every 10 years	Intramuscular/subcutaneous
Varicella (VAR)	Two doses 4–8 weeks apart	Intramuscular/subcutaneous
Recombinant zoster vaccine (RZV)	Two doses 2–6 months apart	Intramuscular
Pneumococcal (PCV, PCV20, and PPSV23)	*If not previously vaccinated*: • One dose of PCV15 or one dose of PCV20 • If PCV15 is used, administer one dose PPSV23 at least 1 year after PCV15 dose (in special situations—8 weeks)	• *PPSV23*: Subcutaneous • *PCV vaccine*: Intramuscular
Hepatitis A (HepA)	Two, three, or four doses depending on the vaccine	Intramuscular
Hepatitis B (HepB)	Two, three, or four doses depending on the vaccine	Intramuscular
Meningococcal A, C, W, Y	One or two doses depending on the indication	Intramuscular
Meningococcal B (men B)	Two or three doses depending on vaccine and indication	Intramuscular
Haemophilus influenzae type b (Hib)	One or three doses depending on the indication	Intramuscular
Mpox		Intramuscular
COVID-19	One or more doses of the updated vaccine	Intramuscular

(CDC: centers for disease control and prevention)

Efficacy of vaccines in older people is summarized in **Table 1** and recommendations are summarized in **Table 2** (CDC, 2024).

CONCLUSION

Vaccination in the elderly is an evidence-based, cost-effective strategy to prevent infections, reduce complications, and maintain quality of life, particularly in regions with a high disease burden such as low- and middle-income countries. Given the challenges of immunosenescence, tailored vaccination schedules, improved vaccine formulations, and proactive healthcare delivery are essential components of geriatric preventive medicine. Greater coverage of vaccine-preventable diseases not only reduces the overall disease burden but also contributes to sustaining longevity, similar to other preventive strategies in older populations.

Take Home Messages

- A major improvement has been made in vaccines for older people in many forms.
- RZV sets the standard for effective vaccines in older individuals by significantly lowering the risk of herpes zoster and postherpetic neuralgia in adults. ZVL remains useful in places where RZV is not available.
- Both conjugate and polysaccharide pneumococcal vaccines show comparable efficacy against pneumococcal disease and pneumococcal pneumonia caused by vaccine serotypes in older adults.
- More good vaccines need to be introduced which could be safely used in immunocompromised patients.
- The emergence of SARS-CoV-2 has hastened the development of new vaccine platforms, which is expected to lead to the creation of vaccines targeting other pathogens in the future.
- As immunization methods continue to advance, there is a growing need for combined vaccines that can reduce the burden of multiple injections.

Self-Assessment Questionnaire

Q1. What is immunosenescence, and how does it affect vaccine efficacy in older adults?

Q2. Distinguish between antigenic drift and antigenic shift in influenza viruses, and explain their relevance to annual vaccination.

Q3. Why is the recombinant herpes zoster vaccine (RZV, Shingrix) preferred over the live attenuated vaccine (ZVL, Zostavax) in elderly populations?

Q4. Compare the mechanisms of protection and immune responses generated by pneumococcal polysaccharide (PPV23) and pneumococcal conjugate (PCV13) vaccines.

Q5. According to CDC 2024 guidelines, what is the recommended vaccination sequence for older adults receiving both PCV15 and PPSV23?

Q6. What are the potential limitations of using live attenuated vaccines in older or immunocompromised individuals?

FURTHER READINGS

1. Halter JB, Ouslander JG, Studenski S. Hazzard's Geriatric Medicine and Gerontology, 8th edition. New York: McGraw Hill; 2022. 1790 p.
2. Osterholm MT, Kelley NS, Sommer A, Belongia EA. Efficacy and effectiveness of influenza vaccines: a systematic review and meta-analysis. Lancet Infect Dis. 2012;12(1):36-44.
3. Chit A, Roiz J, Briquet B, Greenberg DP. Expected cost effectiveness of high-dose trivalent influenza vaccine in US seniors. Vaccine. 2015;33(5):734-41.
4. DiazGranados CA, Dunning AJ, Jordanov E, Landolfi V, Denis M, Talbot HK. High-dose trivalent influenza vaccine compared to standard dose vaccine in elderly adults: safety, immunogenicity and relative efficacy during the 2009–2010 season. Vaccine. 2013;31(6):861-6.
5. Ng TWY, Cowling BJ, Gao HZ, Thompson MG. Comparative immunogenicity of enhanced seasonal influenza vaccines in older adults: a systematic review and meta-analysis. J Infect Dis. 2019;219:1525-35.
6. Cowling BJ, Thompson MG, Ng TWY, Fang VJ, Perera RAPM, Leung NHL, et al. Comparative reactogenicity of enhanced influenza vaccines in older adults. J Infect Dis. 2020;222(8):1383-91.
7. Camilloni B, Basileo M, Valente S, Nunzi E, Iorio AM. Immunogenicity of intramuscular MF59-adjuvanted and intradermal administered influenza enhanced vaccines in subjects aged over 60: a literature review. Hum Vaccin Immunother. 2015;11(3):553-63.
8. Murthy N, Wodi AP, McNally VV, Daley MF, Cineas S. Advisory Committee on Immunization Practices. Recommended adult immunization schedule, United States, 2024. Ann Intern Med. 2024;177(2):221-37.
9. Oxman MN, Levin MJ, Johnson GR, Schmader KE, Straus SE, Gelb LD, et al. A vaccine to prevent herpes zoster and postherpetic neuralgia in older adults. N Engl J Med. 2005;352(22):2271-84.
10. Morrison VA, Johnson GR, Schmader KE, Levin MJ, Zhang JH, Looney DJ, et al. Long-term persistence of zoster vaccine efficacy. Clin Infect Dis. 2015;60(6):900-9.
11. Vermeulen JN, Lange JMA, Tyring SK, Peters PH, Nunez M, Poland G, et al. Safety, tolerability, and immunogenicity after 1 and 2 doses of zoster vaccine in healthy adults ≥60 years of age. Vaccine. 2012;30(5):904-10.
12. Willis ED, Woodward M, Brown E, Popmihajlov Z, Saddier P, Annunziato PW, et al. Herpes zoster vaccine live: A 10 year review of post-marketing safety experience. Vaccine. 2017;35(52):7231-9.
13. Lal H, Cunningham AL, Godeaux O, Chlibek R, Diez-Domingo J, Hwang SJ, et al. Efficacy of an adjuvanted herpes zoster subunit vaccine in older adults. N Engl J Med. 2015;372(22):2087-96.
14. Van Der Poll T, Opal SM. Pathogenesis, treatment, and prevention of pneumococcal pneumonia. Lancet. 2009;374(9700):1543-56.
15. Vadlamudi NK, Parhar K, Malana KLA, Kang A, Marra F. Immunogenicity and safety of the 13-valent pneumococcal conjugate vaccine compared to 23-valent pneumococcal polysaccharide in immunocompetent adults: a systematic review and meta-analysis. Vaccine. 2019;37(8):1021-9.

16. Djennad A, Ramsay ME, Pebody R, Fry NK, Sheppard C, Ladhani SN, et al. Effectiveness of 23-valent polysaccharide pneumococcal vaccine and changes in invasive pneumococcal disease incidence from 2000 to 2017 in those aged 65 and over in England and Wales. EClinicalMedicine. 2018;6:42-50.
17. Bonten MJM, Huijts SM, Bolkenbaas M, Webber C, Patterson S, Gault S, et al. Polysaccharide conjugate vaccine against pneumococcal pneumonia in adults. N Engl J Med. 2015;372(12): 1114-25.
18. Huijts SM, Van Werkhoven CH, Bolkenbaas M, Grobbee DE, Bonten MJM. Post-hoc analysis of a randomized controlled trial: diabetes mellitus modifies the efficacy of the 13-valent pneumococcal conjugate vaccine in elderly. Vaccine. 2017;35(34):4444-9.
19. McLaughlin JM, Jiang Q, Isturiz RE, Sings HL, Swerdlow DL, Gessner BD, et al. Effectiveness of 13-valent pneumococcal conjugate vaccine against hospitalization for community-acquired pneumonia in older US adults: a test-negative design. Clin Infect Dis. 2018;67(10):1498-506.
20. Flannery B, Kondor RJG, Chung JR, Gaglani M, Reis M, Zimmerman RK, et al. Spread of antigenically drifted influenza A(H3N2) viruses and vaccine effectiveness in the United States during the 2018-2019 season. J Infect Dis. 2020;221(1):8-15.
21. Cunningham AL, Lal H, Kovac M, Chlibek R, Hwang SJ, Díez-Domingo J, et al. Efficacy of the herpes zoster subunit vaccine in adults 70 years of age or older. N Engl J Med. 2016;375(11):1019-32.
22. Suzuki M, Dhoubhadel BG, Ishifuji T, Yasunami M, Yaegashi M, Asoh N, et al. Serotype-specific effectiveness of 23-valent pneumococcal polysaccharide vaccine against pneumococcal pneumonia in adults aged 65 years or older: a multicentre, prospective, test-negative design study. Lancet Infect Dis. 2017;17(3):313-21.

CHAPTER 39

Perioperative Assessment

Gevesh Chand Dewangan

CASE VIGNETTES

Case Vignette 1

An 83-year-old woman presented to the preoperative assessment clinic (PAC) prior to an elective total knee replacement. She had a medical history of hypertension, coronary artery disease, with a previous bypass grafting, and atrial fibrillation on chronic anticoagulation. She denied any cardiac symptoms except for mild shortness of breath on exertion. The patient was taking metoprolol, telmisartan, aspirin, rosuvastatin, and apixaban. Her blood pressure was 149/82 mm Hg, heart rate was 71 beats/min, and oxygen saturation was 99% on room air. Her heartbeat was irregularly irregular without murmurs. Her lung sounds were clear. There was no pitting edema. Per the Revised Cardiac Risk Index (RCRI) for preoperative risk, the patient had one risk factor (coronary artery disease) with an expected risk of having a major postsurgical adverse cardiac event of 0.9–1.3%. She underwent total knee replacement with continuation of metoprolol for heart rate control. Perioperatively, she was also bridged with low molecular weight heparin and unfractionated heparin. Her postoperative course was uneventful, and she was discharged on postoperative day (POD) 2 to home with home health services. She returned to the orthopedic clinic 1 month later for surgical follow-up and was found to be doing well without any overt complications.

Case Vignette 2

A 75-year-old man presented to the PAC before his scheduled total knee replacement for severe osteoarthritis. His medical history included hypertension, diabetes, depression, gastroesophageal reflux disease, and irritable bowel syndrome. He was taking telmisartan, amlodipine, metformin, dapagliflozin, sertraline, mirtazapine, atorvastatin, pantoprazole, calcium, and vitamin supplements. He denied any cardiovascular (CV) symptoms. His depression was well-controlled on antidepressant medications and although he has received assistance from a social worker, he was independent in all his activities and instrumental activities of daily living (ADLs and IADLs). In the PAC, his blood pressure was 131/71 mm Hg, heart rate was 78 beats/min, and oxygen saturation was 99% on room air. His heartbeat was regular without murmurs. His lung sounds were clear. There was no pitting edema. Per the RCRI, the patient had no major CV risk factors, and the expected risk of having a major adverse postoperative cardiac event was 0.4–0.5%. He underwent a total knee replacement. His immediate postoperative course was uncomplicated, and he was discharged, accompanied by his daughter, to his home on POD 3, without home health services. Unfortunately, on POD 30, he was admitted to the hospital after sustaining a fall in his apartment and was found to be in delirium. He was found to have a urinary tract infection causing delirium and urinary incontinence. He was managed conservatively with antibiotics and was discharged to a skilled nursing facility.

INTRODUCTION

The aging population is one of the greatest social and medical challenges of the modern world. India is a country that has just entered an era of demographic transition, where the population of older people is on a rapid rise. This increase in the geriatric population has also coincided with the improvement of our knowledge and infrastructure in this ever-evolving field of medicine. This has led to increased longevity and an increased number of surgical patients in the geriatric age group. However, the aging population brings with it the increased burden of various diseases and syndromes, and older patients, especially those with various geriatric syndromes, pose unique challenges in the perioperative settings, making them tricky surgical patients. The older patients often experience a decline in physiological reserve, making them more susceptible to the stress of surgery and anesthesia. Furthermore, age-related changes in pharmacokinetics and pharmacodynamics require careful consideration in the management of medications.

Perioperative care for the geriatric population necessitates a comprehensive, multidisciplinary approach that goes beyond the standard preoperative, intraoperative, and postoperative protocols which have been the cornerstone for perioperative management in the years gone by. The geriatric population often faces a higher risk of medical complications such as postoperative delirium, cognitive dysfunction, functional decline, and social complications such as prolonged hospital stays, increased healthcare costs, and diminished quality of life.

This chapter provides an in-depth exploration of the key aspects of perioperative care in the geriatric population, including preoperative assessment, intraoperative management, postoperative care, and discharge planning. The aim is to equip healthcare providers with the knowledge and tools to optimize surgical outcomes and improve the quality of life for elderly patients.

This chapter delves into the intricacies of perioperative care for the geriatric population with the aim of providing the knowledge and tools to optimize surgical outcomes and improve the well-being and quality of life of older patients.

CHALLENGES IN PERIOPERATIVE CARE OF OLDER PEOPLE

Perioperative care of older adults presents a myriad of challenges due to the intricate interplay of inherent medical and social factors. Several factors can complicate postoperative outcomes and their management in older patients, including multimorbidity, polypharmacy, poor functional status, and frailty among others. Older patients are particularly vulnerable to adverse outcomes, necessitating careful attention and a specialized multidisciplinary approach to ensure safe and effective care and optimization of medical conditions.

Decreased Physiological Reserve

Aging is associated with a decline in organ function and physiological reserve, which reduces the body's ability to cope with the stress of surgery and anesthesia. This diminished reserve can lead to increased susceptibility to complications such as hypotension, hypoxia, and fluid imbalances during and after surgery.

Multimorbidity and Polypharmacy

Older adults typically have multiple chronic medical conditions such as hypertension, diabetes, cardiovascular disease, etc. These comorbidities can complicate surgical procedures and increase the risk of intraoperative and postoperative complications. The management of multiple chronic diseases often involves the use of multiple medications, leading to polypharmacy which further increases the risk of drug interactions and adverse drug reactions, complicating anesthesia and postoperative care. Effective perioperative management requires a comprehensive understanding of each condition and its potential impact on surgical outcomes, careful medication reconciliation, and their adjustments to minimize the risks.

Other Geriatric Syndromes

Geriatric syndromes such as dementia and delirium are common in older adults. These conditions pose significant challenges for perioperative care, affecting informed consent, postoperative recovery, and adherence to treatment plans. Delirium, in particular, is a frequent postoperative complication that can prolong hospital stays and impair recovery. Frailty is another geriatric syndrome that increases vulnerability to adverse outcomes. Frail older adults are at higher risk for postoperative complications, prolonged recovery times, and increased mortality. Preoperative assessment of frailty can help tailor perioperative care plans to mitigate these risks.

Nutritional Status

Malnutrition is prevalent among older adults and can adversely affect wound healing, immune function, and overall recovery. Preoperative nutritional assessment and intervention are essential to optimize surgical outcomes and support postoperative recovery.

Social Factors

Social determinants of health, such as social isolation, lack of support systems, and economic constraints, can impact the ability of older adults to access care, adhere to postoperative instructions, and engage in rehabilitation. Addressing these factors through comprehensive discharge planning and community support services is crucial for successful recovery.

Risk of Postoperative Complications

Older adults are at higher risk for a range of postoperative complications, including infections, venous thromboembolism, and cardiac events. Vigilant monitoring, prophylactic measures, and early intervention are necessary to manage these risks effectively.

Functional Decline

Surgery and anesthesia can lead to temporary or permanent declines in functional status, impacting mobility and independence. Rehabilitation and physical therapy are vital components of perioperative care to restore function and improve quality of life.

Pain Management

Pain management in older adults can be challenging due to altered pain perception, increased sensitivity to opioids, and the risk of side effects such as sedation and respiratory depression. A balanced approach using multimodal analgesia and careful dosing is essential.

Communication Barriers

Hearing loss, visual impairment, and cognitive decline can hinder effective communication between older patients and healthcare providers. Clear communication and the use of aids such as hearing devices and written instructions are important to ensure understanding and adherence to care plans.

Ethical and Legal Issues

Ensuring informed consent and respecting patient autonomy can be complex in the presence of cognitive impairment or decision-making capacity issues. Engaging family members and caregivers in the decision-making process is often necessary.

SURGICAL STRESS RESPONSE AND SURGICAL RISK IN OLDER PEOPLE

In any individual, surgery can have transformative effects that extend beyond the outcomes intended for surgery. In particular, older patients are prone to physical and psychological stress post surgery. It can lead to an imbalance in various physiological systems, including but not limited to cardiovascular, neurological, endocrine, autonomic, and immune functions. Older adults face additional clinical challenges in their postsurgical recovery depending on their preoperative physiologic reserve and comorbid conditions due to age-related changes that can lower the homeostatic threshold, thus increasing their risk of postoperative adverse events and complicating their return to independence after surgery.

The autonomic nervous system, particularly the sympathetic nervous system (SNS), is of paramount importance in stress-like situations, including surgery. The SNS acts by increasing the release of epinephrine from the adrenal medulla and the release of norepinephrine (NE) from presynaptic nerve endings. Norepinephrine further modifies the functions of various organs such as the adrenal cortex, kidneys, pancreas, and liver. The SNS directly acts on myocardium and vasculature resulting in increased blood pressure and heart rate. These cardiovascular changes lead to an increase in myocardial oxygen demand resulting in ischemia in susceptible patients. In patients with preexisting atherosclerotic disease, direct activation of cardiac sympathetic nerves may also trigger coronary vasoconstriction. Furthermore, a hypercoagulable state due to circulating catecholamines may increase the ischemic burden in patients with preexisting coronary artery disease. All these changes along with decreased vascular and left ventricular compliance may impair the maintenance of CV homeostasis during acute surgical illness in older patients.

In addition, increases in anterior and posterior pituitary hormones, aldosterone, cortisol, and glucagon secretion also contribute to the surgical stress response. The hypothalamic–pituitary–adrenal (HPA) axis stimulates the secretion of the growth hormone which stimulates protein synthesis and inhibits protein breakdown, promotes lipolysis, stimulates glycogenolysis in the liver, and has an anti-insulin effect. The HPA axis also stimulates adrenocorticotrophic hormone (ACTH) which results in cortisol secretion from the adrenal cortex promoting protein breakdown and lipolysis, thus increasing the production of gluconeogenic precursors. In contrast, insulin concentrations may fall during surgery, in part due to adrenergic inhibition of pancreatic beta-cell secretion.

Surgical trauma to tissues also contributes to profound inflammatory response near the surgical site resulting in increased release of cellular mediators and cytokines (IL-1, IL-6, TNF-α) leading to systemic changes referred to as the acute-phase response, including fever, granulocytosis, and the production of acute-phase liver proteins such as C-reactive protein (CRP), fibrinogen, and α2-macroglobulin. The release of cellular mediators, cytokines, and acute-phase reactants can activate the HPA axis, thus releasing catecholamines and cortisol. Altogether, these changes cause an imbalance in the Th1/Th2 ratio and postsurgical immunosuppression.

Many of the age-related changes in metabolic responses to surgical illness can also be attributed to significant age- and disease-related reductions in skeletal muscle mass (sarcopenia). The loss of strength that accompanies immobility, starvation, and acute surgical illness may decrease the capacity of the older patient to make a functional recovery. Also, the risk of muscle strength becoming inadequate for respiratory and other vital muscle functions is high in older patients.

Increasing age also results in renal changes such as a decrease in the number of nephrons and decreased sodium and water excretion. It also results in hepatic changes such as decreased blood flow to the liver and microsomal oxidation. These alterations in renal and hepatic metabolism lead to a greater risk of perioperative drug toxicities in older patients. Previously unrecognized cognitive impairment puts older patients at an increased risk of developing acute confusional episodes (delirium), resulting in prolongation of hospital stay and worsening clinical outcomes. A communication gap may remain due to the inability of older patients to adequately communicate concerns or provide clinical history to a healthcare provider. Therefore, it is imperative to ensure the best possible outcomes for older surgical patients by maximizing the communication and data exchange between the surgical team, geriatricians, and other healthcare providers.

The task of geriatricians and clinicians providing services to older adults is to identify underlying hidden illnesses such as geriatric syndromes including frailty, cognitive impairment, risk of falls, and malnutrition in older patients and assess their impact on perioperative risk since normal aging does not account for the bulk of operative risks.

PREOPERATIVE ASSESSMENT

As with any surgical patient, older patients also need to undergo an assessment of current health status and optimization of clinical comorbidities that can impact postoperative outcomes. The preoperative evaluation starts with a basic history and physical examination proceeding to relevant systemic and geriatric evaluation. After an initial assessment, patients might be required to undergo relevant specific investigations based on the findings for the optimization of comorbidities and medications.

History and Physical Examination

Comprehensive history taking, physical examination, and medication review remain the most basic tools to begin with a preoperative assessment in an older patient. It enables geriatricians and clinicians to ascertain and list clinical comorbidities and also helps in identifying diseases with atypical presentations which are common in older patients. Particularly in patients with cognitive impairment, it becomes important to corroborate histories with the patient relatives and caregivers.

A detailed history can also help in identifying the level of social (family and friends) support, cognitive function, and functional status, and along with a physical examination can guide optimal preoperative investigations. It can also guide preoperative evaluation by members of multidisciplinary teams, such as social workers and physical therapists, particularly in those with poor physical function, cognitive impairment, or lack of social support **(Box 1)**.

BOX 1 Points to remember for a geriatric-specific preoperative evaluation.

- Assess current comorbid status
- Screen for substance abuse and alcohol use/dependence
- Take detailed medication review, including over-the-counter drugs and herbal medications
- Assess functional status, including preoperative ADLs and IADLs
- Assess for use of devices such as hearing aids and mobility aids
- Assess for family and social support system
- Assess for frailty and fall risk
- Assess for cognition and nutritional status
- Assess for decision-making capacity
- Determine postoperative risk of cardiac and other system complications using risk assessment tools

(ADLs: activities of daily living; IADLs: instrumental activities of daily living)

Comprehensive Geriatric Assessment

Geriatric syndromes such as frailty, cognitive impairment, and falls are major predictors of mortality and morbidity in older patients. Comprehensive geriatric assessment (CGA) helps in identifying these hidden risk factors or vulnerabilities which can help improve postoperative outcomes. It is a multidimensional, holistic approach involving a multidisciplinary team that evaluates the medical, psychological, and functional status of the patient and delivers an optimal preoperative assessment. CGA can be executed in outpatient clinics or inpatient settings. It can also take place in community settings if required. CGA helps patients, families, caregivers, and treating physicians to engage in discussions about risk management and facilitate shared decision-making. CGA has been found to have demonstrable benefits in improving postoperative outcomes in major surgeries, particularly orthopedic surgeries such as hip fracture surgery and vascular surgery.

- *Functional assessment*: Functional independence remains crucial in living a higher quality of life. Evaluating the patient's functional status is crucial in predicting postoperative recovery and planning rehabilitation. Tools such as the Katz index and Lawton scale can be used to assess the activities of daily living (ADLs) and instrumental activities of daily living (IADLs), respectively. These tools help determine the patient's ability to perform self-care tasks and manage their environment. Assessment of mobility, balance, and frailty is also important as well as determining fall risk. Tools such as the timed up and go test remain a simple and effective screening tool for assessing mobility and balance. Clinical Frailty Scale helps adequately in identifying frailty, and fall risk can be assessed using two-question fall-risk screening: (1) Have you fallen twice or more in the past year or sought medical attention for a fall? (2) If you have not fallen, do you feel unsteady walking?

- *Cognitive assessment*: The presence of dementia, delirium, and/or depression has been shown to increase the risk of postoperative complications and mortality. Screening tools such as the Mini-Mental State Examination (MMSE), the Montreal Cognitive Assessment (MoCA), and Mini-Cog among others can be used to assess for cognitive impairment. The confusion assessment method is useful in identifying patients with delirium in the perioperative period. Screening tools such as Patient Health Questionnaire-2 (PHQ-2) and Geriatric Depression Scale (GDS) can be used to screen for depression preoperatively.
- *Nutritional assessment*: Malnutrition is a significant concern in the elderly and can adversely affect surgical outcomes. The Mini Nutritional Assessment (MNA) and serum albumin levels are useful tools for evaluating nutritional status.

Medication Management

The medication review allows screening for polypharmacy and optimization of medications preoperatively. A complete medication review is essential to prevent perioperative adverse events associated with medications. Since metabolism and elimination of medications and their metabolites may be altered during the perioperative period and there are risks of drug-drug interaction with anesthesia medications, some of the commonly used drugs for various comorbidities need to be carefully managed in the perioperative period.

- *Antiplatelet drugs*: Aspirin, clopidogrel, and other antiplatelets are typically held for a recommended 5–7 days. Aspirin can be safely continued for skin procedures and minor dental surgeries.
- *Anticoagulants*: Warfarin should be stopped at least 5 days before surgery. In patients at a high risk of thromboembolic events (such as recent thromboembolic stroke, mechanical mitral heart valve, and atrial fibrillation with CHA_2DS_2-VASc score of 7 or 8), a bridging therapy with low molecular weight heparins (LMWHs) can be considered in the perioperative period. Direct oral anticoagulants (DOACs) should be discontinued 24–48 hours before surgery and can be restarted 24–48 hours after surgery depending on the bleeding risk (low/moderate or high bleeding risk surgery). Warfarin can be restarted anytime after the surgery, as it may take up to 4 days for international normalized ratio (INR) to reach a therapeutic level after starting warfarin.
- *Cardiovascular and antihypertensive medications*: Most of these medications should be continued on the morning of surgery. If patients on oral beta-blockers are unable to resume oral intake postoperatively, they can be switched to intravenous (IV) metoprolol. As there is a known risk of hypotension upon anesthesia induction, angiotensin-converting enzyme (ACE) inhibitors and angiotensin II receptor blockers (ARBs) are commonly held on the morning of surgery for most patients. However, they can be continued for heart failure or poorly controlled hypertension to avoid the risk of exacerbation of these conditions. Alpha 2 agonists (such as clonidine) should be continued in the perioperative period but not initiated. Transdermal clonidine patches can be used postoperatively if patients are unable to take oral medication.
- *Oral hypoglycemics and insulin*: Most oral hypoglycemics are generally held the night before surgery, to reduce the risk of perioperative hypoglycemia. Sodium-glucose cotransporter 2 (SGLT2) inhibitors (dapagliflozin, etc.) should be stopped 3–4 days before surgery due to the postoperative risk of euglycemic diabetic ketoacidosis. Patients on once-weekly glucagon-like peptide-1 (GLP-1) receptor agonists should discontinue the medication 1 week before the surgery. Patients requiring insulin should receive 50–80% of their usual basal insulin dose on the morning of surgery. Rapid-acting or mealtime insulin is held on the day of surgery as patients remain fasting for surgery.
- *Diuretics*: If not needed to treat excessive volume or symptoms of pulmonary congestion, especially in patients with heart failure, diuretics should be stopped for 24 hours before surgery.
- Oral nonsteroidal anti-inflammatory drugs (NSAIDs) should generally be discontinued at least 3 days before surgery. Ibuprofen can be stopped 24 hours before surgery.
- Medications for seizure disorders, Parkinson's disease, and agents for myasthenia gravis should be continued throughout the perioperative period to minimize the risk of worsening neurologic symptoms.
- Drugs with anticholinergic properties, such as diphenhydramine or meclizine, can increase the

risk of perioperative delirium and should be held or discontinued.

- Psychotropic medications, including tricyclic antidepressants, selective serotonin reuptake inhibitors (SSRIs), serotonin-norepinephrine reuptake inhibitors (SNRIs), and lithium, should be continued. Benzodiazepines and buspirone used chronically for anxiety should generally be continued. However, when possible, these drugs should be tapered to reduce the risk of withdrawal symptoms.

Preoperative Cardiac Evaluation

Cardiac risk evaluation remains at the center of the preoperative surgical evaluation because patients (especially older patients with multiple comorbidities) undergoing noncardiac surgery remain at risk for an adverse cardiovascular event such as myocardial ischemia/infarction, heart failure, arrhythmia, cardiac death, or stroke. The American College of Cardiology (ACA) and the American Heart Association (AHA) have developed a guideline for evaluating cardiac risk before noncardiac surgery. These guidelines formulate a composite risk of perioperative cardiac events based on the preoperative history of cardiovascular events and risk factors. Recommendations have been provided based on the acuity of surgical procedures and the severity of the disease process. The surgical procedures have been classified into major, intermediate, and minor risk procedures, based on the likelihood of postoperative morbidity and mortality associated with them **(Box 2)**.

BOX 2 Cardiac risk stratification for noncardiac surgical procedures.

Major surgical risk: Reported cardiac risk often >5%
- Aortic and other major vascular surgeries
- Large intra-abdominal procedures

Intermediate surgical risk: Reported cardiac risk generally 1–5%
- Intraperitoneal and intrathoracic surgeries
- Carotid endarterectomy
- Head and neck surgery
- Orthopedic surgery
- Prostate surgery

Low surgical risk: Reported cardiac risk generally <1%
- Endoscopic procedures
- Superficial procedure
- Cataract surgery
- Breast surgery
- Ambulatory surgery

Source: Adapted from Bettelli G. Perioperative Care of the Elderly Patient. Cambridge: Cambridge University Press; 2017.

The aggressiveness of cardiac evaluation is determined by the patient's clinical symptoms and surgical time frame or urgency of surgery. An urgent procedure may offer a few more hours for evaluation, whereas an elective procedure offers the best opportunity for preoperative medical optimization. The clinical history, physical examination, and baseline electrocardiogram (ECG) can help identify potentially serious cardiac problems such as a prior myocardial infarction, heart failure, or arrhythmias. To estimate perioperative risk, the ACC/AHA guidelines offer two objective cardiac risk stratification tools:

1. *The Revised Cardiac Risk Index (RCRI) score*: It includes six independent risk factors to calculate a patient's risk of major adverse cardiovascular events (MACE):
   i. Ischemic heart disease
   ii. Heart failure
   iii. Insulin-treated diabetes
   iv. Chronic kidney disease with serum creatinine >2 mg/dL
   v. Stroke/transient ischemic attack (TIA)
   vi. High-risk surgery (defined as intrathoracic, intra-abdominal, or suprainguinal vascular surgery) **(Table 1)**
2. *National Surgical Quality Improvement Program (NSQIP) Calculator*: This is a much more comprehensive tool predicting the risk of cardiac as well as other complications. It has been developed using data from the American College of Surgeons NSQIP database and uses adjusted odds ratios for various risk factors and different surgical sites, thus providing a more detailed procedure-specific risk assessment.

The ACC/AHA guidelines provide a simple flowchart to understand surgical risk and provide management guidance in a stepwise process **(Flowchart 1)**.

Preoperative Pulmonary Evaluation

Older patients are twice as likely to develop pulmonary complications compared with younger patients after controlling for comorbidities which can prolong the

TABLE 1: Revised Cardiac Risk Index.

Number of risk factors	MACE (%)
0	0.4–0.5
1	0.9–1.3
2	4–7
≥3	9–11

Note: Based on this widely used tool, patients with 0 or 1 risk factor would have a low risk of MACE (<1%), whereas those with 2 or more risk factors would be at elevated MACE risk (>1%).

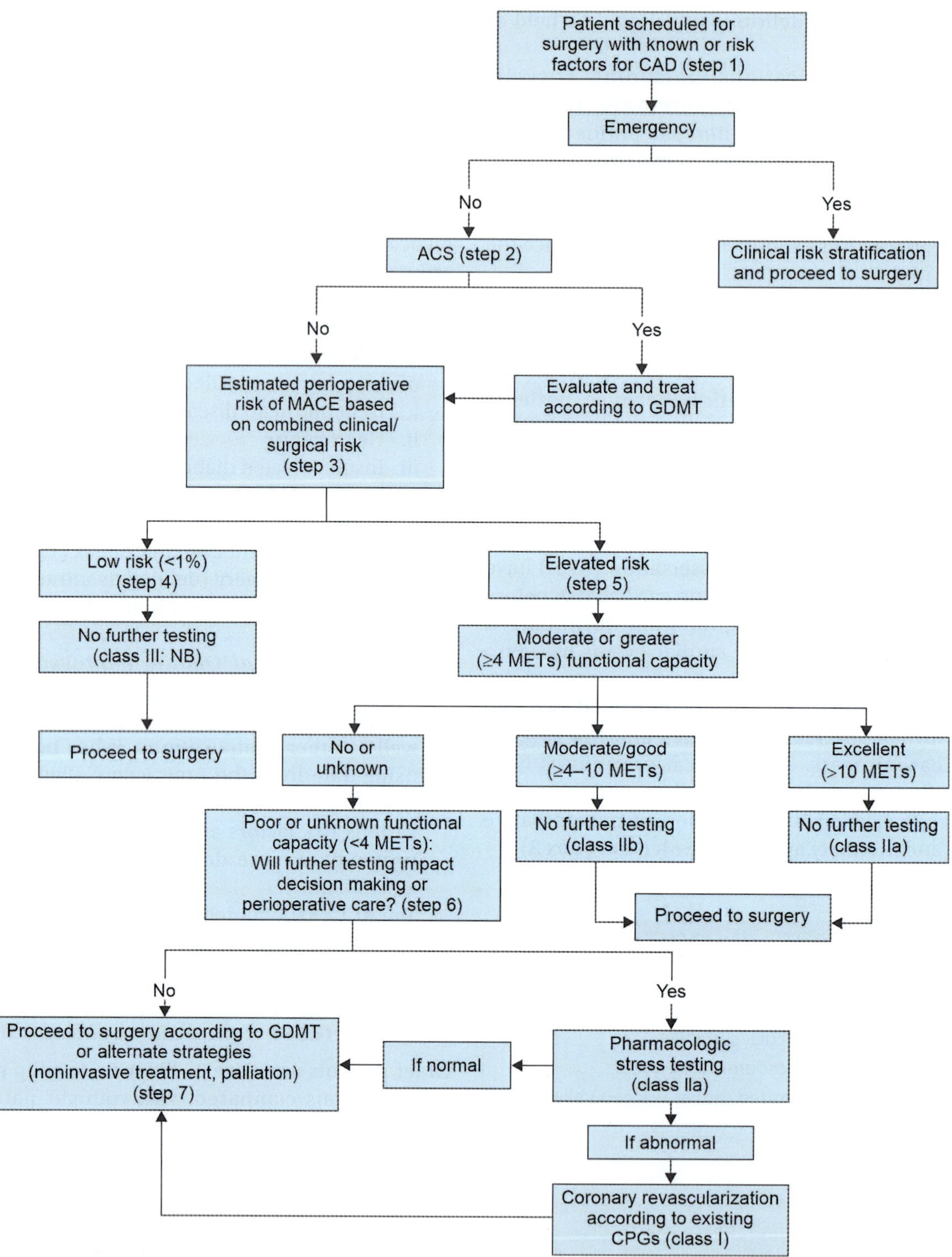

FLOWCHART 1: Preoperative cardiac assessment for patients undergoing noncardiac surgery.

(ACS: acute coronary syndrome; CAD: coronary artery disease; CPG: clinical practice guideline; GDMT: guideline-directed medical therapy; MACE: major adverse cardiac event; MET: metabolic equivalent)

Source: Reproduced from Fleisher LA, Fleischmann KE, Auerbach AD, Barnason SA, Bozkurt B, Davila-Roman VG, et al. 2014 ACC/AHA guideline on perioperative cardiovascular evaluation and management of patients undergoing noncardiac surgery: executive summary. J Am Coll Cardiol. 2014;64(22):2373-405.

hospital stay and contribute to the functional decline and increased morbidity and mortality. Risk factors for pulmonary complications apart from older age include underlying lung diseases such as chronic obstructive pulmonary disease (COPD), functional dependence, tobacco use, altered mental status, weight loss, hypoalbuminemia, and surgical factors such as prolonged or emergency surgery, general anesthesia, and neuromuscular blockage.

A baseline pulmonary function can be determined with a detailed history, examination of the respiratory system and functional capacity, and a 6-minute walk test. Additional investigations such as arterial blood gas, chest X-rays, or pulmonary function tests are not routinely recommended in preoperative evaluation unless indicated for a specific respiratory condition (e.g., COPD) to determine baseline pulmonary function.

Patients should be encouraged regarding smoking cessation long before planned elective procedures and advised to start preoperative breathing exercises. Other evidence-based interventions that reduce postoperative pulmonary complications include incentive spirometry and early ambulation; however, both may be more challenging to implement in older patients.

POSTOPERATIVE EVALUATION AND MANAGEMENT

Older patients in particular are prone to developing various postoperative complications such as delirium, infections, pressure ulcers, and functional decline. Strategies need to be put in place to prevent such complications or to ensure their early identification and adequate management.

Postoperative Delirium

Postoperative delirium is perhaps the most common and significant complication after surgery in older adults with an incidence of 15–25% after major elective surgery and 50% after high-risk surgeries such as cardiac surgery and hip fracture surgery. It is characterized by an acute confusional state and is associated with poor short-term and long-term outcomes. It compromises postoperative care and is one of the most important factors for increased length of stay at the hospital postsurgery. Surgery acts as a precipitating factor, especially in those patients who are already predisposed to developing delirium **(Box 3)**.

The diagnosis of delirium is based on Diagnostic and Statistical Manual of Mental Disorders, Fifth Edition (DSM-5) criteria, and it can be adequately identified using tools such as the Confusion Assessment Method (CAM) in clinical settings. The evaluation of postoperative delirium is similar to delirium in any hospitalized patient, including clinical history, physical and systemic examinations, identification of predisposing and other precipitating factors (such as infection, anemia, and drugs), laboratory tests, and imaging studies. Various strategies can be applied for the prevention and treatment of delirium which take into account both environmental and patient-related factors **(Box 4)**.

BOX 3 Predisposing factors for delirium.

- Advanced age
- Dementia and mild cognitive impairment (MCI)
- History of prior delirium
- Functional disabilities
- Multimorbidity
- Male sex
- Poor vision and hearing
- Depressive symptoms
- Electrolyte imbalance and metabolic abnormalities
- Alcohol abuse

BOX 4 Strategies for the prevention and treatment of postoperative delirium.

Environmental measures:
- Avoidance of physical restraints
- Placement of bedside sitter
- Frequent visitation by family
- Encourage family members to bring in familiar objects from home
- Adequate lighting and avoidance of increased noise

Patient-related measures:
- Reorient patients to time, place, and person (at least three times daily)
- Assess for poor vision and hearing and encourage patients to use eyeglasses and/or hearing aids if needed
- Mobilize patients with assistance and use physical therapy to prevent functional decline
- Implement a nonpharmacologic sleep protocol and sleep hygiene program, and avoid frequent nighttime awakenings (e.g., for measuring vital signs)
- Minimization of patient tethers whenever possible (e.g., Foley catheters, periodic removal of sequential compression devices, ECG cords)
- Identify any acute exacerbations of chronic illness and optimize them
- Identify and treat electrolyte and metabolic derangements, postoperative infections (e.g., catheter-associated), and pressure ulcers
- Adequate pain management and nutrition and fluid repletion
- Use low doses of high-potency antipsychotics (risperidone, olanzapine, haloperidol, and quetiapine) only if needed in agitated patients

Pulmonary Complications

Postoperative pulmonary complications such as hospital-acquired pneumonia, aspiration pneumonia, and atelectasis are more likely to occur in older patients compared to their younger counterparts, increasing the risk of long-term mortality following surgery. Several postoperative strategies can be used to prevent pulmonary complications in the older patient such as:

- Elevation of the head end of the bed, getting out of bed for all meals when possible, and sitting upright while eating and for 1 hour after completing for the prevention of aspiration
- Use of deep breathing exercises, incentive spirometry, and chest physical therapy

Catheter-associated Infections

Urinary tract infections are common due to the use of indwelling catheters for urinary drainage after procedures making it one of the most common postoperative complications. It accounts for 32–40% of all nosocomial infections after surgery. The catheter should be used for a short time and not beyond 48 hours in most cases. If the use of a catheter is projected beyond 48 hours or if there is a risk of urinary retention or bladder distension, then intermittent catheterization should be considered in place of a continued indwelling catheter whenever possible.

The smallest appropriate urine catheter should be used, and the urine drainage bag should be positioned below the bladder and off the floor. Routine catheter irrigation should be avoided, and only closed continuous irrigation should be used if obstruction is anticipated. The use of prophylactic antimicrobials should be discouraged in patients requiring long-term indwelling catheter use.

Functional Decline and Falls

Older patients are at high risk of falls and functional decline in the perioperative period, particularly post surgery due to immobilization and the presence of inherent risk factors such as geriatric syndromes which include incontinence and cognitive impairment. Ongoing assessment of functional status and targeted interventions can help prevent or mitigate functional decline. Regular follow-up with physical and occupational therapists, along with individualized exercise programs, is essential. Strategies that can be applied to prevent functional decline and falls include:

- Early mobilization with or without assistance
- Early use of physical and occupational therapy
- Use of handrails and grab bars
- Keeping patient care areas uncluttered, dry, and nonslippery
- Use large clocks and large calendars
- Use of hospital beds in a low position when the patient is resting and raised to a comfortable height when transferring a patient
- Lock the wheels of the wheelchair when stationary
- Use of nonslip, comfortable, well-fitting footwear
- Use of nightlights or supplemental light using.

Pain Management

Chronic pain can significantly impact the quality of life of older patients. They are inadequately treated for pain because of concerns for adverse events due to potent analgesic medications, making them prone to developing other complications such as delirium. Although the presence of anxiety, fear, cognitive impairment, or depressive symptoms can alter the perception of pain, there is a common misconception that pain sensation is diminished in older age irrespective of other conditions. Adequate pain management should be provided based on the severity of pain calculated using severity scales (e.g., visual analog scale) and anticipated need for pain control rather than as-needed basis. The analgesic medications should be given at frequent intervals with additional doses for breakthrough pain. A multidisciplinary approach involving pain specialists, physical therapists, and psychologists can help manage chronic pain through a combination of medications, physical therapy, and cognitive-behavioral therapy.

Mobilization and Nutrition

Prolonged bed rest after surgery leads to bone and skeletal muscle loss, development of pressure ulcers, atelectasis, aspiration pneumonia, joint contractures, incontinence, and constipation. After surgery, early mobilization from the bed has been shown to decrease the risk of such complications and lead to early recovery and discharge. Patients should be encouraged for early mobilization with or without assistance, and referral to physical therapists should be sought to help with appropriate exercises.

Older patients are at an increased risk of malnutrition due to inherent risk factors such as loss of teeth, comorbidities, and social factors (e.g., isolation) which is further exacerbated by surgery. These patients should have daily evaluations of nutrition and fluid status with a recording of input/output or daily weights post surgery. The use of dentures should be encouraged in patients with a lack of teeth to promote early oral intake if permitted after surgery.

Other Complications

There is also a risk of other complications such as arrhythmia, myocardial infarction, stroke, deep venous thrombosis, and pulmonary embolism in the postoperative period. No active surveillance is recommended for these complications, and they should be managed as identified in the postoperative period due to relevant signs and symptoms. Adequate prophylactic anticoagulation with parenteral anticoagulants (e.g., low molecular weight heparin or unfractionated heparin) may be needed in patients who are immobilized for prolonged periods after surgery and who are at an increased risk of thromboembolic complications due to medical conditions such as atrial fibrillation.

Discharge Planning

Effective discharge planning is crucial for ensuring a smooth transition from the hospital to home or another care setting. It involves comprehensive planning and coordination among the healthcare team, patient, and caregivers and assesses the patient's social and home health support systems before discharge. It has been shown to predict 30-day postoperative morbidity when included in the preoperative assessment of older adults. The American College of Surgeons/American Geriatrics Society guidelines have recommended that a patient's social support systems should be assessed as a critical component of discharge planning.

Comprehensive discharge summary: The discharge summary should include detailed documentation of the surgical procedure, hospital course, medications, follow-up appointments, laboratory, and other diagnostic tests, and any special instructions. It should be communicated to the primary care provider and any involved specialists.

Patient and caregiver education: Education on wound care, medication management, signs of complications, and follow-up appointments is essential. Patients and their caregivers should be educated about all the medications, their dosages, changes in medications post discharge, and expected adverse events. Providing written and verbal instructions, as well as demonstrations, can enhance understanding and adherence.

The rampant advances in medical sciences have undoubtedly increased life expectancy and as a result, adults in the older age group (>65 years) are rising. The life expectancy among women and men is 84 and 79 years, respectively, in the European Union, and the period with comorbidity is approximately 25 and 20 years, respectively. Similarly, in the United States, three out of four older people have multiple comorbidities, and >50% have pain. The provision of good-quality care for the elderly calls for a dedicated interdisciplinary approach to addressing these varied comorbidities.

A geriatrician attends to patients aged > 65 years. However, paying heed to patients of age > 80 years may be quite challenging, as patients are more frail and comorbid and have heavy symptom burdens. The geriatrician's chief goal is to generate a better living standard for the aged by making them more independent and active.

A palliative physician, on the other hand, holistically embraces patients of all age groups and ameliorates their lives by providing not just adequate symptom relief but renders support to their caregivers too. Similarly, palliative physicians are equipped to handle geriatric patients who may need enhanced pain and other symptom management as they are more sensitive and frailer. There is an overlap between the care provided by geriatric and palliative medicine specialties, and their integration can be worthwhile for elderly care.

Palliative care, as defined by the World Health Organization (WHO), is an approach that improves the quality of life of patients and their families facing issues associated with life-threatening illness, by prevention and relief of suffering through early identification, impeccable assessment and treatment of pain and other issues—physical, psychosocial, and spiritual.

CONCEPT OF GERIATRIC PALLIATIVE MEDICINE

Geriatric palliative medicine (GPM) is the provision of medical care and management of elderly patients with advanced diseases and limited prognosis, with care focused on the quality of life. Thus, GPM is a combination of both geriatric medicine and palliative care principles. The principles are given as follows:

- Concentration on comprehensive geriatric assessment, pain, and other physical symptom management and addressing social, emotional, and spiritual issues
- Understanding of symptoms and disease, the need for safe drug prescription, and recognition of the significance of a multidisciplinary tailored approach for the elderly patients and families getting palliative care
- Highlighting the autonomy and involvement of patients in decision-making
- Emphasizes good communication skills while prognosticating and discussing
- Focus on addressing the various concerns of patients and families in various environments such as 41 homes, hospitals, and hospices, as well as special attention during transitions across settings
- Provision of family support during the end-of-life care

DOMAINS OF PALLIATIVE CARE

The National Consensus Project for Quality Palliative Care (NCPQPC) describes eight domains of palliative care: (1) Its structure and processes; (2) physical aspects; (3)

psychological and psychiatric aspects; (4) social aspects; (5) spiritual, religious, and existential aspects; (6) cultural aspects; (7) end-of-life care; and (8) ethical and legal aspects of care.

Structure and Process of Care

Palliative care includes both primary and specialist palliative care. Primary palliative care involves the addressal of initial symptoms and routine discussions regarding prognosis, care goals, etc. Institutions that do not have specialist palliative care access make use of primary palliative care for the general needs of patients who have serious illnesses. Primary palliative care is to be given by the geriatrician in the hospital who is the immediate physician. In order to meet the needs of patients and families, numerous types of palliative care delivery are modeled as per the patient's preferences.

Physical Aspects of Care

Palliative care consultation has been found to attribute to improvement in physical symptom management significantly. Palliative care teams can provide safe and effective treatment recommendations as they are experts in the management of advanced symptoms. Palliative care consultations result in higher patient satisfaction, decreased duration of stay, lower overall costs, and reduced readmission and ICU admission rates. The physical symptoms experienced by older patients are different in terms of prevalence and presentation, thereby making the analysis of symptoms in the elderly all the more challenging. The assessment of Revised Edmonton Symptom Assessment System (ESAS) may be used to measure symptoms. It is important to manage geriatric symptoms such as frailty and comorbidity, as these patients have increased palliative care needs.

Psychological and Psychiatric Aspects of Care

Issues such as mood disorders, anxiety, delirium, substance-use disorders, and posttraumatic stress disorder warrant detailed assessment, which can be done by palliative physicians. Significant patient and family distress can be caused by delirium which may limit a patient's decision-making capacity—this too is addressed by the palliative care team. They also screen patients for depression. Social workers who are focused on palliative care are trained for screening and intervention in psychological issues. Palliative care physicians may seek professional help and refer to psychiatrists, psychologists, or counselors for expert management of the emotional health concerns of patients.

Social Aspects of Care

Palliative care offers heightened social care, including care of the family. Caring for the family with assessment forms a key component of social care in the palliative framework. Bereavement support is also provided by the palliative team. Elderly patients may experience social isolation and have a rise in mortality rates, depression rates, and psychological distress. Subjective well-being, improved quality of life, and physical function can be obtained by better social engagement.

Religious, Spiritual, and Existential Aspects of Care

Spiritual care delivery plays an important role in palliative care among geriatric patients. In older patients, physical functioning and social support are chiefly predicted by religiousness and spirituality. They are associated with fewer depressive symptoms, improved cognition, and better cooperation. Poor quality of life, distress, poor well-being, and confusion may accompany negative religious coping.

Cultural Aspects of Care

Culture can be a complex social structure formed through various factors that confer different values, responsibilities, opportunities, practices, and expectations upon its participants. Cultural differences among geriatric patients from their hospital care teams may be quite different. Cultural problems may prove to be a substantial hinderance to high-quality end-of-life care. Culturally different populations need trust to establish a better healthcare relationship, and hence the significance of specialists attending to cultural needs. A cultural assessment is mandatory for a comprehensive palliative care assessment. Best practices include presence, time, cultural respect, communication, etc. The multidisciplinary palliative care team plays a key role in the provision of cultural care. Palliative care team collaboration helps for a deeper knowledge of culture, and attention is provided to issues of older patients.

End-of-life Care

There is a period of the irreversible decline of functional status prior to death which is defined as the terminal phase. It may last from hours to days and occasionally to weeks. The term end of life is used when patients are expected to die within the next 12 months. During the end of life, the care focus is shifted from treatments aimed at cure or life prolongation to symptom control, comfort measures, dignity, and providing a better quality of life. In the last phase, patients can have various symptoms such as loss of weight, dysphagia, change in breathing pattern, decreased urine output, refractory delirium, cold skin, fatigue, social withdrawal, disinterest, and drowsiness. There should be proper recognition of this phase, an early care plan for the patient, family preparation, conversations involving anticipation of symptoms and control, death place preferences, etc.

Ethical and Legal Aspects of Care

The palliative care team assists with medicolegal issues that happen while caring elderly with serious illnesses. The palliative care team is involved in the ethical or legal aspects, including autonomy, surrogate decision-making, disclosure of information, withholding or withdrawing treatment, artificial nutrition and hydration, and futility of treatment.

APPROACH FOR PALLIATIVE CARE DISCUSSION IN ELDERLY

- Explaining the objectives and goals for the patient.
- To help create advance directives.
- Early discussion involving families, especially in patients with dementia.
- Conducting accurate and clear discussions regarding the pros and cons of aggressive approaches and palliative approaches for the chronic issues of the elderly.
- Describing benefits versus risks of hospitalization, medications, tests, and monitoring the treatment of chronic problems.
- Coordinating care among various providers and doctors.
- Discussion of alternatives to aggressive management.
- Discussion regarding depression, risk of falls, etc.
- Provision of caregiver support.

SYSTEMIC CHANGES IN THE OLD INDIVIDUALS AND THEIR IMPLICATIONS

Cardiovascular System

- Reduced cardiac output leading to slower systemic distribution of drugs.
- Increased blood pressure and atherosclerosis can result in a higher risk of vascular events and other cardiovascular complications requiring treatment and hospitalization.

Genitourinary System

- Decreased renal reserve for recovery from nephrotoxic agents
- Increased incidence of chronic kidney disease (CKD), prostatic enlargement, and atrophy of the uterus, vagina, and breast due to decreased sexual hormone levels
- Increased incidence of stress incontinence
- Less number of nephrons and decreased glomerular filtration rate resulting in decreased excretion of drugs by the kidney requiring cautious monitoring of drugs excreted through the kidney

Neurological System

- Decreased proprioception
- Impairment of cognition and cortical atrophy causing variations in processing and reporting of pain
- Autonomic neuropathy leading to altered responses and injury risks
- Risk of delirium
- Decreased dopamine and acetylcholine stores
- Forgetfulness, depression, Parkinson's disease, insomnia, etc., which may require therapy

Respiratory System

- Decreased respiratory reserve
- Increased incidence of pulmonary diseases

Gastrointestinal and Hepatic System

- Less hepatocytes and decreased hepatic blood flow leading to reduced metabolic drug elimination
- Decreased gastrointestinal transit altering intestinal absorption of medications
- Decreased albumin resulting in increased free drugs and toxicities

Musculoskeletal System

- Muscular atrophy can lead to reduced volume of distribution.
- Increased fat results in a longer duration of action of lipid-soluble drugs.
- The volume of distribution (Vd) of lipophilic drugs gets increased, needing an increased dose and the Vd of hydrophilic drugs gets reduced, needing a lower dose.
- Reduced bone density leading to osteoporosis, fractures, and functional impairment requiring treatment, hospitalization, etc.

Skin Changes and Sensory Functions

- There is a reduction in proteins such as elastin and collagen, leading to decreased skin elasticity
- Thinning of epidermis due to decreased cell renewal
- Decreased sensorial perception, visual acuity, and hearing

BARRIERS AND FACILITATORS FOR COLLABORATION BETWEEN GERIATRIC MEDICINE AND PALLIATIVE CARE

Barriers and facilitators may be at clinical practice, education, training, or policy levels. Less awareness and understanding regarding the other specialties and a lack of communication may be important barriers. Inadequate educational opportunities and shared training, a limited number of academic chairs in both specialties, organization, and financing of health care can also act as barriers to collaboration between geriatric and palliative medicine.

Facilitators may be advanced care planning, sharing of palliative care and geriatric medicine perspectives at platforms such as conferences, mandatory internships within the other disciplines, cross-disciplinary works or multidisciplinary teamwork, expert advice and consultation from the other disciplines, strong leadership, establishing taskforces, etc.

GERIATRIC-SPECIFIC SYNDROMES AND PALLIATIVE CARE

- The major geriatric syndromes are frailty, delirium, dizziness, urinary incontinence, insomnia, falls, malnourishment, pain, and depression.
- Etiology may be multifactorial.
- In clinical practice, geriatric syndromes are associated with poor outcomes and significant morbidity.
- Their prevalence is high in elderly frail patients.

FEW GERIATRIC SYNDROMES: POTENTIAL SCREENING TOOLS AND INTERVENTIONS

Falls

- *Screening tools*: Fall history, timed up and go test, and gait speed assessment
- *Intervention*: Review of medications, visual checkups, monitoring of blood pressure in different positions, footwear checks, evaluation of safety at home, physical and occupational therapies, referral for balance and muscle strength training, exercise programs at home, counseling for prevention of falls, etc.

Cognitive Impairment

- *Screening tools*: Mini-Cog, Blessed Orientation-Memory-Concentration (BOMC) test
- *Intervention*: Review of medications, referral upon the requirement of a comprehensive cognitive assessment, counseling for patients and caregivers regarding the risk of delirium, and assessment of capacity for decision-making

Polypharmacy

- *Screening tools*: STOPP (Screening Tool of Older Persons' Potentially Inappropriate Prescriptions), START () criteria and Beers criteria
- *Intervention*: Brown bag medicine review, active involvement of pharmacists in patient care, and stopping medications that are potentially inappropriate

Depression

- *Screening tools*: Hospital Anxiety and Depression Scale (HADS), GDS, Center for Epidemiology Studies Depression Scale-Revised (CESD-R)
- *Intervention*: Referral for psychological interventions, pharmacologic treatments, problem-solving therapy, cognitive behavioral therapy, etc.

OTHER COMMON SCREENING TOOLS USED IN THE ELDERLY

- Edmonton Symptom Assessment Tool-revised (r-ESAS)
- MD Anderson Symptom Inventory (MDASI)
- European Organization for Research and Treatment of Cancer's Quality of Life Core Questionnaire (EORTC QLQ-C30)
- Memorial Symptom Assessment Tool (MSAS)

ONCOGERIATRICS

As the human population is aging rapidly, it is projected that one in six people will be aged >65 years by 2050. GLOBOCAN data suggest that the cancer cases reported in the elderly population may rise to 18.6 million in 2040, from 9.95 million in 2020. There is a growing need to improve the care standards provided to the geriatric population with cancer in the years to come. As per the World Health Organization, 56.8 million people have the requirement of palliative care each year, and 25.7 million require it in the final year of life. Nearly 40% are aged > 70 years, and it is unfortunate that only about 14% of those who require palliative care are receiving it. Older cancer patients can have various comorbidities, frailty, and reduced cognition which can be challenging for palliative physicians. The healthcare needs of older patients may be complex and need comprehensive assessment. A wise solution would be a collaboration among geriatric and palliative teams as this population carries overlapping concerns for both disciplines **(Fig. 1)**.

Specific Symptom Management in the Elderly with Cancer

Pain

Nearly 25–40% of elderly cancer patients complain of daily pain. Pain amplifies the dependence on daily activities, increases fall risk, depression, and malnutrition risk, and decreases social engagement. Pain can be attributed to the disease itself, its treatment, or due to any comorbid conditions. Pain in geriatric age is usually multifactorial, and a multidisciplinary team approach involving geriatrician, palliative physician, psychiatrist, psychologist, physiotherapist, physiatrist, dietician, etc., would be instrumental.

Barriers to Pain Evaluation and Management

- Impairments in cognition and function
- Poor reporting
- Comorbidities
- Prescription bias
- Polypharmacy
- Administering drugs in the setting of institutional living

Elderly Population—Validated Tools for Pain Assessment

The cancer pain assessment involves a comprehensive evaluation comprising a thorough pain review and physical examination.

- Pain Assessment in Advanced Dementia (PAINAD)
- Pain Assessment Checklist for Seniors with Limited Ability to Communicate (PACSLAC)
- Abbey Pain Scale
- Doloplus-2 Scale

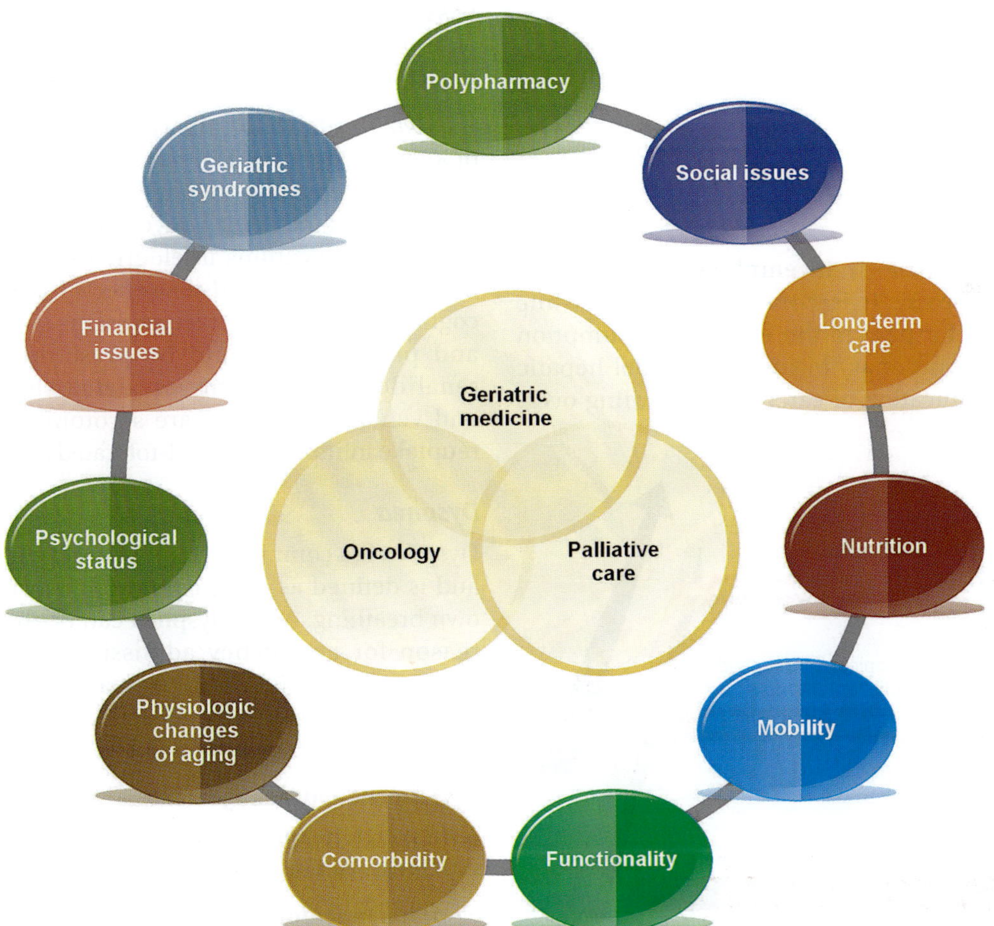

FIG. 1: The complex relationship and overlap between geriatric medicine, palliative care, and oncology.

Source: With permission from Castelo-Loureiro A, Perez-de-Acha A, Torres-Perez AC, Cunha V, García-Valdés P, Cárdenas-Reyes P, et al. Delivering Palliative and Supportive Care for Older Adults with Cancer: Interactions between Palliative Medicine and Geriatrics. Cancers 2023:15(15);3858.

- Rotterdam Elderly Pain Observation Scale (REPOS)
- Pain Assessment in Noncommunicative Elderly Persons (PAINE)
- Elderly Pain Caring Assessment-2 (EPCA-2)
- Certified Nurse Assistant Pain Assessment Tool (CPAT)
- Pain Assessment Tool in Confused Older Adults (PATCOA)
- Pain Assessment for the Demented Elderly (PADE)
- Mahoney Pain Scale
- Checklist of Nonverbal Pain Indicators (CNPI)
- Discomfort Scale (DS-DAT)

Management of Pain

The World Health Organization analgesic ladder forms the backbone of the standard pain management algorithm **(Fig. 2)**. The identification of the etiology of pain is the cornerstone of its management.

Nonpharmacological Interventions

- Relaxation techniques
- Mindfulness
- Massage
- Acupuncture
- Exercises
- Rehabilitation
- Cognitive behavioral therapy—if cognitively intact

Pharmacological Interventions

- *Nonopioids*:
  - *Acetaminophen*: It is employed in mild-to-moderate pain. It is considered the first-line treatment for pain in the elderly. Consumption of >3 g is cautionary owing to potential hepatic toxicity. Education of caregivers regarding over-the-counter drugs and other combination drugs containing acetaminophen is needed.
- *NSAIDs*: These are effective for managing mild-to-moderate pain, particularly bone pain. But there is a risk in the elderly due to the incidence of renal adverse effects, gastrointestinal bleeds, stroke, and myocardial infarction. Side effects associated with NSAIDs are time and dose-dependent; therefore, their usage is advocated for short intervals only, that too along with gastroprotective medications. NSAIDs should be avoided in peptic ulcers, CKD, and heart diseases.

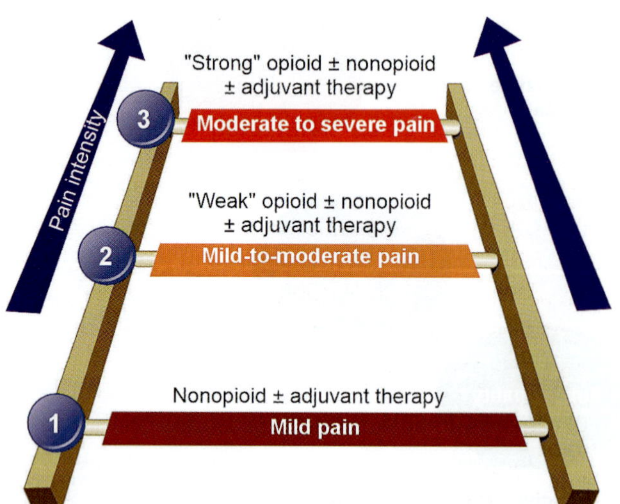

FIG. 2: The new adaptation of the WHO analgesic ladder.

Opioids: These are employed in cancer pain of moderate to severe intensity. Analgesic ceiling dose is absent. Before treatment commencement, evaluation of renal and hepatic function, cognition, social support, and any potential drug reactions is imperative. The opioids commonly used are tramadol, codeine, morphine, fentanyl, and methadone. Common adverse effects related to opioids are sedation, constipation, vomiting, confusion, and hallucinations. A prophylactic bowel regimen is started on patients with opioid prescriptions. Less common side effects associated with opioids in elderly patients with cancer include nausea, pruritus, myoclonus, urinary retention, dry mouth, etc.

Adjuvant medications: They add to the pain relief given by opioids and are primarily used in other indications. These include anticonvulsants, antidepressants, corticosteroids, muscle relaxants, etc. Tricyclic antidepressants (TCAs) have rare indications in elderly cancer patients due to their anticholinergic adverse effects leading to changes in cognition. Common anticonvulsants such as gabapentin and pregabalin should be prescribed according to renal dosages and only escalated slowly. Duloxetine and venlafaxine which are serotonin-norepinephrine reuptake inhibitors are well-tolerated and effective.

Dyspnea

Dyspnea is a common symptom in elderly cancer patients and is defined as an uncomfortable awareness of one's own breathing. Acute dyspnea can be the most common reason for emergency admissions and can result in poor quality of life. Etiology can be effusions, airway obstructions, thick airway secretions, bronchospasms, anemia, anxiety, and other emotional issues.

Assessment and Management

A thorough history, physical examination, imaging, and other tests can be employed to rule out reversible causes.

Nonpharmacological interventions

- Patient repositioning
- Opening windows or using handheld fans to improve air circulation

- Breathing training or relaxation techniques
- Providing reassurance and addressing anxiety

Pharmacological interventions

- Opioids are recommended therapy for dyspnea in palliative care patients. They act by suppressing respiratory awareness effectively. Studies have proven that opioids can be effective and safe in the management of breathlessness in end-stage cancer patients.
- Benzodiazepines can be used to relieve anxiety which worsens dyspnea.
- Treatments with steroids, bronchodilator agents, or diuretics may benefit patients with specific diagnoses.
- In palliative settings, oxygen supplementation may often be unnecessary.

Nausea and Vomiting

These symptoms are commonly found in cancer patients with advanced disease. Among cancer patients, the prevalence ranges from 30 to 70%. Etiologies may be chemotherapy, radiation, opioids, constipation, and intestinal obstruction. A focused history with examination is needed to find out the specific causes. The general principles of management are given as follows:

- Start with round-the-clock dosages of a single agent based on the possible mechanism of nausea.
- Secondary agents may be added to target other classes of receptors if the first agent does not work.
- Adjuvants such as steroids or benzodiazepines can be used in patients who are terminally ill.

If nausea and vomiting are due to:

- Drugs (opioids, antibiotics, anticholinergics) where possible, stop the medications
- Metabolic (uremia, hypercalcemia) correction of the metabolic cause
- *Fear or anxiety*: Anxiolytics, providing reassurance, cognitive behavioral therapy
- *Gastric irritation (NSAIDs)*: Stop drugs, addition of proton-pump inhibitors
- *Cough*: If due to infection, start antibiotics/add cough suppressants.

Management of Nausea and Vomiting

Nonpharmacological interventions

- Small frequent meals
- Preference for patient's choice of food
- Proper intake of fluids
- Relaxation therapy
- Pleasant environment during meals

Pharmacological interventions

Based on the mechanism, different drugs are used:

- Metoclopramide, 5–15 mg before meals, given oral, subcutaneous, or IV
- Domperidone, divided doses before meals to a maximum of 80 mg/day orally
- Diphenhydramine 1 mg/kg/dose q4 hourly, given oral, subcutaneous, or IV
- Haloperidol 0.01–0.05 mg/kg/dose q8 hourly, given oral, subcutaneous, or IV
- Prochlorperazine 0.15 mg/kg/dose q4 hourly, given oral, rectal, or IV
- Ondansetron 0.15 mg/kg/dose q6 hourly, given per oral or IV
- Dexamethasone 2–4 mg q12 hourly to q6 hourly, given oral, subcutaneous, or IV
- Scopolamine 0.5 mg transdermal q72 hourly, given transdermal

Fatigue

Fatigue is one of the most debilitating symptoms experienced by cancer patients. Cancer-related fatigue (CRF) comprises feelings of tiredness and lack of energy. It is associated with distress, anxiety, depression, and poor performance status.

Management of Fatigue

Nonpharmacological interventions

- Aerobic exercise
- Psychological interventions
- Complementary therapies

Pharmacological interventions

- Modafinil
- Corticosteroids
- Methylphenidate
- Antidepressants
- Cholinesterase inhibitors

Delirium

Delirium is a serious neuropsychiatric condition characterized by a disturbance of awareness and attention accompanied by dysfunction of cognition with a decline from baseline. Among cancer patients, it is associated with mortality, morbidity, and increased distress. Delirium has a prevalence of about 20–40% in hospitalized cancer patients and can reach up to 88% in end-stage cancer patients. The etiology of delirium is as follows:

- Medical causes such as organ failure, infections, and paraneoplastic syndromes
- Metabolic causes such as electrolyte abnormalities and uremia
- Uncontrolled pain

- Central nervous system (CNS) causes such as brain metastasis
- Central effects of immune and chemotherapeutic agents
- Medications such as opioids, steroids, antiemetics, and benzodiazepines
- Urinary retention and constipation
- Alcohol withdrawal and use of illicit drugs
- Deprivation of sleep
- Change of environment

Assessment and Management

The assessment of delirium includes a detailed history with a physical examination. Potentially reversible causes must be addressed, and a thorough review of medications and dosages should be made. Routine investigations are to be carried out. Brain imaging can be done to rule out brain metastasis. Diagnosis can be made by Confusion Assessment Method (CAM). For intubated patients, CAM-intensive care unit (CAM-ICU) can be used.

Nonpharmacological interventions

Delirium incidence can be decreased by reducing exposure to the known risk factors.

Pharmacological interventions

Antipsychotics, cholinesterase inhibitors, and alpha-2 agonists may be employed in the prevention and treatment.

Anxiety and Depression

In cancer patients, they are the most common presentation of psychological distress.

Management of Anxiety and Depression

A good history and careful physical examination are important to determine needed interventions.

Nonpharmacological interventions

- Multidisciplinary assessments and psychotherapies
- Relaxation techniques

Pharmacological interventions

- Benzodiazepines are the most important medications in the management of anxiety.
- In case of severe anxiety, antipsychotics such as haloperidol may be used.
- In cases of depression, the initial doses of antidepressant agents should be minimized owing to decreased clearance of drugs leading to adverse effects.
- SSRIs can cause decreased sleepiness and decreased autonomic adverse effects as compared to other antidepressants.
- TCAs can be given at bedtime alone.
- Prompt psychiatry referral is needed if poorly responsive to initial treatment or with a complex initial presentation such as psychosis and suicidal ideation.

ADVANCED CARE PLANNING FOR OLDER ADULTS

It is an approach involving comprehensive communication which assures proper implementation and documentation of patient preferences. It gives patients and their loved ones a platform to discuss their life goals, personal choices, and values regarding future medical care, especially during end of life. Elderly patients with serious illnesses generally want quality of life instead of quantity. The aim of advanced care planning (ACP) is to help patients in getting proper care according to their goals, values, and preferences, thus promoting patient-centered care. Thus, ACP advocates reduced aggressive medical interventions, lower rates of hospital admissions, better communication skills, improved decision-making, and decreased anxiety and depression, resulting in overall decreased cost and better quality of life.

END-OF-LIFE CARE

During the final days or hours of life, patients with terminal illness may confront a variety of symptoms such as pain, vomiting, delirium, anxiety, dyspnea, and distress. Adequate symptomatic management as well as proper caregiver and family support is needed during the care for patients at the end of life.

CONCLUSION

There has been little research in geriatric palliative care although much research has been conducted in palliative medicine to understand the physical, psychological, and social factors associated with patients. The profile of old patients differs from that of younger patients. The elderly may live in institutions and may have impaired functioning, cognitive dysfunction, and associated morbidities that are the main factors in the survival of patients. A team-based multidisciplinary approach can be beneficial to elderly adults in view of their complex medical, social, and psychological needs. Palliative care must be included in the elderly patient's care throughout the disease trajectory. Palliative care is focused on symptomatic management and functional improvement leading to a better quality of life.

To decrease drug interactions and side effects, nonpharmacological interventions have to be an initial consideration in the management plan for the elderly. The timely referral to palliative care reduces patient and caregiver distress greatly.

Self-Assessment Questionnaire

Q1. What are the key physiological changes associated with aging that increase surgical risk in older adults?

Q2. How does multimorbidity and polypharmacy complicate perioperative management in geriatric patients?

Q3. Why is comprehensive geriatric assessment (CGA) important before surgery, and what domains does it typically include?

Q4. What are the most common postoperative complications in elderly patients, and how can they be mitigated?

Q5. How can early mobilization and nutritional support improve postoperative recovery and reduce hospital stay in older patients?

Q6. What are the key elements of discharge planning for older surgical patients to ensure continuity of care and reduce readmissions?

Q7. How do geriatric and palliative care principles overlap in managing older surgical patients with multiple comorbidities and limited physiological reserve?

FURTHER READINGS

1. Makary MA, Segev DL. The aging population and surgical workforce: a looming crisis? J Am Med Assoc. 2010;303(21):2142-3.
2. Fleisher LA, Fleischmann KE, Auerbach AD, Barnason SA, Bozkurt B, Davila-Roman VG, et al. 2014 ACC/AHA guideline on perioperative cardiovascular evaluation and management of patients undergoing noncardiac surgery: executive summary. J Am Coll Cardiol. 2014;64(22):2373-405.
3. Deiner S, Silverstein JH. Postoperative delirium and cognitive dysfunction. Br J Anaesth. 2009;103(suppl_1):i41-6.
4. Mohanty S, Rosenthal RA, Russell MM, Neuman MD, Ko CY, Esnaola NF. Optimal perioperative management of the geriatric patient: a best practices guideline from the American College of Surgeons NSQIP and the American Geriatrics Society. J Am Coll Surg. 2016;222(5):930-47.
5. Robinson TN, Eiseman B. Postoperative delirium in the elderly: diagnosis and management. Clin Interven Aging; 2008;3(2): 351-5.
6. Rich MW, Chyun DA, Skolnick AH, Alexander KP, Forman DE, Kitzman DW, et al. Knowledge gaps in cardiovascular care of the older adult population: a scientific statement from the American Heart Association, American College of Cardiology, and American Geriatrics Society. J Am Coll Cardiol. 2016;67(20): 2419-50.
7. Evered L, Silbert B, Knopman DS, Scott DA, DeKosky ST, Rasmussen LS, et al. Recommendations for the nomenclature of cognitive change associated with anaesthesia and surgery—2018. Br J Anaesth. 2018;121(5):1005-12.
8. Partridge JS, Harari D, Dhesi JK. Frailty in the older surgical patient: a review. Age Ageing. 2012;41(2):142-7.
9. Kehlet H, Wilmore DW. Evidence-based surgical care and the evolution of fast-track surgery. Ann Surg. 2008;248(2):189-98.
10. Sweeney BF, Kwan P. Perioperative management of the geriatric surgical patient. Surg Clin N Am. 2011;91(5):1161-73.
11. Chacko B, Whitley M, Beckmann U, Murray K, Rowley M. Postoperative euglycaemic diabetic ketoacidosis associated with sodium-glucose cotransporter-2 inhibitors (gliflozins): a report of two cases and review of the literature. Anaesth Intens Care. 2018;46(2):215-9.
12. Steinhorn B, Wiener-Kronish J. Dose-dependent relationship between SGLT2 inhibitor hold time and risk for postoperative anion gap acidosis: a single-centre retrospective analysis. Br J Anaesth. 2023;131(4):682-6.
13. Marcantonio ER. Delirium in hospitalized older adults. New Engl J Med. 2017;377(15):1456-66.
14. Hashmi NK, Podgoreanu MV. Stress response to surgery in the elderly. In: Akhtar S, Rosenbaum S (Eds). Principles of Geriatric Critical Care. UK: Cambridge University Press; 2018. pp. 168-86.
15. Mohanty S, Rosenthal RA, Russell MM, Neuman MD, Ko CY, Esnaola NF. Optimal perioperative management of the geriatric patient: a best practices guideline from the American College of Surgeons NSQIP and the American Geriatrics Society. J Am Coll Surg. 2016;222(5):930-47.
16. Partridge JS, Harari D, Martin FC, Dhesi JK. The impact of pre-operative comprehensive geriatric assessment on postoperative outcomes in older patients undergoing scheduled surgery: a systematic review. Anaesthesia. 2014;69(Suppl 1):8-16.
17. Nichani SS, Grant PJ, Malani PN. Perioperative evaluation and management. In: Halter JB, Ouslander JG, Studenski S, High KP, Asthana S, Supiano MA, Ritchie C (Eds). Hazzard's Geriatric Medicine and Gerontology, 7th edition. New York: McGraw-Hill Education; 2017.
18. Manou-Stathopoulou V, Korbonits M, Ackland GL. Redefining the perioperative stress response: a narrative review. Br J Anaesth. 2019;123(5):570-83.
19. Dewan SK, Zheng SB, Xia SJ. Preoperative geriatric assessment: comprehensive, multidisciplinary and proactive. Eur J Inter Med. 2012;23(6):487-94.
20. Kumar C, Salzman B, Colburn J. Preoperative assessment in older adults: a comprehensive approach. Am Fam Physic. 2018;98(4):214-20.
21. Pang CL, Gooneratne M, Partridge JSL. Preoperative assessment of the older patient. BJA Educ. 2021;21(8):314-20.
22. Barnett SR, Neves SE. Perioperative Care of the Elderly Patient. UK: Cambridge University Press; 2018.
23. Starr R, Stefan M. Perioperative assessment of and care for the elderly and frail. Hosp Med Clin. 2016;5:224-41.

CHAPTER 40

Role of Artificial Intelligence in Elderly Care

Raj Kumar Tata

"It is not the most intellectual species nor the strongest species that survive but the one most responsive change."

CASE VIGNETTE

Name: Mrs Sharma

Age: 78-year-old female

Medical history: Hypertension, type 2 diabetes, and history of transient ischemic attacks (TIAs)

Mrs Sharma, a 78-year-old woman with a history of hypertension, type 2 diabetes, and TIAs, lives alone in a suburban neighborhood. Her family had recently equipped her with an artificial intelligence (AI)-powered wearable health monitor designed to track vital signs and provide emergency alerts.

Event: One evening, she was watching television when she suddenly felt dizzy and weak. She tried to stand up but collapsed on the floor, unable to reach her phone to call for help. The AI wearable on her wrist detected the fall and a significant drop in her blood pressure, as well as irregular heart rhythms, suggesting a potential cardiac event.

Artificial intelligence-based wearable response:

- *Fall detection*: The wearable immediately recognized the fall and triggered an alert.
- *Vital signs monitoring*: It continuously monitored her heart rate, blood pressure, and oxygen saturation levels. The data indicated bradycardia (abnormally slow heart rate) and hypotension.
- *Emergency alert*: The device sent an automatic alert to her designated emergency contact—her daughter, who lived 20 minutes away. It also contacted the local emergency medical services (EMS) with Mrs Sharma's location and medical data.

Emergency response:

- Within minutes, paramedics were dispatched to Mrs Sharma's home. The real-time data provided by the AI wearable allowed them to prepare for a potential cardiac event. Upon arrival, they found her unresponsive but breathing.
- The paramedics used the data from the wearable to administer appropriate prehospital care, including intravenous fluids to address hypotension and medications to stabilize her heart rate. She was transported to the nearest hospital, where she received further treatment for a suspected acute myocardial infarction (MI).

Hospital course: In the emergency department, Mrs Sharma was quickly evaluated and treated for an acute MI. The continuous data provided by the AI wearable was instrumental in guiding her initial treatment and monitoring her condition. After receiving stent placement in the cardiac catheterization laboratory, she was admitted to the intensive care unit (ICU) for further monitoring and recovery.

Outcome: She made a full recovery and was discharged from the hospital after a week. Her cardiologist credited the AI wearable with saving her life by ensuring rapid emergency medical attention and providing crucial real-time health data. She continued to use the wearable for ongoing health monitoring, providing peace of mind to her and her family.

This case illustrates the significant impact of AI wearables in managing health emergencies, particularly for elderly individuals living alone. The wearable's ability to detect falls, monitor vital signs, and promptly alert both family and emergency services can be lifesaving. As technology advances, such devices will likely become an integral part of health care, particularly for vulnerable populations.

INTRODUCTION

Technology is set to transform the healthcare needs of the ever-increasing silver population. It is estimated that by 2050, around 2.1 billion people will be above 60 years which is almost two times from 2020 and will constitute about 15–16% population of the world. In India, people aged above 60 years will be around 319 million which will be about 19.5% of the total Indian population; that is, one in every five Indians is likely to be a senior citizen by 2050.

As our population ages, the demand for elderly care continues to grow, presenting both challenges and opportunities for society. In this chapter, we will explore the pivotal role that artificial intelligence (AI) plays in revolutionizing elderly care, enhancing the quality of life for seniors and supporting caregivers.

Where and how should AI be used in elderly health care?

Any revolutionary change at first is hard for people to accept. So, if we are to use AI for elderly health care on a mass level, the first step is to make people understand and believe that it is for their own benefit so that there is acceptance of this new revolutionary change among the masses.

Areas where we can use AI in elderly health care are stated as follows:

- Personalized health care
- Remote monitoring and assistance
- Cognitive support and mental health
- Caregiver support and workforce optimization
- Social engagement and community integration
- Medical imaging and diagnostics
- Predictive analytics and risk stratification
- Drug discovery and development
- Clinical decision support system
- Telemedicine and remote patient monitoring (RPM)
- Healthcare operations and administration
- Ethical and regulatory considerations

We will try to understand all these points in detail in this chapter.

PERSONALIZED HEALTH CARE

Currently, most medical treatments are designed for the "average patients", which may be successful for some but not for others. Precision medicine, also known as personalized medicine, is an innovative approach to tailoring disease prevention and treatment that takes into account differences in people's genes, environments, and lifestyles **(Figs. 1A and B)**.

Personalized medicine has markedly improved the management protocols among the health realms which include:

- Cancer detection
- Cancer treatment
- Pharmacogenetics testing
- Prenatal testing

Cancer Detection

Biomarker testing to detect cancer in asymptomatic individuals is enticing because it could lead to early diagnosis; earlier detection will also reduce the need for more aggressive and more costly therapy, and a greater number of individuals will be cured of the disease.

CancerSEEK is a multianalyte blood test that detects common cancer-associated DNA variants using a panel of 61 amplicons for cancer start "driver" mutation as well as 41 protein biomarkers associated with common cancers. The most common cancers detected were ovary, liver, stomach, pancreas, esophagus, colon/rectum, lung, or breast cancer. Currently, this test is not available in India.

Cancer Treatment

Gene expression profiling helps stratify the need for therapy or the type of therapy in patients with early-stage cancer. Examples include:

- Breast cancer
- Lung cancer
- Colon cancer
- Hematological malignancies

Pharmacogenetics Testing

The earliest implementation of genetic profiling has been in the area of pharmacogenetics. Pharmacogenetics is the study of variability in drug response due to genetic factors; it includes the prediction of two specific therapy toxicity and adverse effects. Pharmacogenetics data help in both the selection of a particular treatment and the individualized dose and dosing schedule for that treatment.

The most notable pharmacogenetics impacts dosing of medications used to treat hematological malignancies and solid tumors; markers are also available for medications used in the treatment of infectious, cardiac, rheumatological, and pulmonary diseases.

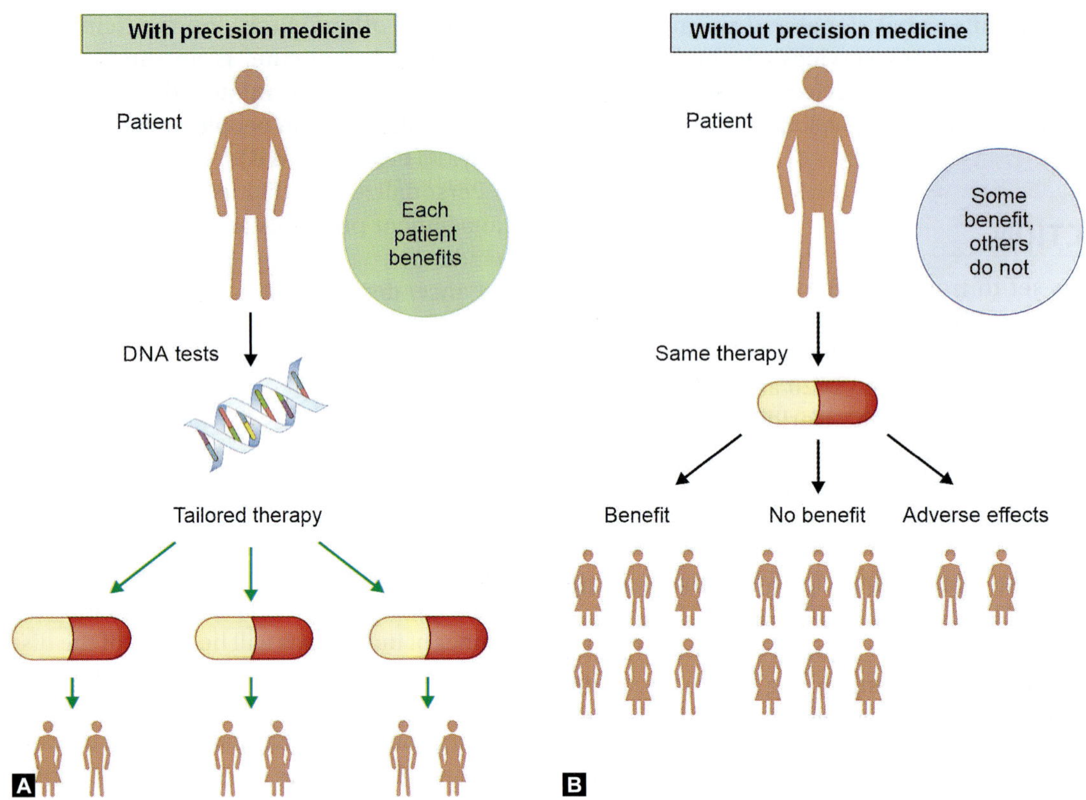

FIGS. 1A AND B: Comparison of treatment benefits (A) with and (B) without the use of precision medicine.

Advantages of Precision Medicine

- Reduced healthcare costs
- Reduction of adverse drug reactions (ADRs)
- Enhanced efficiency of drug action
- Reduces trial-and-error prescribing
- Increased adherence of patients to treatment
- Shift the emphasis in medicine from reaction to prevention
- Predicting susceptibility to disease
- Customizations of disease-prevention strategies
- Reduce the time, cost, and failure rate of pharmaceutical clinical trials
- Designing of new tools for building, analyzing, and sharing large sets of medical data

Obstacles for Implementation

Despite early success in the clinical trial introduction of a limited number of pharmacogenetic assays, multiple barriers preclude the widespread implementation of personalized medicine as standard clinical practice across medicine.

- Limited predictive value of most tests
- *Lack of physician knowledge*: The lack of general knowledge regarding genetics among many medical practitioners is one of the most pressing challenges preventing fraud implementation of personalized medicine.
- *Inadequate informatics infrastructure*: The original recordkeeping was designed for clinical laboratory data. This model of recordkeeping is inadequate to accommodate next-generation sequencing data, and, hence, newer approaches are required to develop or modify the electronic medical record (EMR) to access genetic testing results.
- Information provenance and patient privacy issues
- Inconsistent standardization and oversight of testing
- Reimbursement issues
- Genetic discrimination
- Societal issues and misconceptions

Artificial intelligence algorithms will analyze patients' data to predict health risks and outcomes, leading to early intervention and productive care. This includes predicting disease onset, potential complications, or optimal treatment plans based on the patient's medical history and genetics, and cognitive and physical reserve, especially in the elderly population.

REMOTE MONITORING AND ASSISTANCE

Artificial intelligence-powered monitoring systems, wearable devices, and smart home technologies enable continuous remote monitoring of elderly individuals and help metrics and activities of daily living. These systems can detect emergencies such as falls or sudden health deterioration, and automatically alert caregivers or emergency services, providing *peace of mind* for both seniors and their families.

Telehealthcare: It is the distribution of health-related services and information via electronic information and telecommunication technology. It allows long-distance patient and clinician contact, care, advice, reminders, education, intervention, former monitoring, and remote admission. Delivery of services can occur in four domains:

1. Live video conferencing
2. Storage of patients' data
3. RPM
4. Mobile health

Remote Patient Monitoring

Remote patient monitoring entails using digital technologies for the collection of medical and health data from individuals at one location and electronically transmit that information securely to healthcare providers at a different location for assessment and recommendations. RPM can include monitoring vital signs, chronic disease management, postoperative care, and even mental health.

Key Components of Remote Patient Monitoring

- *Wearable devices*: These include smartwatches, fitness trackers, and specialized medical devices that measure vital signs such as heart rate, blood pressure, and glucose levels.
- *Wireless body area networks (WBANs)*: The new generation of wireless sensor networks is dedicated to healthcare monitoring applications. It aims to ensure continuous monitoring of patients' vital parameters and take immediate steps in case of any abnormalities. Wearable WBANs can be in the form of either devices such as bracelets and watches or other devices based on electronic textiles incorporated into fabrics. Integration of these in a telemedicine system can turn into an alert system when life-threatening conditions occur, thus helping in long-term continuous monitoring that aids in diagnosis and confirms adherence to treatment and drug efficacy **(Figs. 2 and 3)**.

  Other examples are SmartStop, which helps people stop smoking, and Google smart contact lenses for people who suffer from diabetic retinopathy.
- *Epidermal WBANS*: These are placed directly on the skin like tattoos. They are thin biocompatible membranes that adhere firmly to the skin. They can be used to wirelessly monitor temperature without contact in patients **(Figs. 4A to D)**.
- *Mobile health (mHealth) applications*: Apps on smartphones and tablets that help patients track their health data, adhere to medication schedules, and communicate with healthcare providers
- *Home monitoring equipment*: Devices used at home for more detailed monitoring, such as blood pressure cuffs, glucometers, and spirometers
- *Telehealth platforms*: Systems that facilitate remote consultations between patients and healthcare providers through video calls, chat, and secure messaging

Artificial intelligence can analyze complex medical data, recognize patterns, and make predictions, which can significantly enhance the effectiveness of RPM.

Applications of Artificial Intelligence in Remote Patient Monitoring

- *Predictive analytics*: AI algorithms can analyze data from RPM devices to predict potential health issues before they become critical. For example, by monitoring heart rate and activity levels, AI can predict the likelihood of a heart attack or stroke.
- *Personalized medicine*: AI can tailor treatment plans based on individual patient data.
- *Automated alerts*: AI systems can automatically alert healthcare providers and patients to significant changes in health data, such as a sudden spike in blood pressure, allowing for timely intervention.
- *Remote diagnostics*: AI can assist in diagnosing conditions remotely by analyzing medical images, laboratory results, and patient symptoms, thus reducing the need for in-person visits.

Case Studies and Real-world Application

- *Chronic disease management*: Patients with chronic conditions such as diabetes or hypertension can benefit immensely from RPM and AI. For instance, continuous glucose monitors can track blood sugar levels in real time, and AI algorithms can analyze this data to suggest dietary changes or medication adjustments. Healthcare providers can receive alerts if a patient's readings indicate a risk of a hypoglycemic episode, allowing for immediate intervention.
- *Postoperative care*: RPM combined with AI can improve outcomes for patients recovering from surgery. Wearable devices can monitor vital signs such as heart rate and oxygen levels, while AI can analyze this data to detect signs of complications such as infections or blood clots early. This proactive approach can lead to quicker interventions and better recovery rates.
- *Mental health monitoring*: Mental health is another area where RPM and AI are making strides. Wearable

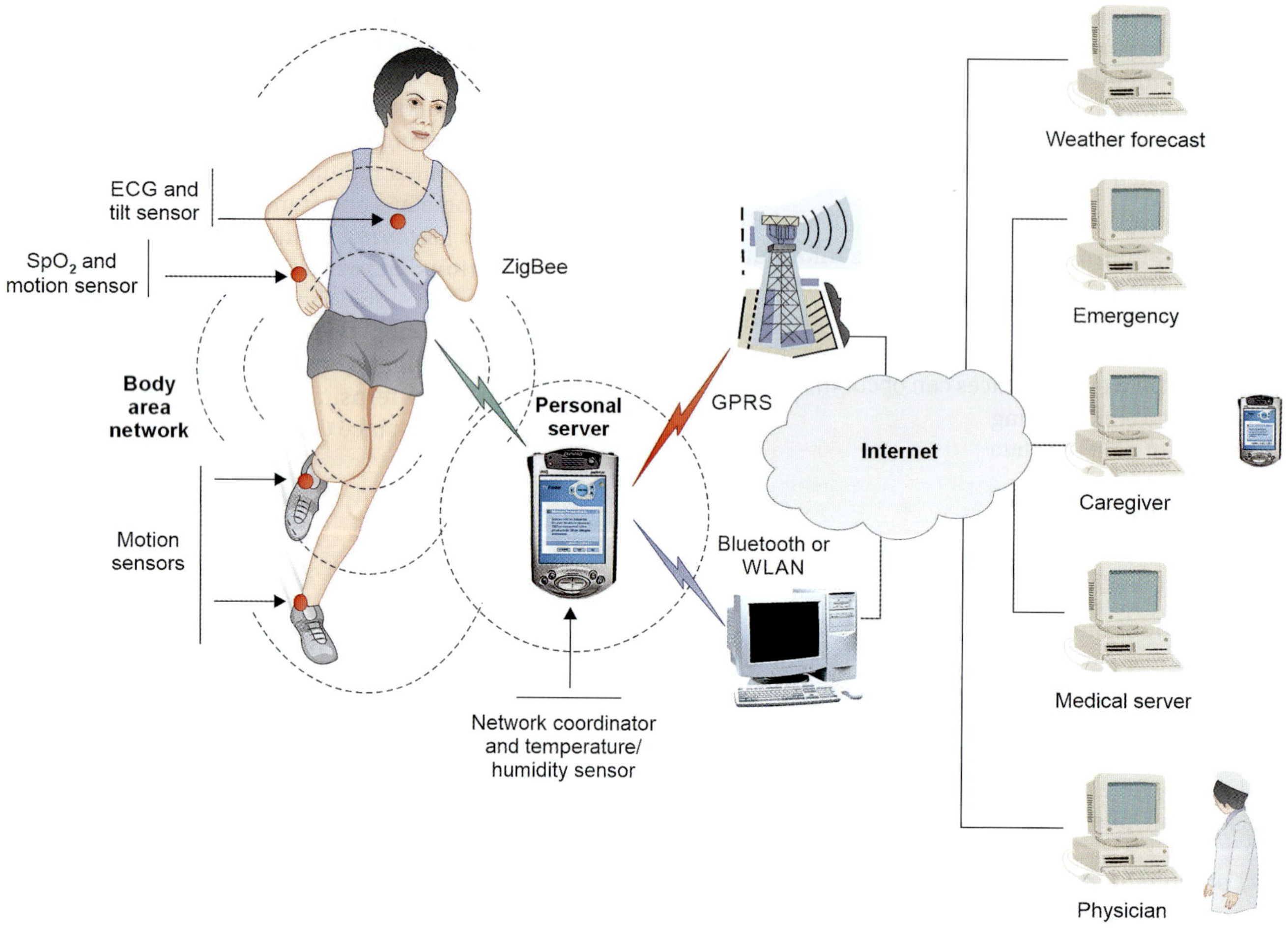

FIG. 2: Wireless body area networks (WBANs).

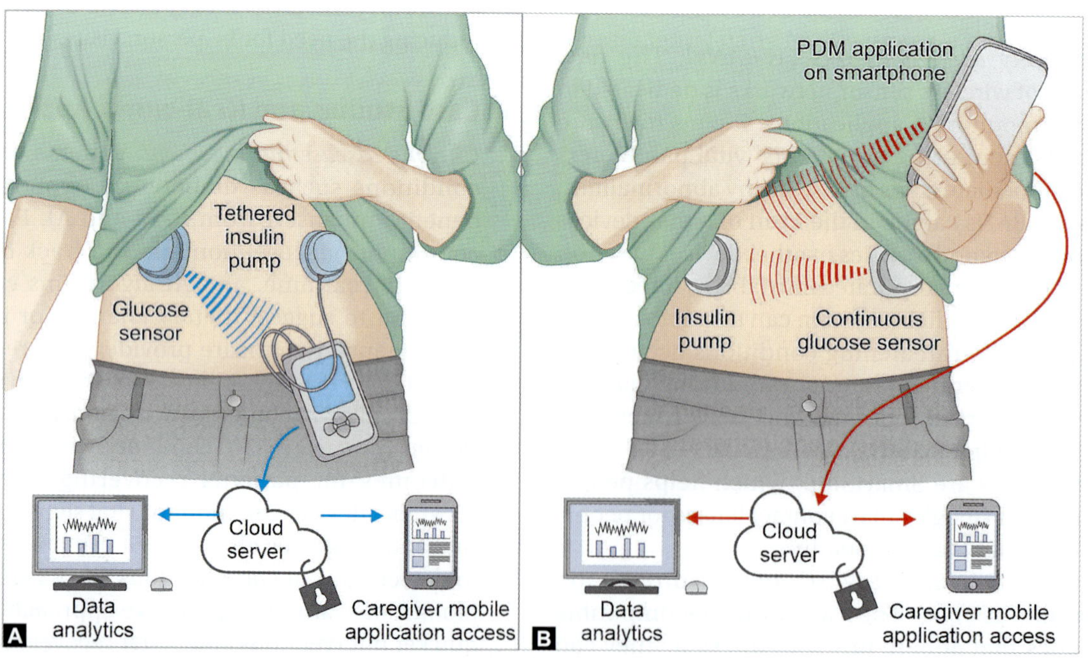

FIGS. 3A AND B: System configuration for automated insulin delivery (AID). (A) A system with a "tethered" insulin pump; and (B) A system using a tubeless or "patch" insulin pump.

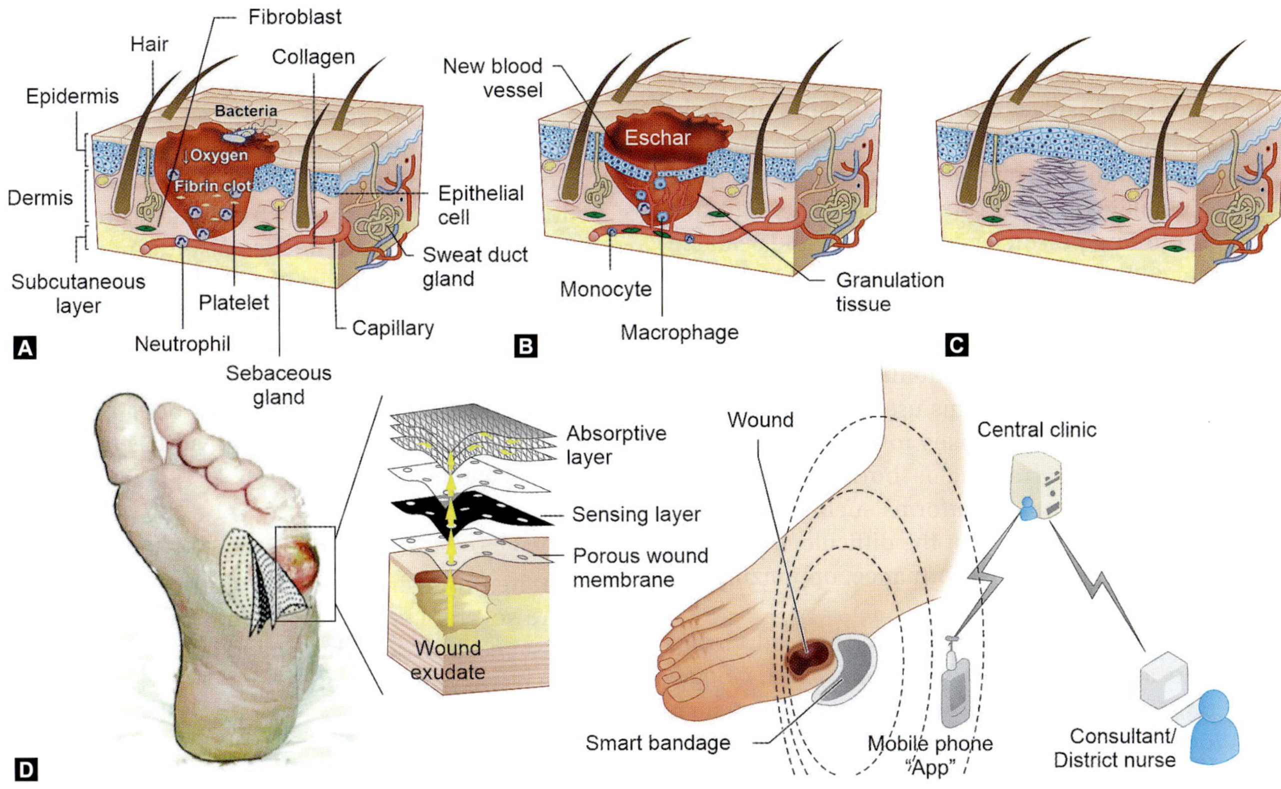

FIGS. 4A TO D: Three wound healing stages: (A) Inflammation; (B) Proliferation; (C) Remodeling; (D) Smart dressing.

devices can track physiological indicators of stress, such as heart rate variability, while mobile apps can monitor mood and behavior. AI can analyze this data to identify patterns and suggest coping strategies or professional interventions when necessary.

Challenges and Ethical Considerations

Despite its potential, the integration of RPM and AI in health care comes with challenges and ethical considerations.

- *Data privacy and security*: The collection and transmission of health data raise concerns about privacy and security. Ensuring that patient data is protected from breaches and unauthorized access is paramount. Compliance with regulations such as the Health Insurance Portability and Accountability Act (HIPAA) in the United States and the General Data Protection Regulation (GDPR) in Europe is essential. India must collaborate with IT giants to develop such security systems.
- *Accuracy and reliability*: The accuracy of AI algorithms is critical. False positives or negatives can lead to unnecessary interventions or missed diagnoses. Continuous validation and improvement of AI models are necessary to maintain their reliability.
- *Patient engagement and compliance*: The success of RPM relies on patient engagement and compliance. Patients need to consistently use their monitoring devices and follow the recommendations provided. Educating patients about the benefits and ease of use of RPM can enhance compliance.
- *Ethical use of AI*: AI systems should be designed and used ethically. This includes ensuring transparency in how AI algorithms make decisions, avoiding biases that could lead to unequal treatment, and maintaining a human element in patient care to ensure compassion and understanding.

MENTAL HEALTH AND COGNITIVE SUPPORT AND ARTIFICIAL INTELLIGENCE

In recent years, the field of mental health has seen significant advancements through the integration of AI. AI technologies are increasingly being used to provide cognitive support and enhance mental health care, offering new ways to diagnose, treat, and manage mental health conditions.

Cognitive Support through Artificial Intelligence

Cognitive support involves tools and strategies that help individuals manage cognitive demands, improve mental processes, and enhance overall mental functioning. AI technologies play a crucial role in providing cognitive support by offering personalized, adaptive, and scalable solutions.

- *AI-based cognitive training*: AI-driven cognitive training programs are designed to enhance cognitive abilities such as memory, attention, and problem-solving skills. These programs use machine-learning algorithms to tailor exercises to individual needs, ensuring that the training is both effective and engaging. For example, platforms such as Lumosity and CogniFit use AI to adapt the difficulty of tasks in real time based on user performance, optimizing the training experience.
- *Virtual assistants and chatbots*: AI-powered virtual assistants and chatbots, such as Apple's Siri, Google Assistant, and specialized mental health bots such as Woebot, provide cognitive support by offering reminders, answering questions, and even delivering cognitive-behavioral therapy (CBT). These tools can help individuals manage daily tasks, reduce cognitive load, and access mental health resources on demand.

Artificial Intelligence in Mental Health Diagnosis and Treatment

- *Predictive analytics*: AI-powered predictive analytics can analyze data from various sources, including electronic health records (EHRs), social media, and wearable devices, to predict the onset or progression of mental health conditions. For instance, machine-learning models can identify early signs of depression or anxiety by analyzing changes in speech patterns, social media activity, or physiological data from wearables. Early detection allows for timely intervention, potentially preventing the condition from worsening.
- *Personalized treatment plans*: AI can help create personalized treatment plans by analyzing patient data and identifying the most effective interventions. For example, AI algorithms can predict how a patient might respond to different medications based on their genetic makeup, medical history, and other factors. This personalized approach increases the likelihood of treatment success and reduces the trial-and-error process often associated with mental health treatment.
- *Enhancing accessibility and reducing stigma*: One of the most significant benefits of AI in mental health is its ability to enhance accessibility to care and reduce stigma associated with seeking help.
- *Teletherapy and remote monitoring*: AI-powered teletherapy platforms, such as Talkspace and BetterHelp, connect patients with licensed therapists through text, audio, or video calls. These platforms often incorporate AI to match patients with therapists who best meet their needs. Additionally, remote monitoring tools using AI can track patient's progress and provide real-time feedback to clinicians, enabling continuous care and support.
- *Anonymous support and self-help tools*: AI-driven mental health apps and chatbots offer anonymous support, making it easier for individuals to seek help without fear of judgment.

Challenges and Ethical Considerations

Despite the promising potential of AI in mental health, there are several challenges and ethical considerations that must be addressed. These include:

- Data privacy and security
- Bias and fairness
- Human–AI interaction

Future Directions

The future of AI in cognitive support and mental health holds exciting possibilities.

- *Integrating AI with neurotechnology*: Integrating AI with neurotechnology, such as brain–computer interfaces (BCIs) and neurofeedback systems, could offer new ways to monitor and treat mental health conditions. For instance, AI algorithms could analyze brain activity in real time to provide personalized neurofeedback, helping individuals manage symptoms of disorders such as attention-deficit/hyperactivity disorder (ADHD) or posttraumatic stress disorder (PTSD).
- *Expanding access to underserved populations*: AI has the potential to expand access to mental health care in underserved and remote areas. mHealth applications and AI-powered platforms can deliver mental health services to individuals who might otherwise have limited access to care due to geographic or socioeconomic barriers.

Artificial intelligence is transforming the landscape of cognitive support and mental health, offering innovative solutions to enhance diagnosis, treatment, and accessibility. While there are challenges and ethical considerations to address, the potential benefits of AI in this field are immense. By leveraging AI technologies responsibly, we can improve mental health outcomes, reduce stigma, and provide more personalized and effective care for individuals worldwide.

MEDICAL IMAGING AND DIAGNOSTIC AND ARTIFICIAL INTELLIGENCE

Artificial intelligence is transforming the field of medical imaging and diagnosis. By harnessing the power of machine-learning and deep-learning algorithms, AI can analyze vast amounts of imaging data quickly and accurately.

Role of Artificial Intelligence in Medical Imaging

Medical imaging is a crucial component of modern health care, aiding in the diagnosis, treatment planning, and monitoring of various conditions. AI technologies enhance the capabilities of medical imaging by providing tools for image acquisition, processing, and interpretation.

- *Image acquisition and preprocessing*: AI algorithms can optimize image acquisition by adjusting parameters in real time to ensure high-quality images while minimizing radiation exposure.
- *Image analysis and interpretation*: The most significant impact of AI in medical imaging is seen in image analysis and interpretation. AI algorithms can analyze images from various modalities, such as X-rays, CT scans, MRI, and ultrasound, to identify abnormalities, segment tissues, and quantify anatomical structures.
- *Detection and diagnosis*: AI systems can detect and diagnose a wide range of conditions, including cancers, cardiovascular diseases, neurological disorders, and musculoskeletal conditions. For instance, AI algorithms have demonstrated high accuracy in detecting lung nodules on chest X-rays and mammographic lesions in breast cancer screening. These systems often outperform human radiologists in certain tasks, offering a second opinion and reducing diagnostic errors.
- *Segmentation and quantification*: AI-driven segmentation tools can delineate organs, tissues, and lesions with high precision. This capability is vital for tasks such as tumor volume measurement, organ contouring for radiation therapy planning, and tracking disease progression. Quantitative analysis provided by AI aids in objective and reproducible assessments, improving treatment planning and monitoring.

Benefits of Artificial Intelligence in Medical Imaging

The integration of AI in medical imaging offers numerous benefits, enhancing the quality, efficiency, and accessibility of health care.

- *Improved diagnostic accuracy*
- *Enhanced efficiency and workflow*: AI can automate time-consuming tasks such as image segmentation, quantification, and reporting. This automation frees up radiologists to focus on more complex cases and clinical decision-making.
- *Increased accessibility to expertise*: AI can democratize access to high-quality diagnostic services, particularly in underserved or remote areas. Cloud-based AI platforms enable healthcare providers to upload images for analysis, receiving expert-level interpretations without the need for on-site radiologists.
- Personalized medicine

Challenges and Ethical Considerations

Despite the promising potential of AI in medical imaging, several challenges and ethical considerations must be addressed.

- *Data quality and diversity*: AI algorithms require large, high-quality datasets for training. Ensuring that these datasets are diverse and representative is crucial to avoid biases that could lead to disparities in diagnostic accuracy across different populations.
- *Interpretability and transparency*: AI algorithms, particularly deep-learning models, often function as "black boxes," making it difficult to understand how they arrive at their conclusions.
- *Regulatory and legal issues*: The use of AI in medical imaging is subject to regulatory approval and oversight to ensure safety and efficacy. Additionally, legal issues related to liability, data privacy, and intellectual property must be carefully navigated.
- *Integration with clinical workflows*: Successful integration of AI into clinical workflows requires careful consideration of existing practices and infrastructure. AI systems should complement, not disrupt, the work of healthcare professionals.

Future Directions

The future of AI in medical imaging and diagnosis is bright, with ongoing research and development aimed at enhancing its capabilities and expanding its applications.

- *Multimodal data integration*: Integrating imaging data with other types of clinical data, such as genomics, pathology, and EHRs, will enable more comprehensive and accurate diagnoses.
- *Real-time analysis and decision support*: Advances in AI and computing power will enable real-time analysis of medical images, providing immediate feedback to clinicians during procedures such as surgeries and interventions. AI-driven decision support systems can assist in intraoperative planning, guiding surgeons with real-time information and recommendations.
- *Collaborative AI and human intelligence*: AI can augment the expertise of radiologists, providing tools

for enhanced visualization, automated measurements, and clinical decision support. This synergy will lead to improved diagnostic accuracy and patient outcomes.

- *AI in medical imaging education*: AI can also play a role in medical imaging education and training. Virtual reality (VR) and augmented reality (AR) platforms powered by AI can simulate clinical scenarios, providing trainees with hands-on experience and feedback. These technologies can enhance learning and skill development, preparing future radiologists for the integration of AI in their practice.

PREDICTIVE ANALYTICS AND RISK STRATIFICATION

Predictive analytics and risk stratification are vital components of modern health care, enabling early detection of diseases, personalized treatment plans, and efficient resource allocation.

Predictive Analytics in Health Care

Predictive analytics involves using historical and real-time data to forecast future outcomes. In health care, it helps predict disease onset, patient outcomes, and treatment responses, among other things.

- *Disease prediction and early detection*: AI algorithms can analyze patient data from EHRs, genetic information, and lifestyle factors to predict the likelihood of developing certain diseases. For instance, AI models can identify individuals at high risk of developing diabetes, cardiovascular diseases, or certain cancers, enabling proactive interventions.
  Case study—diabetes prediction: AI systems can analyze a combination of EHR data, including laboratory results, medication history, and lifestyle factors, to predict the onset of diabetes. By identifying at-risk individuals early, healthcare providers can implement preventive measures such as lifestyle modifications and monitoring, potentially delaying or preventing the disease.
- *Patient outcome prediction*: AI can predict patient outcomes by analyzing clinical data and identifying patterns that indicate likely results of treatments or disease progression.
  Case study—predicting sepsis in intensive care unit (ICU) patients: Sepsis is a life-threatening condition that requires early detection and intervention. AI algorithms can analyze data from ICU monitors, laboratory results, and patient histories to predict the onset of sepsis hours before clinical symptoms become evident. Early prediction allows for timely treatment, reducing mortality rates.
- *Risk stratification with AI:* Risk stratification involves categorizing patients based on their likelihood of experiencing adverse health outcomes. AI enhances risk stratification by providing more accurate and granular risk assessments, enabling targeted interventions and efficient resource allocation.
- *Identifying high-risk patients*: AI models can identify high-risk patients by analyzing various data points, including demographics, medical history, and real-time health data.
  Case study—heart failure risk stratification: For patients with heart failure, AI can analyze data such as EHRs, imaging results, and wearable device data to assess the risk of readmission or adverse events. By identifying high-risk patients, healthcare providers can implement intensive monitoring and tailored interventions, reducing hospital readmissions and improving patient quality of life.
- *Personalized treatment plan*
  Case study—personalized oncology treatment: In oncology, AI can analyze genetic data, tumor characteristics, and patient history to stratify patients based on their risk of treatment failure or relapse. This information allows oncologists to design personalized treatment plans, selecting therapies that are most likely to be effective for each patient, thereby improving outcomes and minimizing side effects.

Benefits of Artificial Intelligence in Predictive Analytics and Risk Stratification

The integration of AI in predictive analytics and risk stratification offers numerous benefits, transforming healthcare delivery and patient outcomes, which include:

- Improved accuracy and efficiency
- Proactive and preventive care
- Optimized resource allocation
- Personalized medicine

Challenges and Ethical Considerations

Despite the promising potential of AI in predictive analytics and risk stratification, several challenges and ethical considerations must be addressed.

- *Data quality and integration*: The accuracy of AI models depends on the quality and comprehensiveness of the data they are trained on. Ensuring high-quality data from diverse sources and integrating disparate datasets are ongoing challenges. Standardizing data formats and improving data-sharing protocols can help address these issues.
- Bias and fairness
- *Privacy and security*: The use of AI in predictive analytics and risk stratification involves handling

sensitive personal health data. Ensuring data privacy and security is paramount to maintaining patient trust and complying with regulations.

- *Interpretability and transparency*: AI models, particularly deep-learning algorithms, often function as "black boxes," making it challenging to understand how they arrive at their predictions.

DRUG DISCOVERY AND DEVELOPMENT

The process of drug discovery and development is complex, costly, and time-consuming, often taking over a decade and billions of dollars to bring a new drug to market. AI has emerged as a transformative force in this field, offering innovative solutions to streamline and enhance various stages of drug discovery and development.

Artificial Intelligence in Drug Discovery

Drug discovery involves identifying potential drug candidates that can modulate biological targets implicated in diseases. AI enhances this process by leveraging machine learning algorithms, deep-learning models, and large datasets to identify promising compounds more efficiently and accurately.

- *Target identification and validation*: Target identification involves discovering biological targets, such as proteins or genes, that are associated with diseases. AI can analyze vast amounts of biomedical data, including genomic, proteomic, and clinical data, to identify and validate potential targets.
  Case study—identifying new drug targets for cancer: AI algorithms can mine genomic and transcriptomic data to identify genes that are overexpressed in cancer cells but not in normal cells. By pinpointing these genes, AI helps researchers identify potential targets for new cancer therapies. For example, IBM Watson for Drug Discovery uses natural language processing (NLP) and machine learning to analyze scientific literature and genomic data, uncovering novel targets for oncology.
- *Drug candidate screening*: Once potential targets are identified, the next step is to screen large libraries of chemical compounds to find those that can interact with the targets. AI accelerates this process by predicting the biological activity of compounds and their interactions with targets.
  Case study—virtual screening for antiviral drugs: During the COVID-19 pandemic, AI-driven virtual screening was used to rapidly identify potential antiviral compounds. Deep-learning models analyzed the structural features of the SARS-CoV-2 virus and screened millions of compounds to predict their binding affinity to viral proteins. This approach significantly reduced the time required to identify promising drug candidates.
- *Drug optimization*: AI can optimize drug candidates by predicting their pharmacokinetic and pharmacodynamic properties, such as absorption, distribution, metabolism, excretion, and toxicity (ADMET). This capability helps researchers design drugs with favorable properties, reducing the risk of failure in later stages.
  Case study—designing safer drugs with AI: Insilico Medicine used AI to design new compounds with improved ADMET properties. Their deep-learning models predicted the toxicity and metabolic stability of compounds, guiding the design of safer and more effective drugs. This approach led to the discovery of novel antifibrotic compounds with reduced toxicity.
- *Preclinical studies*: In preclinical studies, AI can analyze data from in vitro and in vivo experiments to predict the efficacy and safety of drug candidates. AI-driven analysis can identify biomarkers for efficacy and toxicity, guiding the selection of candidates for clinical trials.
  Case study—AI in preclinical toxicology: AI models can predict toxicological outcomes by analyzing data from animal studies and in vitro assays. For instance, companies such as Recursion Pharmaceuticals use AI to analyze cellular images and identify phenotypic changes indicative of toxicity. This approach helps in the early identification of toxic compounds, reducing the risk of failure in clinical trials.
- *Clinical trials*: AI can optimize clinical trial design, patient recruitment, and monitoring, enhancing the efficiency and success rates of trials.
  Case study—AI-driven clinical trial design: AI can analyze historical clinical trial data to design more efficient trials. For example, GNS Healthcare uses machine learning to predict patient responses and stratify patients into subgroups based on their likelihood of responding to treatments. This approach enables more targeted and efficient clinical trials, reducing costs and time to market.

Benefits of Artificial Intelligence in Drug Discovery and Development

- *Accelerated drug discovery*: AI can significantly reduce the time required for target identification, compound screening, and drug optimization.
- *Improved success rates*: AI enhances the accuracy of predictions related to target interactions, drug efficacy, and toxicity. This improvement reduces the likelihood of failures in preclinical and clinical stages, increasing the overall success rate of drug development.

- *Cost reduction*: By streamlining various stages of drug discovery and development, AI helps reduce costs associated with research and development.
- *Personalized medicine*: AI enables the development of personalized therapies by analyzing patient data and predicting individual responses to treatments.

Challenges and Ethical Considerations

Despite the promising potential of AI in drug discovery and development, several challenges and ethical considerations are there:

- Data quality and integration
- Bias and fairness
- Regulatory and legal issues
- Interpretability and transparency

Future Directions

Advances in AI, coupled with increasing access to data and improved understanding of disease mechanisms, will drive innovation and enhance the efficiency and success rates of drug development.

- *Integration with omics data*: Integrating AI with omics data, such as genomics, proteomics, and metabolomics, will enable a deeper understanding of disease mechanisms and identification of novel drug targets.
- *AI-driven drug repurposing*: AI can be used to identify new therapeutic uses for existing drugs, a process known as drug repurposing. By analyzing molecular structures, biological pathways, and clinical data, AI can predict alternative indications for approved drugs, potentially shortening development timelines and reducing costs.
- *Real-time monitoring and adaptive trials*: Advances in AI and real-time data collection will enable adaptive clinical trials that adjust protocols based on ongoing results. AI can analyze real-time patient data to identify trends and make adjustments, improving trial efficiency and success rates.
- *Collaborative AI and human intelligence*: The future of drug discovery and development will likely see increased collaboration between AI and human intelligence. AI can augment the expertise of researchers and clinicians, providing tools for enhanced data analysis, hypothesis generation, and decision-making. This synergy will lead to more efficient and successful drug development.

CLINICAL DECISION SUPPORT SYSTEM

Clinical decision support systems (CDSS) are integral tools in modern health care, designed to aid healthcare professionals in making informed decisions by providing evidence-based information and patient-specific recommendations. AI enhances CDSS by leveraging advanced algorithms and vast amounts of data to deliver more accurate, timely, and personalized support.

Artificial Intelligence in Clinical Decision Support Systems

AI-driven CDSS combine machine learning, NLP, and data analytics to provide clinicians with actionable insights.

- *Diagnosis assistance*: One of the primary applications of AI in CDSS is assisting in diagnosis. AI algorithms can analyze patient data, including symptoms, medical history, laboratory results, and imaging studies, to suggest potential diagnoses and differential diagnoses.
  Case study—IBM Watson for oncology: IBM Watson for oncology uses NLP and machine learning to analyze patient data and provide oncologists with evidence-based treatment recommendations. The system reviews vast amounts of medical literature and clinical guidelines to suggest personalized treatment options, improving the accuracy and speed of cancer diagnosis and treatment planning.
- *Treatment recommendations*: AI-driven CDSS can recommend personalized treatment plans based on patient-specific data and clinical guidelines. These recommendations consider factors such as comorbidities, medication interactions, and patient preferences, ensuring that treatment plans are tailored to individual needs.
  Case study—treatment pathways in diabetes management: AI-based CDSS can assist in managing chronic conditions such as diabetes, by analyzing patient data and recommending treatment adjustments. For example, an AI system might suggest changes in insulin dosage based on real-time glucose monitoring data, improving glycemic control and reducing the risk of complications.
- *Prognostic predictions*: AI algorithms can predict patient outcomes by analyzing clinical data and identifying risk factors. These predictions help clinicians anticipate potential complications and intervene early to improve patient outcomes.
  Case study—predicting hospital readmissions: AI-driven CDSS can analyze EHR data to predict the likelihood of hospital readmissions for patients with chronic conditions. By identifying high-risk patients, healthcare providers can implement targeted interventions, such as follow-up appointments and patient education, to reduce readmission rates and improve care quality.
- *Workflow optimization*: AI can optimize clinical workflows by automating routine tasks, prioritizing

patient care based on urgency, and providing decision support at the point of care. This optimization enhances efficiency and allows clinicians to focus on complex cases and patient interactions.

Case study—triage in emergency departments: AI-based triage systems can analyze patient symptoms and vital signs to prioritize cases in emergency departments. These systems help ensure that patients with the most critical conditions receive timely care, improving outcomes and reducing wait times.

TELEMEDICINE

Telemedicine has revolutionized health care by providing remote access to medical services, reducing the need for in-person visits, and expanding the reach of healthcare providers.

Artificial Intelligence in Telemedicine

AI-driven telemedicine leverages machine learning, NLP, and data analytics to improve patient care and streamline healthcare delivery. By integrating AI with telemedicine platforms, healthcare providers can offer more accurate, efficient, and personalized care to patients regardless of their location.

- *Remote diagnostics*: AI algorithms can analyze patient data, including medical history, symptoms, and diagnostic tests, to provide remote diagnostic support. This capability is particularly valuable in telemedicine, where physical examinations are limited.
  Case study—AI in dermatology: AI-powered tools such as SkinVision and DermAI can analyze images of skin lesions uploaded by patients through telemedicine platforms. This approach enables early detection and timely intervention, even when in-person dermatology visits are not feasible.
- *Personalized treatment recommendations*: AI can offer personalized treatment recommendations based on patient-specific data, including medical history, genetic information, and lifestyle factors. Telemedicine platforms can integrate these recommendations to provide tailored care plans during virtual consultations.
- *Virtual health assistants*: AI-powered virtual health assistants can interact with patients through telemedicine platforms, providing information, answering questions, and assisting with routine tasks. These assistants enhance patient engagement and support self-management of health conditions.
  Case study—chatbots for mental health support: AI chatbots such as Woebot and Wysa offer mental health support through telemedicine platforms by engaging in natural language conversations with users. These chatbots use AI to provide CBT techniques, mood tracking, and coping strategies, offering immediate support and resources to individuals experiencing mental health challenges.
- *Predictive analytics and risk stratification*: AI can analyze patient data to predict health outcomes and stratify patients based on their risk of developing certain conditions. Telemedicine platforms can use these insights to prioritize care and allocate resources effectively.

Future Directions

Advances in AI, coupled with increasing access to data and improved connectivity, will drive innovation and enhance the capabilities of telemedicine platforms.

- *Integration with wearable devices and Internet of Things (IoT)*: Integrating AI with wearable devices and the IoT will provide real-time health monitoring and decision support. Wearable devices can collect continuous data on vital signs, physical activity, and other health metrics, enabling AI to deliver real-time recommendations and alerts. This integration will enhance RPM and proactive care.
- *Advanced predictive analytics*: Advances in AI and machine learning will enable more sophisticated predictive analytics, allowing telemedicine platforms to provide even more accurate and timely predictions. These improvements will enhance early detection of diseases, risk stratification, and personalized treatment planning.
- *Collaborative AI and human intelligence*: The future of telemedicine will likely see increased collaboration between AI and human intelligence. AI can augment the expertise of healthcare providers, providing tools for enhanced data analysis, hypothesis generation, and decision-making. This synergy will lead to more efficient and effective care delivery.
- *Telemedicine for specialized care*: AI-driven telemedicine will expand its applications to specialized care areas, such as cardiology, neurology, and pediatrics. AI tools can assist specialists by providing advanced diagnostic support, treatment recommendations, and patient monitoring, improving care quality and outcomes in these fields.

HEALTHCARE ADMINISTRATION

Healthcare operations and administration encompass a wide range of activities, including patient management, resource allocation, scheduling, billing, and overall organizational efficiency. AI has the potential to revolutionize these aspects by automating routine tasks, optimizing resource use, enhancing decision making, and improving patient outcomes.

- *Patient management*: AI-driven systems can streamline patient management by automating administrative tasks, managing patient flow, and personalizing care.
  Case study—patient scheduling: AI algorithms can optimize patient scheduling by analyzing appointment types, clinician availability, and patient preferences. For example, AI tools such as Zocdoc use machine learning to match patients with the best available appointment slots, reducing wait times and no-show rates. This leads to more efficient use of clinical resources and improved patient satisfaction.
  Case study—patient flow optimization: In hospital settings, AI can predict patient admissions, discharges, and transfers to manage bed occupancy and reduce overcrowding. Tools such as Qventus use AI to analyze real-time data from EHRs and other sources to predict patient flow and suggest interventions, improving overall hospital efficiency.
- *Resource allocation*: AI can optimize the allocation of healthcare resources, such as staffing, equipment, and facilities, ensuring that they are used efficiently and effectively.
  Case study—staff scheduling: AI-driven workforce management systems can create optimal staff schedules by considering factors such as staff availability, skill sets, and patient demand. Tools like Kronos use AI to predict staffing needs and automate schedule creation, reducing administrative burden and improving staff satisfaction.
  Case study—equipment utilization: AI can analyze data on the use of medical equipment to identify patterns and optimize utilization. For instance, AI systems can predict when imaging machines or surgical suites will be needed, ensuring that they are available when required and reducing downtime.
- *Workflow optimization*: AI can streamline workflows by automating routine tasks and enhancing decision-making processes.
  Case study—automated billing and coding: AI-powered billing and coding systems can analyze clinical notes and automatically generate accurate billing codes, reducing errors and administrative workload. Companies such as Olive use AI to automate revenue cycle management, ensuring timely and accurate billing.
  Case study—clinical documentation: NLP algorithms can assist with clinical documentation by transcribing and summarizing patient interactions. Tools such as Nuance's Dragon Medical One use NLP to convert speech into structured EHR entries, allowing clinicians to focus more on patient care and less on paperwork.
- *AI in healthcare administration*: AI applications in healthcare administration focus on improving decision-making, enhancing strategic planning, and optimizing organizational performance.
- *Decision support*: AI can provide administrators with data-driven insights to inform decision-making and strategic planning.
  Case study—predictive analytics for decision-making: AI-driven predictive analytics can help administrators forecast trends, such as patient demand, financial performance, and operational efficiency. For example, health systems can use AI to predict seasonal variations in patient volume and adjust staffing and resource allocation accordingly.
- *Strategic planning*: AI can assist with strategic planning by analyzing large datasets to identify opportunities for improvement and innovation.
  Case study—population health management: AI can analyze population health data to identify at-risk groups and inform interventions. For instance, AI tools can identify trends in chronic disease prevalence and suggest community health initiatives to address these issues, guiding strategic planning and resource allocation.
- *Performance optimization*: AI can monitor and evaluate organizational performance, identifying areas for improvement and suggesting actionable insights.
  Case study—operational efficiency: AI-driven dashboards can provide real-time insights into key performance indicators (KPIs), such as patient satisfaction, staff productivity, and financial metrics. Administrators can use these insights to identify inefficiencies and implement targeted improvements.

Benefits of Artificial Intelligence in Healthcare Operations and Administration

The integration of AI in healthcare operations and administration offers numerous benefits, including enhanced efficiency, cost reduction, improved patient outcomes, and better resource management.

Future Directions

- *Advanced predictive analytics*: Advances in AI and machine learning will enable more sophisticated predictive analytics, allowing healthcare administrators to anticipate trends and make data-driven decisions. These improvements will enhance strategic planning, resource allocation, and operational efficiency.
- *Integration with IoT and wearable devices*: Integrating AI with the IoT and wearable devices will provide real-time data for operational decision-making.

For example, IoT-enabled equipment can provide data on usage patterns, maintenance needs, and availability, allowing for more efficient resource management.

- *Collaborative AI and human intelligence*: AI can augment the expertise of healthcare administrators, providing tools for enhanced data analysis, hypothesis generation, and decision-making. This synergy will lead to more efficient and effective healthcare delivery.
- *AI in healthcare policy and regulation*: AI can also play a role in shaping healthcare policy and regulation by providing insights into healthcare trends, outcomes, and best practices. Policymakers can use AI-driven analytics to inform decisions and develop evidence-based policies that improve healthcare systems.

SMART HOME AND INDEPENDENT LIVING FOR ELDERLY

Smart homes are homes with technologically advanced systems to enable domestic task automation, easier communication, and higher security. As the global population ages, the demand for effective elderly care solutions has become increasingly important. Smart home technology offers a promising avenue to enhance the quality of life for older adults, promoting independence, safety, and health. This section explores the various smart home technologies that can support elderly care, examining their benefits, applications, and considerations.

Enhancing Safety and Security

Safety is a primary concern in elderly care, and smart home technology offers several solutions to address this **(Figs. 5A and B)**:

- *Fall detection sensors*: Falls are a common risk for older adults and can lead to severe injuries. Fall detection sensors use advanced algorithms and motion detection to identify falls and automatically alert emergency services or family members.
- *Smart locks and doorbells*: Smart locks allow caregivers and family members to remotely control and monitor access to the home. Video doorbells provide real-time footage of visitors, enhancing security and reducing the risk of unwanted intrusions.
- *Motion sensors*: Motion sensors can track daily activity patterns and send alerts if there is an unusual lack of movement, potentially indicating a problem. These sensors can also trigger automated lighting to prevent accidents in the dark.

Health Monitoring

Maintaining health and managing medical conditions are crucial aspects of elderly care. Smart home devices can assist in these areas:

- *Smart medical devices*: Devices such as blood pressure monitors, glucose monitors, and heart rate monitors can automatically record health metrics and share data with healthcare providers. This continuous monitoring helps in the early detection of health issues.
- *Medication reminders*: Smart medication dispensers and reminder systems ensure that medications are taken on time. These systems can send alerts to caregivers if a dose is missed.

Enhancing Convenience

Smart home technology can simplify daily tasks, making life easier for elderly individuals:

- *Voice assistants*: Voice-activated assistants such as Amazon Echo and Google Home can provide reminders, control other smart devices, and make calls. These assistants can also answer questions and play music, providing companionship and entertainment.
- *Smart lighting*: Automated lighting systems can be programmed to turn lights on and off at specific times, ensuring that the home is well lit when needed and conserving energy when it is not.

Social Connection

Maintaining social connections is vital for mental and emotional well-being. Smart home devices can help:

- *Video calling*: Smart displays and tablets with video calling capabilities make it easy for elderly individuals to stay in touch with family and friends. Regular face-to-face interaction, even virtually, can reduce feelings of isolation.
- *Social robots*: Some advanced social robots are designed to provide companionship and assist with simple tasks. These robots can interact with users, play games, and even remind them to take their medications.

Energy Management

Energy management not only contributes to a comfortable living environment but also helps in cost savings:

- *Smart thermostats*: Smart thermostats can learn user preferences and adjust the temperature to maintain comfort while optimizing energy usage. Remote control features allow caregivers to adjust settings as needed.

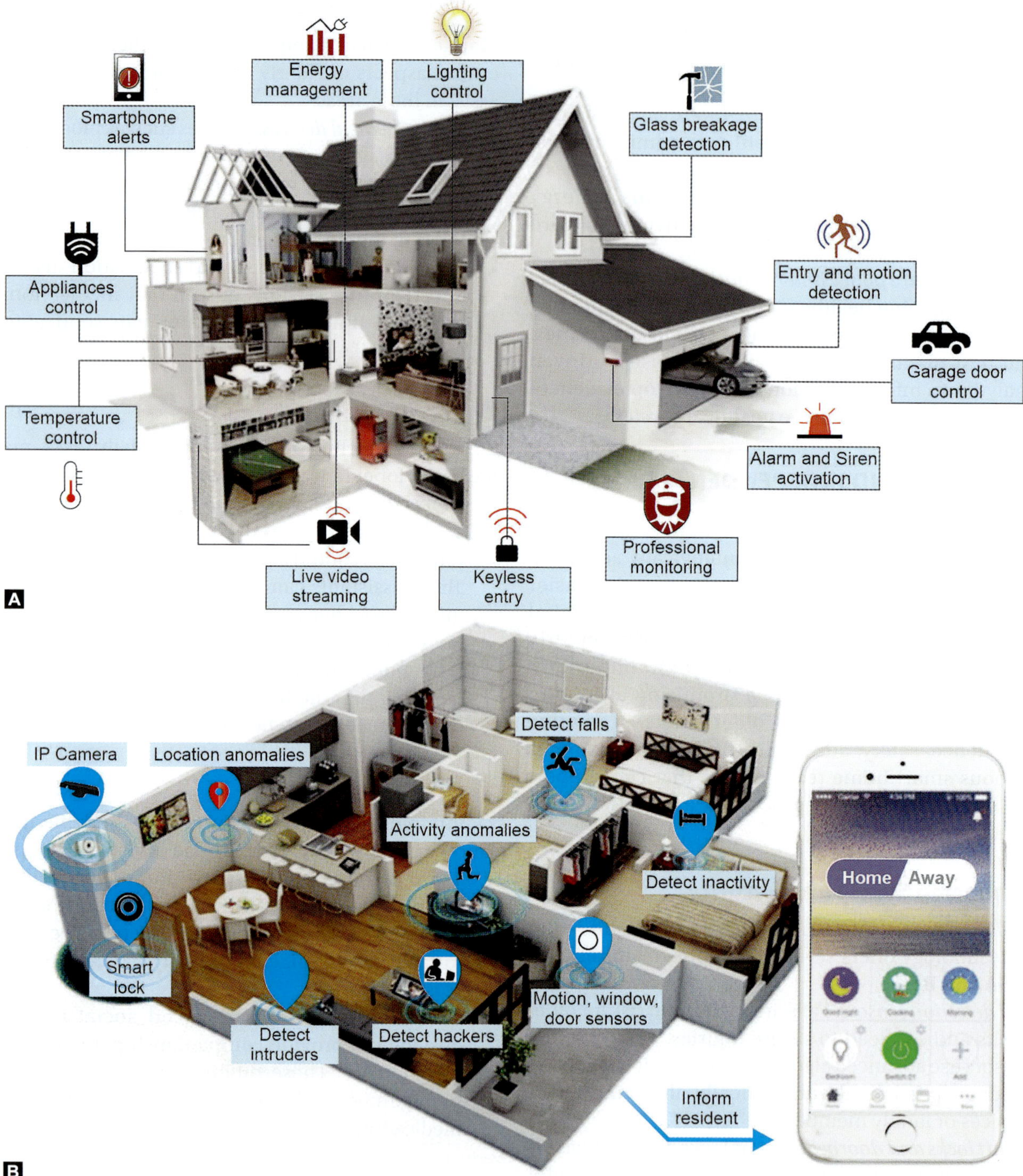

FIGS. 5A AND B: (A) General overview of smart home infrastructure; and (B) Artificial intelligence-driven monitoring with mobile interface integration for activity and safety management.

- *Smart plugs*: Smart plugs enable remote control of appliances, ensuring that devices are turned off when not in use, preventing potential hazards and saving energy.

Home Automation

Automation of daily routines can significantly enhance the quality of life for elderly individuals:

Routine automation: Schedules can be set for various devices, such as lights, coffee machines, and blinds. Automation of these routines reduces the physical effort required and helps maintain a consistent daily schedule.

Considerations and Challenges

While smart home technology offers many benefits, there are also considerations and challenges to address:

- *Privacy and security*: Data privacy and security are paramount. Ensuring that devices are secure from hacking and that personal data is protected is essential.
- *Usability*: The usability of smart home devices is crucial. They must be easy to set up and operate, especially for individuals who may not be tech-savvy.
- *Cost*: The cost of smart home devices can be a barrier for some. Evaluating the cost-benefit ratio and exploring options for financial assistance can help mitigate this challenge.

Smart home technology holds significant potential to transform elderly care, promoting safety, health, and independence. By thoughtfully integrating these technologies, caregivers can provide better support, and elderly individuals can enjoy a higher quality of life. As technology continues to advance, the capabilities and accessibility of smart home solutions for elderly care are likely to expand, offering even greater benefits in the future.

CONCLUSION

Artificial intelligence has the potential in revolutionizing elderly healthcare by offering personalized health solutions, enhanced remote monitoring, and rapid emergency interventions. AI integration has been initiated in few important domains like early detection and accurate assessments, cognitive training, personalized rehabilitation, to enhance quality care. There is substantial work is going on predictive analytics and risk stratification for proactive and preventive care, optimizing resources and customizing treatments for individuals. Smart home technologies along with remote monitoring would be a great help to the older adults to live independently and safely, but maintaining privacy.

Self-Assessment Questionnaire

Q1. How can artificial intelligence enhance the independence and safety of elderly individuals living alone?

Q2. How precision medicine differ from conventional medical treatment approaches, and how does AI support its implementation?

Q3. How do AI-based remote monitoring systems improve outcomes for elderly patients with chronic conditions?

Q4. What ethical challenges must be addressed when integrating AI into healthcare, especially concerning privacy and data security for older adults?

Q5. How can AI tools contribute to mental health and cognitive support for the elderly population?

Q6. What are the key benefits and potential pitfalls of using AI for predictive analytics and risk stratification in older adults?

Q7. What roles do telemedicine and smart home technologies play in promoting healthy and independent aging?

CHAPTER 41

Palliative Care in Geriatric Care

Sushma Bhatnagar, Neethu Susan Abraham

INTRODUCTION

There is an increasing life expectancy with advancements in medical science, and as a result, adults in the older age group (>65 years) are rising. They may have multiple comorbidities that need an interdisciplinary team approach for providing better care. The life expectancy among women and men is 84 and 79 years, respectively, in the European Union, and the period with comorbidity is approximately 25 and 20 years, respectively. Similarly, in the United States, three out of four older people have multiple comorbidities, and >50% have pain.

A geriatrician attends to patients of age more than 65 years. However, attending to patients of age more than 80 years may be challenging, as patients are more frail, have heavy symptom burdens, and have multiple comorbidities. The geriatrician's chief goal is to generate a better living standard for older individuals to make them active and less dependent.

A palliative physician deals with all patients irrespective of their age and provide holistic care, symptom management, caregiver support, and improvement of quality of life. Geriatric patients may need better pain and other symptom management as they are more sensitive and frail which palliative physicians can provide. There is an overlap between the care provided by geriatric and palliative medicine specialties, and their integration can help in providing better care to older patients.

Palliative care is defined by World Health Organization (WHO) as an approach that improves the quality of life of patients and their families facing issues associated with life-threatening illness, by prevention and relief of suffering through early identification, impeccable assessment and treatment of pain and other issues—physical, psychosocial, and spiritual.

CONCEPT OF GERIATRIC PALLIATIVE MEDICINE

Geriatric palliative medicine (GPM) is the provision of medical care and management of elderly patients with advanced diseases and limited prognosis, with care focused on the quality of life. Thus, GPM is a combination of both geriatric medicine and palliative care principles. The principles are given as follows:

- Concentration on comprehensive geriatric assessment, pain, and other physical symptom management, and addressing social, emotional, and spiritual issues
- Understanding of symptoms and disease, the need for safe drug prescription, and recognition of the significance of a multidisciplinary tailored approach for older patients and their families getting palliative care
- Highlighting the autonomy and involvement of patients in decision-making
- Emphasizes good communication skills while prognostication and discussion
- Focus on addressing the various concerns of patients and families in various environments such as homes, hospitals, and hospices, as well as special attention during transitions across settings
- Provision of family support during the end-of-life care

DOMAINS OF PALLIATIVE CARE

The National Consensus Project for Quality Palliative Care (NCPQPC) describes eight domains of palliative care: (1) Its structure and processes; (2) physical aspects; (3) psychological and psychiatric aspects; (4) social aspects; (5) spiritual, religious, and existential aspects; (6) cultural aspects; (7) end-of-life care; and (8) ethical and legal aspects of care.

Structure and Process of Care

Palliative care includes both primary and specialist palliative care. Primary palliative care involves the initial addressal of symptoms and routine discussions regarding prognosis, care goals, etc. Institutions that do not have specialist palliative care access make use of primary palliative care for the general needs of patients who have serious illnesses. Primary palliative care is to be given by the geriatrics team in the hospital who is the immediate physician. In order to meet the needs of patients and families, various models of palliative care delivery are employed according to patient conditions and preferences.

Physical Aspects of Care

Palliative care consultation has been shown to make improvements in the management of physical symptoms. Palliative care teams can provide safe and effective treatment recommendations as they are experts in the management of advanced symptoms. Palliative care consultations result in higher patient satisfaction, decreased duration of stay, lower overall costs, and reduced readmission and intensive care unit (ICU) admission rates. The physical symptoms experienced by older patients are different in terms of prevalence and presentation. The assessment of symptoms may be challenging for the elderly. The Edmonton Symptom Assessment Tool-Revised (r-ESAS) may be used to measure symptoms. It is important to manage geriatric symptoms such as frailty and comorbidity, as these patients have more chances for increased palliative care needs.

Psychological and Psychiatric Aspects of Care

Issues such as mood disorders, anxiety, delirium, substance-use disorders, and post-traumatic stress disorder need assessment, and addressal can be done by palliative physicians. Significant patient and family distress can be caused by delirium which may limit patients' capacity for decision-making and may be addressed by the palliative care team. They also screen patients for depression. Social workers who are focused on palliative care are trained for screening and intervention in psychological issues. Palliative care physicians may seek professional help and refer to psychiatrists, psychologists, or counselors for expert management of the emotional health concerns of patients.

Social Aspects of Care

Palliative care offers quality social care, including care of the family. Caring for the family following assessment forms a key component of social care in the palliative framework. Bereavement support is also provided by the palliative team. Elderly patients may experience social isolation and have a rise in mortality rates, depression rates, and psychological distress. Subjective well-being, improved quality of life, and physical function can be obtained by better social engagement.

Religious, Spiritual, and Existential Aspects of Care

Spiritual care delivery plays an important role in palliative care among geriatric patients. In older patients, physical functioning and social support are chiefly predicted by religiousness and spirituality. They are associated with fewer depressive symptoms, improved cognition, and better cooperation. Poor quality of life, distress, poor well-being, and confusion may accompany negative religious coping.

Cultural Aspects of Care

Culture can be a complex social structure formed through various factors that confer different values, responsibilities, opportunities, practices, and expectations upon its participants. Cultural differences are more common among geriatric patients from their hospital care teams. Cultural problems may be significant barriers to patients getting high-quality end-of-life care. Culturally different populations might need trust to establish a better healthcare relationship, and hence the significance of specialists attending to cultural needs. A cultural assessment is mandatory for a comprehensive palliative care assessment. Best practices include presence, time, cultural respect, communication, etc. The multidisciplinary palliative care team plays a key role in the provision of cultural care. Palliative care team collaboration helps for a deeper knowledge of culture, and attention is provided to issues of older patients.

End-of-life Care

There is a period of the irreversible decline of functional status prior to death which is defined as the terminal phase. It may last from hours to days and occasionally to weeks. When patients are expected to die within the next 12 months, their end of life is approaching. During the end of life, the focus of care is shifted from treatments aimed at cure or life prolongation to symptom control, comfort measures, dignity, and providing a better quality of life. In the last phase, patients can have various symptoms such as loss of weight, dysphagia, change in breathing pattern, decreased urine output, refractory delirium, cold skin, fatigue, social withdrawal, disinterest, and drowsiness. There should be proper recognition of this phase, an early care plan for the patient, family preparation, conversations involving anticipation of symptoms and control, death place preferences, etc.

Ethical and Legal Aspects of Care

The palliative care team assists with medicolegal issues that happen while caring for elderly with serious illnesses. The palliative care team is involved in the ethical or legal aspects, including autonomy, surrogate decision-making, disclosure of information, withholding or withdrawing treatment, artificial nutrition and hydration, and futility of treatment.

APPROACH FOR PALLIATIVE CARE DISCUSSION IN ELDERLY

- Explaining the objectives and goals for the patient
- To help create advance directives
- Early discussion involving families, especially in patients with dementia
- Conducting accurate and clear discussions on the pros and cons of aggressive approaches and palliative approaches for the chronic issues of the elderly
- Describing benefits versus risks of hospitalization, medications, tests, and monitoring in the treatment of chronic problems
- Coordinating care among various providers and doctors
- Discussion of alternatives to aggressive management
- Discussion regarding depression, risk of falls, etc.
- Provision of caregiver support

SYSTEMIC CHANGES IN THE OLD INDIVIDUALS AND THEIR IMPLICATIONS

Cardiovascular System

- Reduced cardiac output leading to slower body distribution of medications
- Increased blood pressure and atherosclerosis can result in a higher risk of vascular events and other cardiovascular complications requiring treatment and hospitalization

Genitourinary System

- Decreased renal reserve for recovery from nephrotoxic agents
- Increased incidence of chronic kidney disease (CKD), prostatic enlargement, and atrophy of the uterus, vagina, and breast, due to decreased hormone levels
- Increased incidence of stress incontinence
- Less number of nephrons and decreased glomerular filtration rate, resulting in decreased excretion of drugs by the kidney, requiring cautious monitoring of drugs excreted through the kidney

Neurological System

- Decreased proprioception
- Impairment of cognition and cortical atrophy causing variations in processing and reporting of pain
- Autonomic neuropathy leading to altered responses and injury risks
- Risk of delirium
- Decreased stores of choline and dopamine
- Forgetfulness, depression, Parkinson's disease, insomnia, etc., which may require therapy

Respiratory System

- Decreased respiratory reserve
- Increased incidence of pulmonary diseases

Gastrointestinal and Hepatic System

- Less hepatocytes and decreased hepatic blood flow leading to reduced metabolic drug elimination
- Decreased gastrointestinal transit altering intestinal absorption of medications
- Decreased albumin levels resulting in increased free drugs and toxicities

Musculoskeletal System

- Muscular atrophy can lead to reduced volume of distribution (Vd).
- Increased fat results in a longer duration of action of lipid-soluble drugs.
- The Vd of lipophilic drugs gets increased needing an increased dose and the Vd of hydrophilic drugs gets reduced needing a low dose.
- Reduced bone density leading to osteoporosis, fractures, and functional impairment requiring treatment, hospitalization, etc.

Skin Changes and Sensory Functions

- There is a reduction in proteins such as elastin and collagen, leading to decreased skin elasticity
- Thinning of epidermis due to decreased cell renewal
- Decreased sensorial perception, visual acuity, and hearing

BARRIERS AND FACILITATORS FOR COLLABORATION BETWEEN GERIATRIC MEDICINE AND PALLIATIVE CARE

Barriers and facilitators may be at clinical practice, education, training, or policy levels. Less awareness and understanding regarding the other specialties and lack of communication may be an important barrier. Inadequate educational opportunities and shared training, a limited number of academic chairs in both specialties, organization, and financing of health care can also act as barriers to collaboration between geriatric and palliative medicine.

Facilitators may be advance care planning, sharing of palliative care and geriatric medicine perspectives at platforms such as conferences, mandatory internships within the other disciplines, cross-disciplinary works, multidisciplinary teamwork, expert advice and consultation from the other disciplines, strong leadership, and establishing taskforces.

GERIATRIC-SPECIFIC SYNDROMES AND PALLIATIVE CARE

- The major geriatric syndromes are frailty, delirium, dizziness, urinary incontinence, insomnia, falls, malnourishment, pain, and depression.
- Etiology may be multifactorial.
- In clinical practice, geriatric syndromes are associated with poor outcomes and significant morbidity.
- Their prevalence is high in elderly frail patients.

FEW GERIATRIC SYNDROMES: POTENTIAL SCREENING TOOLS AND INTERVENTIONS

Falls

Screening tools: Fall history, timed up and go test, gait speed assessment.

Intervention: Review of medications, visual checkups, monitoring of blood pressure in different positions, footwear checks, evaluation of safety at home, physical and occupational therapies, referral for balance and muscle strength training, exercise programs at home, counseling for prevention of falls, etc.

Cognitive Impairment

Screening tools: Mini-Cog, Blessed Orientation-Memory-Concentration (BOMC) test.

Intervention: Review of medications, referral upon the requirement of a comprehensive cognitive assessment, counseling for patients and caregivers regarding the risk of delirium, and assessment of capacity for decision making.

Polypharmacy

Screening tools: STOPP (screening tool of older persons potentially inappropriate prescriptions) and START (Screening tool to alert doctors to right treatment) criteria and Beers criteria.

Intervention: Brown bag medicine review, active involvement of pharmacists in patient care, and stopping medications that are potentially inappropriate.

Depression

Screening tools: Hospital Anxiety and Depression Scale (HADS), Geriatric Depression Scale (GDS), and Center for Epidemiology Studies Depression Scale-Revised (CESD-R).

Intervention: Referral for psychological interventions, pharmacologic treatments, problem-solving therapy, cognitive behavioral therapy, etc.

OTHER COMMON SCREENING TOOLS USED IN THE ELDERLY

- Edmonton Symptom Assessment Tool-revised
- MD Anderson Symptom Inventory (MDASI)
- European Organization for Research and Treatment of Cancer's Quality of Life Core Questionnaire (EORTC QLQ-C30)
- Memorial Symptom Assessment Tool (MSAS)

ONCOGERIATRICS

As the human population is aging rapidly, it is projected that one in six people will be aged >65 years by 2050. GLOBOCAN data suggest that the cancer cases reported in the elderly population may rise to 18.6 million in 2040, from 9.95 million in 2020. There is a growing need to improve the standards of care provided to the geriatric population with cancer in the years to come. As per the WHO, 56.8 million people have the requirement of palliative care each year, and 25.7 million require it in the final year of life. Nearly 40% are aged >70 years, and it is unfortunate that only about 14% of those who require palliative care are receiving it. Older cancer patients can have various comorbidities, frailty, and reduced cognition which can be challenging for palliative physicians. The healthcare needs of older patients may be complex and need a comprehensive assessment. A wise solution may be a collaboration among geriatric and palliative teams, as this population carries overlapping concerns for both disciplines **(Fig. 1)**.

SPECIFIC SYMPTOM MANAGEMENT IN THE ELDERLY WITH CANCER

Pain

Twenty-five to forty percent of elderly cancer patients complain of daily pain. Pain may accompany more dependence on daily activities, increased fall risk, more depression, decreased social engagement, malnutrition, etc. Pain can be attributed to the disease itself, its treatment, or due to any comorbid conditions. Pain in geriatric age is usually multifactorial, and a multidisciplinary team approach is beneficial, including geriatrician, palliative physician, psychiatrist, psychologist, physiotherapist, physiatrist, and dietician.

Barriers to Pain Evaluation and Management

- Impairments in cognition and function
- Poor reporting
- Comorbidities
- Prescription bias
- Polypharmacy
- Administering drugs in the setting of institutional living

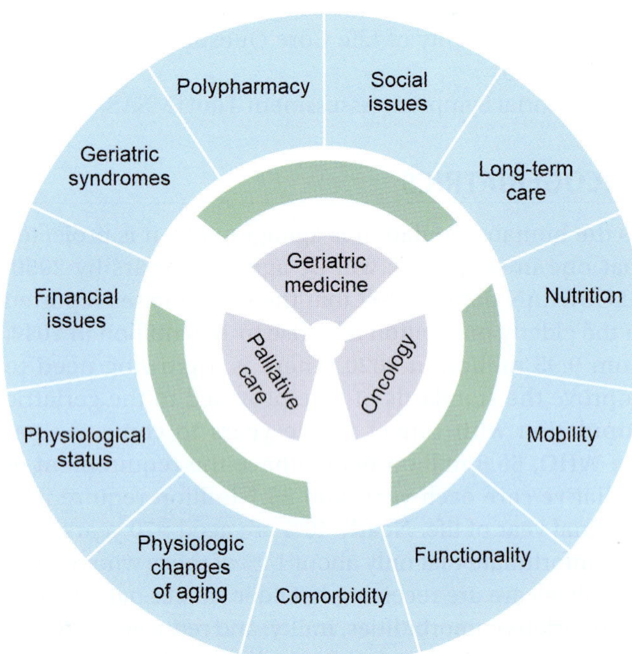

FIG. 1: The complex relationship and overlap between geriatric medicine, palliative care, and oncology.

Elderly Population—Validated Tools for Pain Assessment

The cancer pain assessment involves a comprehensive evaluation comprising a thorough pain review and physical examination.

- PAINAD (Pain Assessment in Advanced Dementia)
- PACSLAC (Pain Assessment Checklist for Seniors with Limited Ability to Communicate)
- Abbey Pain Scale
- Doloplus-2 Scale
- REPOS (Rotterdam Elderly Pain Observation Scale)
- PAINE (Pain Assessment in Noncommunicative Elderly Persons)
- EPCA-2 (Elderly Pain Caring Assessment-2)
- CPAT (Certified Nurse Assistant Pain Assessment Tool)
- PATCOA (Pain Assessment Tool in Confused Older Adults)
- PADE (Pain Assessment for the Demented Elderly)
- Mahoney Pain Scale
- CNPI (Checklist of Nonverbal Pain Indicators)
- DS-DAT (Discomfort Scale)

Management of Pain

The WHO analgesic ladder forms the backbone of the standard pain management algorithm **(Fig. 2)**. The identification of the etiology of pain is the cornerstone of its management.

- *Nonpharmacological interventions*:
  - Relaxation techniques
  - Mindfulness
  - Massage
  - Acupuncture

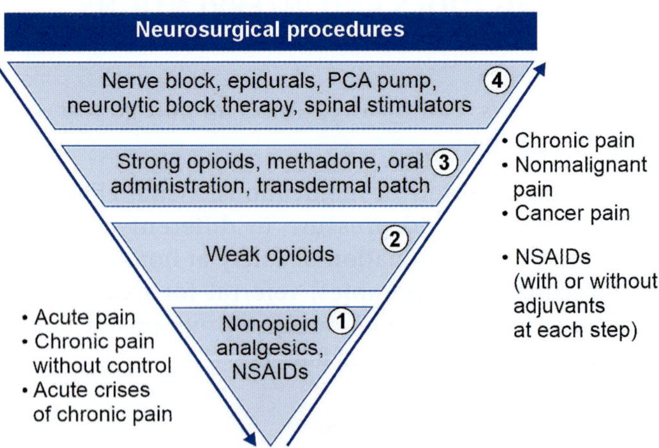

FIG. 2: The new adaptation of the WHO analgesic ladder.
(NSAIDs: nonsteroidal anti-inflammatory drugs; PCA: patient-controlled analgesia; WHO: World Health Organization)

- Exercises
- Rehabilitation
- Cognitive behavioral therapy—if cognitively intact

- *Pharmacological interventions*:
  - *Nonopioids*:
    - *Acetaminophen*: This is employed in mild-to-moderate pain. It is considered the first-line treatment for pain in the elderly. Consumption of >3 g is cautionary owing to potential hepatic toxicity. Education of caregivers regarding over-the-counter drugs and other combination drugs containing acetaminophen is needed.
  - *Nonsteroidal anti-inflammatory drugs (NSAIDs)*: These are effective for managing mild-to-moderate pain, particularly bone pain but are risky in the elderly due to the incidence of renal adverse effects, gastrointestinal bleeds, stroke, and myocardial infarction. Side effects associated with NSAIDs are time and dose-dependent, so their usage is advocated for short intervals only, that too along with gastroprotective medications. NSAIDs should be avoided in peptic ulcers, CKD, and heart diseases.
  - *Opioids*: These are employed in cancer pain of moderate-to-severe intensity. Analgesic ceiling dose is absent. Before treatment commencement, evaluation of renal and hepatic function, cognition, social support, and any potential drug reactions is imperative. The opioids commonly used are tramadol, codeine, morphine, fentanyl, and methadone. Common adverse effects related to opioids are sedation, constipation, vomiting, confusion, and hallucinations. A prophylactic bowel regimen is started on patients with opioid prescriptions. Less common side effects associated with opioids in elderly patients with cancer include nausea, pruritus, myoclonus, urinary retention, dry mouth.
  - *Adjuvant medications*: They add to the pain relief given by opioids and are primarily used in other indications. These include anticonvulsants, antidepressants, corticosteroids, muscle relaxants, etc. Tricyclic antidepressants have rare indications in elderly cancer patients due to their anticholinergic adverse effects, leading to changes in cognition. Common anticonvulsants such as gabapentin and pregabalin should be prescribed according to renal dosages and only escalated slowly. Duloxetine and venlafaxine which are serotonin–norepinephrine reuptake inhibitors are well-tolerated and effective.

Dyspnea

Dyspnea is a common symptom in elderly cancer patients and is defined as an uncomfortable awareness of one's own breathing. Acute dyspnea can be the most common reason for emergency admissions and can result in poor quality of life. Etiology can be effusions, airway obstructions, thick airway secretions, bronchospasms, anemia, anxiety, and other emotional issues.

Assessment and Management

A thorough history, physical examination, imaging, and other tests can be employed to rule out reversible causes.

- *Nonpharmacological interventions*:
  - Patient repositioning
  - Opening windows or using handheld fans to improve air circulation
  - Breathing training or relaxation techniques
  - Providing reassurance and addressing anxiety
- *Pharmacological interventions*:
  - Opioids are recommended therapy for dyspnea in palliative care patients. They act by suppressing respiratory awareness effectively. Studies have proven that opioids can be effective and safe in the management of breathlessness in end-stage cancer patients.
  - Benzodiazepines can be used to relieve anxiety which worsens dyspnea.
  - Treatments with steroids, bronchodilator agents, or diuretics may benefit patients with specific diagnoses.
  - In palliative settings, oxygen supplementation may often be unnecessary.

Nausea and Vomiting

These symptoms are commonly found in cancer patients with advanced disease. Among cancer patients, the prevalence ranges from 30 to 70%. Etiologies may be chemotherapy, radiation, opioids, constipation, and intestinal obstruction. A focused history with examination is needed to find out the specific causes. The general principles of management are given as follows:

- Start with round-the-clock dosages of a single agent based on the possible mechanism of nausea.
- Secondary agents may be added to target other classes of receptors if the first agent does not work.
- Adjuvants such as steroids or benzodiazepines can be used in patients who are terminally ill.
- *If nausea and vomiting are due to*:
  - Drugs (opioids, antibiotics, anticholinergics) → where possible, stop the medications

- Metabolic (uremia, hypercalcemia) → correction of the metabolic cause
- Fear or anxiety → anxiolytics, providing reassurance, and cognitive behavioral therapy
- Gastric irritation (NSAIDs) → stop drugs and addition of proton-pump inhibitors
- Cough → if due to infection, start antibiotics/add cough suppressants

Management of Nausea and Vomiting

- *Nonpharmacological interventions*:
  - Small and frequent meals
  - Preference for patient's choice of food
  - Proper intake of fluids
  - Relaxation therapy
  - Pleasant environment during meals
- *Pharmacological interventions*:
  Based on the mechanism, different drugs are used:
  - Metoclopramide, 5–15 mg before meals, given oral, subcutaneous, or intravenous (IV)
  - Domperidone, divided doses before meals to a maximum of 80 mg/day orally
  - Diphenhydramine 1 mg/kg/dose q4 hourly, given oral, subcutaneous, or IV
  - Haloperidol 0.01–0.05 mg/kg/dose q8 hourly, given oral, subcutaneous, or IV
  - Prochlorperazine 0.15 mg/kg/dose q4 hourly, given oral, rectal, or IV
  - Ondansetron 0.15 mg/kg/dose q6 hourly, given peroral or IV
  - Dexamethasone 2–4 mg q12 hourly to q6 hourly, given oral, subcutaneous, or IV
  - Scopolamine 0.5 mg transdermal q72 hourly, given transdermal

Fatigue

Fatigue is one of the most debilitating symptoms experienced by cancer patients. Cancer-related fatigue (CRF) comprises feelings of tiredness and lack of energy. It is associated with distress, anxiety, depression, and poor performance status.

Management of Fatigue

- *Nonpharmacological interventions*:
  - Aerobic exercise
  - Psychological interventions
  - Complementary therapies
- *Pharmacological interventions*:
  - Modafinil
  - Corticosteroids
  - Methylphenidate
  - Antidepressants
  - Cholinesterase inhibitors

Delirium

Delirium is a serious neuropsychiatric condition characterized by a disturbance of awareness and attention accompanied by dysfunction of cognition with a decline from baseline. Among cancer patients, it is associated with mortality, morbidity, and increased distress. Delirium has a prevalence of about 20–40% in hospitalized cancer patients and can reach up to 88% in end-stage cancer patients. The etiology of delirium is as follows:

- Medical causes such as organ failure, infections, and paraneoplastic syndromes
- Metabolic causes such as electrolyte abnormalities and uremia
- Uncontrolled pain
- Central nervous system (CNS) causes such as brain metastasis
- Central effects of immune and chemotherapeutic agents
- Medications such as opioids, steroids, antiemetics, and benzodiazepines
- Urinary retention and constipation
- Alcohol withdrawal and use of illicit drugs
- Deprivation of sleep
- Change of environment

Assessment and Management

The assessment of delirium includes a detailed history with a physical examination. Potentially reversible causes must be addressed, and a thorough review of medications and dosages should be made. Routine investigations are to be carried out. Brain imaging can be done to rule out brain metastasis. Diagnosis can be made by the Confusion Assessment Method (CAM). For intubated patients, CAM-ICU can be used.

- *Nonpharmacological interventions*: Delirium incidence can be decreased by reducing exposure to the risk factors that are known.
- *Pharmacological interventions*: Antipsychotics, cholinesterase inhibitors, and alpha-2 agonists may be employed in the prevention and treatment.

Anxiety and Depression

In cancer patients, anxiety and depression are the most common presentations of psychological distress.

Management of Anxiety and Depression

A good history and careful physical examination are important to determine needed interventions.

- *Nonpharmacological interventions*:
  - Multidisciplinary assessments and psychotherapies
  - Relaxation techniques

- *Pharmacological interventions*:
  - Benzodiazepines are the most important medications in the management of anxiety.
  - In case of severe anxiety, antipsychotics such as haloperidol may be used.
  - In cases of depression, the initial doses of antidepressant agents should be minimized owing to decreased clearance of drugs, leading to adverse effects.
  - Selective serotonin reuptake inhibitors can cause decreased sleepiness and decreased autonomic adverse effects as compared to other antidepressants.
  - TCAs can be given at bedtime alone.
  - Prompt psychiatry referral is needed if poorly responsive to initial treatment or with a complex initial presentation such as psychosis and suicidal ideation.

ADVANCED CARE PLANNING FOR OLDER ADULTS

It is an approach involving comprehensive communication which assures proper implementation and documentation of patient preferences. It gives patients and their loved ones a platform to discuss their life goals, personal choices, and values regarding future medical care, especially during end of life. Elderly patients with serious illnesses generally want quality of life instead of quantity. The aim of advanced care planning (ACP) is to help patients in getting proper care according to their goals, values, and preferences, thus promoting patient-centered care. Thus, ACP advocates reduced aggressive medical interventions, lower rates of hospital admissions, better communication skills, improved decision making, and decreased anxiety and depression, resulting in overall decreased cost and better quality of life.

END-OF-LIFE CARE

During the final days or hours of life, patients with terminal illness may confront a variety of symptoms such as pain, vomiting, delirium, anxiety, dyspnea, and distress. Adequate symptomatic management as well as proper caregiver and family support is needed during the care for patients at the end of life.

CONCLUSION

There has been little research in geriatric palliative care, although much research has been conducted in palliative medicine to understand the physical, psychological, and social factors associated with patients. The profile of old patients differs from that of younger patients. The elderly may live in institutions and may have impaired functioning, cognitive dysfunction, and associated morbidities that are the main factors in the survival of patients. A team-based multidisciplinary approach can be beneficial to elderly adults in view of their complex medical, social, and psychological needs. Palliative care must be included in the elderly patient's care throughout the disease trajectory. Palliative care is focused on symptomatic management and functional improvement, leading to a better quality of life.

To decrease drug interactions and side effects, nonpharmacologic interventions have to be an initial consideration in the management plan for the elderly. The timely referral to palliative care reduces patient and caregiver distress greatly.

Self-Assessment Questionnaire

Q1. What are the eight domains of palliative care described by the National Consensus Project for Quality Palliative Care (NCPQPC)?

Q2. How can a comprehensive geriatric assessment improve symptom management and quality of life in elderly patients receiving palliative care?

Q3. What are common physical, psychological, and social issues faced by older adults requiring palliative care, and how should each be addressed?

Q4. Which screening tools are used to detect geriatric syndromes (falls, cognitive impairment, polypharmacy, depression) in palliative-care settings?

Q5. How does pain assessment differ in elderly cancer patients, and what are validated tools and principles for safe analgesic use?

Q6. What are the goals and benefits of advance-care planning (ACP) for older adults with serious illnesses?

Q7. Why should palliative care be initiated early in the disease trajectory of elderly patients rather than reserved only for end-of-life situations?

FURTHER READINGS

1. Jagger C, Weston C, Cambois E, Van Oyen H, Nusselder W, Doblhammer G, et al. Inequalities in health expectancies at older ages in the European Union: findings from the Survey of Health and Retirement in Europe (SHARE). J Epidemiol Community Health. 2011;65(11):1030-5.
2. Gerteis J, Izrael D, Deitz D, LeRoy L, Ricciardi R, Miller T, et al. Multiple chronic conditions chartbook. Rockville (MD): Agency for Healthcare Research and Quality; 2014.
3. Abdulla A, Adams N, Bone M, Elliott AM, Gaffin J, Jones D, et al. Guidance on the management of pain in older people. Age Ageing. 2013;42:i1-57.
4. Rodriguez-Manas L, Fried LP. Frailty in the clinical scenario. Lancet. 2015;385(9968):e7-9.
5. World Health Organization. (2023). Palliative care. [online] Available from https://www.who.int/news-room/fact-sheets/detail/palliative-care. [Last accessed June, 2025].
6. World Health Organization. (2010). WHO definition of palliative care. [online] Available from https://www.who.int/news-room/fact-sheets/detail/palliative-care. [Last accessed June, 2025].
7. Marengoni A, Angleman S, Meinow B, Santoni G, Mangialasche F, Rizzuto D, et al. Coexisting chronic conditions in the older population: variation by health indicators. Eur J Intern Med. 2016;31:29-34.
8. Davies E, Higginson IJ. (2004). Better Palliative Care for Older People. [online] Available from https://iris.who.int/handle/10665/107563. [Last accessed June, 2025].
9. Duursma S, Castleden M, Cherubini A, Cruz Jentoft A, Pitkala K, Rainfray M, et al. European Union Geriatric Medicine Society. Position statement on geriatric medicine and the provision of health care services to older people. J Nutr Health Aging. 2004;8:190-5.
10. Sepulveda C, Marlin A, Yoshida T, Ullrich A. Palliative care: the World Health Organization's global perspective. J Pain Symptom Manage. 2002;24:91-6.
11. Ferrell BR, Twaddle ML, Melnick A, Meier DE. National consensus project clinical practice guidelines for quality palliative care guidelines. J Palliat Med. 2018;21(12):1684-9.
12. Connor SR. Development of hospice and palliative care in the United States. Omega (Westport). 2008;56(1):89-99.
13. Centers for Medicare and Medicaid Services. (2004) Coverage of Hospice Services under Hospital Insurance. [online] Available from https://www.cms.gov/regulations-and-guidance/guidance/manuals/downloads/bp102c09.pdf. [Last Accessed June, 2025].
14. Brownlee S, Lazris A. Curing Medicare: A Doctor's View on How Our Health Care System is Failing Older Americans and How We Can Fix It. Ithaca, NY: Cornell University Press; 2016.
15. Rajan J, Behrends M. Acute pain in older adults: recommendations for assessment and treatment. Anesthesiol Clin. 2019;37:50-20.
16. Eckhart L, Tschachler E, Gruber F. Autophagic control of skin aging. Frontiers in cell and developmental biology. 2019;7:143.
17. Albers G, Froggatt K, Van den Block L, Gambassi G, Vanden Berghe P, Pautex S, et al. A qualitative exploration of the collaborative working between palliative care and geriatric medicine: barriers and facilitators from a European Perspective. BMC Palliative Care. 2016;15:47.
18. Eyigor S. Geriatric syndromes. Turk J Phys Med Rehab. 2009;55(Suppl 2):57-61.
19. Magnuson A, Sattar S, Nightingale G, Saracino R, Skonecki E, Trevino KM. A practical guide to geriatric syndromes in older adults with cancer: a focus on falls, cognition, polypharmacy, and depression. Am Soc Clin Oncol Educ Book. 2019;39:e96-109.
20. Browner IS, Smith TJ. Symptom assessment in elderly cancer patients receiving palliative care. Ann oncol. 2013;24:vii25-9.
21. Castelo-Loureiro A, Perez-de-Acha A, Torres-Perez AC, Cunha V, García-Valdés P, Cárdenas-Reyes P, et al. Delivering palliative and supportive care for older adults with cancer: interactions between palliative medicine and geriatrics. Cancers. 2023;15(15):3858.
22. Ferlay J, Laversanne M, Ervik M, Lam F, Colombet M, Mery L, et al. Global cancer observatory: cancer tomorrow. Int Agency Res Cancer. 2020;3:2019.
23. Rosa WE, Bhadelia A, Knaul FM, Travers JL, Metheny N, Fulmer T. A longevity society requires integrated palliative care models for historically excluded older people. Lancet Healthy Longev. 2022;3:e227-8.
24. World Health Organization. Palliative care [Internet]. 2023 [cited 2025 Jun]. Available from: https://www.who.int/news-room/fact-sheets/detail/palliativecare
25. Hadjistavropoulos T, Herr K, Turk DC, Fine PG, Dworkin RH, Helme R, et al. An interdisciplinary expert consensus statement on assessment of pain in older persons. Clin J Pain. 2007;23:S1-43.
26. Makris UE, Abrams RC, Gurland B, Reid MC. Management of persistent pain in the older patient: a clinical review. Jama. 2014;312:825-36.
27. Rodriguez CS. The management of persistent pain in older persons. J Am Geriatr Soc. 2002;50:S205-24.
28. Rittberg R, Sutherland J, Huynh E, Green S, Wiens A, Stirling M, et al. Assessing the learning needs of the multidisciplinary team on geriatric oncology and frailty. J Geriatr Oncol. 2019;10:829-31.
29. Alexander K, Goldberg J, Korc-Grodzicki B. Palliative care and symptom management in older patients with cancer. Clin Geriatr Med. 2016;32(1):45-62.
30. Zech DF, Grond S, Lynch J, Hertel D, Lehmann KA. Validation of World Health Organization Guidelines for cancer pain relief: a 10-year prospective study. Pain. 1995;63:65-76.
31. Taylor R Jr, Lemtouni S, Weiss K, Pergolizzi JV Jr. Pain management in the elderly: an FDA safe use initiative expert panel's view on preventable harm associated with NSAID therapy. Current Gerontology and Geriatrics Research. 2012;2012:196159.
32. Medlock S, Eslami S, Askari M, Taherzadeh Z, Opondo D, De Rooij SE, et al. Co-prescription of gastroprotective agents and their efficacy in elderly patients taking nonsteroidal anti-inflammatory drugs: a systematic review of observational studies. Clin Gastroenterol Hepatol. 2013;11(10):1259-69.
33. Marinangeli F, Ciccozzi A, Leonardis M, Aloisio L, Mazzei A, Paladini A, et al. Use of strong opioids in advanced cancer pain: a randomized trial. J Pain Symptom Manage. 2004;27:409-16.
34. Schrijvers D, van Fraeyenhove F. Emergencies in palliative care. Cancer J. 2010;16:514-20.
35. Wiese CH, Barrels UE, Graf BM, Hanekop GG. Out-of-hospital opioid therapy of palliative care patients with "acute dyspnoea": a retrospective multicenter investigation. J Opioid Manag. 2009;5:115-22.
36. Lopez-Saca JM, Centeno C. Opioids prescription for symptoms relief and the impact on respiratory function: updated evidence. Cur Opin Support Palliat Care. 2014;8:383-90.
37. Herrstedt J, Lindberg S, Petersen PC. Prevention of chemotherapy-induced nausea and vomiting in the older patient: optimizing outcomes. Drugs Aging. 2022;39:1-21.
38. Yennurajalingam S, Frisbee-Hume S, Palmer JL, Delgado-Guay MO, Bull J, Phan AT, et al. Reduction of cancer-related fatigue with

dexamethasone: a double-blind, randomized, placebo-controlled trial in patients with advanced cancer. J Clin Oncol. 2013;31:3076-82.

39. Gong S, Sheng P, Jin H, He H, Qi E, Chen W, et al. Effect of methylphenidate in patients with cancer-related fatigue: a systematic review and meta-analysis. PloS One. 2014;9:e84391.
40. Breitbart W, Alici Y. Pharmacologic treatment options for cancer-related fatigue: current state of clinical research. Clin J Oncol Nurs. 2008;12:27-36.
41. Bruera E, El Osta B, Valero V, Driver LC, Pei BL, Shen L, et al. Donepezil for cancer fatigue: a double-blind, randomized, placebo-controlled trial. J Clin Oncol. 2007;25:3475-81.
42. Inouye SK, Westendorp RG, Saczynski JS. Delirium in elderly people. Lancet. 2014;383:911-22.
43. Ely EW, Inouye SK, Bernard GR, Gordon S, Francis J, May L, et al. Delirium in mechanically ventilated patients: validity and reliability of the confusion assessment method for the intensive care unit (CAM-ICU). JAMA. 2001;286:2703-10.
44. Hshieh TT, Yue J, Oh E, Puelle M, Dowal S, Travison T, et al. Effectiveness of multicomponent nonpharmacological delirium interventions: a meta-analysis. JAMA Intern Med. 2015;175(4): 512-20.
45. Derogatis LR, Morrow GR, Fetting J, Penman D, Piasetsky S, Schmale AM, et al. The prevalence of psychiatric disorders among cancer patients. JAMA. 1983;249:751-7.
46. Brown AJ, Shen MJ, Ramondetta LM, Bodurka DC, Giuntoli RL 2nd, Diaz-Montes T. Does death anxiety affect end-of-life care discussions? Int J Gynecol Cancer. 2014;24:1521-6.
47. Tang ST, Chen JS, Chou WC, Lin KC, Chang WC, Hsieh CH, et al. Prevalence of severe depressive symptoms increases as death approaches and is associated with disease burden, tangible social support, and high self-perceived burden to others. Support Care Cancer. 2016;24:83-91.
48. Janberidze E, Pereira SM, Hjermstad MJ, Knudsen AK, Kaasa S, van der Heide A, et al. Depressive symptoms in the last days of life of patients with cancer: a nationwide retrospective mortality study. BMJ Supportive & Palliative Care. 2016;6(2):201-9.
49. Pautex S, Herrmann FR, Zulian GB. Role of advance directives in palliative care units: a prospective study. Palliat Med. 2008;22:835-41.
50. Vonnes C, Parrish L, El-Rady R, Patterson D, Mason TM. "What matters most" to older adults with cancer: advance care planning. J Hosp Palliat Nurs. 2022;24:240-6.
51. Weathers E, O'Caoimh R, Cornally N, Fitzgerald C, Kearns T, Coffey A, et al. Advance care planning: a systematic review of randomised controlled trials conducted with older adults. Maturitas. 2016;91:101-9.
52. Robinson L, Dickinson C, Rousseau N, Beyer F, Clark A, Hughes J, et al. A systematic review of the effectiveness of advance care planning interventions for people with cognitive impairment and dementia. Age Ageing. 2012;41(2):263-9.
53. Oxford Textbook of Palliative Medicine.
54. Morrison RS, Meier DE (Eds). Geriatric palliative care. 1st edition. New York: Oxford University Press; 2003.
55. Oxford American Handbook of Hospice and Palliative Medicine and Supportive Care.

CHAPTER 42

Geriatric Oncology

Abhijith Rajaram Rao

CASE VIGNETTES

Case Vignette 1

A 68-year-old male with metastatic nonsmall cell lung cancer (NSCLC) is planned for chemotherapy and undergoes a geriatric oncological assessment. His basic and instrumental activities of daily living (BADLs and IADLs) are intact, and the Mini Nutritional Assessment (MNA) indicates he is at risk of malnutrition. His Cancer and Aging Research Group (CARG) score is 4, placing him at low risk for severe toxicity. He desires a good quality of life. Following the assessment, he is evaluated by a dietitian and starts nutritional intervention while awaiting chemotherapy. The oncologist decides to proceed with full-dose chemotherapy.

Case Vignette 2

A 66-year-old male smoker with metastatic NSCLC has impaired IADL but maintained BADL. His timed up and go test is 24 seconds (indicating slow mobility), and the MNA reveals malnutrition. His CARG score is 7, indicating a moderate risk of severe toxicity. He is referred to a physiotherapist and a dietitian for further interventions. The oncologist decides to start reduced-dose chemotherapy.

Despite having the same disease, the interventions and treatment plans for these two cases differ due to variations in their geriatric assessments.

INTRODUCTION

Geriatric oncology in India is still developing. Most older cancer patients are evaluated based on clinical judgment rather than validated geriatric assessments (GA). This is due to a lack of trained professionals and dedicated geriatric oncology units. Western-developed GA tools are often unsuitable for older Indian patients because of cultural differences and varying literacy levels. Functional status, crucial for maintaining independence, declines with age, leading to variations in treatment and outcomes. The traditional Eastern Cooperative Oncology Group (ECOG) performance status cannot replace a formal GA, which is rarely offered in Indian centers. Additionally, there is a lack of educational programs and research focused on older cancer patients in India. Addressing these issues could improve care for older Indian cancer patients and inspire the development of geriatric oncology services and centers of excellence.

EPIDEMIOLOGY OF OLDER ADULTS IN INDIA

In 2010, 524 million people worldwide were aged 65 years or older, and by 2050, this number is projected to reach 1.5 billion, with 80% living in low- and middle-income countries. In India, older adults constituted 8.6% of the population in 2011, expected to rise to 19.5% by 2050. Aging is a major risk factor for cancer, with those over 65 years accounting for 60% of new cancer cases and 70% of cancer deaths, primarily from cancers of the breast, lung, prostate, cervix, esophagus, and ovary. The Indian Council of Medical Research (ICMR) estimates a rise in cancer diagnoses from 1.39 million in 2020 to 1.57 million by 2050, indicating a significant increase in older cancer patients in India.

MULTIDISCIPLINARY TEAM FOR GERIATRIC ONCOLOGY CLINIC

The GA of older patients with cancer should involve healthcare professionals from various departments, including oncologists, geriatricians, pharmacologists, physiotherapists, occupational therapists, dietitians, and social workers. Each member plays a vital role in evaluating, planning, and implementing individualized care plans for these older patients.

SCREENING TOOLS USED IN GERIATRIC ONCOLOGY

In geriatric oncology, screening tools such as the G8 and the Vulnerable Elders Survey-13 (VES-13) are widely used to identify older adults at risk of frailty and adverse outcomes. The G8 is a screening tool specifically designed for older cancer patients, consisting of eight items that assess multiple domains such as nutritional status, mobility, neuropsychological problems, polypharmacy, and self-perceived health status. A G8 score of ≤14 suggests that a full GA is warranted, indicating potential vulnerabilities that may influence treatment decisions and outcomes. This tool is quick and easy to administer, making it highly valuable in busy clinical settings where comprehensive assessments may not be feasible for all patients.

The VES-13 is another widely used tool that identifies older adults at risk of health deterioration. It includes 13 items covering age, self-rated health, physical function, and functional disabilities. A score of ≥3 on the VES-13 indicates a higher risk of health decline and mortality, suggesting the need for a more detailed GA. Both the G8 and VES-13 have been validated in various settings and are effective in predicting adverse outcomes, such as mortality and treatment-related toxicity, in older cancer patients. By utilizing these screening tools, healthcare providers can better stratify patients based on their frailty status, ensuring that those who require more intensive assessment and tailored interventions receive appropriate care.

GERIATRIC ASSESSMENT

The GA can be divided into the following components: Overall assessment, nononcologic domain assessment, assessment of risk of chemotherapy-related toxicity, and evaluation of patients' and caregivers' goals of therapy.

- *Overall assessment*: Patients are evaluated for geriatric syndromes such as constipation, insomnia, lower urinary tract symptoms, urinary incontinence, osteoporosis, pressure sores, falls, visual and hearing impairment, voice, and oral health.
- *Nononcologic domain*: This includes assessment of function, nutrition, comorbidities, medications, cognition, psychological domain, quality of life, and financial burden.
- *Assessment of chemotherapy-related toxicity*: The tools which can be used include CARG (Cancer and Aging Research Group) and CRASH (Chemotherapy Risk Assessment Scale for High-age Patients) score.

Table 1 gives an example of domains, the tools used, and the cutoff scores.

TABLE 1: Details of tools, questionnaires as part of GA, and their cutoff scores.

GA tools	Scale	Cutoff to define an abnormal value (vulnerability in the GA)
Function		
Activities of daily living (ADL)	Katz ADL	<6
IADL	Lawton IADL	• Men < 5 • Women < 8
Performance-based assay	Timed up and go	>10 seconds
Risk of falls	*Single question*: "How many falls have you had in the past 1 year?"	≥1
Nutrition		
Body mass index	Weight (kg)/height (m^2)	<18.5 kg/m^2
Unintentional weight loss	Proportion of weight lost as compared to the preillness baseline	>10%
Nutritional status	MNA	<24 (24–30: Normal nutrition, 17–23.5: At risk of malnutrition, and <17: Malnourished)
Comorbidities		
Presence of comorbidities	Hypertension, diabetes, chronic airway disease, coronary artery disease, any other comorbidity	Specific comorbidity is documented

Continued

Continued

GA tools	Scale	Cutoff to define an abnormal value (vulnerability in the GA)
Validated comorbidity tools	Charlson Comorbidity Index	≥2
Validated comorbidity tools	CIRS-G	• ≥4 • *Any category score*: 3–4 • Severity index (total score/number of scales with score >0) >2
Cognition		
Literate patients	MMSE	<24 (24–30: No cognitive impairment, 18–23: Mild cognitive impairment, 0–17: Severe cognitive impairment)
Illiterate patients	Hindi Mental Status Examination	
Mood		
Depression	GDS-short form	>4 (5–8: Mild depression, 9–11: Moderate depression, 12–15: Severe depression)
Anxiety	GAD-7	≥10 (0–4: Minimal anxiety, 5–9: Mild anxiety, 10–14: Moderate anxiety, >15: Severe anxiety)
Medications		
Polypharmacy	Number of regular medications	≥5 medications
PIM	American Geriatrics Society Beers Criteria	Any PIM
Social support		
Validated tool	Older Americans' resources and services, medical social support	≥1 (in questions 2–4)
Living situation	Resident of Mumbai/staying with a relative, in a rented room, a hotel/guest house, or ashram/homeless/staying on the footpath	Homeless or staying on the footpath
Number of caregivers	"How many persons are available to care for you all the time, or most of the time, or at the times that you need a caregiver?"	0
Screening tools		
	Geriatric 8 (G8)	<12
	Vulnerable Elders Survey-13 (VES-13)	≥3
	Rockwood Clinical Frailty Scale	≥5
Chemotherapy toxicity risk prediction score	CARG Chemotoxicity Calculator	Low risk (30%): 0–5, intermediate risk (52%): 6–9, high risk (83%): ≥10
Noncancer life expectancy	ePrognosis (Lee and Schonberg indices)	Estimate of the 5- and 10-year mortality (noncancer-related) and the life expectancy in years
QoL	The European Organization for Research and Treatment of Cancer QLQ-C30, v3.0	Higher score indicates a better QoL
	EORTC QLQ-ELD14	Higher scores on "Maintaining purpose" scale and "Family support" item indicate a high level of functioning; higher scores for "Mobility," "Worries about others," "Future worries," "Burden of illness," and "Joint stiffness" indicate a poor QoL
Caregiver QoL	(Frontotemporal lobe disorders) Caregiver Burden Scale	>20 (0–20: Little or no burden, 21–40: Mild-to-moderate burden, 41–60: Moderate-to-severe burden, and 61–88: Severe burden)

Continued

Continued

GA tools	Scale	Cutoff to define an abnormal value (vulnerability in the GA)
General assessments		
Vision		
Distant vision	Snellen chart	6/18 or worse
Near vision	Landolt C chart	N/18 or worse
Hearing		
Questionnaire	Hearing Handicap Index	>10 (0–8: No handicap, 10–24: Mild-to-moderate handicap, 26–40: Severe handicap)
Voice	Voice Handicap Index	>11
Oral health	Geriatric Oral Health Assessment Index	Total score: 12–60; higher scores indicate better perception of oral-dental health
Cancer-related symptoms	Edmonton Symptom Assessment Scale	Any score ≥4
Financial burden		
	Comprehensive Score for Financial Toxicity-Functional Assessment of Chronic Illness Therapy (COST-FACIT)	<12 [≥26: No impact on QoL (grade 0), 14–25: Mild impact (grade 1), 1–13: Moderate impact (grade 2), 0: High impact (grade 3)]
	Consumer Financial Protection Bureau Financial Well-being Scale	Range: 0–100 points; lower scores represent worse financial well-being
Patients' and caregivers' viewpoint regarding disclosure	Does the patient/caregiver want the treating team to disclose and discuss the diagnosis and prognosis?	Based on the patients' and caregivers' viewpoints, the results of the GA, the curability/treatability of the cancer, and the potential toxicity of the therapy, a discussion occurs
Patients' expectations from treatment	• *If curative*: Complete cure/symptom control/improvement in present status/improved QoL or prolongation of life • *If palliative*: Improved QoL/prolongation of life/immediate symptom relief	
Blood tests		
	eGFR	Based on the kidney function, a decision will be taken
	NLR	NLR < 3.4 = Poor prognosis
Vaccination status	Uptake of pneumococcal, influenza, and COVID-19 vaccines	If not received, patients are advised these vaccines

(CARG: Cancer and Aging Research Group; CIRS-G: Cumulative Illness Rating Scale-Geriatric; eGFR: estimated glomerular filtration rate; EORTC: European Organization for Research and Treatment of Cancer; GA: geriatric assessment; GAD: generalized anxiety disorder; GDS: Geriatric Depression Scale; IADL: instrumental activities of daily living; MMSE: Mini-Mental State Examination; MNA: Mini Nutritional Assessment; NLR: neutrophil-lymphocyte ratio; PIM: potentially inappropriate medicines; QLQ: Quality of Life Questionnaire; QoL: quality of life)

Source: Reproduced with permission from Noronha V, Rao AR, Ramaswamy A, Kumar A, Pillai A, Dhekale R, et al. The current status of geriatric oncology in India. Ecancermedicalscience. 2023;17:1595.

Benefits of Geriatric Assessment

Geriatric assessment in older patients with cancer provides a comprehensive evaluation that goes beyond traditional oncologic assessment, ensuring that the unique needs of elderly patients are addressed. This multidimensional tool assesses a variety of domains, including functional status, comorbidities, cognition, psychological state, social support, nutritional status, and polypharmacy. By evaluating these areas, healthcare providers can gain a holistic understanding of an older patient's health and functional abilities, allowing for the creation of personalized treatment plans that consider the complexities of aging. This tailored approach helps in identifying patients who are more likely to benefit from aggressive cancer treatments and those who may require modified or less intensive therapies due to vulnerabilities.

Additionally, GA can significantly enhance the management of older cancer patients by identifying issues that may not be evident through standard oncologic evaluations. For instance, it can uncover geriatric syndromes such as frailty, falls, or depression, which may impact treatment tolerance and outcomes. By addressing these issues proactively, healthcare providers can implement interventions to improve overall health and quality of life, reduce treatment-related toxicities, and potentially improve survival rates. Furthermore, involving a multidisciplinary team in the assessment process fosters a more coordinated and comprehensive approach to care, ensuring that all aspects of a patient's health are considered and managed appropriately. This not only optimizes cancer treatment outcomes but also enhances the overall well-being of older adults navigating the complexities of cancer care.

Impact of Geriatric Assessment on Systemic Therapy Plan

Globally, it is well-recognized that systematic evaluation of older patients with cancer through GA is valuable and leads to better treatment choices, lowers toxicity, and improves communication. At one institution, the GA led to a change in the cancer-directed systemic therapy plan in 38.7% of cases, with the most common change being treatment deintensification in 32.1% of patients. Thus, a significant proportion of older patients with cancer are over-treated when a GA is not performed.

Correlation with Overall Survival

A study aimed to assess the impact of GA on survival in older Indian patients with cancer and to identify factors associated with survival. Among the patients evaluated, those classified as frail had a median overall survival of 11.2 months, while fit patients had a median survival of 24.3 months. Another study investigating frailty in older Indian cancer patients found that those fit on the Clinical Frailty Scale (CFS) had a median survival of 28.02 months, prefrail patients had 13.24 months, and frail patients had 7.79 months. Abnormal G8 and VES-13 scores were also associated with significantly lower median survival. Identifying frailty through GA and appropriate tools allows for better-tailored treatment plans, improving outcomes and survival in older cancer patients.

CONCLUSION

Geriatric oncology is a burgeoning field that addresses the unique challenges of treating older adults with cancer. The case vignettes demonstrate how individualized treatment plans based on comprehensive GA can significantly impact therapeutic decisions and outcomes. A multidisciplinary team approach, incorporating oncologists, geriatricians, pharmacologists, physiotherapists, occupational therapists, dietitians, and social workers, is essential to provide holistic care for older cancer patients.

The GA, encompassing overall assessment, non-oncologic domain evaluation, and risk assessment for chemotherapy-related toxicity, plays a crucial role in optimizing treatment plans. Despite the resource-intensive nature of GA, its benefits in improving treatment choices, reducing toxicity, and enhancing communication are well-documented. Studies show that frail patients, identified through GA, have significantly lower median overall survival compared to fit patients, underscoring the importance of GA in tailoring interventions.

As the population of older adults with cancer continues to grow, it is imperative to integrate GA into routine oncology practice. This will ensure that treatment plans are personalized, addressing the multifaceted needs of older patients, thereby improving their quality of life and survival outcomes. The establishment of dedicated geriatric oncology services and centers of excellence in India can lead to better care and inspire further advancements in this vital field.

Self-Assessment Questionnaire

Q1. How can we best assess an older adult patient's fitness for cancer treatment?

Q2. How do we modify cancer treatment regimens for older adults to optimize efficacy and minimize side effects?

Q3. What role does a multidisciplinary approach play in geriatric oncology care?

Q4. How can we manage geriatric syndromes alongside cancer treatment?

Q5. What are the ethical considerations in geriatric oncology, particularly regarding treatment goals and patient autonomy?

FURTHER READINGS

1. Balducci L, Extermann M. Management of cancer in the older person: A practical approach. The Oncologist. 2000;5(3):224-37.
2. Hurria A, Kayo Togawa K, Mohile SG, et al. Validation of a prediction tool for chemotherapy toxicity in older adults with cancer: The Cancer and Aging Research Group (CARG) score. J Clin Oncol. 2011;29(25):3457-65.
3. Wildiers H, Heeren P, Puts M, et al. International Society of Geriatric Oncology (SIOG) consensus on geriatric assessment in older patients with cancer. J Clin Oncol. 2014;32(24):2595-03.
4. Mohile SG, Dale W, Somerfield MR, et al. Practical assessment and management of vulnerabilities in older patients receiving chemotherapy: ASCO guideline. J Clin Oncol. 2018;36(22):2326-47.
5. Extermann M, Hurria A. Comprehensive geriatric assessment for older patients with cancer. J Clin Oncol. 2007;25(14):1824-31.
6. Puts MTE, Hardt J, Monette J et al. The use of geriatric assessment for older adults in oncology: A systematic review. J Natl Cancer Inst. 2012;104(16):1133-1163.
7. Kumar S, Balachandar R, Rao AR. Geriatric oncology in low- and middle-income countries: Indian perspectives and challenges. Curr Opin Support Palliat Care. 2022;16(4):180-187.

Constipation in Older Adults: Assessment, Management, and Special Considerations

Abhijith Rajaram Rao

CASE VIGNETTES

Case Vignette 1

Mrs S is a 75-year-old woman living independently. She presents to her primary care physician with complaints of bloating, abdominal discomfort, and difficulty passing stools over the past few months. She mentions that she typically has fewer than three bowel movements a week and often feels that her stools are hard and incomplete. Her medical history includes hypertension and mild osteoarthritis. She takes amlodipine for her blood pressure and nonsteroidal anti-inflammatory drugs (NSAIDs) for joint pain. Mrs S is also less active than she used to be and admits that her fluid intake has decreased recently.

Case Vignette 2

Mr R, an 82-year-old man with advanced Parkinson's disease, is brought to the clinic by his caregiver. He has a long-standing history of constipation, which has worsened over the past 6 months. Mr R has difficulty passing stools despite using over-the-counter laxatives, and he experiences occasional fecal incontinence. His caregiver reports that he spends extended periods straining during defecation. He takes multiple medications, including levodopa, anticholinergics, and opioids for his chronic pain. His diet is low in fiber, and he is mostly sedentary due to his physical limitations.

INTRODUCTION

Constipation is a frequent yet underreported issue in older adults, significantly impacting their quality of life, overall health, and functioning. While constipation is not exclusive to aging, older individuals are disproportionately affected due to a complex interplay of physiological, lifestyle, and medical factors. Defined by the Rome IV criteria as infrequent bowel movements (fewer than three per week) and/or difficult passage of stools (e.g., straining, hard stools, sensation of incomplete evacuation), constipation can manifest in various ways and is often subjective. Many older adults experience symptoms that range from mild discomfort to severe abdominal pain, bloating, and even fecal incontinence.

The prevalence of constipation in older adults varies widely depending on the population studied. It is estimated that 20–40% of community-dwelling older adults report symptoms of constipation, with this rate increasing to as much as 50% or more in institutionalized or nursing home populations. Aging itself does not directly cause constipation but contributes to the vulnerability through multiple mechanisms, including reduced colonic motility, impaired defecation reflexes, and weakened abdominal and pelvic floor muscles. Moreover, many older adults have comorbidities and take medications that further predispose them to constipation.

In older adults, constipation is more than just an uncomfortable inconvenience—it can lead to serious complications if not addressed appropriately. Chronic constipation is associated with increased risks of fecal impaction, hemorrhoids, anal fissures, rectal prolapse, and even urinary retention due to the close anatomical relationship between the rectum and the bladder. Additionally, severe cases may contribute to delirium, malnutrition, or functional decline, especially in frail older individuals.

Despite its high prevalence and potential consequences, constipation in older adults is often overlooked or dismissed as a normal part of aging. This misconception can delay diagnosis and appropriate management, allowing symptoms to worsen and complications to develop. Older adults may also feel reluctant to discuss bowel problems with healthcare providers, further complicating timely intervention. As a result, it is crucial for clinicians to proactively screen for constipation during routine assessments and to adopt a holistic approach to management that considers the unique needs and challenges faced by older individuals.

The management of constipation in older adults poses additional challenges. First, older adults often have multiple chronic conditions (multimorbidity) that complicate treatment decisions. Second, polypharmacy is common in this population, and many medications, including opioids, calcium channel blockers, and anticholinergic agents, can exacerbate constipation. Finally, functional limitations such as mobility issues, cognitive impairment, and frailty may hinder an older person's ability to engage in lifestyle interventions that are crucial for preventing and treating constipation, such as increasing fiber intake, physical activity, and fluid consumption.

This chapter delves into the complex issue of constipation in older adults, focusing on its underlying causes, assessment methods, and therapeutic strategies. In addition to the physiological changes associated with aging, this chapter will explore other key factors, such as the role of medications, the impact of neurological and metabolic conditions, and the importance of dietary and lifestyle modifications. A detailed discussion on pharmacological treatments, including laxatives and newer agents such as prokinetics and opioid antagonists, will also be provided. Special attention will be given to vulnerable populations, such as those with frailty, dementia, or Parkinson's disease (PD), where constipation may present unique management challenges. Ultimately, this chapter aims to equip healthcare providers with the knowledge and tools necessary to address constipation in older adults effectively, ensuring a better quality of life for this growing segment of the population.

Through proactive assessment, early intervention, and tailored management, constipation in older adults can be better controlled, improving not only gastrointestinal (GI) health but also overall well-being and functional independence.

PATHOPHYSIOLOGY

Understanding the pathophysiology of constipation in older adults requires a multifaceted approach, as several interconnected biological, anatomical, and lifestyle factors contribute to the condition. The aging process itself brings about numerous physiological changes that can adversely affect GI motility and stool passage. The key elements influencing the pathophysiology of constipation are given in the following text.

Colonic Motility Changes

As individuals age, there is a natural decline in colonic motility. This reduction manifests as decreased peristaltic activity in the colon, leading to slower transit times. Key factors contributing to this decline include the following:

- *Muscle changes*: The smooth muscle cells in the colonic wall may undergo structural changes, including loss of elasticity and a decrease in the number of functioning muscle fibers. This can impair the colon's ability to contract effectively, leading to delayed bowel movements.
- *Hormonal changes*: Aging alters the levels of GI hormones such as motilin and ghrelin, which play roles in stimulating bowel motility. A decrease in these hormones can contribute to slower intestinal transit.
- *Neural changes*: Age-related degeneration of enteric neurons, which coordinate GI motility, may impair peristalsis and disrupt the normal reflexes involved in bowel movements.

Alterations in Rectal Sensitivity and Defecation Reflexes

The rectum serves as a crucial sensory organ that detects the presence of stool and triggers the urge to defecate. Several age-related changes can impair rectal sensitivity:

- *Decreased sensitivity*: Aging can lead to a reduced ability to sense the presence of stool in the rectum, which can delay the urge to defecate. This diminished sensitivity can result in infrequent bowel movements and the feeling of incomplete evacuation.
- *Impaired reflexes*: The coordinated reflex actions required for effective defecation may become less efficient with age. The anal sphincter muscles may weaken, making it more difficult to initiate a bowel movement, leading to straining and increased discomfort.

Pelvic Floor Dysfunction

The pelvic floor muscles and their coordination are essential for proper bowel function. Age-related changes can lead to the following:

- *Weakened musculature*: Loss of muscle tone and strength in the pelvic floor can contribute to difficulties in bowel evacuation. Conditions such as pelvic organ prolapse can further complicate this issue, particularly in women.
- *Coordination issues*: The ability to coordinate abdominal and pelvic floor muscles during defecation can decline with age. This loss of coordination may lead to straining and the sensation of incomplete evacuation.

Dietary and Lifestyle Factors

Dietary habits and lifestyle choices have a significant impact on bowel health given as follows:

- *Low fiber intake*: Many older adults consume diets low in fiber, which is crucial for promoting bowel regularity. A fiber-deficient diet contributes to hard stools and decreased stool bulk, making it harder to pass.
- *Dehydration*: Aging often leads to decreased thirst perception and lower fluid intake. Inadequate hydration can result in harder stools and increased straining during defecation.
- *Sedentary lifestyle*: Physical activity is essential for maintaining healthy bowel function. Reduced mobility due to age-related conditions (e.g., arthritis, frailty) can lead to decreased intestinal motility and constipation.

Comorbidities and Medications

Several common comorbidities and medications prevalent in older adults exacerbate constipation as follows:

- *Neurological disorders*: Conditions such as PD, multiple sclerosis, and dementia can significantly impair bowel motility and the defecation process. These disorders can affect both the autonomic nervous system, which regulates involuntary bodily functions, and the enteric nervous system, which controls GI motility.
- *Metabolic and endocrine disorders*: Hypothyroidism, diabetes mellitus, and other metabolic disorders can affect intestinal function. For instance, hypothyroidism slows metabolism, which may decrease bowel motility.
- *Medication side effects*: Many medications commonly prescribed to older adults, such as opioids, anticholinergics, calcium channel blockers, and iron supplements, can contribute to constipation by affecting bowel motility and stool consistency. Opioids, e.g., inhibit peristalsis and reduce GI secretions, leading to harder stools and prolonged transit time.

Psychological Factors

Psychosocial factors can also play a role in the development and persistence of constipation:

- *Cognitive impairment*: Dementia and cognitive decline can interfere with the awareness of bowel habits and the ability to act on the urge to defecate. Individuals may forget to go to the bathroom or may not recognize the need to do so.
- *Mood disorders*: Depression and anxiety are prevalent in older adults and can negatively affect appetite, dietary habits, and motivation to engage in physical activity, all of which can contribute to constipation.

The pathophysiology of constipation in older adults is complex and multifactorial, involving interactions between physiological aging processes, lifestyle factors, comorbidities, and medication use. Recognizing these contributing factors is crucial for effective assessment and management of constipation in this population. A thorough understanding of the underlying mechanisms enables healthcare providers to tailor interventions that address both the physical and psychosocial aspects of this common yet often neglected condition. By focusing on individualized care and prevention strategies, clinicians can significantly improve the quality of life for older adults experiencing constipation.

COMMON RISK FACTORS

Constipation in older adults is influenced by a wide range of risk factors that can be broadly categorized into dietary and lifestyle factors, medication-related factors, comorbidities, and psychosocial factors. Understanding these risk factors is essential for developing effective prevention and management strategies.

Dietary and Lifestyle Factors

Low Fiber Intake

Dietary fiber is crucial for promoting regular bowel movements by increasing stool bulk and moisture content. Older adults often have diets that lack sufficient fiber due to preferences for low-fiber foods, limited access to fresh fruits and vegetables, or dietary restrictions. A fiber intake of 20–30 g/day is generally recommended for older adults, yet many fall short of this target, leading to harder, less voluminous stools that are difficult to pass.

Inadequate Fluid Intake

Dehydration is common among older adults, partly due to decreased thirst perception and the tendency to limit fluid intake for various health reasons (e.g., heart failure). Inadequate hydration can lead to constipation by causing stool to become dry and hard, making it more challenging to pass. It is essential for older adults to consume adequate fluids (generally 1.5–2 L daily) unless contraindicated by specific medical conditions.

Sedentary Lifestyle

Physical activity stimulates intestinal motility and promotes bowel regularity. Many older adults may lead sedentary lifestyles due to mobility issues, fear of falling, or chronic pain. This inactivity can slow down the digestive process and contribute to constipation. Encouraging regular, moderate physical activity tailored to an individual's capabilities can help improve bowel function.

Changes in Routine

Life changes such as relocation to a nursing home or hospitalization can disrupt established routines, including those related to diet and bowel habits. These disruptions can contribute to constipation, especially if individuals are not provided with adequate access to food, fluids, and opportunities for physical activity.

Medication-related Factors

Older adults often take multiple medications, a situation known as polypharmacy, which increases the likelihood of drug-related constipation. Common classes of medications that can contribute to constipation include:

- *Opioids*: Medications used to manage pain, particularly opioids, are notorious for causing constipation due to their effects on the central nervous system and GI motility. Opioids reduce peristalsis and secretions in the intestines, leading to slower transit times and harder stools.
- *Anticholinergics*: These medications, often prescribed for conditions such as overactive bladder and respiratory disorders, block the action of acetylcholine, which is necessary for bowel contractions. Examples include antihistamines, tricyclic antidepressants, and certain medications for PD.
- *Calcium channel blockers*: Commonly used to treat hypertension and cardiac conditions, calcium channel blockers can cause constipation by relaxing smooth muscle in the GI tract, leading to reduced peristalsis.
- *Iron supplements*: Iron supplements, particularly ferrous sulfate, can lead to constipation by causing GI irritation and altering stool consistency.
- *Diuretics*: While primarily used to manage fluid retention and hypertension, diuretics can lead to dehydration, further increasing the risk of constipation.
- *Antidepressants*: Certain classes of antidepressants, particularly tricyclic antidepressants, can have anticholinergic effects that contribute to constipation.

Comorbidities

Older adults often have multiple chronic conditions, which can complicate the management of constipation. Key comorbidities include the following:

- *Neurological disorders*: Conditions such as PD, multiple sclerosis, stroke, and dementia can disrupt normal bowel function. These disorders can impair the autonomic nervous system, which regulates GI motility, and affect the coordination of the muscles involved in defecation.
- *Metabolic disorders*: Endocrine conditions such as hypothyroidism can lead to decreased metabolism and reduced bowel motility, contributing to constipation. Diabetes mellitus can also affect bowel function, with potential nerve damage (diabetic neuropathy) impairing gut motility.
- *Gastrointestinal disorders*: Chronic conditions such as irritable bowel syndrome (IBS), diverticulitis, and colorectal cancer can alter bowel habits and contribute to constipation. Inflammatory bowel disease (IBD) may cause changes in bowel motility and stool consistency, complicating constipation management.
- *Psychiatric disorders*: Depression, anxiety, and cognitive decline can impact appetite, dietary choices, and motivation to engage in physical activity, all of which can contribute to constipation. Cognitive impairment can further complicate the recognition of the urge to defecate, leading to delays in responding.

Psychosocial Factors

Cognitive Impairment

Dementia and other cognitive disorders can lead to forgetfulness regarding bowel habits, reduced awareness of the need to defecate, and difficulty following dietary recommendations. This impairment can significantly increase the risk of constipation.

Mood Disorders

Depression is prevalent among older adults and is associated with changes in dietary habits, physical activity, and overall motivation. The feelings of fatigue and low energy often seen in depression can contribute to a sedentary lifestyle, exacerbating constipation.

Social Isolation

Older adults who are socially isolated may have limited access to nutritious foods, healthcare, and social support. Isolation can lead to a lack of motivation to maintain healthy habits, further increasing the risk of constipation.

Fear of Incontinence or Pain

Many older adults may experience anxiety related to bowel movements, especially if they have previously experienced pain during defecation or are fearful of fecal incontinence. This fear can lead to withholding of bowel movements, contributing to constipation.

CLINICAL ASSESSMENT

A comprehensive clinical assessment is vital for understanding the underlying causes of constipation in older adults and tailoring appropriate management strategies. This process involves a systematic approach that encompasses patient history, physical examination, and relevant diagnostic investigations. The key components of a thorough clinical assessment for constipation are as follows.

Detailed History

Bowel Habits

Gathering detailed information about the patient's bowel habits is crucial. Key questions include the following:

- *Frequency*: How often do you have bowel movements? Is this different from your normal pattern?
- *Consistency*: How would you describe your stools? Are they hard, lumpy, or watery? Using the Bristol stool chart can help patients identify stool consistency more easily.
- *Effort*: Do you experience difficulty or straining when trying to pass stool? How long does it usually take?
- *Sensation of incomplete evacuation*: Do you feel that you have completely emptied your bowels after a movement?

Dietary and Fluid Intake

Understanding the patient's diet is essential. Key aspects to explore include the following:

- *Fiber intake*: How often do you consume fruits, vegetables, whole grains, and legumes? Are you familiar with dietary fiber recommendations?
- *Fluid consumption*: How much fluid do you drink daily? Are there specific reasons for reduced fluid intake, such as medical conditions?

Medications

A thorough medication review is necessary to identify any drugs that may contribute to constipation. Important points to consider include the following:

- *Current medications*: List all prescription and over-the-counter medications. Focus particularly on known constipating agents (e.g., opioids, anticholinergics, and calcium channel blockers).
- *Recent changes*: Have there been any recent changes in medication regimens or dosages that could coincide with the onset of constipation?

Associated Symptoms

Assessing for additional GI or systemic symptoms is crucial. Important questions include the following:

- *Abdominal symptoms*: Do you experience abdominal pain, bloating, or cramping? Have there been any changes in appetite or weight?
- *Rectal symptoms*: Are there any signs of rectal bleeding, fissures, or hemorrhoids?
- *General symptoms*: Have you experienced any fatigue, weakness, or other systemic signs that could indicate underlying issues?

Quality of Life

Understanding the impact of constipation on daily activities and psychological well-being is important. Questions to explore include the following:

- *Impact on daily life*: How does constipation affect your daily routine and social interactions? Are you avoiding activities due to bowel issues?
- *Psychosocial factors*: Are there any feelings of embarrassment, anxiety, or distress related to your bowel habits?

Physical Examination

A focused physical examination can provide valuable insights into potential causes of constipation. Key components of the examination include:

- *Abdominal examination*:
    - *Inspection*: Look for signs of distension or tenderness.
    - *Palpation*: Assess for abdominal tenderness, masses, or palpable stool (indicating fecal impaction).
    - *Auscultation*: Listen for bowel sounds, which can provide information about motility.
- *Rectal examination*: A rectal examination is often a crucial component of the assessment, particularly if there are concerns about fecal impaction or other rectal issues. Important points to note include:
    - *Anal tone*: Assess the tone of the anal sphincter, which can provide insights into pelvic floor function.
    - *Presence of hemorrhoids*: Check for external or internal hemorrhoids that could contribute to discomfort during bowel movements.
    - *Fecal impaction*: Evaluate for palpable fecal matter within the rectum, which may require manual disimpaction.

Laboratory Tests

While laboratory tests are not always necessary in the initial evaluation of constipation, they can be helpful in ruling out underlying conditions or identifying contributing factors. Common tests may include the following:

- *Complete blood count (CBC)*: This test can help identify anemia, which may be indicative of chronic blood loss from GI sources or an underlying malignancy.
- *Serum electrolytes*: Electrolyte levels, including sodium, potassium, and calcium, should be evaluated to rule

out metabolic causes of constipation. Hypercalcemia, for example, can slow intestinal motility.

- *Thyroid function tests*: Assessing thyroid function [thyroid-stimulating hormone (TSH) and T4] is essential, as hypothyroidism can lead to decreased bowel motility and constipation.
- *Blood glucose levels*: Checking blood glucose levels is important, particularly in patients with a history of diabetes, as diabetic neuropathy can contribute to bowel dysfunction.

Diagnostic Imaging

In certain cases, imaging studies may be necessary to rule out structural abnormalities or other significant conditions contributing to constipation. Options include the following:

- *Abdominal X-rays*: An X-ray can help identify fecal impaction or obstructions. It can also provide information about colonic gas patterns.
- *Colonoscopy*: If there are red flags (e.g., rectal bleeding, significant weight loss, or changes in bowel habits), a colonoscopy may be warranted to evaluate for colorectal cancer, IBD, or other abnormalities.
- *Defecography or anorectal manometry*: These specialized tests may be considered for individuals with ongoing symptoms despite treatment, particularly if there are concerns about pelvic floor dysfunction or rectal outlet obstruction.

RED FLAG SIGNS IN CONSTIPATION

When assessing constipation in older adults, it is crucial to be vigilant for "red flag" signs that may indicate more serious underlying conditions. Identifying these signs can prompt further investigation and intervention, ensuring timely diagnosis and treatment. Key red flag signs include the following:

- *Unexplained weight loss*: Significant or unexplained weight loss (e.g., >5% of body weight over 6–12 months) can be indicative of underlying malignancy, particularly colorectal cancer, or other serious health issues.
- *Rectal bleeding*: Any rectal bleeding, whether bright red blood or darker stools (melena), warrants immediate evaluation. This may suggest bleeding from hemorrhoids, anal fissures, diverticular disease, or malignancy.
- *Anemia*: Signs of anemia, such as fatigue, pallor, or shortness of breath, can suggest chronic blood loss due to GI bleeding. A CBC should be performed to assess hemoglobin levels.
- *Change in bowel habits*: A sudden change in bowel habits, such as a shift from diarrhea to constipation or changes in the frequency and consistency of stools, can indicate underlying GI disorders, including IBD or malignancy.
- *Severe abdominal pain*: Severe or persistent abdominal pain, especially if accompanied by distension, may suggest bowel obstruction, severe constipation (fecal impaction), or other acute abdominal conditions.
- *New-onset constipation*: New-onset constipation in older adults, particularly if it occurs after the age of 50 years, can be concerning. This may warrant further evaluation for structural or pathological changes in the colon.
- *Nausea and vomiting*: The presence of nausea and vomiting, particularly if associated with abdominal pain or distension, may indicate bowel obstruction or significant GI pathology.
- *Incontinence or neurological symptoms*: New or worsening fecal incontinence, changes in urinary patterns, or neurological symptoms (e.g., weakness, sensory loss) may suggest spinal cord lesions or other neurological conditions that require urgent evaluation.
- *History of cancer or IBD*: A personal or family history of colorectal cancer or IBD heightens the suspicion of serious underlying pathology in patients presenting with constipation.
- *Failure to respond to standard treatment*: Constipation that is refractory to standard treatments, including lifestyle modifications, increased fiber intake, and over-the-counter laxatives, may warrant further investigation to identify underlying causes.

ROME IV CRITERIA FOR FUNCTIONAL CONSTIPATION

To be diagnosed with functional constipation, patients must meet the following criteria:

- *At least two of the following symptoms must be present for the past 3 months* (with symptoms onset at least 6 months prior to diagnosis):
  - Fewer than three bowel movements per week.
  - More than 25% of bowel movements with one or more of the following:
    - Straining during defecation
    - Lumpy or hard stools (Bristol Stool Form Scale types 1 or 2)
    - Sensation of incomplete evacuation
    - Sensation of anorectal obstruction/blockage
    - Manual maneuvers to facilitate defecation (e.g., digital evacuation, support of the pelvic floor)

- *The symptoms are not attributable to another medical condition* (e.g., IBD, colorectal cancer, and medication effects) and do not occur exclusively during episodes of diarrhea.
- *The symptoms should occur at least 1 in every 4 weeks* during the last 3 months.

NOTE ON SUBTYPES OF CONSTIPATION

Based on the patient's bowel habits and characteristics of their stool, functional constipation can be further classified into subtypes, including:

- *Normal transit constipation*: The most common type, where patients may report constipation but have normal colonic transit times upon investigation.
- *Slow transit constipation*: Characterized by prolonged colonic transit times, often associated with decreased bowel motility.
- *Outlet dysfunction*: Involves difficulty in evacuating stool due to pelvic floor dysfunction or anorectal obstruction.

MANAGEMENT STRATEGIES

Effective management of constipation in older adults involves a multifaceted approach that combines dietary and lifestyle modifications, pharmacological interventions, and consideration of underlying medical conditions. The strategies should be tailored to the individual's needs, preferences, and any specific risk factors identified during the clinical assessment. Key management strategies for addressing constipation in this population are given in the following text.

Dietary Modifications

Increased Fiber Intake

- *Dietary recommendations*: Encourage a gradual increase in dietary fiber, aiming for 20–30 g/day. This can be achieved through the inclusion of fruits, vegetables, whole grains, legumes, and nuts. High-fiber foods include beans, lentils, broccoli, berries, whole-grain bread, and cereals.
- *Fiber supplements*: For individuals who struggle to meet fiber intake through diet alone, fiber supplements such as psyllium (Metamucil), methylcellulose (Citrucel), or wheat dextrin (Benefiber) may be recommended. These supplements can help increase stool bulk and facilitate easier passage.

Hydration

- *Fluid intake*: Encourage adequate fluid intake (1.5–2 L daily) to help soften stools and improve bowel function. Adjustments may be necessary based on individual medical conditions (e.g., heart failure, renal issues) that might limit fluid intake.
- *Monitor caffeine and alcohol*: Advise moderation of caffeinated and alcoholic beverages, as excessive consumption can contribute to dehydration.

Lifestyle Modifications

Physical Activity

- *Encourage regular exercise*: Promote regular physical activity tailored to the individual's abilities. Activities such as walking, stretching, and resistance exercises can stimulate bowel motility and reduce constipation.
- *Structured programs*: Consider referral to physical therapy or exercise programs designed for older adults, which can enhance strength and balance, promoting greater mobility and independence.

Bowel Habits

- *Establish a routine*: Encourage patients to establish a regular time for bowel movements, ideally after meals when the gastrocolic reflex is strongest.
- *Respond to urges*: Advise patients to respond promptly to the urge to defecate to prevent withholding, which can exacerbate constipation.

Pharmacological Interventions

When dietary and lifestyle modifications are insufficient in managing constipation, pharmacological interventions can be beneficial. The choice of medication should be individualized based on the patient's clinical presentation, underlying conditions, and response to previous treatments. An expanded overview of various pharmacological options available for managing constipation in older adults is given in the following text.

Laxatives

Osmotic Laxatives

Osmotic laxatives are among the most commonly used agents for treating constipation. They work by drawing water into the intestines, softening stools, and promoting bowel movements.

- *Polyethylene glycol (PEG)*:
  - *Brand names*: MiraLAX and GoLYTELY (in higher doses for bowel preparation).
  - *Dosage*: Typically, 17 g is dissolved in 4–8 ounces of water once daily.
  - *Mechanism*: Increases osmotic pressure in the intestinal lumen, resulting in enhanced water retention in the stool, leading to softer stools and increased bowel frequency.

- *Considerations*: Generally well-tolerated with minimal side effects. Adequate hydration is important to maximize effectiveness.

- *Lactulose*:
  - *Brand names*: Enulose and Kristalose.
  - *Dosage*: Start with 15–30 mL daily, which can be adjusted based on response.
  - *Mechanism*: A synthetic disaccharide that is not absorbed in the intestines. It is fermented by colonic bacteria, producing organic acids that draw water into the bowel.
  - *Considerations*: May cause gas, bloating, or abdominal discomfort, especially at higher doses.
- *Magnesium hydroxide*:
  - *Brand names*: Phillips' Milk of Magnesia
  - *Dosage*: 30–60 mL orally, usually at bedtime
  - *Mechanism*: Increases water in the intestinal lumen via osmotic effects
  - *Considerations*: Use cautiously in patients with renal impairment due to the risk of hypermagnesemia

Stimulant Laxatives

Stimulant laxatives promote bowel movements by directly stimulating the enteric nervous system and increasing peristalsis.

- *Senna*:
  - *Brand names*: Senokot and Ex-Lax
  - *Dosage*: 8.6–17.2 mg taken once daily or in divided doses
  - *Mechanism*: Increases colonic motility and alters electrolyte secretion in the intestines
  - *Considerations*: Generally safe for short-term use. Prolonged use can lead to dependence or tolerance
- *Bisacodyl*:
  - *Brand names*: Dulcolax
  - *Dosage*: 5–10 mg orally or 10 mg rectally as needed
  - *Mechanism*: Stimulates colonic mucosal nerve endings, increasing peristalsis
  - *Considerations*: Can cause abdominal cramps and diarrhea. Avoid in patients with GI obstruction.

Bulk-forming Laxatives

Bulk-forming laxatives increase stool bulk, promoting regular bowel movements through a natural mechanism.

- *Psyllium*:
  - *Brand names*: Metamucil
  - *Dosage*: One tablespoon in 8 ounces of water, taken one to three times daily
  - *Mechanism*: Absorbs water in the intestines to form a gel-like substance, adding bulk to the stool
  - *Considerations*: Must be taken with adequate fluids to prevent choking or obstruction. Generally well tolerated
- *Methylcellulose*:
  - *Brand names*: Citrucel
  - *Dosage*: One tablespoon in 8 ounces of water, taken one to three times daily
  - *Mechanism*: Similar to psyllium, it absorbs water to increase stool bulk
  - *Considerations*: Safe for long-term use but can cause bloating or gas

Prokinetic Agents

- *Prucalopride*:
  - *Brand names*: Resolor
  - *Dosage*: 2 mg orally once daily (adjustable to 1 mg for older adults or those with renal impairment)
  - *Mechanism*: A selective serotonin 5-HT4 receptor agonist that enhances GI motility
  - *Considerations*: Effective in treating chronic constipation, particularly in cases of slow transit. Side effects may include headache, nausea, and abdominal pain.

Secretagogues

- *Lubiprostone*:
  - *Brand names*: Amitiza
  - *Dosage*: 24 µg taken orally twice daily
  - *Mechanism*: A chloride channel activator that increases intestinal fluid secretion and enhances motility
  - *Considerations*: Used for chronic idiopathic constipation and IBS-C. May cause nausea, diarrhea, and abdominal discomfort
- *Linaclotide*:
  - *Brand names*: Linzess
  - *Dosage*: 145 µg taken orally once daily, typically on an empty stomach
  - *Mechanism*: A guanylate cyclase-C agonist that increases intestinal fluid secretion and transit
  - *Considerations*: Effective for chronic constipation and IBS-C. Common side effects include diarrhea and abdominal pain.

Enemas and Rectal Agents

- *Saline enemas*:
  - *Indications*: Often used for immediate relief of constipation or bowel preparation
  - *Mechanism*: Osmotic effect draws water into the bowel, facilitating evacuation
  - *Considerations*: Can be administered at home but may cause discomfort or electrolyte imbalances with excessive use
- *Glycerin suppositories*:
  - *Mechanism*: Lubricates the stool and stimulates rectal contractions

- *Considerations*: Useful for quick relief but should not be used regularly due to potential for dependence

Management of Underlying Conditions

Addressing any underlying medical conditions contributing to constipation is crucial for effective management. This may include the following:

- *Reviewing medications*: Conduct a thorough review of the patient's medication list, identifying any drugs that may be contributing to constipation. Consider adjusting dosages or switching to alternative medications when possible.
- *Management of chronic conditions*: Addressing chronic conditions such as diabetes, hypothyroidism, or neurological disorders can help improve bowel function. Collaborate with other healthcare providers as necessary to optimize management of these comorbidities.

Patient Education and Support

Education

Provide patients and caregivers with clear information about constipation, its causes, and treatment options. Education can empower patients to take an active role in managing their symptoms.

Support Groups

Encourage participation in support groups or educational sessions focused on GI health, which can provide additional resources and foster social connections.

Follow-up and Reassessment

Regular follow-up is essential to assess the effectiveness of the management plan and make necessary adjustments. Key aspects of follow-up include the following:

- *Monitoring symptoms*: Regularly evaluate the patient's bowel habits, dietary changes, and the effectiveness of any pharmacological treatments. Assess for any new red flag symptoms that may arise.
- *Adjusting treatment plans*: Be prepared to modify the management plan based on the patient's response. If constipation persists despite initial interventions, consider further diagnostic evaluations or referral to a gastroenterologist.

SPECIAL CONSIDERATIONS IN THE MANAGEMENT OF CONSTIPATION

When managing constipation in older adults, it is crucial to account for the unique challenges presented by certain populations, particularly those who are frail, have cognitive impairments such as dementia, or have neurodegenerative disorders such as PD. These conditions can complicate the presentation and management of constipation, necessitating tailored strategies. The key special considerations for these vulnerable populations are given in the following text.

Frailty

Frailty is a common syndrome in older adults characterized by decreased physiological reserve and increased vulnerability to stressors. Patients with frailty may experience multiple comorbidities, polypharmacy, and reduced functional capacity, all of which can contribute to constipation.

- *Management challenges*:
    - *Increased sensitivity to medications*: Frail patients may be more sensitive to the side effects of laxatives, necessitating cautious dosing and close monitoring.
    - *Dietary challenges*: Individuals with frailty may have difficulty maintaining adequate nutrition and hydration, leading to insufficient fiber and fluid intake.
    - *Mobility issues*: Reduced physical activity can impair bowel motility, making regular exercise and mobility support critical components of management.
- *Management strategies*:
    - Prioritize nonpharmacological approaches, such as dietary modifications and encouraging physical activity within the patient's capabilities.
    - Regularly assess medication regimens for potential constipating agents and adjust as necessary.
    - Foster an environment that promotes independence and dignity, such as providing adaptive aids for mobility.

Dementia

Patients with dementia often experience challenges that can complicate the management of constipation, including difficulties in communication, reduced insight into their condition, and behavioral changes.

- *Management challenges*:
    - *Cognitive impairment*: Patients may not recognize the urge to defecate, leading to stool retention and worsening constipation.
    - *Dietary preferences*: Changes in appetite and food preferences can limit fiber and fluid intake, exacerbating constipation.
    - *Increased dependence*: Patients may require assistance with toileting, dietary choices, and

medication management, making caregiver education essential.

- *Management strategies*:
  - Establish a regular toileting schedule to encourage routine bowel habits and respond to cues.
  - Work with caregivers to create supportive environments that facilitate access to the bathroom and adequate hydration and nutrition.
  - Use simple, clear communication and visual cues to help patients understand dietary changes and medication regimens.

Parkinson's Disease

Parkinson's disease is a neurodegenerative disorder that can significantly impact GI function, leading to constipation as a common nonmotor symptom.

- *Management challenges*:
  - *GI dysmotility*: Patients with PD may experience slowed gastric emptying and decreased colonic motility due to autonomic dysfunction, leading to constipation.
  - *Medication effects*: Dopaminergic medications, while beneficial for motor symptoms, can contribute to constipation as a side effect.
  - *Postural changes*: Patients with PD may have postural issues that complicate bowel movements, making access to the toilet challenging.
- *Management strategies*:
  - Regularly assess the patient's medication regimen, considering the balance between managing PD symptoms and minimizing constipation.
  - Encourage dietary modifications, including increased fiber and hydration, and consider fiber supplements if necessary.
  - Promote physical activity and encourage exercises that focus on core strength and flexibility to enhance mobility and bowel function.
  - Collaborate with a multidisciplinary team, including physical therapists and occupational therapists, to create individualized care plans that address mobility and access issues.

Polypharmacy Considerations

Older adults frequently take multiple medications for various chronic conditions, increasing the risk of constipation due to drug interactions and side effects.

- *Management challenges*:
  - Many common medications, including opioids, anticholinergics, diuretics, and certain antidepressants, can lead to constipation.
  - The complexity of managing multiple medications can lead to confusion, adherence issues, and adverse effects.
- *Management strategies*:
  - Conduct a thorough medication review to identify potential constipating agents and consider alternatives when appropriate.
  - Educate patients and caregivers about the importance of reporting new-onset constipation and the potential roles of their medications.
  - Involve a pharmacist in care coordination to optimize medication regimens and minimize adverse effects.

Cultural and Socioeconomic Factors

Cultural beliefs and socioeconomic status can significantly influence dietary choices, access to healthcare, and overall management of constipation.

- *Management challenges*:
  - Dietary preferences and beliefs may affect the acceptance of recommended dietary changes.
  - Limited access to healthcare resources can impede timely interventions and follow-up care.
- *Management strategies*:
  - Engage with patients and caregivers to understand cultural perspectives and dietary practices, ensuring that recommendations align with their beliefs.
  - Provide education on affordable dietary sources of fiber and hydration, considering community resources or programs that may assist with access to healthy foods.
  - Explore local resources that offer support services or transportation options to facilitate access to medical care.

CONCLUSION

Constipation in older adults is a common yet often underrecognized condition with multifactorial origins, including age-related physiological changes, comorbidities, polypharmacy, and functional or cognitive impairments. Effective management requires a holistic approach that combines lifestyle modifications, dietary interventions, and judicious use of pharmacological agents tailored to individual needs. Special attention must be given to vulnerable populations such as those with dementia or Parkinson's disease. By prioritizing early identification, personalized care, and regular medication review, clinicians can significantly improve bowel health, comfort, and overall quality of life in the elderly.

Self-Assessment Questionnaire

Q1. What are the key physiological changes in older adults that contribute to an increased prevalence of constipation?

Q2. How does polypharmacy in older adults complicate the management of constipation, and what strategies can be employed to mitigate these challenges?

Q3. What are the Rome IV criteria for diagnosing functional constipation, and why are they important in the geriatric population?

Q4. Discuss the role of dietary modifications in the management of constipation in older adults. What specific recommendations would you provide?

Q5. What pharmacological options are available for treating constipation in older adults, and how would you decide which to use?

Q6. What special considerations should be taken into account when managing constipation in older adults with dementia or Parkinson's disease?

FURTHER READINGS

1. Rao SSC, Go JT. Constipation in older adults: Stepwise approach to keep things moving. Cleveland Clinic J Med. 2012;79(9):699-705.
2. Joseph A, Monaghan T, O'Donnell MJ. Understanding constipation as a geriatric syndrome. J Geriatr Med. 2025.
3. Rao AR, Shetty CN, Shenoy JS. Management of constipation in older adults. Am Fam Physician. 2015;92(6):500-506.
4. Camilleri M, Bharucha AE. Pathophysiology of constipation in the older adult. J Gerontol Med Sci. 2008;63(6):619-625.
5. Talley NJ, Fleming KC, Evans JM. Constipation. StatPearlsTreasure Island StatPearls Publishing; 2023.

CHAPTER 44

Prehabilitation and Postoperative Rehabilitation among the Elderly Patients: Recent Advances and Future Prospectives

Arun Kumar Choudhary

CASE VIGNETTE

Mrs Suman Gupta, a 72-year-old retired school teacher, presents to the outpatient department for a preoperative assessment. She is scheduled for elective surgery for a right-sided hemicolectomy due to a recently diagnosed colonic adenocarcinoma. Her medical history includes hypertension controlled with amlodipine, type 2 diabetes mellitus on metformin, and mild osteoarthritis of the knees. She has a 28 kg/m^2 body mass index (BMI), reports low physical activity, and recently experienced fatigue and mild weight loss.

Baseline functional assessment:

- *Gait speed*: 0.8 m/s (slow gait speed)
- *Handgrip strength*: 18 kg (low for age and sex)
- *Short Physical Performance Battery (SPPB) score*: 7/12 (indicating moderate physical impairment)

Nutritional status:

- Mildly malnourished (serum albumin 3.2 g/dL)
- Recent dietary recall reveals reduced protein intake (~0.6 g/kg/day).

Psychosocial context: Mrs Gupta lives with her son and daughter-in-law but feels socially isolated due to limited engagement in activities and a lack of peer interaction. She expresses anxiety about surgery and concerns about postoperative recovery.

Prehabilitation strategy: The surgical and geriatric teams collaboratively design a tailored 4-week prehabilitation program given as follows:

- *Physical prehabilitation*: Supervised resistance training and aerobic exercises, including progressive walking and lower-limb strengthening.
- *Nutritional optimization*: High-protein diet with supplementation (whey protein) to meet protein requirements (~1.2–1.5 g/kg/day).
- *Psychological support*: Counseling sessions and relaxation techniques to address anxiety and build resilience.

Postoperative rehabilitation plan: After a successful surgery, Mrs Gupta's recovery plan involves:

- *Early mobilization*: Initiating physical therapy (PT) within 24 hours postsurgery to prevent deconditioning.
- *Nutritional continuity*: Continued emphasis on protein-rich diets to support wound healing and muscle recovery.
- *Cognitive engagement*: Monitoring for delirium and providing activities to promote cognitive function.
- *Comprehensive follow-up:* Regular visits to address functional, nutritional, and psychosocial needs.

Outcome: At the 3-month follow-up, Mrs Gupta demonstrates significant improvement given as follows:

- Gait speed: 1.1 m/s
- *SPPB score*: 10/12
- Increased confidence in daily activities and participation in a local yoga group.

This case highlights the critical role of prehabilitation and postoperative rehabilitation in optimizing outcomes for elderly surgical patients.

INTRODUCTION

Geriatric rehabilitation focuses on the unique needs of aging individuals, primarily those aged 65 years and above. It emphasizes distinguishing normal aging from the sequelae of prolonged illness. Aging is associated with multiple physiological changes, including decreased muscle mass, slower gait speed, declines in vision and hearing, and diminished adaptive and protective reflexes necessary to maintain balance and coordination.

According to the World Health Organization, rehabilitation medicine aims to maximize function and minimize activity limitations and participation restrictions resulting from underlying impairments or diseases. Geriatric rehabilitation is inherently multidisciplinary, involving a team of physiatrists, therapists (physical, occupational, and speech), nurses, prosthetists, orthotists (a healthcare professional who creates and fits orthotic devices, or orthoses to support and protect a patient's musculoskeletal system), psychologists or psychiatrists, dieticians, and social workers. This collaborative approach ensures comprehensive care tailored to the needs of older adults.

Geriatric rehabilitation plays a critical role in improving the functional status and quality of life (QoL) of elderly patients. It includes two major components: (1) prehabilitation—aimed at optimizing functional capacity before surgery to help patients withstand the physiological stress of surgical interventions—and (2) postoperative rehabilitation, which focuses on recovery, minimizing complications, and reducing mortality rates after surgery.

Elderly patients admitted to hospitals, particularly for surgical interventions, are especially vulnerable to functional decline, reduced endurance, and loss of muscle strength. Studies show that up to 50% of hospitalized older adults experience functional decline before admission due to reduced baseline capacity. During hospitalization, 80% of the elderly spend their time in bed, leading to complications such as decreased aerobic capacity, lower extremity muscle strength, and bone mineral density.

Rehabilitation management for elderly patients is thus broadly categorized into preoperative interventions—designed to enhance functional capacity and resilience to withstand surgery—and postoperative interventions, which aim to facilitate recovery, restore functionality, and minimize complications. Emerging clinical evidence underscores the effectiveness of interdisciplinary rehabilitation strategies, both preoperatively and postoperatively, in improving functional capacity, physical performance, and QoL among elderly patients.

SOCIODEMOGRAPHIC FACTORS AND FRAILTY

With the present change in sociodemographics, operative teams are dealing with a more significant number of older patients. Between 1999 and 2015, the number of patients over 70–75 undergoing surgery has nearly doubled. The future projections predict that, by 2030, one fifth of surgical procedures will be conducted in this age cohort. In older patients, their conditions have been significantly influenced by the disease itself, surgery, long treatment cycles, aging, and psychological stress, all of which make the phenomenon of frailty outstanding and common among them.

Frailty is defined as a state of physiological susceptibility that varies with age due to system instability, decreased physiological reserve capacity, and reduced ability to resolve stressful situations, making it more difficult for patients to recover from surgery. The process of frailty is dynamic and ever-changing and is characterized by several systemic dysfunctions, including immune system dysfunction.

Frailty has been established as a valid and independent predictor of postoperative morbidity, mortality, and complications. Enhanced recovery after surgery (ERAS) can enhance surgical safety by minimizing stress responses in frail patients, enabling surgeons to discharge patients earlier. Continued research and multidisciplinary collaboration will be essential to refine and optimize protocols for surgical care in frail older adults. Rehabilitation performed before surgery (prehabilitation) is used to improve the results of surgical treatment. However, the results of studies have not unquestionably confirmed the effectiveness of preoperative rehabilitation and its impact on the outcome of surgery.

An in-depth and early knowledge of factors that influence length of stay (LOS) in hospital may enable the multidisciplinary team to plan a patient-tailored rehabilitation program and better allocate resources to maximize patients' functional recovery while reducing LOS and the overall cost of the procedure. Evidence suggests that patients receiving inpatient rehabilitation following a TKA or THA experience similar outcomes as those with rehabilitation in other settings. Using kinesiotaping early in postoperative rehabilitation could be a useful modality for reducing pain and increasing the range of knee flexion. However, the certainty of evidence is very low.

The state of nutrition of elderly patients with intertrochanteric fracture of the femur before the operation affects the patient's tolerance to the operation, body recovery, healing of the wound, and clinical prognosis. For these patients, the poor state of nutrition may lengthen the hospital stay and lead to poor hip recovery and clinical outcomes.

Preoperative Assessment of Elderly Patients

In addition to a comprehensive history and physical examination, the following assessments are recommended for elderly patients undergoing surgery:

- *Cognitive assessment*: Evaluate for cognitive impairment, including dementia or mild cognitive decline.
- *Screen for depression*: Use validated tools to identify depressive symptoms that may affect recovery.

- *Assessment of risk factors for postoperative delirium*: Identify modifiable and nonmodifiable risk factors for delirium.
- *Screen for alcohol or drug abuse/dependence*: Assess and manage substance use that could complicate perioperative care.
- *Preoperative cardiac evaluation*: Follow the American College of Cardiology/American Heart Association (ACC/AHA) guidelines for cardiac risk assessment in noncardiac surgery.
- *Prevention of postoperative pulmonary complications*: Incorporate pulmonary rehabilitation strategies, including inspiratory muscle training, especially in patients with pre-existing respiratory conditions.
- *Functional status assessment*: Evaluate the patient's baseline mobility and independence in activities of daily living.
- *History of falls*: Document details of previous falls and assess for balance or gait issues.
- *Baseline frailty score*: Measure frailty using validated tools such as the Fried Frailty Phenotype or Clinical Frailty Scale.
- *Nutritional status assessment*: Assess for malnutrition and plan for nutritional optimization preoperatively.
- *Medication history and polypharmacy*: Review all medications and identify potentially inappropriate prescriptions.
- *Goal setting*: Define short-term and long-term treatment goals, incorporating the patient's and family's expectations.

A detailed preoperative assessment allows for the design of a customized rehabilitation plan, addressing reversible alterations in systems such as cardiovascular, pulmonary, gastrointestinal, nervous, and musculoskeletal. This comprehensive approach positively impacts postoperative outcomes and recovery in older patients.

Preoperative Malnutrition in Elderly Patients

Malnutrition in elderly patients undergoing surgery, such as those with intertrochanteric fractures, has significant adverse effects (AEs), including:

- Poor postoperative hip function recovery.
- Reduced 1-year postoperative survival rates.

Nutritional optimization through dietary interventions and supplementation is essential to improve surgical outcomes and enhance recovery.

Delirium in Elderly Patients

Delirium is a critical concern in elderly surgical patients, associated with:

- Increased morbidity and mortality.
- Prolonged hospital stays, especially after hip fractures.

Key insights:

- *Preoperative delirium*: Associated with distinct risk factors, poorer prognosis, and higher mortality compared to postoperative delirium.
- Patients with risk factors for preoperative delirium require close monitoring and interventions to mitigate their heightened risk of adverse outcomes.

Prehabilitation in Colorectal Cancer Surgery

Prehabilitation before colorectal cancer (CRC) surgery offers significant benefits:

- Reduces postoperative complications.
- Enhances recovery of functional performance.

This approach is particularly effective in:

- Patients aged 70 years or older.
- Patients with an American Society of Anesthesiologists (ASA) physical status classification of 3–4, where surgery poses higher risks.

Implementing prehabilitation in these high-risk groups minimizes long-term functional decline and improves overall surgical outcomes.

Postoperative Rehabilitation of Elderly Patients

Postoperative rehabilitation includes various interventions that have several positive outcomes among elderly individuals while recovering from postsurgical procedures. Many studies claimed that exercises such as mobilization, endurance, and progressive resistive exercises have significantly increased strength and functional and motor performance among elderly patients and may also improve balance coordination. In this phase, it is beneficial for the rehabilitation team to counsel patients and their families regarding the expected outcomes. The prescription of an appropriate customized postoperative rehabilitation program tailored according to the individual elderly patient's needs is part of a multidisciplinary postoperative rehabilitation program.

Many high-quality studies have claimed that early mobilization is the fundamental ingredient of the postoperative rehabilitation program in elderly patients.

A study claimed that patients receiving early physical training and occupational therapy showed better functional outcomes when they were discharged.

In many studies that included elderly patients, it was demonstrated that early physical training after surgery is feasible, safe, and tolerable, resulting in improvement of QoL, physical fitness and overall well-being. Elderly patients should receive the rehabilitation specialist's advice on the first postoperative day, followed by close monitoring and supervising the graded increase in the exercise program. In order to improve the mobility of elderly patients who underwent surgery, portable suction drains must be used. Portable exercise devices must be used for elderly patients who are unable to leave their bed space. Patients must be encouraged to perform the individually tailored mobilization program, with an increase in a graded manner.

During the postoperative mobilization program, elderly patients are encouraged to perform a customized exercise program at least three to four times daily. The training intensities are predominately based on heart rate reserve and rated perceived exertion using commonly the modified Borg scale. It is postulated that posture and arm exercises may significantly reduce shoulder dysfunction and regain functional independence in activities of daily living (ADL). Various training modalities such as endurance, resistive, and interval training must be integral to any exercise program for postoperative rehabilitation of elderly patients. Several studies showed that such training modalities can potentially improve the musculoskeletal, cardiovascular, and pulmonary function of elderly individuals.

Other important components such as adequate pain management and dietary modifications are incorporated in current postoperative rehabilitation programs for elderly patients. Pain management is of paramount importance for the rehabilitation team to achieve better participation of the elderly patients in the program, and rehabilitation team may control pain using various modalities, such as pharmacological (analgesic medications, opioids) and nonpharmacological measures such as transcutaneous electrical nerve stimulation (TENS), and various heat and cold modalities.

A careful discharge plan must be executed, and before discharge elderly surgical patients are checked for functional independence, functional capacity, pain, balance, independent walking, need for assistive devices, grip strength, and overall general well-being. An individual customized postoperative rehabilitation program is designed and to be followed after discharge in order to achieve the best possible outcomes and better QoL of the elderly patients.

RECENT ADVANCES AND FUTURE PROSPECTIVES

Virtual Reality in Rehabilitation for Orthopedic Surgery Patients

The effectiveness of virtual reality (VR)-based interventions in orthopedic surgery patients has been examined in several studies. While some demonstrate improved patient-reported outcomes and satisfaction, others show mixed results, with comparable or varied outcomes compared to traditional rehabilitation methods. However, VR-based rehabilitation has shown positive impacts on proprioception, pain management, and balance, particularly in elderly patients.

It is concluded that VR-based rehabilitation complements, rather than replaces, conventional rehabilitation approaches. It has the potential to aid in pain reduction and functional improvement, presenting a dynamic and engaging method for enhancing recovery after orthopedic surgery.

Prehabilitation in Cardiac and Pulmonary Rehabilitation

Studies indicate that participation in cardiac or pulmonary rehabilitation programs is associated with reduced frailty compared to patients who do not engage in such programs. These findings highlight the potential benefits of prehabilitation for patients awaiting heart or lung transplantation, improving their resilience and readiness for surgery.

Sarcopenia and Surgical Outcomes in Adult Spinal Deformity Surgery

Sarcopenia, defined by a low normalized total psoas area (NTPA), is a predictor of poor perioperative outcomes following adult spinal deformity (ASD) surgery. Evidence linking the benefits of PT to sarcopenic patients remains limited. However, sarcopenic patients may benefit from structured preoperative PT, which could:

- Improve early postoperative mobility.
- Reduce AEs.
- Decrease LOS in the hospital.

Incorporating PT into the preoperative management of sarcopenic patients is a promising strategy to enhance surgical outcomes.

Functional Decline and Rehabilitation after Cardiac Surgery in Elderly Patients

Advances in surgical technology and perioperative cardiac surgery management now enable surgeries in elderly patients over 65 years old and those with comorbidities. Despite these advancements, *20–30% of elderly patients undergoing cardiac surgery experience postoperative physical functional decline*, a significant predictor of long-term impairment or mortality.

Key insights on functional decline:

- Prolonged intensive care unit (ICU) stays are associated with poor outcomes, including a heightened risk of physical functional decline.
- ICU-acquired weakness (ICU-AW) syndrome develops in approximately *40% of critically ill patients,* significantly impairing physical function and health-related QoL (HRQoL) over an extended period.

Factors influencing physical function at hospital discharge after cardiac surgery include:

- Age
- Preoperative gait speed
- Cognitive function
- Quality and timing of postoperative rehabilitation

Rehabilitation strategies: Early mobilization and targeted rehabilitation are critical to mitigating functional decline and improving long-term outcomes in elderly cardiac surgery patients.

Clinical Implications for Rehabilitation

Prehabilitation has been promoted to improve postoperative outcomes and shorten recovery periods after total knee/hip arthroplasty (TKA/THA) for osteoarthritis. Prehabilitation improved relevant self-report and performance-based outcomes after TKA surgery. More high-quality research is required before recommending the implementation of prehabilitation programs in clinical practice for people awaiting TKA/THA. Participants adhered well to the nonoperative interventions, and their HRQoL improved. Participant and health professional feedback were extremely positive. Early rehabilitation of post-distal radius fracture (DRF) surgery with palmar plating has been found to be beneficial in enhancing upper limb functionality and back extension mobility, and in reducing pain levels. Nevertheless, no significant impact was observed regarding wrist function and complications.

KEY NOTES

The multimodal prehabilitation may decrease complications in upper abdominal surgery and associated diseases among the older people in the world. Prehabilitation improves short-term functional outcome and reduces postoperative complications in elderly patients. Elderly patients undergoing THA/TKA had several benefits from prehabilitation and tailormade postoperative rehabilitation programs. Future research direction should investigate on customized the program in different disease cohorts and exploring integrating technological advances and artificial intelligence (AI) along with telerehabilitation and its cost-effectiveness.

CONCLUSION

The importance of prehabilitation is now well established along with postoperative rehabilitation in enhancing outcomes of surgery in older patients. The combination of holistic multidisciplinary care of cognitive, psychological, frailty status before and after surgery is not only helping older adults to recover their overall capacity faster through preventing complications, but also improving overall quality of life.

As populations age and frailty increases, ongoing research and innovation are crucial to define protocols and integrate artificial intelligence, prehabilitation, rehabilitation, and telerehabilitation into geriatric surgical care for better health outcomes.

Self-Assessment Questionnaire

Q1. What are the major goals of prehabilitation in elderly surgical patients, and how do they differ from postoperative rehabilitation goals?

Q2. How does frailty influence surgical outcomes and postoperative recovery in older adults?

Q3. In the case vignette of Mrs. Suman Gupta, which interventions contributed most to her improved postoperative recovery?

Q4. Why is a multidisciplinary approach crucial in geriatric rehabilitation?

Q5. What are the main predictors of postoperative functional decline after cardiac surgery in elderly patients?

Q6. How can emerging technologies such as virtual reality, wearable robotics, or AI enhance geriatric rehabilitation outcomes?

Q7. How can prehabilitation programs be customized for patients with sarcopenia or multiple comorbidities?

Q8. Based on current evidence, what future directions should research in geriatric prehabilitation and postoperative rehabilitation focus on?

FURTHER READINGS

1. Wang SK, Wang QJ, Wang P, Li XY, Cui P, Wang DF, et al. The impact of frailty on clinical outcomes of older patients undergoing enhanced recovery after lumbar fusion surgery: a prospective cohort study. Int J Surg. 2024;110(8):4785-95.
2. Zdziechowski A, Zdziechowska M, Rysz J, Woldańska-Okońska M. The effectiveness of pre-operative outpatient and home rehabilitation and the impact on the results of hip arthroplasty: introductory report. Healthcare. 2024;12(3):327.
3. She KY, Huang L, Zhang HT, Gao Y, Yao KR, Luo Q, et al. Effect of prehabilitation on postoperative outcomes in the frail older people: a systematic review and meta-analysis. Geriatr Nurs. 2024;55:79-88.
4. Tornese D, Robustelli A, Ricci G, Rancoita PM, Maffulli N, Peretti GM. Predictors of postoperative hospital length of stay after total knee arthroplasty. Singapore Med J. 2024;65(2):68-73.
5. An KR, Seijas V, Xu MS, Grüßer L, Humar S, Moreno AA, et al. Does prehabilitation before esophagectomy improve postoperative outcomes? A systematic review and meta-analysis. Dis Esophag. 2024;37(3):doad066.
6. Yu Y, Gong X, Wan W, Hu X, Xiong L, Gui S, et al. Evaluation of the clinical effect of a multimodal pre-rehabilitation program guided by the behaviour change wheel in elderly women with breast cancer. Geriatr Nurs. 2024;58:44-51.
7. Osundolire S, Mbrah A, Liu SH, Lapane KL. Association between patient and facility characteristics and rehabilitation outcomes after joint replacement surgery in different rehabilitation settings for older adults: a systematic review. J Geriatr Phys Ther. 2024;47(1):E1-8.
8. Wong HM, Qi D, Ma BH, Hou PY, Kwong CK, Lee A, et al. Multidisciplinary prehabilitation to improve frailty and functional capacity in high-risk elective surgical patients: a retrospective pilot study. Perioper Med. 2024;13(1):6.
9. Lan D, Li Y, Liu J, Wei S, Li L, Xu H. Effect of pre-operative nutritional status on postoperative functional recovery of hip joint in elderly patients with intertrochanteric fractures. Altern Ther Health Med. 2024;30(2):140-5.
10. Adebero T, Omana H, Somerville L, Lanting B, Hunter SW. Effectiveness of prehabilitation on outcomes following total knee and hip arthroplasty for osteoarthritis: a systematic review and meta-analysis of randomised controlled trials. Disab Rehab. 2024; 46(24):5771-90.
11. Groen LC, van Gestel T, Daams F, van den Heuvel B, Taveirne A, Bruns ER, et al. Community-based prehabilitation in older patients and high-risk patients undergoing colorectal cancer surgery. Eur J Surg Oncol. 2024;50(1):107293.
12. Ickert EC, Griswold D, Ross O, Dudash S, Duchon C, Learman K. Effects of kinesiotaping during early post-operative rehabilitation in individuals who underwent a total knee arthroplasty: a systematic review and meta-analysis of randomised control trials. Clin Rehab. 2024;38(6):732-48.
13. van Dijk M, Allegaert P, Locus M, Saenen L, Breuls S, Michiels D, et al. In-hospital rehabilitation with the Geriatric Activation Program Pellenberg improves functional performance in a heterogeneous geriatric population. Physiother Theory Prac. 2024;40(4):755-66.
14. Dinesh V, Pierce R, Hespe L, Thakkar S, Wong M, El Sabbagh L, et al. The relationship between rehabilitation and frailty in advanced heart or lung disease. Transplant Direct. 2024;10(4): e1606.
15. Hirase T, Lovecchio F, Allen M, Achebe CC, Mazzucco M, Uzzo RN, et al. Pre-operative physical therapy is associated with decreased length of stay and improved postoperative mobility in patients with sarcopenia undergoing adult spinal deformity surgery. Spine. 2025;50(3):172-8.
16. Honda Y, Honma K, Nishimura S, Nakao S, Sasanuma N, Manabe E, et al. Predictors of postoperative physical functional decline at hospital discharge in elderly patients with prolonged intensive care unit stay after cardiac surgery. Heart Lung. 2024;64:86-92.
17. Zhou Z, Li X, Wu X, Wang X. Impact of early rehabilitation therapy on functional outcomes in patients post distal radius fracture surgery: a systematic review and meta-analysis. BMC Musculoskel Disord. 2024;25(1):198.
18. Ma H, Huang S, You M, Yang J, Zong R, Zhang C. Effect of early rehabilitation exercise on lower limb function and psychological state after coronary artery bypass grafting: a randomized controlled trial. Heart Surg Forum. 2024;27(5):E520-7.
19. Kristensen MT, Turabi R, Sheehan KJ. The relationship between extent of mobilisation within the first postoperative day and 30-day mortality after hip fracture surgery. Clin Rehab. 2024;38(7):990-7.
20. Milton-Cole R, Kazeem K, Gibson A, Guerra S, Sheehan KJ. Effectiveness of exercise rehabilitation interventions on depressive symptoms in older adults post hip fracture: a systematic review and meta-analysis. Osteoporosis Int. 2024;35(2):227-42.
21. Bottomley JM, Lewis CB. Pathological manifestations of aging. In: Clinical Approach to Geriatric Rehabilitation. New York: Routledge; 2024. pp. 74-108.
22. de Almeida Alcantara DA, Dos Santos FN, de Almeida Ferreira JJ, de Noronha M, de Andrade PR. The effect of kinesiotaping on edema: a systematic review and meta-analysis. Musculoskelet Sci Prac. 2024;74:103168.
23. Núñez-Cortés R, López-Bueno L, Besoain-Saldaña Á, Cruz-Montecinos C, Solís-Navarro L, Suso-Martí L, et al. Comorbidity burden and nutritional status are associated with short-term improvement in functional independence and pain intensity after hip fracture surgery in older adults with in-hospital rehabilitation. Geriatr Nurs. 2024;59:223-7.
24. Pires DP, Monte FA, Monteiro LF, Soares FR, Faria JL. Updates in the treatment of knee osteoarthritis. Revista Brasileira de Ortopedia. 2024;59(3):337-48.
25. Tabet CG, Pacheco RL, Martimbianco AL, Riera R, Hernandez AJ, Bueno DF, et al. Advanced therapy with mesenchymal stromal cells for knee osteoarthritis: Systematic review and meta-analysis of randomised controlled trials. J Orthopaed Transl. 2024;48: 176-89.
26. Pabla P, Jones EJ, Piasecki M, Phillips BE. Skeletal muscle dysfunction with advancing age. Clin Sci. 2024;138(14):863-82.
27. Chang H, Luan C, Li C. Effect of comprehensive rehabilitation training based on balance function on postoperative recovery and function of hip fracture in the elderly: a systematic review and meta-analysis. Geriatr Orthopaed Surg Rehab. 2024;15:21514593241261506.
28. Wang F, Zhang J, Guan Y, Xie J. The effect of pre-operative education on postoperative pain and function after orthopedic surgery: A systematic review and meta-analysis. Patient Educ Counsel. 2024;128:108406.
29. Özden F, Sarı Z. The effect of mobile application-based rehabilitation in patients with total knee arthroplasty: a systematic review and meta-analysis. Arch Gerontol Geriatr. 2023;113:105058.
30. Mazzolai L, Belch J, Venermo M, Aboyans V, Brodmann M, Bura-Rivière A, et al. Exercise therapy for chronic symptomatic peripheral artery disease: a clinical consensus document of the

European Society of Cardiology Working Group on aorta and peripheral vascular diseases in collaboration with the European Society of Vascular Medicine and the European Society for Vascular Surgery. Eur Heart J. 2024;45(15):1303-21.

31. Lo WT, Brodie MA, Tsang WWN, Yan CH, Lam PL, Chan CM, et al. Acceptability and feasibility of a community-based strength, balance, and Tai Chi rehabilitation program in improving physical function and balance of patients after total knee arthroplasty: study protocol for a pilot randomized controlled trial. Trials. 2021;22(1):129.
32. Lingampally PK, Ramanathan KC, Shanmugam R, Cepova L, Salunkhe S. Wearable assistive rehabilitation robotic devices—a comprehensive review. Machines. 2024;12(6):415.
33. Ehioghae M, Montoya A, Keshav R, Vippa TK, Manuk-Hakobyan H, Hasoon J, et al. Effectiveness of virtual reality–based rehabilitation interventions in improving postoperative outcomes for orthopedic surgery patients. Curr Pain Headache Rep. 2024;28(1): 37-45.
34. Medenica V, Ivanovic L, Milosevic N. Applicability of artificial intelligence in neuropsychological rehabilitation of patients with brain injury. Appl Neuropsychol Adult. 2024:1-28.
35. Ng MS, Low SS, Tay WX, Lee P, Liau ZQ. Enhanced recovery after surgery protocol improves postoperative pain and shortens length of stay among patients undergoing primary total knee arthroplasty. J Orthopaed. 2024;47:63-6.
36. Zhou W, Chu S, Zhou Y, Huang Y. Enhanced recovery after surgery for hip and knee arthroplasty: A systematic review and meta-analysis on randomised control trials. Geriatr Nurs. 2024;60: 249-57.
37. Pace V, Marzano F, Carriero B, Filippi N, Antonucci A, Topa D, et al. Enhanced recovery after surgery (ERAS) in hip and knee replacement surgery: current concepts and future trends. IntechOpen; 2024.
38. Smoor RM, van Dongen EP, Daeter EJ, Emmelot-Vonk MH, Cremer OL, Vernooij LM, et al. The association between preoperative multidisciplinary team care and patient outcome in frail patients undergoing cardiac surgery. J Thorac Cardiovasc Surg. 2024;168(2):608-16.
39. Jenkins H, Elkilany I, Guler E, Cummins K, Ayyat K, Pennacchio C, et al. Predictors and outcomes of discharge to long-term acute care facilities after cardiac surgery. J Thorac Cardiovasc Surg. 2024;168(4):1155-64.e1.
40. Malvindi PG, Bifulco O, Berretta P, Galeazzi M, Alfonsi J, Cefarelli M, et al. The enhanced recovery after surgery approach in heart valve surgery: a systematic review of clinical studies. J Clin Med. 2024;13(10):2903.
41. Master H, Pennings JS, Coronado RA, Henry AL, O'Brien MT, Haug CM, et al. Physical performance tests provide distinct information in both predicting and assessing patient-reported outcomes following lumbar spine surgery. Spine. 2020;45(23): E1556-63.
42. Devasenapathy N, Maddison R, Malhotra R, Zodepy S, Sharma S, Belavy DL. Pre-operative quadriceps muscle strength and functional ability predict performance-based outcomes 6 months after total knee arthroplasty: a systematic review. Phys Ther. 2019;99(1):46-61.
43. Thomas B, Morgan S, Smith JM. Impact of early mobilisation within the intensive care unit after coronary artery bypass grafting: a systematic review. Cardiopulm Phys Ther J. 2024;35(2):56-70.
44. Yang Q, Wang L, Zhang X, Lu P, Pan D, Li S, et al. Impact of an enhanced recovery after surgery program integrating cardiopulmonary rehabilitation on post-operative prognosis of patients treated with CABG: protocol of the ERAS-CaRe randomised controlled trial. BMC Pulmon Med. 2024;24(1):512.
45. Sahar W, Elengoe A, Batool SA, Bashir A, Shan A, Jalal A. The role of pre-operative breathing exercises in reducing postoperative respiratory complications in coronary artery bypass grafting: a comparative review of on-pump and off-pump techniques. Pak Heart J. 2024;57(3):179-87.
46. Shen Y, Cong Z, Ge Q, Huang H, Wei W, Wang C, et al. Effect of nutrition-based prehabilitation on the postoperative outcomes of patients with esophagogastric cancer undergoing surgery: a systematic review and meta-analysis. Canc Med. 2024; 13(14):e70023.
47. Wobith M, Hill A, Fischer M, Weimann A. Nutritional prehabilitation in patients undergoing abdominal surgery—a narrative review. Nutrients. 2024;16(14):2235.
48. Lydom LN, Jensen SA, Lauridsen SV, Rasmussen M, Christensen R, Joensen UN, et al. Impact on postoperative complications of combined prehabilitation targeting co-existing smoking, malnutrition, obesity, alcohol drinking, and physical inactivity: a systematic review and meta-analysis of randomised trials. F1000Research. 2024;13:694.
49. Guerra-Londono CE, Cata JP, Nowak K, Gottumukkala V. Prehabilitation in adults undergoing cancer surgery: a comprehensive review on rationale, methodology, and measures of effectiveness. Curr Oncol. 2024;31(4):2185-200.
50. Bargnes III V, Davidson S, Talbot L, Jin Z, Poppers J, Bergese SD. Start strong, finish strong: a review of prehabilitation in cardiac surgery. Life. 2024;14(7):832.
51. Cruz Mosquera FE, Murillo SR, Naranjo Rojas A, Perlaza CL, Castro Osorio D, Liscano Y. Effect of exercise and pulmonary rehabilitation in pre-and post-surgical patients with lung cancer: systematic review and meta-analysis. Medicina. 2024;60(11):1725.
52. Lai Y, Dong Y, Tian L, Li H, Ye X, Che G. The optimal time of high-intensity pre-rehabilitation for surgical lung cancer patients: a retrospective cohort study with 4452 patients. Ann Surg Oncol. 2025;32(1):265-73.
53. Tao W, Huang J, Jin Y, Peng K, Zhou J. Effect of pulmonary rehabilitation exercise on lung volume and respiratory muscle recovery in lung cancer patients undergoing lobectomy. Altern Ther Health Med. 2024;30(2):90-6.
54. Wei G, Shang Z, Li Y, Wu Y, Zhang L. Effects of lower-limb active resistance exercise on mobility, physical function, knee strength and pain intensity in patients with total knee arthroplasty: a systematic review and meta-analysis. BMC Musculoskel Disord. 2024;25(1):730.
55. El-Boghdadly K, Levy NA, Fawcett WJ, Knaggs RD, Laycock H, Baird E, et al. Peri-operative pain management in adults: a multidisciplinary consensus statement from the Association of Anaesthetists and the British Pain Society. Anaesthesia. 2024;79(11):1220-36.
56. Namusisi HN. Pharmacological and lifestyle interventions for managing osteoarthritis pain in elderly patients. IDOSR J Sci Res. 2024;9(3):33-7.
57. Skorus-Zadęcka U, Miążek A, Zmysłowska N, Kupniewski K, Kenig J. Comorbidity assessment methods and their significance in predicting the results of treatment of older patients undergoing elective abdominal surgeries for cancer–A scoping review. Cancer Epidemiol. 2024;91:102597.
58. Theodorakis N, Nikolaou M, Hitas C, Anagnostou D, Kreouzi M, Kalantzi S, et al. Comprehensive peri-operative risk assessment and management of geriatric patients. Diagnostics. 2024;14(19): 2153.
59. Khalil MI, El-Monshed AH, Shaala RS, El-Sherif SM, Mousa EF. Home-based transitional cardiac telerehabilitation in older adults post coronary artery bypass grafting: a randomised controlled trial. Geriatr Nurs. 2024;59:139-49.

CHAPTER 45

Introduction to Orthogeriatrics

Sahil Batra, Rajesh Malhotra

INTRODUCTION

Orthogeriatrics is a specialized field of medicine that bridges the gap between orthopedic surgery and geriatric medicine. It focuses on the comprehensive care of older adults with musculoskeletal disorders, particularly those requiring surgical intervention. This interdisciplinary approach recognizes the unique challenges posed by the physiological changes of aging and the complex medical comorbidities often present in elderly patients.

HISTORICAL CONTEXT

The concept of orthogeriatrics emerged in the 1950s and gained momentum in the 1960s and 1970s as healthcare providers recognized the need for specialized care for elderly patients with orthopedic injuries. The field has since evolved significantly, with the development of dedicated orthogeriatric units and the implementation of collaborative care models.

IMPORTANCE IN MODERN HEALTHCARE

As the global population ages, the relevance of orthogeriatrics continues to grow. The World Health Organization projects that by 2050, the proportion of the world's population over 60 years will nearly double from 12 to 22%. This demographic shift underscores the critical need for specialized orthogeriatric care to address the increasing prevalence of age-related musculoskeletal conditions and injuries.

KEY CHALLENGES

Orthogeriatric care faces several unique challenges given as follows:
- Multiple comorbidities
- Increased risk of perioperative complications
- Cognitive impairment and delirium
- Frailty and reduced physiological reserve
- Polypharmacy and medication management
- Social and psychological factors affecting recovery

PATIENT POPULATION

The typical orthogeriatric patient is over 65-years-old and presents with:
- Fragility fractures (e.g., hip, spine, wrist)
- Osteoarthritis requiring joint replacement
- Falls and related injuries
- Osteoporosis and its complications
- Degenerative spine

GOALS OF ORTHOGERIATRIC MANAGEMENT

The primary objectives of orthogeriatric care include:
- Providing comprehensive geriatric assessment (CGA) vand management
- Optimizing patients for surgery and minimizing complications
- Expediting functional recovery and independence
- Preventing future falls and fractures
- Improving long-term outcomes and quality of life
- Reducing mortality rates and healthcare costs

COMMON ORTHOPEDIC CONDITIONS IN THE ELDERLY

Older adults are susceptible to a variety of orthopedic conditions due to age-related changes in bone density, muscle mass, and joint function. This section outlines the most prevalent conditions encountered in orthogeriatric practice.
- *Fragility fractures*:
  - Hip fractures
  - Vertebral compression fractures
  - Distal radius (wrist) fractures

- Osteoarthritis
- Osteoporosis
- *Spinal conditions*:
  - Spinal stenosis
  - Degenerative disk disease
  - Rotator cuff pathology
- Foot and ankle disorders
- Paget's disease of bone
- *Osteosarcopenia*: Age-related loss of bone, muscle mass, and strength

Understanding these common conditions is crucial for effective orthogeriatric care. Each presents unique challenges in diagnosis, treatment, and rehabilitation, often complicated by the physiological changes of aging and comorbidities typical in the elderly population.

COMPREHENSIVE GERIATRIC ASSESSMENT IN ORTHOGERIATRIC CARE

Comprehensive geriatric assessment is a multidimensional, interdisciplinary diagnostic process used to determine an elderly person's medical, psychological, and functional capabilities. In orthogeriatric care, CGA plays a pivotal role in optimizing patient outcomes and tailoring treatment approaches.

Medical assessment involves reviewing acute and chronic medical conditions, optimizing medications, evaluating nutritional status, and assessing pain management strategies.

Functional assessment focuses on evaluating the patient's ability to perform activities of daily livings (ADLs) and instrumental ADLs (IADLs), assessing mobility and gait, using standardized tools such as the Barthel Index or Functional Independence Measure (FIM), and evaluating sensory function, including vision and hearing.

Cognitive assessment includes screening for delirium and dementia using validated tools, such as the Mini-Mental State Examination (MMSE) or the Montreal Cognitive Assessment, and assessing the patient's decision-making capacity.

Psychological assessment screens for depression and anxiety while evaluating the patient's coping mechanisms and resilience.

The social assessment examines the patient's living situation, availability of social support and caregivers, and their financial resources and access to healthcare.

Comprehensive Geriatric Assessment Process in Orthogeriatric Settings

Preoperative Assessment

- Conducted as soon as possible after admission
- *CGA*:
  - Functional status evaluation
  - Cognitive assessment
  - Nutritional status
  - Social support assessment
- *Medical history*:
  - Focus on comorbidities common in older adults
  - Medication review, including polypharmacy concerns
- *Physical examination*:
  - Cardiovascular and respiratory systems
  - Neurological assessment
  - Musculoskeletal evaluation
  - Risk of deep vein thrombosis (DVT)
- *Laboratory and diagnostic tests*:
  - Complete blood count
  - Renal and liver function tests
  - Coagulation studies
  - ECG and chest X-ray
- *Frailty assessment*:
  - Use of validated frailty scales
  - Evaluation of sarcopenia
- *Cognitive screening*: Use of tools such as MMSE
- *Nutritional evaluation*:
  - Albumin levels
  - Body mass index (BMI)
  - Malnutrition screening tools
- *Functional capacity assessment*: ADLs
- *IADLs*: Gait and balance assessment
- *Pain assessment*: Use of age-appropriate pain scales
- *Anesthesia risk assessment*:
  - American Society of Anesthesiologists (ASA) physical status classification system
  - Consideration of regional versus general anesthesia
- *Perioperative risk stratification*:
  - Cardiac risk assessment
  - Pulmonary risk assessment
- *Medication management*:
  - Evaluation of medications that may increase surgical risk
  - Planning for perioperative medication adjustments
- *Delirium risk assessment*: Identification of predisposing and precipitating factors
- *Discharge planning*:
  - Early assessment of postoperative care needs
  - Evaluation of home environment and support systems

Postoperative Assessment

- Monitors recovery and identifies new issues
- Guides ongoing care and rehabilitation plans

Follow-up Assessment

- Evaluates progress and adjusts care plans
- Assesses long-term outcomes and quality of life

Interdisciplinary Team Involvement

- Geriatricians
- Orthopedic surgeons
- Anesthesiologists
- Specialized nurses
- Physiotherapists and occupational therapists
- Social workers
- Nutritionists
- Pharmacists

Challenges in Implementing Comprehensive Geriatric Assessment

- Time constraints in acute care settings
- Resource availability, especially in smaller hospitals
- Need for specialized training in geriatric assessment
- Coordination among multiple specialties

Comprehensive geriatric assessment is an essential tool in orthogeriatric care, providing a holistic view of the patient and informing personalized care strategies. Its systematic application can significantly improve outcomes, reduce complications, and enhance the quality of life for elderly patients with orthopedic conditions.

PERIOPERATIVE MANAGEMENT IN ORTHOGERIATRIC CARE

Perioperative management in orthogeriatric care is a complex and critical process that demands a comprehensive, multidisciplinary approach to optimize outcomes for elderly patients undergoing orthopedic procedures.

In the preoperative phase, thorough medical optimization is paramount, encompassing a detailed assessment and management of cardiovascular and pulmonary health, chronic conditions such as diabetes and renal insufficiency, and nutritional status. This often involves collaboration with specialists to fine-tune management of comorbidities. Medication reconciliation is crucial, with particular attention to anticoagulation management and the implications of polypharmacy. Cognitive assessment plays a vital role, as it influences anesthetic choices and postoperative care strategies. Functional evaluation, including frailty assessment, guides realistic goal-setting and tailored rehabilitation plans. Preoperative physiotherapy and patient education are often employed to enhance postoperative recovery.

Intraoperatively, anesthetic management requires a delicate balance between ensuring adequate depth for surgical conditions and maintaining physiological stability, with close monitoring of cerebral perfusion and temperature regulation. Surgical techniques may be adapted for the elderly population, often favoring less invasive approaches when feasible, and employing strategies to minimize blood loss and operative time. Careful fluid management is essential, considering the reduced physiological reserve and potential for fluid overload or dehydration in older patients.

The immediate postoperative period focuses on multimodal pain management, tailored to the individual's needs and tolerances, often incorporating regional anesthesia techniques. Early mobilization protocols, implemented in collaboration with physiotherapy and nursing staff, are crucial for preventing complications and promoting functional recovery. Vigilant monitoring for postoperative delirium is essential, with proactive implementation of preventive strategies and prompt management when it occurs. Thromboprophylaxis strategies are initiated early, balancing the risk of venous thromboembolism against bleeding risks. Wound care and infection-prevention measures are meticulously applied, recognizing the increased susceptibility to infections in the elderly. Nutritional support is optimized to promote healing and maintain muscle mass.

Throughout the perioperative journey, clear communication and coordinated care between orthopedic surgeons, geriatricians, anesthesiologists, specialized nurses, physiotherapists, and other allied health professionals are fundamental to addressing the complex needs of orthogeriatric patients. This integrated approach extends to discharge planning, ensuring a smooth transition to postacute care settings or home with appropriate support. By comprehensively addressing these multifaceted aspects of perioperative care, tailored to the unique needs of the elderly population, healthcare providers can significantly enhance recovery, reduce complications, and improve overall outcomes in orthogeriatric surgery.

POSTOPERATIVE CARE AND REHABILITATION

Postoperative care and rehabilitation play a crucial role in orthogeriatric patient management, significantly influencing recovery outcomes, functional status, and overall quality of life.

In the immediate postoperative phase, pain management is essential, with multimodal analgesia and regular pain assessments using age-appropriate scales. Close monitoring for potential side effects from pain medications is also necessary. Effective wound care and infection prevention involve regular wound inspections, dressing changes, and early recognition of surgical site infections, along with patient and caregiver education on proper wound care techniques. Thromboembolism prophylaxis, both mechanical and pharmacological, must be continued, with early mobilization emphasized as a key preventive strategy.

In addition, early resumption of oral intake is encouraged when safe, with nutritional supplementation provided as needed. Monitoring the patient's fluid balance and electrolytes ensures appropriate hydration and prevents complications. Early mobilization protocols are implemented gradually, progressing from bed mobility to ambulation with the use of assistive devices as needed. Physical therapy programs are individualized, focusing on strength, balance, and functional activities, while occupational therapy addresses ADLs, environmental adaptations, and the promotion of independence. Special consideration is given to patients with cognitive impairments, with adaptations made to rehabilitation techniques to accommodate their needs.

Furthermore, vigilant monitoring for postoperative complications, such as delirium and medical issues such as cardiac, pulmonary, and renal complications, is essential. Nonpharmacological interventions are preferred for delirium, with careful use of medications when necessary. Preventing falls is a priority, incorporating multifactorial prevention strategies, environmental modifications, and education for both patients and caregivers. Comprehensive discharge planning is also crucial, involving functional assessments, home environment evaluations, and careful consideration of the patient's cognitive status. Clear communication with primary care providers, medication reconciliation, and arrangement of appropriate follow-up appointments ensure smooth care transitions.

Long-term rehabilitation focuses on functional goals and the return to preinjury status, with rehabilitation plans adapted as the patient progresses. Secondary prevention strategies, such as osteoporosis management and ongoing falls risk assessment, are integral, as is the management of underlying medical conditions. Psychological support addressing anxiety, depression, and fear of falling is also provided to promote social engagement and improve quality of life. Special considerations in orthogeriatric rehabilitation include adapting strategies for patients with dementia, frailty, and multimorbidity, with a focus on tailored rehabilitation approaches and coordinated management of chronic conditions. Lastly, outcome measures and quality improvement initiatives are implemented to continually assess and enhance patient care, using standardized tools such as the FIM and the Barthel Index.

In summary, effective postoperative care and rehabilitation for orthogeriatric patients require a patient-centered, comprehensive approach that addresses the complex needs of older adults. Early mobilization, prevention of complications, and tailored rehabilitation strategies optimize recovery and enhance functional outcomes following orthopedic surgery.

FALL PREVENTION STRATEGIES IN ORTHOGERIATRIC PATIENTS

Falls are a major health concern for older adults, often leading to severe injuries such as hip fractures, reduced mobility, loss of independence, and increased mortality. In orthogeriatric care, fall prevention is critical for both patients recovering from fall-related injuries and those at risk of future falls.

A comprehensive approach to fall prevention begins with a thorough risk assessment using standardized tools such as the Morse Fall Scale, STRATIFY, and Berg Balance Scale. This is supplemented by a CGA that evaluates cognitive function, vision, hearing, gait, and balance, alongside a review of medications that may contribute to fall risk. An environmental assessment is also necessary to identify potential hazards both at home and in healthcare settings.

Multifactorial interventions are essential in reducing fall risk. Exercise programs that focus on strength and balance, such as tai chi, are tailored to individual patient capabilities. Medication reviews aim to reduce or discontinue psychoactive drugs and manage medications affecting blood pressure, with vitamin D supplementation provided when needed. Vision correction through regular eye examinations and appropriate corrective lenses, along with the management of conditions such as cataracts, is another crucial element. Proper footwear and assistive devices, such as well-fitting shoes and walking aids, help enhance stability, and regular maintenance of these devices is important to ensure their effectiveness.

Environmental modifications play a key role in fall prevention. Home modifications, such as the installation of handrails, grab bars, improved lighting, and the removal of trip hazards such as loose rugs and clutter, are essential. In hospitals and care facilities, interventions include the use of low beds, fall mats, nonslip flooring, and clear pathways to reduce the risk of falls.

Education and behavioral interventions further support fall prevention efforts. Patients are educated about fall risks, the correct use of assistive devices, and the importance of maintaining physical activity. Caregivers are trained in safe transfer techniques, fall risk recognition, and home safety measures. In healthcare settings, staff education focuses on fall risk assessment, implementation of prevention protocols, and the proper use of bed alarms and other monitoring devices.

Technology and innovation offer additional tools for fall prevention. Wearable devices with accelerometers and gyroscopes analyze gait, while personal emergency response systems can provide immediate assistance. Smart home technologies, such as motion sensors and automated lighting, enhance safety, and fall detection systems can alert caregivers in case of an incident. Virtual reality training provides a safe, simulated environment for balance and gait training, and cognitive-motor dual-task exercises further improve coordination.

In the event of a fall, immediate response protocols prioritize the quick assessment of injuries and the use of safe lifting techniques. Root cause analysis helps to identify the circumstances and contributing factors, leading to adjustments in the patient's care plan and the intensification of interventions where necessary.

Special considerations in orthogeriatric patients include postoperative fall prevention strategies, such as early mobilization with appropriate support, pain management to facilitate safe movement, and the adaptation of strategies to specific surgical procedures. For patients with cognitive impairment, increased supervision, simplified routines, and the use of bed and chair alarms can enhance safety. Osteoporosis management, including bone health assessments, pharmacological interventions, and fracture risk assessments using the Fracture Risk Assessment (FRAX) tool, is also crucial in reducing fall-related injuries.

Organizational approaches to fall prevention involve the implementation of evidence-based fall prevention programs, regular staff training, and continuous quality improvement initiatives. Interdisciplinary collaboration ensures coordinated care among healthcare providers, with regular case conferences to discuss high-risk patients. Institutions develop policies on fall risk assessment and prevention, with standardized reporting and documentation of falls.

To measure the effectiveness of these strategies, outcome measures such as fall rates, severity of fall-related injuries, functional independence, and quality of life assessments are tracked. Process measures, including adherence to fall prevention protocols, completion rates of fall risk assessments, and the implementation of recommended interventions, help ensure the consistency and efficacy of fall prevention efforts.

OSTEOPOROSIS MANAGEMENT IN ORTHOGERIATRIC CARE

Osteoporosis, a skeletal disorder characterized by compromised bone strength, significantly increases the risk of fractures in older adults. In orthogeriatric care, managing osteoporosis is essential for both primary and secondary fracture prevention.

Effective management begins with the diagnosis and assessment, primarily through bone mineral density (BMD) testing using dual-energy X-ray absorptiometry (DXA) scans, where T-scores and Z-scores are interpreted to evaluate bone health. The frequency of follow-up scans is individualized based on the patient's risk factors. Additionally, fracture risk assessments using tools such as the FRAX® tool incorporate clinical risk factors beyond BMD. Laboratory testing, including serum calcium and vitamin D levels and markers of bone turnover, is essential for identifying secondary causes of osteoporosis.

Nonpharmacological interventions play a crucial role in osteoporosis management. Regular weight-bearing exercises, resistance training, and balance exercises are recommended to improve bone strength and coordination. Nutritional interventions focus on a calcium-rich diet, adequate vitamin D supplementation, and sufficient protein intake to support muscle strength and bone health. Fall prevention strategies, which integrate home safety assessments and balance training, are also vital for reducing fracture risk.

Pharmacological management forms a cornerstone of osteoporosis treatment. First-line treatments typically include bisphosphonates (e.g., alendronate, zoledronic acid), which reduce bone resorption and improve bone density, though their route of administration must be carefully considered in elderly patients. Alternative treatments, such as denosumab, are particularly useful in patients with chronic kidney disease, while anabolic agents such as teriparatide and abaloparatide are reserved for severe osteoporosis. Emerging therapies, including romosozumab, offer dual action by both increasing bone formation and reducing resorption.

Special considerations in orthogeriatric patients include perioperative management, where the timing of osteoporosis treatment initiation post fracture is critical. Frailty also affects treatment decisions, requiring a careful balance of risks and benefits in very elderly patients. For those with cognitive impairment, strategies to ensure medication adherence often involve caregivers, who play a key role in managing treatment plans.

Secondary fracture prevention is enhanced through Fracture Liaison Services (FLS), which coordinate care between orthopedic and osteoporosis teams, ensuring timely initiation of treatment and appropriate follow-up. Postfracture care pathways further support this coordination, helping to optimize both orthopedic outcomes and long-term bone health.

Monitoring and long-term management of osteoporosis include strategies to improve treatment adherence, such as patient education and regular follow-up. Bisphosphonate drug holidays may be considered based on individualized fracture risk, and treatment efficacy is monitored through serial DXA scans and bone turnover markers. Nutritional aspects, including calcium supplementation and vitamin D management, are fundamental to maintaining bone health. Adequate protein intake is also emphasized for its role in supporting both bone and muscle strength.

Patient education is an essential component of osteoporosis management. Providing patient-friendly explanations of the disease and its implications encourages adherence to treatment. Lifestyle modifications, such as smoking cessation, alcohol moderation, and safe exercise practices, are critical for long-term bone health.

An interdisciplinary approach is necessary for effective osteoporosis management in orthogeriatric settings. Collaboration between orthopedic surgeons, geriatricians, endocrinologists, and rheumatologists ensures that care plans are coordinated and tailored to the individual needs of the patient. Clear communication between specialties supports shared decision-making and optimized patient outcomes.

Looking to the future, personalized medicine approaches, such as the use of genetic markers for fracture risk and tailoring treatments based on bone turnover markers, hold promise. Novel drug delivery systems, including long-acting injectable and transdermal formulations, may enhance treatment adherence. Additionally, advanced bone quality assessments using tools such as the trabecular bone score (TBS) and high-resolution peripheral quantitative computed tomography (HR-pQCT) offer insights beyond traditional BMD.

Effective osteoporosis management in orthogeriatric care requires a comprehensive approach that addresses both fracture care and long-term bone health. Implementing these strategies can significantly reduce the risk of both initial and subsequent fractures, improve outcomes after orthopedic interventions, and enhance the overall quality of life for elderly patients with osteoporosis.

ETHICAL CONSIDERATIONS IN ORTHOGERIATRIC CARE

Orthogeriatric care often involves complex ethical dilemmas due to the vulnerability of elderly patients, the presence of multiple comorbidities, and the potential impact on quality of life. Healthcare providers must navigate these challenges by addressing several key ethical principles.

Autonomy and informed consent are central, beginning with the careful assessment of decision-making capacity in elderly patients, which may fluctuate. Providers need to adapt how information is delivered, ensuring patients understand the risks, benefits, and alternatives of their treatment. Family members and caregivers often play a role in this process, particularly when patients face challenges in making informed decisions. Advance directives are important tools in guiding care, though ethical challenges arise when a directive conflicts with a patient's current best interests.

Beneficence and nonmaleficence are also essential considerations, requiring a careful risk–benefit analysis, especially in frail or physiologically vulnerable patients. Providers must balance the potential for improved longevity with quality of life, considering patient-centered goals of care. In some cases, integrating palliative care principles can help manage end-of-life issues, requiring ethical reflection on withholding or withdrawing treatment.

Justice and resource allocation in healthcare highlight the need to address ageism and ensure that treatment decisions are based on individual patient needs rather than generalized age-based algorithms. With increasing demands on healthcare systems, there are ethical dilemmas in balancing individual patient care with societal resource constraints, and healthcare providers must consider disparities in access to care, particularly for those in underserved regions. The rise of telemedicine introduces additional ethical challenges, particularly regarding equitable access to remote care for orthogeriatric patients.

Shared decision-making emphasizes the importance of including both the patient and their family in treatment decisions, especially when preferences differ. A multidisciplinary team approach can help resolve conflicts, ensuring that ethical case discussions guide patient care. In *research ethics,* it is essential to address the underrepresentation of elderly patients in clinical trials, ensuring they are included while carefully balancing the risks and benefits of innovative treatments.

As patients approach the end of life, ethical issues become even more pronounced. *End-of-life care* in orthogeriatric settings requires recognizing when a transition from curative to palliative care is appropriate, particularly in managing artificial nutrition, hydration, and aggressive pain management. Ethical considerations arise in decisions to withdraw or withhold treatments, especially in patients with advanced dementia. Cultural and religious beliefs must be respected in care planning, and healthcare providers must navigate potential conflicts between cultural or religious practices and medical recommendations.

For patients with *cognitive impairment,* including dementia, ethical concerns around patient safety, autonomy, and the use of restraints demand careful attention. Providers should explore alternatives to restrictive practices while ensuring patient safety. Professional ethics also require healthcare providers to maintain boundaries and address moral distress when ethical conflicts arise within healthcare teams, particularly in high-pressure or long-term care environments.

Looking to the future, ethical challenges in orthogeriatric care will evolve with aging populations and emerging technologies. *Artificial intelligence (AI)-assisted decision-making* and monitoring technologies raise concerns about privacy and autonomy, while life extension technologies spark debates about the balance between natural aging and medical intervention. Addressing these future ethical challenges will require ongoing reflection, ensuring that care for elderly patients remains not only medically appropriate but also ethically sound and respectful of their dignity and wishes. By engaging in ethical discourse, healthcare providers can navigate these challenges and deliver compassionate, patient-centered care.

FUTURE DIRECTIONS IN ORTHOGERIATRIC CARE

As the global population ages and medical technology advances, orthogeriatrics is poised for significant transformation. Emerging trends in technology, personalized medicine, and integrated care will shape the future of this field.

Technological advancements such as AI and machine learning will enable AI-assisted diagnosis, predictive models for complications, and automated image analysis, while robotics will enhance surgical precision, particularly through minimally invasive techniques tailored for frail elderly patients. Telemedicine and wearable devices will offer virtual consultations, continuous health monitoring, and fall prevention solutions. *Personalized medicine* will be increasingly driven by genomics, with genetic profiling informing fracture risk assessments and pharmacological interventions, while precision rehabilitation will integrate virtual and augmented reality for individualized exercise programs.

The development of *advanced materials and implants* will see bioactive materials that resist infection and promote bone healing, along with nanotechnology for improved implant longevity and targeted drug delivery. *Integrated care models* will focus on seamless coordination between acute orthopedic care and long-term geriatric management, supported by interdisciplinary teams that include geriatric psychiatrists and specialized pharmacists. *Preventive strategies* will evolve with the use of AI-powered fall prevention tools, exoskeletons, and novel therapies for bone health, including stem cell treatments for bone regeneration.

Education and training will be revolutionized through virtual and augmented reality, offering immersive surgical simulations and specialized orthogeriatric fellowship programs.

The future of orthogeriatrics promises to be dynamic and transformative, driven by technological innovations and a commitment to personalized, ethical, and equitable care for the growing elderly population.

CONCLUSION

As we conclude this comprehensive exploration of orthogeriatric care, it becomes evident that this field stands at the intersection of multiple medical disciplines, embodying the essence of patient-centered, multidisciplinary healthcare. The complexity of managing elderly patients with orthopedic conditions necessitates a holistic approach that goes beyond traditional boundaries of orthopedic surgery and geriatric medicine.

Throughout this chapter, we have examined several crucial aspects of orthogeriatric care:

- The foundational principles and historical development of orthogeriatrics highlight the recognition of unique needs in elderly orthopedic patients.
- Common orthopedic conditions in the elderly underscore the diverse challenges faced by clinicians in this field.
- CGA plays a critical role in tailoring care plans and optimizing outcomes
- Perioperative management strategies that address the complexities of surgical interventions in older adults
- The importance of specialized postoperative care and rehabilitation in maximizing functional recovery
- The indispensable nature of a multidisciplinary team approach in providing comprehensive care
- Fall prevention strategies as a cornerstone of both primary and secondary prevention in orthogeriatrics
- The integral role of osteoporosis management in fracture prevention and overall bone health
- Ethical considerations that permeate decision-making processes in orthogeriatric care
- Future directions that promise to revolutionize care delivery through technological advancements and personalized medicine approaches

The field of orthogeriatrics continues to evolve rapidly, driven by demographic shifts toward an aging population and technological innovations.

As healthcare providers, researchers, and policymakers, we must remain adaptable and forward-thinking in our approach to orthogeriatric care. The challenges are significant, but so too are the opportunities to improve the quality of life for our aging population. By embracing interdisciplinary collaboration, evidence-based practices, and patient-centered care principles, we can ensure that orthogeriatric care continues to meet the evolving needs of elderly patients with musculoskeletal conditions.

Ultimately, the goal of orthogeriatric care extends beyond merely treating fractures or managing osteoporosis. It aspires to maintain and restore the functional independence, dignity, and quality of life of older adults facing orthopedic challenges. As we advance in this field, let us carry forward the core principles of compassionate, comprehensive, and collaborative care that define the essence of orthogeriatrics.

Self-Assessment Questionnaire

Q1. What are the key principles that define orthogeriatric care, and how does it differ from traditional orthopedic or geriatric management?

Q2. Why is a comprehensive geriatric assessment (CGA) considered the cornerstone of orthogeriatric care?

Q3. List the common orthopedic conditions encountered in elderly patients and explain why they present unique challenges.

Q4. How do frailty and multimorbidity influence perioperative management in older adults undergoing orthopedic surgery?

Q5. Discuss the importance of fall prevention strategies and identify key interventions to minimize fall risk.

Q6. Outline the multidisciplinary team roles in optimizing outcomes for orthogeriatric patients.

Q7. What are the current pharmacological and nonpharmacological approaches to osteoporosis management in elderly populations?

Q8. How might advances in artificial intelligence, telemedicine, and personalized medicine shape the future of orthogeriatric care?

FURTHER READINGS

1. McCarthy J, Davis A. Diagnosis and management of vertebral compression fractures. Am Fam Physician. 2016;94(1):44-50.
2. Minetto MA, Giannini A, McConnell R, Busso C, Torre G, Massazza G. Common musculoskeletal disorders in the elderly: the star triad. J Clin Med. 2020;9(4):1216.
3. Pilotto A, Cella A, Pilotto A, Daragjati J, Veronese N, Musacchio C, et al. Three decades of comprehensive geriatric assessment: evidence coming from different healthcare settings and specific clinical conditions. J Am Med Dir Assoc. 2017;18(2):e1-192
4. Sainsbury A, Seebass G, Bansal A, Young JB. Reliability of the Barthel Index when used with older people. Age ageing. 2005;34(3):228-32.
5. Linacre JM, Heinemann JW, Wright BD, Granger CV, Hamilton BB. The structure and stability of the functional independence measure. Arch Phys Med Rehabil. 1994;75:127-32.
6. Francisco I, Nunes C, Pereira F, Travassos R, Ribeiro MP, Marques F, et al. Bone mineral density through DEXA and CBCT: a systematic review with meta-analysis. Applied Sciences. 2023;13(10):5962.
7. Kanis JA, Hans D, Cooper C, Baim S, Bilezikian JP, Binkley N, et al. Interpretation and use of FRAX in clinical practice. Osteoporos int. 2011;22:2395-411.
8. American Academy of Orthopedic Surgeons. (2020). Exercise and bone health. [online] Available from https://orthoinfo.aaos.org/en/staying-healthy/exercise-and-bone-health. [Last accessed June, 2025].
9. Wu CH, Tu ST, Chang YF, Chan DC, Chien JT, Lin CH, et al. Fracture liaison services improve outcomes of patients with osteoporosis-related fractures: a systematic literature review and meta-analysis. Bone. 2018;111:92-100.
10. Yu J, Brown D, Kodner IJ, Ray S. Looking beyond the crystal ball: an ethical dilemma in advance directive implementation in multidisciplinary patient care. Surgery. 2015;158(5):1389-94.
11. Randhawa SS, Varghese D. Geriatric evaluation and treatment of age-related cognitive decline. Treasure Island (FL): StatPearls Publishing; 2025.
12. Subramaniam S, Faisal AI, Deen MJ. Wearable sensor systems for fall risk assessment: a review. Front Digit Health. 2022;4:921506.
13. Van Heghe A, Mordant G, Dupont J, Dejaeger M, Laurent MR, Gielen E. Effects of orthogeriatric care models on outcomes of hip fracture patients: a systematic review and meta-analysis. Calcif Tissue Int. 2022;110(2):162-84.
14. Lachance CC, Jurkowski MP, Dymarz AC, Robinovitch SN, Feldman F, Laing AC, et al. Compliant flooring to prevent fall-related injuries in older adults: a scoping review of biomechanical efficacy, clinical effectiveness, cost-effectiveness, and workplace safety. PLoS One. 2017;12(2):e0171652.
15. Ministry of Health and Family Welfare. (2021). Operational Guidelines for Elderly Care at Health and Wellness Centres. [online] Available from https://nhsrcindia.org/sites/default/files/2021-06/Operational%20Guidelines%20for%20Elderly%20Care%20at%20HWC.pdf. [Last accessed June, 2025].
16. Figueiro MG. Light, sleep, and circadian rhythms in older adults with Alzheimer's disease and related dementias. Neurodegener Dis Manag. 2017;7(2):119-45.

CHAPTER 46

Planning and Designing Age Friendly Health Care Facility

Namrata Makkar, Tilotma Jamwal

INTRODUCTION

Background and Significance of Geriatric Health Care

In India, the elderly population is estimated to be around 138 million, and the age of 60 years is regarded as the threshold for old age. According to a source, this figure is expected to exceed 170 million by 2026. Although India's elderly population is increasing in size and proportion, the ability to get high-quality health care remains a major obstacle. The main cause responsible for this issue is a lack of knowledge about geriatric care, which is a specialized field of medicine that provides healthcare services to elderly adults, focusing on their physical and emotional well-being, as well as the management of age-related conditions such as diabetes and arthritis. The primary objective of geriatric care is to consistently deliver integrated care across different healthcare settings **(Fig. 1)**.

OBJECTIVES OF BUILDING AN AGE-FRIENDLY HEALTHCARE SETUP

The primary objective of building an age-friendly healthcare setup is to ensure that older adults receive the highest quality of care in an environment that minimizes healthcare-related harms, enhances patient satisfaction, and optimizes resource use.

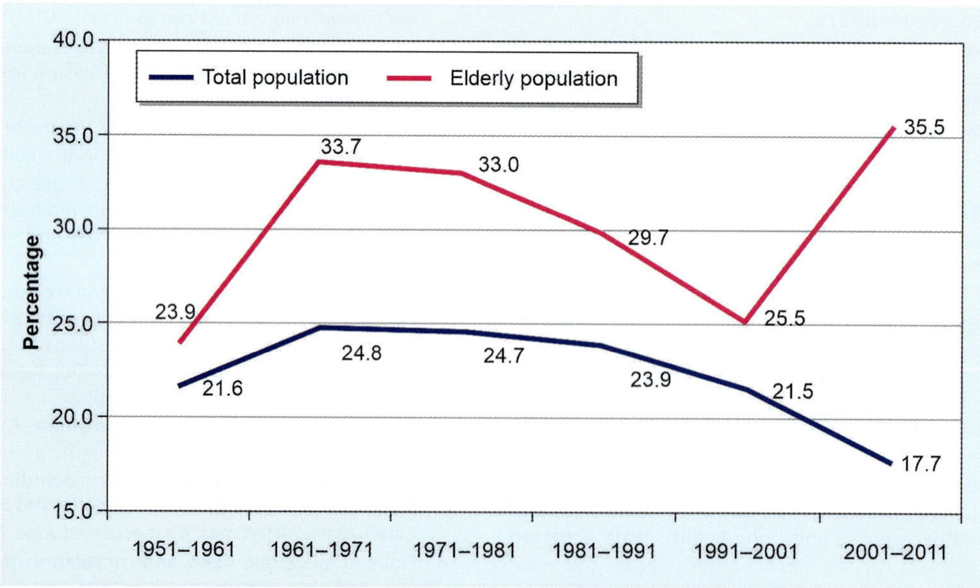

FIG. 1: Decadal growth in elderly population vis-à-vis that of total population.

Safe design process: This is a collaborative risk management process implemented at the design stage of any product (including healthcare facility, both external and internal aspects). The owner initiates the safe design process through the procurement process, identifies and assembles a risk management team, collates information about risks associated with all stages of the product's life cycle, reviews the design to identify health and safety risks, and considers redesign options to eliminate or minimize the identified risks. Additionally, the process involves establishing a residual risk register to record details of risks not eliminated, reviewing the process, updating the register, and informing the designer. Designs should be targeted at three primary groups: Direct care workers who handle patients, managers, and designers, as well as the design and layout of inpatient areas within the hospital.

Providing Evidence-based Care

Evidence-based care ensures that treatments and interventions are effective and tailored to the unique needs of older adults. This involves training healthcare professionals specifically in geriatric care and incorporating a wide range of community-based services. These services can help support the elderly in their homes, reducing the need for hospitalization and institutional care.

Engaging Older Adults and Their Families

Engaging older adults and their families in the care process is critical for personalized and satisfactory health care. This engagement means actively involving them in decision-making about their care plans, respecting their preferences, and ensuring they understand their health conditions and treatment options.

Proactive Health Management

Proactive health management involves anticipating and addressing health issues before they become severe. This includes regular health screenings, vaccinations, and early interventions for chronic conditions. By taking a proactive approach, healthcare providers can prevent complications, reduce hospital admissions, and improve the quality of life for older adults. Additionally, end-of-life care should be managed with sensitivity and respect, ensuring that patients' wishes are honored and that they receive compassionate care during their final days.

Supporting Family Caregivers

Family caregivers play a crucial role in the care of older adults, often providing daily assistance and emotional support. It is essential to support these caregivers by offering resources, education, and respite care. Providing support to caregivers helps to alleviate their burden, reduces caregiver stress, and ensures that they can continue to provide effective care for their loved ones.

Comprehensive and Coordinated Services

Developing a comprehensive and coordinated healthcare system is vital for managing the complex health needs of the elderly. This system should integrate numerous services, including outpatient care, inpatient care, rehabilitation, and palliative care.

Addressing Social and Economic Challenges

The social and economic challenges faced by older adults, such as financial insecurity, social isolation, and elder abuse, must also be addressed. Providing social services, financial support, and community programs can help to alleviate these issues. For instance, the National Programme for Healthcare of Elderly (NPHCE) in India aims to provide accessible and affordable health care to the elderly, especially those from low socioeconomic backgrounds, by creating a supportive and enabling environment.

Creating an Age-friendly Environment

An age-friendly healthcare setup should include physical environments that are safe, accessible, and comfortable for older adults. This involves designing facilities with features such as nonslip flooring, handrails, good lighting, and easy-to-read signage. Such design considerations help to prevent accidents, reduce confusion, and ensure that older adults can navigate the healthcare facility independently and safely.

LOCATION AND ACCESSIBILITY

Selecting an appropriate location for a geriatric healthcare facility is crucial to ensure that it is easily accessible to older adults and their families. The facility should be situated in a place with good transportation links, including public transport and ample parking facilities. Proximity to other medical facilities and emergency services is also essential to providing comprehensive care. Additionally, the location should be in a safe, quiet neighborhood that is conducive to healing and relaxation.

Space Planning and Layout Considerations

Effective space planning and layout are essential to creating a functional and comfortable environment for elderly patients. The design should prioritize open, clutter-free spaces that are easy to navigate with clear signage and wayfinding aids. Corridors should be wide enough to accommodate wheelchairs and walkers, with resting spots at regular intervals. Shared areas should be designed to encourage social interaction, and private areas should offer tranquility and privacy. The layout should facilitate smooth transitions between different care areas, such as examination rooms, treatment areas, and patient rooms. Have a dedicated "May I Help You Desk" for assisting patients.

Integration of Local Architecture and Aesthetics

Incorporating elements of local architecture and aesthetics can make the facility feel more familiar and comfortable for patients.

Creating a Home-like, Noninstitutional Environment

Creating a home-like, noninstitutional environment is essential to promoting the well-being and comfort of elderly patients. This can be achieved by using warm colors, allowing ample sunlight, using comfortable and ergonomic furniture, and a residential-style decor to ensure a design that maintains dignity. Common areas should be inviting and designed to encourage socialization and activities. The overall aim is to reduce the clinical atmosphere and create a space that feels safe, welcoming, and familiar.

Safety and Security Features

Safety and security are paramount in a geriatric healthcare facility. Features such as nonslip flooring, handrails, and grab bars should be standard throughout the facility to prevent falls and accidents. Emergency call systems should be easily accessible in all patient areas. Security measures, such as controlled access points and surveillance systems, help protect patients from potential harm and ensure a safe environment. Fire safety systems, including alarms, sprinklers, and clear evacuation routes, must also be in place and regularly maintained.

Integration of Technology for Health Care and Assistance

Integrating modern technology can significantly enhance the quality of care and the efficiency of a geriatric healthcare facility. Telehealth services allow for remote consultations and continuous monitoring of patients with chronic conditions. Wearable devices can track vital signs and alert healthcare providers to any changes in a patient's condition. Smart home technologies, such as sensor-based motion detecting/automated lighting and temperature control/climate regulation system, can improve comfort and safety for patients. Additionally, electronic health records (EHRs) facilitate better coordination of care and quick access to patient information for healthcare providers.

IMPORTANT DESIGNING DETAILS

Ergonomic design: Designing a geriatric healthcare facility requires careful attention to ergonomics to ensure comfort, safety, and accessibility for older adults. The following elements are critical:

- *Distinctive doorways*: Ensure visibly distinctive doorways and bed areas for easy recognition.
- *Direct sight lines*: Maintain a direct sight line to washrooms from the bed.
- *Call bells*: Use remote voice-activated call bells or ones fixed to the bedside with large, easily activated buttons.
- *Telephones*: Provide black phones with large white push buttons, located within easy reach of the bed, with volume control suitable for use with hearing aids.

Furniture and Fixtures

Beds

- *Electric adjustable height*: Beds should be adjustable to a low height of 18 inches to facilitate safe and easy transfers for patients with mobility issues.
- *Simple technology controller*: Controls should have large, easily identifiable buttons to ensure user-friendliness, particularly for patients with limited dexterity or vision impairments.
- *Pressure-relieving mattress*: These mattresses help prevent pressure ulcers, which are common among bedridden elderly patients.
- *Avoid side railings that fold down to the floor*: Side railings should be stable and secure to prevent falls if they inadvertently fold down.

Tables

- *Sturdy four-legged tables*: Tables should be robust and stable, ensuring that they do not tip over easily, and providing support for elderly patients who might need to lean on them.
- *Rounded corners*: To minimize the risk of injury from bumps and falls, tables should have rounded corners instead of sharp edges.
- *Contrasting color borders*: Edges defined with contrasting colors can enhance depth perception,

making it easier for elderly patients to navigate and use tables safely.

- *Matte tabletop*: A matte finish helps prevent glare, which can be disorienting or uncomfortable for older adults.
- *Contrast table settings*: Using contrasting colors for table settings assists with depth perception and makes it easier for elderly patients to identify items on the table.

Chairs

- *Seat dimensions*: Chairs should have a seat height of 18–19 inches and a depth of 18–20 inches with firm cushioning to provide comfort and support.
- *Extended armrests:* Armrests should extend to the front edge of the chair, about 10 inches above the seat height, to assist patients in standing up and sitting down.
- *Lumbar support*: Proper lumbar support is crucial for reducing back strain and providing comfort.
- *Nonslip, easily cleaned fabric*: The upholstery should be nonslip to prevent patients from sliding off and easy to clean to maintain hygiene.
- *Clearance under front of seat*: There should be enough clearance under the front of the seat to allow feet to tuck under, aiding in standing up.
- *Stable/tip-free design*: Chairs should be designed to be stable and tip-free to ensure safety.
- *Minimal back recline and backward seat tilt*: The chair should have minimal back recline and backward tilt to provide stable and comfortable seating.

Electrical and Mechanical Fittings

Electrical and mechanical fittings should be strategically located to minimize hazards and enhance functionality as follows:

- *Avoid trailing cables*: Electrical cords should not trail across circulation areas as they can cause tripping hazards or impede the movement of wheeled equipment.
- *Appropriate location of fittings*: Electrical outlets and mechanical fittings should be positioned for easy access, reducing the need for bending or stretching. This includes placing light switches, plug outlets, and cabling inaccessible locations.
- *Climate control systems*: Air conditioning, heating, and ventilation systems should be designed to maintain a comfortable environment. The systems should be easy to control and maintain.
- *Power outlets*: Provide sufficient individual power outlets to avoid the need for extension cords or double adaptors.

Flooring and Surfaces

Shock-absorbent flooring: The use of shock-absorbent flooring materials can significantly reduce the impact of falls, which are common among elderly patients. Vinyl flooring with cushioned backing, rubber flooring, and carpet tiles are ideal choices as they provide a balance of comfort and durability. These materials should be nonslip to prevent accidents, especially in areas such as bathrooms and dining rooms where spills are more likely.

Doors and Windows

- *Sensor doors*: Provide hands-free entrance, automatic opening, and sliding glazed doors at the front entry, with all door openings at a clear minimum of 920 mm wide.
- *Window design*: Use domestic-scale transparent glass windows with sills at chair-rail height, ensuring that they are easy to open and close. Open windows should have insect screens.

EN SUITES AND ASSISTED TOILETS

Design and Layout

- *Toilet location*: Ideally, the toilet is to be located opposite the door. Provide minimum access space called functional space around the toilet for carers, the person, and equipment.
- *Storage*: Include storage for wheelchairs and walking frames and ensure access to basins.

Sanitary Ware and Equipment

- *Support arms*: Ensure support arms are on both sides of the toilet.
- *Taps*: Use taps that are easy to operate, mostly sensor-based taps.

Considerations of Use

- *Carers and equipment*: Allow for carers and family members to assist with transfers and personal care. Various equipment may be used, requiring sufficient space.
- *Surface hazards*: Avoid slippery or wet floors, space restrictions, poor lighting, and inadequate ventilation. Ensure personal emergency doors can be unlocked and avoid visual problems such as light pooling and contrast patterns.

LIGHTING AND COLOR SCHEMES

Natural and artificial lighting: Lighting in geriatric facilities should mimic natural light as much as possible to help regulate circadian rhythms and improve mood. Large windows and skylights can be used to maximize natural light during the day. For artificial lighting, a combination of ambient, task, and accent lighting can create a comfortable and functional environment.

Proper lighting is critical in geriatric healthcare facilities to ensure safety and comfort for elderly patients. Key considerations include the following:

- *Increased light requirements*: Seniors require 30% more light for equivalent vision and up to five times brighter light in areas for reading and task completion. Ensuring no glare and using light-emitting diode (LED) lights can help meet these needs.
- *Cove lighting*: Cove lighting, a form of indirect lighting built into ledges, recesses, or valences in a ceiling or high on the walls of a room, is ideal. It hides the fixtures and provides even, warm light, reducing glare and shadows. Direct illumination on vertical surfaces and avoiding highly polished surfaces can also help reduce glare.
- *Consistent lighting levels*: Providing night lighting in patient washrooms and footlights helps prevent falls. Focused light on signs and wayfinding cues, consistent brightness levels in adjacent areas, and gradual changes in light levels when coming indoors from outdoors are crucial for patient safety and comfort.
- *Remote-controlled lighting*: Remote audio-controlled lighting systems can enhance convenience for both patients and staff, allowing easy adjustments without physical effort.
- *Lighting control*: Provide capability to reduce light levels automatically at night and during daylight hours. Ensure pathways are well-lit, with additional focused lighting on signs and way-finding cues.

ACOUSTIC CONSIDERATIONS

Noise-reduction strategies: Noise levels can impact the comfort and well-being of elderly patients. Using sound-absorbing materials such as acoustic ceiling tiles, carpets, and wall panels can help reduce ambient noise and create a more peaceful environment.

Strategic spatial design can help manage noise levels effectively. For example, placing noisy areas such as kitchens and laundry rooms away from patient rooms and quiet zones helps to reduce noise pollution. Incorporating sound barriers and creating separate zones for different activities can also help in managing noise levels.

High noise levels can lead to anxiety, confusion, and fatigue among elderly patients. Effective noise-control strategies include reducing the use of public address systems, particularly in patient bedrooms, and combining visual displays to inform patients in waiting areas can help minimize noise.

Providing hearing amplifiers in all patient-contact areas can help those with hearing impairments understand what is being said, reducing miscommunication and improving patient satisfaction.

HALLWAYS

- *Pathways*: Clear, unimpeded pathways wide enough for wheelchair/walker and caregiver in each direction (larger than minimum wheelchair access standard)
- *Surface*: Avoid shiny surfaces with glare. Use nonslip materials to prevent falls.
- *Seating*: Provide seating areas at regular intervals along long hallways to offer rest spots for elderly patients.
- *Handrails*: Hand railings in hallways should be 1.5 inches in diameter with a 2-inch hand clearance, easy grip rounded style. Ensure handrails extend beyond top and bottom landings.
- *Steps*: Conventional steps should have 6-inch risers and 12-inch treads. Highlight step edges with a contrasting color, such as yellow, to enhance visibility.
- *Ramps*: Avoid ramps if possible. If required, ensure a 5–8% slope with rest areas every 30 feet. Mark the top and bottom of the ramps with a yellow strip.

FUNCTIONAL AREAS AND THEIR DESIGN

Specific Spatial Requirements Inside the Building

Waiting Area

Waiting areas should be designed to provide a welcoming and comfortable environment as follows:

- *Size and function*: An indicative size would typically be around 30 m^2, including the waiting area. The entry may be through a front porch, hall lobby, or foyer space, allowing for easy wheelchair access and room for family groups.
- *Location*: Positioned near the entrance to serve as the arrival and departure point. It should provide clean, dry access for ambulatory or disabled persons.
- *Colors*: Bright, welcoming colors create a caring atmosphere. Use colors that are easy on the eyes and avoid harsh contrasts that can cause visual discomfort.
- *Allowance for seating*: Ensure sufficient lounge chairs, recliners, and tables to accommodate all residents and visitors comfortably.
- *Activity separation*: Design the layout to separate passive activities (such as reading) from active ones (such as group exercises).

Access and Mobility

- *Design for frail and disabled*: Ensure the design caters to frail, disabled, and ambulatory persons.
- *Weather protection*: Provide protection from the elements with a covered porch overhang at the entrance.
- *Direct access*: Ensure direct access to public telephones and toilets for visitors and proximity to street pedestrian access and onsite parking.

Visibility and Navigation

- *Visual access*: Ensure visual access to the main circulation corridor, reception, office, and meeting rooms. The reception counter should be clearly identifiable from the entrance door.
- *Signage*: Use clear, large, and contrasting lettered signage for easy navigation, including tactile signage for the visually impaired.
- *Wayfinding aids*: Include a "You are Here" map or directory board at the entrance and directions to toilets and telephones.
- *Floors and floor finishes*: Floors should intercept grit, mud, water, and other debris, and be easily cleaned. They should also be nonslip to prevent falls.
- *Ceilings*: Ceilings should be light and reflective, with a height that is in scale with the space, providing a noninstitutional appearance.
- *Furniture placement*: Ensure furniture is placed to allow clear walkways, especially for those using wheelchairs or walking frames.

Lighting and Environment

- *Natural light and ventilation*: Incorporate large, clear windows with insect screens for natural light and ventilation.
- *Noninstitutional lighting*: Use noninstitutional lighting centered over walkways and consider table lamps to create a warm ambience. Place ceiling fans to avoid flicker and ensure air circulation.
- *Visual and acoustic privacy*: Ensuring visual and acoustic privacy in the waiting areas is crucial for maintaining confidentiality and reducing stress. Visual privacy can be achieved through partitions or screens, while acoustic privacy can be enhanced using sound-absorbing materials and designing the layout to separate noisy areas from quiet ones.

Communication and Data Access

The waiting area should be equipped with modern communication tools such as wi-fi, charging stations, and public telephones. Digital information displays can provide updates on wait times and general information about the facility, ensuring that patients and their families stay informed and connected while waiting.

Common Rooms Design

Common rooms should be multipurpose spaces for activities and relaxation, designed with the following guidelines:

- *Indicative size*: The room should be approximately 30 m^2, including the waiting area.
- *Entry points*: The entry may be through a front porch, hall lobby, or foyer space.
- *Accessibility*: The design should accommodate wheelchair access, particularly at the reception counter. There should be room for family groups to pause near the entry door, within easy sight of wayfinding cues.
- *Security and mobility*: One entry point should be provided with security design for access and mobility for frail, disabled, and ambulatory persons.
- *Weather protection*: The entrance should have a covered porch overhang to protect from the elements, with direct access to the reception area from the door.
- *Additional amenities*: Provide direct access to public telephones and toilets for visitors, and ensure the facility is close to street pedestrian access and onsite parking.

Examination and Treatment Rooms

Examination and treatment rooms must be designed for efficiency, privacy, and comfort. They should be easily accessible from the waiting area and spacious enough to accommodate medical equipment and caregivers. Adjustable lighting is crucial for medical examinations, while soundproofing ensures privacy. Climate control is essential to maintaining a comfortable environment. Each room should be equipped with ergonomic furniture, nonslip flooring, and accessible storage for medical supplies and equipment.

Inpatient Rooms and Wards

Inpatient rooms and wards should provide a homely atmosphere to promote healing and comfort. Each room should be spacious enough to accommodate mobility aids and medical equipment, with large windows for natural light. Adjustable beds, comfortable seating for visitors, and easy access to bathrooms are essential. Privacy can be ensured with curtains or partitions. Safety features such as handrails, nonslip flooring, and emergency call systems are crucial to ensuring the safety and well-being of elderly patients.

Rehabilitation and Therapy Areas

Rehabilitation and therapy areas should be designed to facilitate various therapeutic activities. These areas need to be spacious, with equipment for physiotherapy, occupational therapy, and other rehabilitation services.

Equipment and Aids Storage

Proper storage for medical equipment and mobility aids is essential to maintaining an organized and efficient facility. Storage areas should be easily accessible to staff and located close to the areas where the equipment is most often used. Shelving and storage units should be clearly labeled and organized to ensure quick access. Secure storage for sensitive or expensive equipment is also important to prevent loss or damage.

SECURITY

The security of patients, visitors, and staff in a geriatric healthcare facility must be carefully balanced to ensure safety without compromising ease of access and egress. The following security concepts and design principles should be incorporated:

- *Balanced approach*: Security measures must balance safety with accessibility, ensuring that patients, visitors, and staff can move freely while being protected from potential threats.
- *Latest security initiatives*: Incorporating the latest security technologies and practices is essential. This includes surveillance systems, electronic access control, and emergency response protocols. Advanced security systems such as biometric access control, CCTV surveillance, and automated alarm systems can enhance safety without being obtrusive.
- *Clear delineation between public and controlled areas*: There should be a clear distinction between public areas and restricted zones to prevent unauthorized access. Controlled areas should be accessible only to authorized personnel, using keycard systems or biometric scanners. This helps protect sensitive areas such as patient rooms, medical records, and medication storage.
- *Avoidance of unobserved areas and hiding places*: The facility's design should minimize unobserved areas and potential hiding places that could pose security risks. Strategic placement of security cameras and the use of mirrors in blind spots can help monitor all areas effectively. Landscaping should be planned to avoid creating concealed spots near the building.
- *Subtle security design*: Security features should be integrated seamlessly into the facility's design to avoid creating a fortress-like atmosphere. Natural barriers such as hedges, bollards, and decorative fences can provide security without being intimidating. Access control points should be designed to blend with the overall architecture of the building.

INFECTION-CONTROL CONSIDERATIONS

Infection control is a critical aspect of managing a healthcare facility, especially for vulnerable elderly populations as follows:

- *Biomedical waste management*: According to the Biomedical Waste Management and Handling Rules of 2016, clinical waste must be segregated at source, contained securely, and transported carefully. This involves using designated waste containers, proper labeling, and secure storage areas.
- *Waste disposal facilities*: Clear access to waste disposal facilities is necessary, including sluices and storage areas for clean items. These areas should be designed to prevent exposure to vapors, splashes, or aerosols during waste handling procedures and must be dedicated.
- *Hand washing and equipment cleaning*: Clinical hand basins should be available in all areas where patient treatment occurs, equipped with hot and cold water, nontouch taps, liquid soap, and disposable paper towels. Equipment washing areas should have adequate lighting, ventilation, and appropriate receptacles for waste disposal.
- *Ultrasonic cleaning and reprocessing*: Specialized cleaning areas for medical instruments should include ultrasonic cleaners and sufficient space for reprocessing. These areas must adhere to strict hygiene standards to prevent contamination and ensure the safety of both patients and staff.
- *Clinical hand basins*: All areas where resident treatment occurs must have clinical hand basins equipped with hot and cold water, nontouch taps, supplies of liquid handwash, and disposable paper towels. Antisplash devices on taps are necessary to prevent water from spreading germs.

Catering

Catering facilities need to provide both staff and patients with nutritious meals in a comfortable setting. Key points include the following:

- *Central kitchen facility*: A central kitchen facility with satellite areas in each of the units ensures efficient meal preparation and distribution. If a central kitchen is not feasible, individual kitchens will be needed in many units.

- *Dining environment*: Dining areas should be designed to be welcoming and comfortable, with furniture that is easy to clean and maintain.

Nutrition

Nutritional considerations are vital in a geriatric healthcare setup to maintain or improve the nutritional intake of patients and a diet plan designed by a qualified dietician:

- *Quality mealtime experience*: Mealtimes should foster dignity and pleasure in eating, respecting cultural and personal preferences. The adequate intake of nutrients is necessary to maintain physical and emotional health.
- *Social components*: Mealtimes provide an opportunity not only to ingest nutrients but also to maintain critical social aspects of life. Observing mealtime rituals, cultural norms, and food preferences can enhance the dining experience.
- *Encouraging self-feeding*: Patients should be encouraged and assisted to self-feed for as long as possible. Those who depend on assistance for eating should be helped with dignity, ensuring that their independence is maintained as much as possible.

CONCLUSION

Building an age-friendly healthcare setup underscores the pressing need for specialized geriatric care amidst the global trend of an aging population. In India, where the elderly demographic is expanding rapidly, the challenges of providing high-quality health care to older adults are multifaceted. The lack of awareness and specialized facilities for geriatric care highlights the urgency for comprehensive strategies to meet the unique needs of this population.

Geriatric health care must adopt a holistic approach, integrating physical, mental, and social aspects of well-being. Addressing the common health challenges faced by the elderly, such as chronic conditions and functional decline, requires a coordinated and proactive health management strategy.

Designing an age-friendly environment involves thoughtful consideration of space planning, lighting, acoustics, and safety features. Functional areas such as waiting rooms, common rooms, examination and treatment rooms, and inpatient wards must be designed to cater to the specific needs of elderly patients. Infection control, security, and environmental systems play critical roles in maintaining a safe and sustainable healthcare environment.

In conclusion, creating an age-friendly healthcare setup is a complex but essential task that requires a multidisciplinary approach. It involves not only medical and healthcare interventions but also the integration of social services, environmental design, and community support. As the population ages, the importance of geriatric care will continue to grow, making it imperative for healthcare systems to adapt and evolve to meet the needs of older adults.

Self-Assessment Questionnaire

Q1. What are the primary objectives of creating an age-friendly healthcare setup?

Q2. How does evidence-based care improve the quality of healthcare delivery for older adults?

Q3. Why is it important to engage both older adults and their families in the care process?

Q4. Describe the design features that make a healthcare facility physically safe and comfortable for elderly patients.

Q5. What are the key considerations in location and accessibility when planning a geriatric healthcare facility?

Q6. Discuss the ergonomic principles that should guide the selection of furniture and fixtures in a geriatric ward.

Q7. What measures are essential to ensure infection control in facilities catering to older adults?

Q8. How can integration of modern technology enhance care delivery and safety in an age-friendly healthcare setup?

Q9. Why is a multidisciplinary approach critical for successfully planning and managing an age-friendly healthcare facility?

FURTHER READINGS

1. Ministry of Statistics and Programme Implementation. (2021). Elderly in India 2021. [online] Available from https://mospi.gov.in/sites/default/files/publication_reports/Elderly%20in%20India%202021.pdf. [Last accessed June, 2025].
2. NITI Aayog. (2024). Senior Care Reforms in India. [online] Available from https://www.niti.gov.in/sites/default/files/2024-02/Senior%20Care%20Reforms%20in%20India%20FINAL%20FOR%20WEBSITE_compressed.pdf. [Last accessed June, 2025].

3. Abdi S, Spann A, Borilovic J, de Witte L, Hawley M. Understanding the care and support needs of older people: a scoping review and categorisation using the WHO international classification of functioning, disability, and health framework (ICF). BMC Geriatr. 2019;19:195.
4. AbdulRaheem Y. Unveiling the significance and challenges of integrating prevention levels in healthcare practice. J Prim Care Community Health. 2023;14:21501319231186500.
5. Agency for Healthcare Research and Quality. (2012). Coordinating Care for Adults with Complex Care Needs in the Patient-Centered Medical Home: Challenges and Solutions. [online] Available from https://www.ahrq.gov/sites/default/files/wysiwyg/ncepcr/tools/PCMH/coordinating-care-for-adults-with-complex-care-needs-white-paper.pdf. [Last accessed June, 2025].
6. Liu B, Qiu N, Zhang T. Accessibility of elderly care facilities based on social stratification: a case study in Tianjin, China. Sustainability. 2023;15:1507.
7. Kuligowski E, Peacock R, Wiess E, Hoskins B. Stair evacuation of older adults and people with mobility impairments. Fire Saf J. 2013;62:230-7.
8. Singh S. The impact of architecture in the process of healing & well-being. Int J Res Appl Sci Eng Technol. 2021;9(3):202-22.
9. WION News. (2023). 10 expert-approved tips to create a safe and comfortable home environment for elderly care. [online] Available from https://www.wionews.com/entertainment/lifestyle/news-_0-expert-approved-tips-to-create-a-safe-and-comfortable-home-environment-for-elderly-care-629101. [Last accessed June, 2025].
10. Bouricha D, Kammoun D. Upgrading the living space of the elderly person: towards a healthcare design. J Salutog Architect. 2023;2:85-103.
11. Debnath S. Integrating information technology in healthcare: recent developments, challenges, and future prospects for urban and regional health. World J Adv Res Rev. 2023;19(01):455-63.
12. Regional Geriatric Program of Eastern Ontario (RGPEO). (2025). Regional Geriatric Rounds 2025. [online] Available from https://www.rgpeo.com. [Last accessed June, 2025].
13. Australian Commission on Safety and Quality in Health Care. (2004). Guidelines for Safe and Effective Care in Residential Aged Care Facilities. [online] Available from https://www.safetyandquality.gov.au/sites/default/files/migrated/Guidelines-RACF.pdf. [Last accessed June, 2025].
14. Hiray AA, Kulkarni N. Design and development of automatic position adjustable bed cum stretcher to improve patients comfort and safety. IEEE Bombay Sect Signat Conf. 2020;74-8.
15. Blackler A, Brophy C, O'Reilly M, Chamorro-Koc M. Seating in aged care: physical fit, independence, and comfort. SAGE Open Med. 2018;6:2050312117744925.
16. Hencová M, Kotradyová V. Colour in the environment for older adults. Architecture Pap Fac Archit Des STU. 2023;28:15-23.
17. Ceiling and Interior Systems Construction Association. (2017). Acoustics in Healthcare Environments. [online] Available from https://www.cisca.org/files/public/Acoustics%20in%20Healthcare%20Environments_CISCA.pdf. [Last accessed June, 2025].
18. Australian Government Department of Health. (2024). National Aged Care Design Principles and Guidelines. [online] Available from https://www.health.gov.au. [Last accessed June, 2025].
19. Geriatric and Gerontology Development Agency (GGDA). Grangegorman histories. [online] Available from https://www.ggda.ie. [Last accessed June, 2025].
20. Ministry of Health and Family Welfare, Government of India. (2022). Indian Public Health Standards (IPHS) Guidelines for Primary Health Centres. [online] Available from https://nhm.gov.in/images/pdf/guidelines/iphs/iphs-revised-guidlines-2022/03_PHC_IPHS_Guidelines-2022.pdf. [Last accessed June, 2025].
21. Minemura T, Hanzawa Y, Dutta S. Planning facilities for elderly patients care examination room. Comput Ind Eng. 1992;23(1-4):191-4.
22. Health Facility Guidelines India. (2014). Part B: Inpatient Accommodation Unit. [online] Available from https://india.healthfacilityguidelines.com/Guidelines/ViewPDF/HFG-India/part_b_inpatient_accommodation_unit. [Last accessed June, 2025].
23. Rand S, Smith N, Jones K, Dargan A, Hogan H. Measuring safety in older adult care homes: a scoping review of the international literature. BMJ Open. 2021;11(3).
24. Bouza E, Navarro JAG, Alonso S, Alonso JCD, Escobar C, Gómez BJF, et al. Infection control in long term care institutions for the elderly: a reflection document on the situation in Spain. Rev Esp Quimioter. 2023;36(4):346-79.
25. British Dietetic Association. (2024). The first menu planning and food service guideline for care homes for older adults launches. [online] Available from https://www.bda.uk.com/resource/the-first-menu-planning-and-food-service-guideline-for-care-homes-for-older-adults-launches.html. [Last accessed June, 2025].

INDEX

Page numbers followed by *b* refer to box, *f* refer to figure, *fc* refer to flowchart, and *t* refer to table.

A

B

D

E

I

J

K

L

M

N

O

P

Q

R

S